BSAVA Manual of
Practical Veterinary Nursing

Formerly BSAVA Manual of Veterinary Nursing

Editors:

Elizabeth Mullineaux
BVM&S CertSHP MRCVS
Quantock Veterinary Hospital, Quantock Terrace,
The Drove, Bridgewater, Somerset TA6 4BA

and

Marie Jones
BSc(Hons) DipAVN(Med) CertEd VN
College of Animal Welfare, Bolton's Park Farm,
Potters Bar, Herts EN6 1NB

Consulting Editor – Exotics:

AJ Pearson
BA VetMB MRCVS
Cambridge Veterinary Group,
89A Cherry Hinton Road, Cambridge CB1 7BS

Published by:

British Small Animal Veterinary Association
Woodrow House, 1 Telford Way, Waterwells Business Park,
Quedgeley, Gloucester GL2 2AB

A Company Limited by Guarantee in England.
Registered Company No. 2837793.
Registered as a Charity.

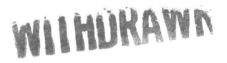

Other veterinary nursing titles from BSAVA:

Manual of Advanced Veterinary Nursing
Manual of Practical Animal Care
Textbook of Veterinary Nursing (formerly Jones's Animal Nursing)

Other titles in the BSAVA Manuals series:

Manual of Canine & Feline Abdominal Surgery
Manual of Canine & Feline Anaesthesia and Analgesia
Manual of Canine & Feline Behavioural Medicine
Manual of Canine & Feline Clinical Pathology
Manual of Canine & Feline Dentistry
Manual of Canine & Feline Emergency and Critical Care
Manual of Canine & Feline Endocrinology
Manual of Canine & Feline Gastroenterology
Manual of Canine & Feline Haematology and Transfusion Medicine
Manual of Canine & Feline Head, Neck and Thoracic Surgery
Manual of Canine & Feline Infectious Diseases
Manual of Canine & Feline Musculoskeletal Disorders
Manual of Canine & Feline Musculoskeletal Imaging
Manual of Canine & Feline Nephrology and Urology
Manual of Canine & Feline Neurology
Manual of Canine & Feline Oncology
Manual of Canine & Feline Wound Management and Reconstruction
Manual of Exotic Pets
Manual of Ornamental Fish
Manual of Psittacine Birds
Manual of Rabbit Medicine and Surgery
Manual of Raptors, Pigeons and Waterfowl
Manual of Reptiles
Manual of Small Animal Cardiorespiratory Medicine and Surgery
Manual of Small Animal Dermatology
Manual of Small Animal Diagnostic Imaging
Manual of Small Animal Fracture Repair and Management
Manual of Small Animal Ophthalmology
Manual of Small Animal Reproduction and Neonatology
Manual of Wildlife Casualties

For information on these and all BSAVA publications please visit our website: www.bsava.com

Contents

Contributors

Belinda Andrews-Jones VTS (ECC) DipAVN(Surg) VN
Queen Mother Hospital for Animals, Royal Veterinary College, Hawkshead Lane,
North Mymms, Hatfield AL9 7TA

Sally Anne Argyle MVB PhD CertSAC EBVC MRCVS
Royal (Dick) School of Veterinary Studies, Roslin, Midlothian EH25 9RG

Amanda Boag MA VetMB DipACVIM DipACVECC FHEA MRCVS
Lecturer in Emergency and Critical Care, Department of Veterinary Clinical Science,
Royal Veterinary College, Hawkshead Lane, North Mymms, Hatfield AL9 7TA

Clare Bryant CertEd VN
Deputy Programme Leader, The Royal (Dick) School of Veterinary Studies, College of Animal Welfare,
1 Summerhall Square, Edinburgh EH9 1QH

Sue Dallas CertEd VN
Walford and North Shropshire College, Baschurch, Shrewsbury, Shropshire

Carole Davis RGN BA(Hons) MSc PGCert(HE)
School of Arts & Education, Middlesex University, Trent Park, Bramley Road, London N14 4YZ

Sarah Heath BVSc DipECVBM MRCVS
Behavioural Referrals Veterinary Practice, 11 Cotebrook Drive, Upton, Chester, Cheshire CH2 1RA

Alasdair Hotston Moore MA VetMB CertSAC CertVR CertSAS MRCVS
Department of Clinical Veterinary Science, University of Bristol, Langford House, Langford,
Bristol BS40 5DU

Paula Hotston Moore CertEd VN
University of Bristol, Langford House, Langford, Bristol BS40 5DU

Marie Jones BSc(Hons) DipAVN(Med) CertEd VN
College of Animal Welfare, Bolton's Park Farm, Hawkshead Road, Potters Bar EN6 1NB

Clare M Knottenbelt BVSc MSc DSAM MRCVS
Senior Lecturer in Internal Medicine, Division of Companion Animal Sciences,
University of Glasgow Veterinary School, Bearsden, Glasgow G61 1QH

Rachel Lumbis BSc(Hons) VN
College of Animal Welfare, Royal Veterinary College, Bolton's Park Farm, Hawkshead Road,
Potters Bar EN6 1NB

Annaliese Magee DipAVN(Surg) VN
Stainland, Halifax

Elizabeth Mullineaux BVM&S CertSHP MRCVS
Quantock Veterinary Hospital, Quantock Terrace, The Drove, Bridgwater TA6 4BA

Laura Nicholls VN
Quantock Veterinary Hospital, Quantock Terrace, The Drove, Bridgwater TA6 4BA

Dominic SM Phillips BVM&S BSc MBA MRCVS
Quantock Veterinary Hospital, Quantock Terrace, The Drove, Bridgwater TA6 4BA

John Prior VetMB MA CertSAO MRCVS
Suffolk

Heather Roberts BSc(Hons) VN
Mypetstop Pet Resort & Care Centre, Topcliffe Close, Capitol Park, Tingley WF3 1BU

Karen Scott DipAVN(Surg) VN
The Royal (Dick) School of Veterinary Studies, 1 Summerhall Square, Edinburgh EH9 1QH

Freda Scott-Park BVM&S PhD MRCVS
Portnellan Trian, Gartocharn, Alexandria, Dunbartonshire G83 8NL

Maggie Shilcock BSc PGDipLib CMS
The Old Rectory, Anmer PE31 6RN

Garry Stanway BVSc CertVA MSc MRCVS
Cheshire

Anne Ward BSc DipAVN(Surg) VN
Lecturer in Veterinary Nursing, The Royal (Dick) School of Veterinary Studies,
College of Animal Welfare, 1 Summerhall Square, Edinburgh EH9 1QH

Foreword

Veterinary nursing has developed considerably since BSAVA first published the 'little green book' *Practical Veterinary Nursing* edited by Colin Price in 1985. At that time the original RANAs (Royal Animal Nursing Auxilliaries) wore dresses and starched aprons, and nurses in training were trainee veterinary nurses. RANAs are now VNs, trainees are student veterinary nurses, and both now wear more suitable uniforms. Training and textbooks have mirrored these changes. The BSAVA recognized the changes and accepted the challenge to produce not one but three books for ancilliary staff – two books for student nurses (*BSAVA Manual of Veterinary Care* and *BSAVA Manual of Veterinary Nursing*) and one written especially for qualified veterinary nurses and those working towards further qualification (*BSAVA Manual of Advanced Veterinary Nursing*). Being considerably involved in veterinary nurse education and having worked with BSAVA on the concept of the three book series, I was privileged to act as Series Editor. I found the project extremely rewarding and enjoyed overseeing all three books. The series has laid the pathway for this new edition.

The *BSAVA Manual of Practical Veterinary Nursing* returns to the original title but has developed the themes first introduced in the *BSAVA Manual of Veterinary Nursing*. This new edition is a welcome development, progressing the concepts of the first edition but placing more emphasis on practical aspects. It is intended that this new edition should become the practical companion to the *BSAVA Textbook of Veterinary Nursing* and relate more directly to the S/NVQ occupational standards.

As with all new editions of BSAVA Manuals there is significant revision and extension to cover new developments. The tables and illustrations, along with the numerous colour photographs, make this book a useful resource for everyone in the practice as well as an excellent study guide for the student veterinary nurse. Above all, this is a practical guide for the veterinary care team of the twentyfirst century.

Gillian Simpson BVM&S MRCVS
June 2007

Preface

The profession of veterinary nursing is moving forward with strength and confidence. Veterinary practice has changed dramatically over the years, not only in technical advances but also in the way veterinary nurses are employed. In years past, veterinary nurses were largely underused; today veterinary nurses have become an indispensable part of the veterinary care team and true professionals in their own right. The number and diversity of skills required of veterinary nurses has greatly expanded since the previous edition of this manual. Therefore the need for a new BSAVA Manual, which can be used by qualified and student veterinary nurses to meet today's requirements in veterinary practice.

This Manual offers a practical and easily accessible guide to common procedures and nursing skills used within general practice. It represents an effort to collect the broad scope of information required by veterinary nurses to satisfy the practical Occupational Standards of veterinary nurse training, while the *BSAVA Textbook of Veterinary Nursing* provides the more theoretical components. The Manual also aims to provide additional information for the newly qualified veterinary nurse in his/her first few years in a modern practice.

The Manual updates core chapters in the previous edition, whilst adding new stand-alone chapters on Fluid therapy and Wounds and bandaging. There is increased information on the care and treatment of exotic pets. Also new for this addition is a chapter on Nursing models, which introduces the reader to the concepts of this subject and shows how standard human nursing models can be adapted to construct care plans for veterinary patients.

We would like to thank our group of authors for sharing their expertise, clinical experience and hard work in getting this Manual to print. Also a huge thankyou goes to BSAVA for making the Manual possible.

It is our hope that this new edition will become an essential reference in daily use within practice and a useful teaching aid in the training of veterinary nurses.

Elizabeth Mullineaux
Marie Jones

June 2007

Professional responsibilities of the veterinary nurse

Maggie Shilcock

This chapter is designed to give information on:

- Professional responsibilities of the veterinary nurse
- General health and safety

Professional responsibilities

The veterinary nurse is a professional whose name, if they qualified from September 2007 onwards, is entered in the Royal College of Veterinary Surgeons' Register of Veterinary Nurses. (Nurses who entered the previous unregulated RCVS list on or after 1st January 2003 were automatically transferred to the new Register, while nurses qualifying before 2003 may register voluntarily.) A Guide to Professional Conduct and new Bye–laws for veterinary nurses provide a framework within which regulated nurses will be expected to work. Included in this framework is a responsibility to the practice, clients and themselves. The nurse must be seen to be acting in a professional manner at all times.

Personal performance

As professionals, nurses must always be aware of the importance of maintaining a high level of personal performance in all that they do within the practice. All nurses should have a detailed job description that outlines their roles and responsibilities and identifies the specific tasks required of the job. Nurses should always be mindful of the content of their job description and aim to fulfil the requirements to the best of their ability. It is also important to be aware of the limits of job responsibility; if there is any doubt regarding this, nurses should seek advice from their supervisor and next in command.

Chain of command

There will usually be a 'chain of command' within the practice. This enables employees to go to the right

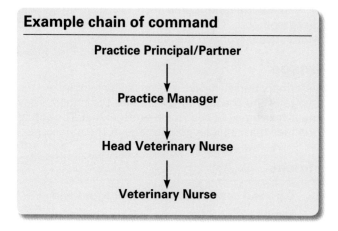

Example chain of command

Practice Principal/Partner

↓

Practice Manager

↓

Head Veterinary Nurse

↓

Veterinary Nurse

person for the right advice and it should always be adhered to. This may be in the first instance the Head Nurse but, depending on the advice required, could be a Practice Manager or Practice Principal.

Failure to seek advice about how to carry out tasks or activities can, in the worst case, lead to serious damage to an animal's health – for example, if incorrect medication is administered. This is possibly life-threatening for the animal, upsetting for the owner and could lead to an insurance claim against the practice.

Appraising performance

It is important that nurses agree and understand the personal performance targets required of them; this is often discussed during an annual appraisal. Personal development needs and how they will be achieved (for example, training courses, individual learning, extra responsibility) are set at the appraisal. The appraiser will usually be the Head Nurse or Practice Manager. It is helpful to set targets for achieving new developmental goals, as this gives the nurse something to aim for. At agreed intervals there should be meetings to discuss how well the nurse is progressing towards the set targets, any problems and what help may be required.

Working relationships

Nurses must be able to develop and maintain good and effective working relationships with their colleagues. Poor working relationships lead to poor communication within the practice and stress for the staff. This will be reflected in the quality of work and the client care that the practice provides. This situation can quickly lead to dissatisfied clients, complaints and loss of business, and poorer care for the animals.

Teamwork

Teamwork is the key to successful working relationships. Teamwork requires all members of the team to cooperate with, communicate with and support each other. Everyone has to contribute to the team effort and there should be no competition between members; everyone should share successes and failures and work together to produce the best animal and client care possible. Team meetings are a good and effective way to discuss issues and problems and they give everyone an opportunity to make suggestions and iron out difficulties and disagreements. This sort of communication helps to motivate everyone in the team.

Image

Veterinary nurses have a responsibility to maintain the image of the practice to clients and the public. They must at all times be seen to be professional. The sort of qualities that reflect a good image of the nurse are:

Image
■ **Care and consideration for colleagues and clients**
■ **Politeness**
■ **Efficiency**
■ **Personal smartness**
■ **Helpfulness**
■ **Friendly manner**

Nurses represent the practice at all times, especially when in uniform. This means that while outside the practice, on lunch breaks, on the way home or shopping in the supermarket, nurses must still be conscious of the image they portray.

Conduct

Good conduct is expected at all times. Most veterinary practices have disciplinary rules that lay out the conduct expected from all staff and the disciplinary procedures that take place if conduct is deemed to be unacceptable. Figure 1.1 lists examples of what most practices would consider unacceptable conduct.

Misconduct
Poor attendance for reasons other than sickness
Poor work standards
Non-compliance with health and safety rules
Breach of confidentiality
Refusal to carry out instructions
Unacceptable behaviour (e.g. rudeness to clients or other staff)
Non-cooperation
Unacceptable off-duty behaviour

Gross misconduct
Theft
Falsification of records
Fraud
Assault
Malicious damage
Drunkenness
Drug abuse
Serious negligence

1.1 Unacceptable conduct.

Anyone breaking the practice's disciplinary rules is likely to receive an official warning which, if the bad conduct continues, can lead to dismissal. Gross misconduct will usually result in immediate dismissal.

Confidentiality and data protection

Confidentiality

The treatment given to clients' animals, the health problems they may have, and the financial costs and payment of bills are all totally confidential matters between the client and the veterinary practice. Under no circumstances should any of this information be discussed with other clients or with anyone outside the practice. In addition, staff home and mobile telephone numbers and addresses should never be given to clients or to anyone over the telephone. Figure 1.2 lists examples of the types of information that should be considered confidential.

Laboratory tests
Animal treatments
X-ray results
Medication prescribed
Client information (e.g. address, etc.)
An animal's diagnosis
An animal's prognosis
Conversations with clients
Staff addresses and home or mobile telephone numbers

1.2 Confidential information.

Data protection

Clients' records contain large amounts of personal details and information which the veterinary practice must keep secure and confidential. Records will contain the sort of information listed below.

Client record information

- Client's name and address
- Telephone number
- E-mail
- Insurance details
- Name and details of pet
- Vaccination dates
- Flea and worm treatments
- Weight
- Treatment details
- Client's financial details

The collection, storage and use of these data are controlled by the Data Protection Act 1998 (DPA). The Act has two main requirements:

- Users of personal data should notify the Information Commissioner that personal data are being held
- Users must comply with the eight principles of data protection (Figure 1.3).

Data must be:
- Fairly and lawfully processed
- Processed for limited purposes
- Adequate, relevant and not excessive
- Accurate and up to date
- Not kept longer than necessary
- Processed in accordance with the individual's rights
- Secure
- Not transferred to countries outside the European Economic Area without adequate protection

1.3   The principles of data protection.

The DPA gives individuals certain rights regarding information held about them (Figure 1.4).

- The right to find out what information is held about them
- The right to request that damaging or distressing information is not processed
- The right to prevent personal information being used for direct marketing
- The right to request that decisions based on their data are not made solely by automated means, e.g. automatic credit ratings
- The right to claim compensation for damage or distress caused by any breach of the Act
- The right to request destruction of personal details if they are inaccurate
- The right to request an assessment of their personal information if they believe it has not been processed in accordance with the Act

1.4   Client rights under the Data Protection Act.

All users of client data must comply with the DPA. In practical terms this means that data held about clients and their animals must be accurate, no more detailed than necessary, not held for longer than is necessary and held securely. To ensure that data are held securely, computer screens in the reception area and consulting rooms should be placed in such a position that clients and other visitors cannot read the information displayed (Figure 1.5).

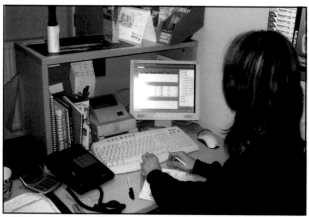

1.5   The confidentiality of client records must apply at all times.

Clients have the right to request a description of the data held about them. This information should be supplied in a permanent form and explanations of the information given if necessary. It should be borne in mind that veterinary practices often make coded notes on owners' records and that the right to inspect records will also cover these coded notes. Nurses should speak to a partner before passing such information on to a client.

Legislation and the veterinary nurse

Veterinary nurses, like anyone else, may give first aid and look after animals in ways that do not involve acts of veterinary surgery. In addition, veterinary nurses may carry out procedures specified in paragraphs 6 and 7 of Schedule 3 of the Veterinary Surgeons Act 1966 (Schedule 3 Amendment) Order 2002.

Schedule 3 lists the treatments and operations that may be carried out by non-veterinary surgeons and those that may only be performed by veterinary surgeons. Additionally it outlines the treatments that may be carried out by listed veterinary nurses and student veterinary nurses.

Listed Veterinary Nurses

Paragraph 6 of Schedule 3 applies to qualified veterinary nurses whose names are entered on the list maintained by the RCVS. It allows such veterinary nurses to carry out any medical treatment or any minor surgery (not involving entry into the body cavity) to any animal if the following conditions apply:

- The animal is, for the time being, under the care of a veterinary surgeon and the medical treatment or minor surgery is carried out by the veterinary nurse at the veterinary surgeon's direction
- The veterinary surgeon is the employer or is acting on behalf of the employer of the veterinary nurse
- The directing veterinary surgeon is satisfied that the veterinary nurse is qualified to carry out the treatment or surgery.

The Act does not define what constitutes medical treatment or minor surgery. This is left to the discretion of the veterinary surgeon, who must decide:

- Whether the nurse has the necessary qualifications and/or experience
- The difficulty of the procedure
- How available the veterinary surgeon would be to respond to any request for assistance
- How confident the veterinary nurse is in their capabilities.

The directing veterinary surgeon is always ultimately responsible for the actions of the veterinary nurse, although VNs do carry some legal responsibility under the new regulations.

Species covered by Schedule 3

All listed veterinary nurses (VNs) are qualified to administer medical treatment or minor surgery (not involving entry into a body cavity), under veterinary direction, to all the species that are commonly kept as companion animals, including exotic species so kept. Unless they are suitably trained or hold further qualifications, where such qualifications exist, they are not qualified to treat the equine species, wild animals or farm animals. Listed veterinary nurses who hold the RCVS Certificate in Equine Veterinary Nursing (EVNs) are qualified to administer medical treatment or minor surgery (not involving entry into a body cavity), under veterinary direction, to any of the equine species – horses, asses and zebras.

Procedures covered by Schedule 3

The procedures that veterinary nurses are specifically trained to carry out and that are listed in the RCVS advice to veterinary nurses on Schedule 3 are shown in Figure 1.6.

Administer medication
By mouth
Topically
By rectum
By inhalation
By subcutaneous injection
By intramuscular injection
By intravenous injection
Administer treatments
By oral, intravenous and subcutaneous injection
By fluid therapy
By catheterization
By cleaning and dressing of surgical wounds
By treatment of abscesses and ulcers
By application of external casts
By holding and handling of viscera when assisting in operations and cutaneous suturing
Prepare animals for anaesthesia and assist in the administration and termination of anaesthesia, including premedication, analgesia and intubation
Collect samples of blood, urine, faeces, skin and hair
Radiography: obtain X-ray images

1.6 Procedures that may be carried out by veterinary nurses.

Anaesthesia

Only a veterinary surgeon may assess the animal to be anaesthetized, select the premedication and anaesthetic regime, and administer anaesthetic if the induction dose is either incremental or to effect (this applies to most intravenous drugs). Provided that the veterinary surgeon is present and available for consultation, a listed veterinary nurse may:

- Administer a selected sedative, analgesic or other agent before and after the operation
- Administer non-incremental anaesthetic agents on veterinary instruction
- Monitor clinical signs and maintain an anaesthetic record
- Maintain anaesthesia by administering supplementary incremental doses of intravenous anaesthetic or adjusting the delivered concentration of anaesthetic agents under the direction of the veterinary surgeon.

Student veterinary nurses

Paragraph 7 of Schedule 3 applies to student veterinary nurses who are enrolled for the purpose of training as a veterinary nurse at an approved training and assessment centre (VNAC) or at a veterinary training practice (TP) approved by such a centre. It allows such veterinary nurses to carry out any medical treatment or any minor surgery (not involving entry into the body cavity), as outlined above, to any animal if the following conditions apply:

- The animal is, for the time being, under the care of the veterinary surgeon and the medical treatment or minor surgery is carried out by the student veterinary nurse at the surgeon's direction and in the course of the student veterinary nurse's training
- The treatment or surgery is supervised by a veterinary surgeon or listed veterinary nurse and, in the case of surgery, the supervision is direct, continuous and personal
- The veterinary surgeon is the employer or is acting on behalf of the employer of the student veterinary nurse.

In the view of the RCVS, a veterinary surgeon or listed veterinary nurse can only be said to be supervising if they are present on the premises and able to respond to a request for assistance.

Health and safety

Health and safety form an integral part of work in a veterinary practice. Veterinary nurses should be aware of health and safety issues in all the activities they undertake and in the situations they have to deal with. The Health and Safety at Work etc. Act 1974 requires an employer to ensure the health and safety of the staff they employ, as well as that of visitors and contractors who enter or work on the premises. In order to comply with the Act an employer must carry out risk assessments for all areas of their premises and the work that is carried out there (i.e. 'tasks') so that any potential dangers to employees, visitors or contractors are identified and then eliminated or controlled. Examples of typical 'task' and 'area' risk assessment forms are shown in Figures 1.7 and 1.8. These include instructions and references to data sheets for the use of agents that may be hazardous to health (e.g. biological agents, cleaning agents, drugs); these are COSHH (Control of Substances Hazardous to Health) assessments.

Risk assessments should be reviewed on a regular basis, usually annually, to ensure that any changes in the hazards are adequately controlled.

THE BENCHMARK VETERINARY SURGERY

TASK C.O.S.H.H. ASSESSMENT RECORD

Task No. 3	CLEANING UP OF ANIMAL FAECES, URINE ETC.	Record No. 1
Description:	Removal of animal faeces, urine, body fluids etc. & cleaning and disinfection.	
Location:	All animal handling areas of practice.	

Hazardous substances in use or that may be present or produced:

Name of substance	Nature of Hazard	Data Sheet No. or reference
Cleaning agents/disinfectants	May be toxic, irritant or corrosive. Potentially harmful by ingestion, inhalation of aerosols, skin and eye contact. Particularly if sensitive.	General Safety Data Sheets 4A, 4B & 4C in **Section E** of the **H&S Manual** and Specific Data Sheets:–
a. **Parvocide (EXAMPLE)**	Contains **glutaraldehyde** which is very harmful & has a very low exposure limit. Strong irritant by skin/eye contact and inhalation. Skin & respiratory sensitiser.	No. P45 **(EXAMPLE)**
c. **Virkon (EXAMPLE)**	Liquid is mild irritant. Powder irritant & may cause sensitisation by inhalation.	No. .V19 **(EXAMPLE)**
Micro-organisms from animal faeces, body fluids and tissue.	Zoonoses/infection. Potentially harmful by ingestion, skin/eye contact and via cuts and abrasions.	**Zoonoses Notes** in **Section E** of **H&S Manual**.

Frequency of task & duration:	Occasional short periods.

Control Measures CURRENTLY IN OPERATION/COMMENTS:

Staff are (**must be**) formally instructed in the methods for the safe handling and use of the various products, as specified in the Safety Data Sheets, and the procedures to follow in the event of spillage or personal exposure.

All necessary protective clothing is available and is (**must be**) used in accordance with instructions:
Minimum of gloves and waterproof apron for all cleaning tasks.
Disposable gloves must be worn to prevent contact with animal excreta/body fluids/tissue.
Eye protection and face masks may be required for some concentrated or spray products.

In the event of   **skin contact**:– wash off with cold water and remove contaminated clothing.
                    eye contact:– rinse with copious running water or eye wash & seek medical attention.
                    ingestion:– rinse mouth with water and consult specific data sheet. Seek medical attention.
                    inhalation:– move to fresh air. Seek medical attention if irritation or other symptoms develop.

Employees must not handle products if they are known to be sensitive or have allergies to them.
No "home made" mixtures of cleaning agents are to be used. Don't mix products as harmful fumes may be given off.
All cleaning agents/disinfectants must be kept in their original labelled containers. The containers must be discarded if the labels become unreadable.
No cleaning agents or materials are to be left within reach of clients, especially children.
Strict adherence to Codes Of Practice especially regarding personal hygiene is required.
Every care must be taken to prevent exposing clients to the hazardous substances (e.g. from spills/splashes).
This task must be performed by staff only, NEVER by the clients.

Assessment of personal exposure and RISKS TO HEALTH:
Generally LOW – provided that the control measures are implemented.
Potentially high risks associated with products containing glutaraldehyde. **Additional controls required** – see below.

Actions required:	Responsible persons:	When:
1. Carry out & record periodic spot-checks (as described and detailed in the H&S Manual) to ensure control measures, as stated, are routinely and fully implemented.	Relevant Area Safety Officers.	Every six months
2. **Discontinue use of Parvocide. Use alternative product.**	**Practice Safety Officer**	NOW

Signed:	**Date:**
Date for next assessment:	**Implement action 2 and review assessment record ASAP.** Fully re-assess this task June 2008 – or sooner if circumstances change.

1.7 An example of a health and safety task assessment form. (© Salus Q.P. Ltd)

THE BENCHMARK VETERINARY SURGERY

AREA C.O.S.H.H. ASSESSMENT RECORD

Area No. 1	WAITING ROOM / RECEPTION	Record No. 1

Description/Location:	Gnd floor. Reception desk in centre of rear wall (closed to public). Access to/from Cons Rms, corridor to rear of practice, staff/client WC (disabled). Ventilation via windows/doors. Vinyl flooring. See the schematic site plan.

Tasks & Activities carried out:	For safety information & procedures refer to:
T1 General Cleaning	Task COSHH Assessment No. 1 in **Section D** of **H&S Manual**
T2 Cleaning Surfaces	Task Assessment No. 2 "
T3 Cleaning up of Animal Faeces, Urine etc.	Task COSHH Assessment No. 3 "
T10 Handling & Storage of Packaged Drugs & Chemicals	Task COSHH Assessment No. 10 "
A2 Animal Handling	COPs re Handling of Animals in **Section B** of **H&S Manual**
A7 General Office Work	COPs re COSHH, Work Equipment in **Section B** of **H&S Manual**

Hazardous substances in use or that may be present or produced:

T/A	Name of substance	Nature of Hazard	Data Sheet No. or reference
T1,2,3	Cleaning Agents	May be toxic, caustic, irritant or harmful by ingestion, inhalation, skin & eye contact (particularly if sensitive).	Specific Task COSHH Assessments and **General Safety Data Sheets 4A & 4B** in **Section E** of **H&S Manual.**
T10	Medicinal and Veterinary products and chemicals	Various. May be harmful by ingestion, inhalation, skin/eye contact. **Exposure only likely in event of** damage to packaging or poor working practice.	**General Safety Data Sheets** in **Section E** of **H&S Manual** and the **NOAH compendium.**
A2	Micro-organisms from faeces, urine, blood, bites, scratches.	Zoonoses/Infection. Potentially harmful by ingestion, inhalation, eye contact & via cuts and abrasions.	**Zoonoses Notes** in **Section E** of **H&S Manual.**
A7	Small quantities of office chemicals	Toxic, irritant. Potentially harmful by ingestion, inhalation, skin/eye contact	Product labels & General COPs

Who may be exposed, and for how long:	All staff & clients (**inc children**). Short periods daily. Max time (staff) 1 full day.

FACILITIES/SYSTEMS	ASSESSMENT	FACILITIES/SYSTEMS	ASSESSMENT
Ventilation (re need vs ability to extract)? **PASSIVE**	OK	Nearest Hand-Wash facilities? **Cons Rooms**	OK
Flooring (re ease to clean/disinfect)? **VINYL, good**	OK	Access (who is vs needs to be there – Staff/Clients)?	OK
Segregation (re **Haz:Non-H** areas/tasks/people)?	OK	Re Eating/drinking (i.e. **how bug/drug/chem free**)?	Not Suitable

Control Measures CURRENTLY IN OPERATION/COMMENTS:
The "General Site" control measures also apply (see the General Site, Area 0, COSHH Assessment Record).

Staff receive training in, and strictly adhere to, good hygiene and work practices (**confirmed by regular spot checks**).
Veterinary and medical products are not (**must not be**) displayed within the reach of children.
Only those medicinal and veterinary products required on a regular basis are (allowed to be) stored in the Reception area – and **only** in their packaged form.
Cleaning agents/chemicals are not (**must not be**) left within the reach of clients, especially children, in the Waiting Room or in the WC used by clients.
Faeces/urine are (**must be**) cleaned up promptly – by staff NOT by clients (see Task 3 COSHH Assessment Record).
Clients and visitors are not (**must not be**) left unsupervised in this area.

Assessment of personal exposure and RISKS TO HEALTH:
LOW – provided that the control measures are fully implemented.

Actions required:	Responsible persons:	When:
1. Carry out & record periodic spot-checks (as described and detailed in the H&S Manual) to ensure the control measures, as stated, are routinely & fully implemented. 2.	Area Safety Officer.	Every six months

Signed:	Date:

Date for next assessment:	**June 2008** – or sooner if circumstances change

1.8 An example of a health and safety area risk assessment for waiting areas and reception. (© Salus Q.P. Ltd)

As employees of the veterinary practice, veterinary nurses have a legal responsibility under the Act to take reasonable care with regard to their own and others' health and safety and to follow the health and safety instructions and guidance provided by their employer. They must also report to the Health and Safety Officer any concerns they may have about health and safety

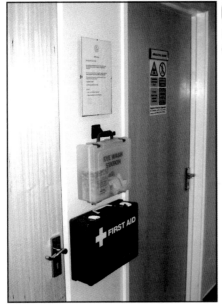

1.9

Human first aid equipment.

– for example, procedures not followed or equipment that is broken or faulty. There should be formal health and safety induction for all staff who join the practice. This will usually be given by a designated Health and Safety Officer.

'Health and Safety' is sometimes mistakenly seen as an 'added extra' to the working day, but should be an integral part of the nurse's job. Everything that is done should carry an awareness of maintaining safety.

Each practice will have designated 'First Aiders' with suitable qualifications and access to first aid equipment (Figure 1.9). In the absence of the designated First Aider, staff must be aware of the practice's policy and have basic skills for dealing with human accident and injury.

Health and safety in reception

Although no significant veterinary procedures are carried out in the reception area, there are still a number of possible hazards to staff and clients to be considered. Typical control measures that might be put in place to reduce the potential hazards in the reception area are shown in Figures 1.8 and 1.10. Nurses should be aware of the possible hazards in the reception area and the control measures that the practice has in place to remove or reduce the likelihood of danger to staff and clients. It is important that these control measures are followed for the safety of both staff and clients.

Hazard	Control measures
Staff and clients being bitten by animals	Staff training in animal handling All cats must be in cat boxes and dogs on a lead First Aider available
Slipping on wet floors	'Wet floor' notices Clean floors at least busy times
Fire	Fire extinguishers Fire procedures training Fire rules
Lifting heavy bags of food or heavy animals	Staff training in animal and manual handling Provision of handling equipment
Trailing wires and cables	Staff training in good safety practice
Unsafe equipment	Equipment checks
Unsafe use of equipment	Staff training in equipment use
Contamination from biological agents (e.g. blood, faeces)	COSHH (Control of Substances Hazardous to Health) risk assessment
Contact with drugs	Staff training COSHH risk assessment
Lone working	Staff training Lone worker protocols Personal alarms for staff
Excessive use of computer screens	Staff training in use of equipment Protocol for use of computer equipment
Contamination from cleaning materials	Staff training COSHH risk assessment (see Figure 1.7)

1.10 Examples of potential hazards and control measures in the reception area.

Health and safety in the consulting room

The consulting room poses a greater health and safety risk, simply because of the nature of the work carried out there. Animals are being examined and treated and are therefore more stressed and likely to cause injury to the veterinary surgeon, nurse or client. Drugs are being used and injections given, some of which are potentially hazardous, and clinical waste is often being generated. Typical control measures that might be in place to reduce the potential hazards in the consulting room are shown in Figures 1.7, 1.11 and 1.12.

Hazard	Control measures
Staff and clients being bitten by animals	Staff training in animal handling Only nurses or veterinary surgeons to hold animals on consulting table, or a sign advising owners to ask for assistance (Figure 1.12) First Aider available Muzzle available
Slipping on wet floors	'Wet floor' notices
Fire	Fire extinguishers Fire procedures training Fire rules
Lifting heavy animals	Staff training in animal and manual handling Provision of handling equipment
Trailing wires and cables	Staff training in good safety practice
Unsafe equipment	Equipment checks
Unsafe use of equipment	Staff training in equipment use
Contamination from biological agents (e.g. blood, faeces)	COSHH (Control of Substances Hazardous to Health) risk assessment
Contact with drugs	Staff training COSHH risk assessment
Lone working causing danger from attack or accident	Staff training Lone worker protocols Personal alarms for staff
Clients' children coming into contact with drugs placed at child height	All drugs kept out of reach of children
Self-injection	Good working practices COSHH risk assessment
Clinical waste contamination	Staff training in waste disposal Protocol for disposal of different types of waste COSHH risk assessment
Sharp injuries causing cuts and lacerations	Good working practices
Contamination from cleaning materials causing adverse reactions	Staff training COSHH risk assessment (see Figure 1.7)

1.11 Examples of potential hazards and control measures in the consulting room.

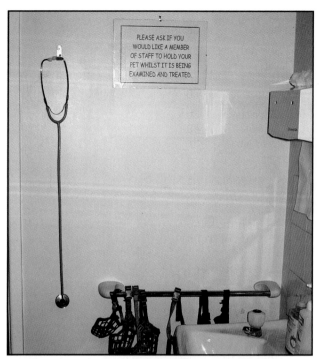

1.12 A notice in the consulting room advises clients on the availability of assistance in handling pets, with easy access to muzzles.

Nurses should be aware of the possible hazards in the consulting room and the control measures that the practice has in place to reduce the likelihood of danger to staff and clients. It is important that these control measures are followed for the safety of both staff and clients.

Health and safety in the kennels

Kennels pose particular hazards for nursing staff. Not only is there the possibility of scratches and bites from caged animals but there is also the possibility of contamination from biological hazards while handling the animals or while cleaning out cages. Typical control measures that might be in place to reduce the potential hazards in kennels are shown in Figure 1.13.

Hazard	Control measures
Staff and clients being bitten by animals	Staff training in animal handling First Aider available Muzzle available
Slipping on wet floors	'Wet floor' notices
Fire	Fire extinguishers Fire procedures training Fire rules
Lifting heavy animals	Staff training in animal and manual handling Provision of handling equipment
Contamination from biological agents (e.g. blood, faeces)	Staff training COSHH (Control of Substances Hazardous to Health) risk assessment (see Figure 1.7)

1.13 Examples of potential hazards and control measures in kennels. (continues) ▶

Hazard	Control measures
Clinical waste contamination	Staff training in waste disposal Protocol for disposal of different types of waste COSHH risk assessment
Contamination from cleaning materials causing adverse reactions	Staff training COSHH risk assessment
Noise from barking dogs	Ear protection

1.13 (continued) Examples of potential hazards and control measures in kennels.

Nurses should be aware of the possible hazards in the kennels and the control measures that the practice has in place to reduce the likelihood of danger to staff and also to clients, should they be visiting their hospitalized pets. It is important that these control measures are followed for the safety of both staff and clients.

Health and safety in the theatre and 'prep' room

The theatre and 'prep' (preparation) room probably pose the greatest health and safety risk to staff (Figure 1.14). Animals are being examined, treated, anaesthetized and operated upon. There are a large variety of instruments, many different types of equipment and the use of anaesthetics (see Chapter 12). Drugs are being used and injections given, some of which are potentially hazardous, and clinical waste is being generated. Typical control measures that might be in place to reduce the potential hazards in the theatre and 'prep' room are shown in Figure 1.15.

Nurses should be aware of the possible hazards in the theatre and prep room and the control measures that the practice has in place to reduce the likelihood of danger to staff. It is important that these control measures are followed for the safety of staff.

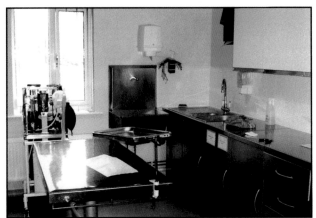

1.14 The theatre and preparation areas have many hazards. How many can you recognize?

Radiation

Radiation is a very important health hazard in veterinary practice and is dealt with in Chapter 11.

Hazard	Control measures
Clinical waste contamination	Staff training in waste disposal Protocol for disposal of different types of waste COSHH (Control of Substances Hazardous to Health) risk assessment
Sharp injuries causing cuts and lacerations	Good working practice
Contamination from cleaning materials causing adverse reactions	Staff training COSHH risk assessment
Self-injection	Good working practices COSHH risk assessment
Unsafe equipment	Equipment checks
Unsafe use of equipment	Staff training in equipment use
Contamination from biological agents (e.g. blood, faeces)	Staff training COSHH risk assessment (see Figure 1.7)
Contact with drugs	Staff training COSHH risk assessment
Staff being bitten by animals	Staff training in animal handling First Aider available Muzzle available
Slipping on wet floors	'Wet floor' notices
Fire	Fire extinguishers Fire procedures training Fire rules
Lifting heavy animals	Staff training in animal and manual handling Provision of handling equipment
Inhalation of anaesthetic gases	Staff training in use of anaesthetic equipment COSHH risk assessment Gas scavenging
Use of general operating equipment (e.g. dental machine, clippers, autoclave)	Staff training in use of equipment Personal protective equipment (PPE) Equipment checks

1.15 Examples of potential hazards and control measures in the theatre and 'prep' room.

Further reading and useful websites

Data Protection Act 1998
Health and Safety Executive (HSE) *An Introduction to Health and Safety.*
Health and Safety Executive (HSE) *Five Steps to Risk Assessment.*
Health and Safety Executive website: www.hse.gov.uk
RCVS (2006) *Guide to Professional Conduct.* RCVS, London (also available online at www.rcvs.org.uk)

2

Client communication and advice

Laura Nicholls, Maggie Shilcock, Sarah Heath and Freda Scott-Park

---

This chapter is designed to give information on:

- Communicating with clients
- Advising clients on buying pets
- Advising clients on pet behaviour, including puppy parties; nutrition and feeding; obesity and weight clinics; pet reproduction; neutering of pets; control of infectious diseases; vaccination; overseas travel with pets, and pet passports; management of parasitic infections
- Preparing the client for euthanasia of a pet; the grief sequence and dealing with bereavement
- Admission and discharge of patients
- The processing of payments from clients

Principles of client communication

Communicating well and effectively with clients is an essential part of the service provided by veterinary practice staff. The veterinary nurse plays a very important role in client communication at many different levels, from greeting clients in reception to holding nurse clinics, discharging patients and explaining treatments. The veterinary practice and its staff must create a good working relationship with clients so that the client feels that they are part of the practice and that the practice staff really care about them and their animals. A good relationship of this kind is key to bonding with and retaining clients. Clients are looking for convenience, confidence, help, advice, understanding and care when they come to the practice. Nurses are often the first point of contact for a client either on the telephone, in the reception area, when an animal is admitted, or at a nurse's clinic, and the nurse's communication skills can have a great effect on the client's first impressions of the practice.

Meeting and greeting clients

The greeting is the first point of contact the client has with the practice and it is very important that they are made to feel welcome and confident that the practice is going to help them and their pet. How a client is greeted can make or break the impression they gain of the practice. Many clients come to the veterinary practice worried and anxious; the nurse should always aim to put them at their ease by being friendly, helpful, sympathetic and, above all, professional.

When a client enters the practice they should be acknowledged immediately. It takes only a few seconds for a client to feel ignored.

- Smile and establish eye contact with the client and greet them and their pet by name whenever possible. Even if the nurse is on the telephone it is still possible to smile at the client and indicate that they should take a seat.
- Always check the client's appointment time when they arrive and inform them if the veterinary surgeon's consultation times are running late.

- Check the appointment details, the animal's name and the reason for the appointment and make sure that all the correct details are available for the veterinary surgeon.
- Make sure that the client understands the appointment procedure. Be aware that some clients will require a more complete explanation of practice procedures than others and that clients with disabilities (e.g. hard of hearing, visually impaired or with mobility problems) will require extra help from the nursing staff.

Being professional

First impressions count. The nurse should always appear smartly and tidily dressed in a clean uniform. The reception desk should be kept tidy and orderly. Food and drink should be consumed in the staff room, never at the reception desk.

Confidentiality

Clients' records contain large amounts of personal details that the veterinary practice must keep secure and confidential (see Chapter 1).

Computer screens in the reception area should be placed in such a position that clients and other visitors to the surgery cannot read the information displayed and any confidential paperwork should be kept out of sight of other clients. Client details should never be discussed in front of other clients, or with other clients or members of the public or outside the practice.

The reception area

This is the first part of the practice that the client sees and it should be clean and tidy at all times. An untidy, smelly or dirty reception area suggests to the client an untidy and dirty practice and immediately they will start to worry about the care of their animal.

Magazines and leaflets should be kept in tidy piles or in racks; posters should look attractive; and notice boards should be uncluttered and have no out-of-date information on them. Floors should be cleaned on a regular basis; any urine or faeces should be removed immediately and the area cleaned using the correct disinfectant. Gloves should always be worn to do this and the waste should be disposed of as clinical waste.

Restraint of animals in the reception area

For the safety of clients, their animals and the veterinary staff, all dogs should be kept on leads in the reception area and all cats should be kept in cat baskets. All other types of animal should be suitably restrained. It helps if there is a notice in the reception area requiring clients to restrain their pets.

Making appointments

Some practices will have a computerized appointments diary; others will use an appointments book. When a client phones for or asks to make an appointment for a consultation, the client should be asked for the information shown in the box below.

Making appointments

Ask the client for the following information:

- **Client's name**
- **Address**
- **Name and type of animal**
- **How many animals the client is bringing**
- **Reason for wanting appointment**
- **History of condition, if any**
- **Current situation**
- **Vet last seen**
- **Vet client wishes to see.**

If the owner considers that their animal is very ill or is suffering, an appointment should be made as soon as possible. If the call is an emergency (Figure 2.1) the client should be asked to bring their animal to the surgery immediately. See Chapter 7 for more information on telephone triage.

Road traffic accidents (RTAs)
Breathing/respiratory problems
Collapse
Insect stings, especially around or in the mouth
Snake bites, especially around or in the mouth
Major (arterial) bleeding
Long-term problems with whelping

2.1 Examples of emergencies.

For less urgent and routine visits, appointments should be offered to the client that are convenient to them but also to the practice, i.e. that fit in with the consulting pattern required for the day. For example, if there are appointments booked from 2 pm to 3 pm and then from 4 pm to 5.30 pm, the client should be offered a time at the end of the first set of appointments or the beginning of the second, rather than at 3.30 pm. Organizing appointments in this way gives the veterinary surgeon time to make phone calls and catch up on paperwork. It should be checked that the client is bringing only one animal; if they are bringing more than one animal, a double appointment should be booked. Some procedures will require the booking of a double appointment (e.g. first vaccinations) and the practice's policy for making appointments of this kind should be checked.

Providing information

Part of the nurse's role is to ensure that clients are informed of all the services the practice offers to enable them to keep their animal fit and healthy. This client education is an important part of good client care provided by the practice.

The nurse should talk to the client about services that would benefit their animal and offer the advice necessary. This may be information about nurse's clinics, or advice on matters such as feeding, worming or microchipping. The client must not be pressurized into agreeing to treatments or buying products, as this would be unprofessional.

Nurses need to be aware which veterinary products they can legally discuss with clients. For example, under the current new medicines directives, veterinary nurses can only discuss AVM–GSL products with clients. (For more information on drug classification, see Chapter 3.)

Non-verbal communication

A large proportion of communication is non-verbal. People do not need to speak to show how they feel – their actions, expressions and body language can do this for them. When dealing with clients face to face, it is important to be aware of the non-verbal signals that clients are sending and being given. Clients need to be given positive non-verbal messages, to show that practice staff are listening to them and care about them. Figure 2.2 gives some examples of positive and negative body language.

Positive body language	Negative body language
Smiling	Not smiling, but frowning or looking glum
Eye contact, but not staring	Not making eye contact
Facing the person	Turning away
Open and relaxed body position	Arms folded Clenched fists
No fiddling or fidgeting	Fiddling or fidgeting
Nodding in agreement	Foot or hand tapping

2.2   Body language.

Recognizing basic positive and negative body language can help in dealing with difficult situations and in judging how likely a client is to accept suggestions or agree to treatment. For example, a client who continues to exhibit negative body language after having the reasons for diet food explained to them is less likely to purchase the food than the client who is smiling and showing positive body language.

Telephone manner

The telephone is a major method of communication in veterinary practice (Figure 2.3). It is often the first point of contact that a client or potential client has with the practice and the impression they receive from the person answering the phone must be good. The nurse who picks up the phone must make the very best use of their communication skills.

Answering the telephone

Number of rings

Normally the telephone should be answered after three or four rings. If it rings too many times it suggests that the practice is not interested in the call or is simply too busy to reply. In either case the client may give up and contact another practice.

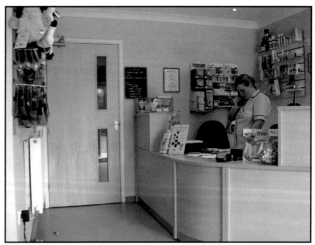

2.3   The telephone is an important means of client communication.

The greeting

The greeting given to the client will have been decided by the practice, but generally a greeting such as 'Good morning' or 'Good afternoon' should be given, followed by the name of the practice. It is polite to ask how the practice can help the client and some practices also require receptionists to give their name to the client in the greeting.

Speaking clearly

It is important to speak clearly and not too fast, to sound welcoming and never to use slang, such as 'OK'. The tone of voice is very important, because it is the only means of communicating with the client. The client cannot see the person at the other end of the telephone or any of their body language, so what is said can sometimes be less important that how it is said. A grumpy or disinterested voice could easily cause the client to feel unwanted or a nuisance.

Identifying the caller and the problem

Details should be taken of the caller's name and address, the name of their animal and its illness, or the treatment or service required, so that the veterinary surgeon can prepare for the consultation.

- Listen carefully and make sure that all the facts about the animal have been taken and fully understood. It can help to repeat the symptoms back to the client just to make sure that there have been no misunderstandings if the case is complicated.
- If the call is a request for advice, provide the necessary information or pass the caller on to a member of staff who can help.

The phone as priority

A phone call can mean an emergency and so even if a client is already being dealt with the phone must be answered. Apologies should be made to the client at the reception desk, with an explanation if necessary that the phone call could be a life or death situation. Most clients will be understanding – after all, it might be them making the call one day.

Putting on hold

There will be times when it is necessary to put a caller on hold.

- If this is the case, always ask the client whether it is all right to put them on hold.
- Wait for their answer (remember that the call could be an emergency, in which case being put on hold would not be acceptable).
- Return to the client at regular intervals and do not leave them on hold for intervals of more than 30 seconds.
- Then ask if they are still happy to remain on hold.
- If they are not happy, or it is clear that they will have to wait a long time, offer to phone them back.

Busy times

The nurse should try not to sound harassed at busy times: the client will hear the stress in their voice and this is not a good advertisement for the practice, as it suggests bad organization. At busy times it may be appropriate to offer to phone back a client who has a particularly complicated query that cannot be dealt with easily when phones are constantly ringing.

Taking messages

It will often be necessary to take detailed messages from clients or other veterinary practices or organizations.

- Always have a pen and paper available.
- Make careful, clear, detailed notes of any message.
- Remember to take a contact name and telephone number.
- Be sure who the message was for.
- If any of the message is unclear, ask for it to be repeated.
- If the practice has a computer message system, send a message straight away – before it is forgotten or the paper message becomes lost.

Difficult clients

Dealing with difficult clients is occasionally part of the nurse's role and it is important that communication with these clients reduces rather than increases their difficult behaviour. Clients can be difficult for a variety of reasons. They may be anxious or upset or having a stressful day. Sometimes it is because the practice has upset them in some way. Or they may just always behave in this way. The steps to follow when dealing with a difficult client are shown in the box below.

Dealing with a difficult client

- **Listen carefully to what they are saying and make sure their problem or complaint is understood.**
- **Be patient. Sometimes the client needs to get the problem off their chest and the situation is then diffused.**
- **Remain calm and use a normal tone of voice with the client.**
- **Never become angry or defensive. This will only worsen the situation, making the client even more difficult to deal with.**
- **Do not pass blame or make excuses. The client will simply not be interested.**
- **Sort the problem out (if this is possible) quickly and in a positive manner.**
- **If the client is causing embarrassment, consider asking them to move to a separate room where their problem can be discussed in private. (For personal safety, do *not* do this with an aggressive or really angry client.)**
- **If unable to sort out the problem easily, seek help from someone in authority (e.g. the Practice Manager) and pass the client on to them so that other waiting clients can be dealt with.**

Aggressive clients

There are occasions when clients become aggressive or abusive and need to be dealt with even more carefully. Their behaviour can sometimes be because of drink or drugs, and this kind of client is not acting in a reasonable manner. The steps to follow when dealing with an aggressive client are shown in the box below.

Dealing with the aggressive client

- **Listen carefully.**
- **Stay calm; do not argue or become defensive.**
- **Remain polite at all times.**
- **Avoid any prolonged eye contact (as this can be seen as threatening or challenging).**
- **Take action by sorting out the problem quickly or by seeking help from a more senior member of staff.**
- **Keep your distance from the client – they may be unpredictable. Never make any physical contact with them.**
- **If the client is likely to be a danger to staff or other clients, call the police.**

Whatever the outcome of dealing with a difficult client, the encounter should not be taken personally. The client has no personal grudge – they simply took out their feelings or anger on the first person they came across in reception.

Advice on buying pets and on pet behaviour

Advice on selecting a pet

When working with prospective pet owners, the main objective is to meet their requirements and offer them the best potential for a long and mutually rewarding relationship between themselves and their pet.

Prospective owners may not have fully considered and evaluated their reasons for selecting a particular species, breed, age or sex. Asking the right questions can help to avoid mismatches between owner and pet. Questions to ask prospective owners include the following:

- How much time can be spent with a pet?
- Are there any children in the household? What are their ages?
- Are the owners disabled or elderly?
- Are the family working full time?
- Is there anyone in the family with known allergies?
- Are there any other animals currently at home?
- What is the size of the garden, if any?
- What is the availability of local dog walking?
- What size is the house?
- What are the anticipated costs and available finance?

Advice on new pets

When an owner has chosen their new pet, it is an essential time for the veterinary nurse to be able to provide them with a range of useful information. Subjects on which owners will require advice include:

- Importance of socialization of the pet
- Vaccinations
- Flea and worm treatments
- Neutering
- Insurance
- Microchipping
- Diet
- Toilet training
- Understanding of natural behaviour of the species concerned.

Information on these subjects is given below or elsewhere in this chapter.

Socializing puppies and kittens

Introduction to complexity in both the physical and social environment is essential for appropriate emotional development. The aim is for the early rearing environment to match as closely as possible the environment in which the animal will live as an adult. Research has shown that puppies are most receptive to complexity between 4 and 8 weeks of age, while kittens benefit most from appropriate interactions and environments between the ages of 2 and 7 weeks. The important learning processes during this important phase of development are referred to as socialization and habituation. Figure 2.4 gives a checklist for clients to refer to when trying to give their pets a full range of experiences in those first few weeks but it is also important to ensure that puppies and kittens have received adequate socialization and habituation at the breeder's premises. Examples of the sorts of experiences that puppies need to receive are:

- Different surfaces to walk on
- Different sounds
- Different animals
- Different people's appearances
- A range of different everyday human activities.

Places to go
Veterinary clinic
Other people's houses
Recreation area
Roadside
Railway stations and bus depots
Rural environment
Towns and cities
Lifts and escalators

People to meet
Men
Women
Children and babies
Elderly people
Disabled people
Delivery people, e.g. milkman, postman
People on bicycles, pushing prams, jogging
People who differ significantly in appearance from the family members
Veterinary practice staff and others in distinctive clothing

Animals to meet
Dogs
Cats
Other domestic pets
Livestock

Things to encounter
Domestic appliances
Vehicles
Children's toys
Pushchairs

2.4   Checklist for socialization and habituation.

Once a puppy is fully vaccinated (see later), the level of exposure can be further increased as it can be taken out on a lead into a variety of different environments.

Puppy parties

Puppy parties are a good way to socialize puppies to people and other dogs. They offer advice on preventive healthcare and correct dietary requirements and also allow discussion relating to the prevention of the most common unwanted behaviours. Any obvious signs of inappropriate behaviour can be identified and behavioural advice can be sought whilst the puppy is still young. The parties also benefit the practice, by introducing new clients to the practice and ensuring that owners fully understand how to care for their pets. Puppy parties also raise the profile of the practice nurse within the practice.

Puppy parties can be advertised by:

- Notice boards in waiting rooms and consultation rooms
- Letters/invitations sent to owners
- Reception staff making clients aware
- Local press advertisements
- Leaflets.

Running puppy parties in veterinary practices

Appropriate interactions with puppies at this young age are crucial to successful behavioural development. If a veterinary practice does not have the correct facilities to run puppy parties well, it is better to advise clients to seek alternative sources of early socialization and training, such as through a local reputable puppy school or training club. If practices do not feel able to provide the correct environment or staff ratio to carry out a successful puppy party with puppies present, they can still offer client education evenings in which they can talk to clients and offer them important advice about their pet's development.

When puppy parties are offered, the best time of day for them to take place is often the evening, when people have finished work and the practice is closed so that very few interruptions should occur. Most puppy parties are run in the reception/waiting room area to allow easy cleaning. The size of room available will determine what can take place during the party. It is important that the nurse is able to see what is happening everywhere in the room to ensure that all puppies have a good experience (especially during the puppy play) and the nurse can still be in control. Figure 2.5 shows a puppy party in progress after normal surgery hours in the waiting room of a veterinary hospital.

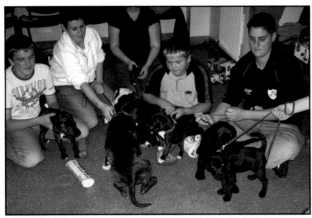

2.5 A puppy party in a veterinary hospital waiting room.

Creating a party atmosphere is essential for the enjoyment of owners and puppies. However, it is important to retain a degree of control and avoid situations where puppy parties become a free for all of poorly supervised interaction between the puppies. For the puppy, the main aims of the parties are:

- Socialization – getting used to other humans and animals
- Habituation – getting used to the non-living part of the environment, made up of different sights, sounds, smells and experiences (including getting used to coming to the veterinary surgery).

An example of a puppy class plan is given in Figure 2.6. It is set over 4 weeks on a particular night of the week to suit the practice.

For more information on basic training, see the *BSAVA Textbook of Veterinary Nursing.*

Week 1	Week 2
Nutrition talk Puppy play Vaccine talk Fun game	Talk on fleas and worms Puppy play Fun game
Week 3	**Week 4**
Microchip night Puppy play Dentistry talk Fun game	Training talk Puppy play Fun game Passing out

2.6 Example of a plan for 4-week puppy parties.

Recognizing behaviour problems

Many owners will not seek advice about behaviour and it is the responsibility of the practice to encourage owners to ask for help before behavioural problems become too serious. Reasons why clients may not ask for help include the following:

- They may not realize that a veterinary surgeon or veterinary nurse can help with this sort of problem
- They do not realize that something can be done to correct the unwanted behaviour
- They blame themselves for being poor owners
- They are embarrassed to admit that they have a problem
- They are frightened that others will find the situation amusing and even trivial.

Clients may react in a number of ways when their pet begins to display unusual behaviour patterns. They might:

- Accept and even encourage the behaviour
- Tolerate the behaviour
- Consider returning the pet to the breeder
- Consider rehoming
- Consider euthanasia
- Actively seek advice and help from a veterinary practice or other source.

Tolerant owners or those considering rehoming or euthanasia can be identified by the veterinary practice. Through offering advice and assistance, it is often possible to alter their perception of the problem and encourage them to seek appropriate help.

Identifying potential behavioural cases relies on skills of observation and listening. For example, a dog's behaviour can be determined by the way it enters the waiting room with its owner and the interaction between owner and pet whilst waiting for an appointment.

- Does a dog charge into the waiting room ahead of the owner?
- Does an owner carry a dog in while partially hiding it under a coat or blanket?
- Where does the owner choose to sit? Is it close to the door for easy exit, or in a quiet corner where they will not be disturbed?

Carefully observing the owner and the pet is a good way to understand their relationship. Mismatches between people and their pets may be evident, but in most cases it is too late to correct these. The advice that is given to owners needs to be tactful, relevant and practical.

Possible behavioural problems in dogs

- **Control problems, either at home or on walks**
- **Toileting problems**
- **Destructive behaviour**
- **Aggression to people or animals**
- **Separation-related problems**
- **Fears and phobias**
- **Geriatric behavioural changes**
- **Medically based behavioural problems**
- **Behavioural pathologies**

Possible behavioural problems in cats

- **Elimination problems (urinating or defecating in inappropriate places)**
- **Inappropriate marking behaviours**
- **Aggression to people or animals**
- **Pica (eating non-food items)**
- **Fears and phobias**
- **Geriatric behavioural changes**
- **Medically based behavioural problems**
- **Behavioural pathologies**

Owner's response to pet's behaviour

Knowledge of the owner's response to behavioural problems will help to determine whether owner involvement has had any effect on the progression of the problem. For example, a dog that growls defensively when someone attempts to remove a valued object from its possession may have been punished by the owner for doing so. The behaviour may subsequently have developed into a more generalized aggression to the owner, because the dog is fearful that further negative interactions might occur in the future.

Questions to ask owners about their pet's behaviour might include the following:

- Describe the behavioural problem in detail.
- When did it start?
- What were the circumstances of the first occurrence?
- How has the behaviour developed since the first incidence?
- How often does it occur?
- When does it occur?
- Where does it occur?
- How do the owners rate the severity?
- What attempts have been made to deal with the behaviour?
- How do the owners react?

Specialist advice

Some behavioural problems can be dealt with successfully in the veterinary practice; others may require referral to someone with more experience in the field. Behavioural medicine is a specialized veterinary discipline, and the offering of behavioural advice is a specialist area of veterinary nursing that requires specific training. Incorrect advice may lead to the problem becoming worse for both the pet and the owner. Until experienced in this field, veterinary nurses should seek advice from others with specialist training. For further information see the *BSAVA Manual of Canine and Feline Behavioural Medicine*.

Advice on feeding and nutrition

Feeding healthy pets

In veterinary practices it is often the role of the veterinary nurse to provide clients with guidance on feeding their pets. It is important to help clients meet the unique and changing nutritional requirements of their pet at each stage of its life. It is also important to advise clients correctly to avoid the dangers of feeding an incorrect or deficient diet. Clients are often knowledgeable in this area and will need well informed advice. Additional details of nutrients and the principles of nutrition can be found in the *BSAVA Textbook of Veterinary Nursing*.

Feeding requirements for life

The dietary requirements of pets are usually based around their energy requirements, which vary with growth, age and other influencing factors such as pregnancy, lactation, disease and exercise. The calculation of the maintenance energy requirement (MER) for dogs, cats and exotics is discussed in Chapter 9. As well as energy, animals require a variable protein, vitamin and mineral content in their diet at different stages of life.

Life stages are broadly defined for dogs and cats as:

- Kittens and puppies: weaning to 1 year of age
- Adult cat or dog: between 1 and 7 years of age
- Senior cat or dog: over 7 years of age.

The breed of pet is an additional influencing factor; for example, larger-breed dogs require suitable nutrition for a protracted growing period and tend to 'age' earlier than smaller breeds.

Life-stage nutrition for dogs and cats is described in Figure 2.7.

Diet types and formulations

Because of the difficulties in formulating homemade diets to meet energy and other nutritional requirements and avoid deficiencies and excesses, most veterinary practices recommend manufactured commercial foods. These come in many formulations (e.g. complete, complementary) and various physical forms (e.g. dried, tinned), some of which are described in Figure 2.8.

Life stage/activity	Advice to clients
Growth	*Pre-weaning* Ideally the bitch's or queen's milk, if this is not possible then fostering is the next best approach. If kittens or puppies are to be hand-reared then a proprietary milk substitute is required in the long term as both cow's and goat's milk give inadequate levels of nutrients. *Post-weaning* Most puppies attain 50% of their adult weight by 5–6 months, but maximal growth does not mean optimal growth. The energy demands of a growing puppy are high and need to be met by frequent meals to enable the necessary volume to be consumed (e.g. a 20 kg, 12-week-old puppy needs about 2.5 kg of wet food per day). Puppy feeds need to be energy dense, and highly digestible, with a suitable amount and balance of vitamins and minerals, particularly calcium and phosphorus. Kittens, unlike puppies, are better fed *ad libitum*. Energy requirements/kg peak at about 10 weeks of age but tend to be lower than those of puppies, as the percentage increases over birth weights are smaller, though they achieve a higher percentage of adult weight (75%) by 6 months of age. Various types of commercial foods are available for this life stage. Puppy foods may be specific to a range of breeds (e.g. 'large breed puppy') and may include a 'junior' version for older puppies where energy requirements are lower but calcium and phosphorus ratios are maintained. Selection should therefore be made based on age, breed and size. Kitten foods in a variety of types are suitable for all kittens.
Maintenance	There are few requirements for maintenance except a balanced diet. Cats and small dogs have achieved adult requirements by 12 months of age, medium-sized dogs mature at around 15–18 months and giant breeds 18–24 months. Various commercial adult dog and cat foods are available and in healthy adult pets client and pet preference are the greatest determining factors. In the majority of dogs, overfeeding (causing obesity) is the major concern. Owners should be encouraged to weigh their pets regularly and restrict their food as necessary or use a less energy-dense product.
Gestation (pregnancy)	Most fetal weight gain occurs in the last 3 weeks of canine pregnancy. To this point little extra feeding is required. A palatable balanced maintenance diet is suitable, fed at normal rates. From the fifth week onwards, the ration should be increased by 15% per week. In late pregnancy, feeding small meals of higher density diets may be required due to the reduced space available in the abdomen for the stomach to expand. Cats tend to require a steady increase in food intake from conception. As they rarely overeat, *ad lib* feeding can occur. Alternatively a 4–5% increase in ration can be given weekly. Commercial puppy and kitten diets are suitable and often formulated for feeding adult animals in late gestation and lactation.
Lactation	This is the biggest nutritional test of a bitch or queen. Energy requirements depend on litter size, with the maximum demand occurring 4 weeks after the litter is born. Small meals of highly palatable, highly digestible food are required for bitches; *ad lib* feeding of queens is recommended. Supplementation of vitamins and minerals is not necessary if a balanced diet is used. In general it is necessary to feed a diet that is more tightly formulated than for maintenance, preferably one specifically designed for lactation (increased energy density). Commercial puppy and kitten diets are suitable and often formulated for feeding adult animals in late gestation and lactation.
Activity	Few dogs, despite many owners' beliefs, are truly active. A 5 km run will increase a dog's daily requirements by around 10%. Maximum demand occurs in dogs travelling long distances in cold conditions, where they may have an energy requirement of 4–5 times maintenance. Diets should meet the needs for muscular work and stress. For short-burst athletic dogs such as greyhounds, increased carbohydrates are required; for sustained effort, particularly at low temperatures, energy needs are best met through high-fat, low-carbohydrate diets. There is no evidence that an increase in dietary protein is required. It has been suggested that working dogs may have a higher requirement for iron, vitamin E and selenium. Generally working dogs need a highly palatable, energy-dense, highly digestible and nutritionally balanced diet. A good quality fixed formula adult diet is probably the most appropriate for this group of animals. Specific 'performance' or 'working breed' diets are also available.
Old age	The requirements for ageing cats and dogs are poorly defined. Intestinal function starts to decline from around 8 years of age. It is general felt that lower nutritional density is desirable. Energy demands also decrease, due to reduced levels of activity and a lower lean body mass. The requirement for vitamins, particularly water soluble (B and C) vitamins, may be increased, due to increased water turnover. A decrease in energy requirement and nutrient density needs to be balanced against the tendency to poorer appetite. A compromise of a highly palatable diet with mildly reduced nutrient density and increased vitamin levels is currently recommended. Increasing the number of feeds per day is also desirable. A wide variety of commercial 'senior' diets is available for this group. Animals in older age should have blood parameters monitored to ensure that additional dietary considerations are not indicated (see Chapter 9).

2.7 Life-stage nutrition.

Complete diets

Formulated to meet all the nutritional requirements of the animal. Usually life stage-oriented (puppy/kitten, adult or senior) and must be fed appropriately. 'Fixed formula' diets are usually made to specific 'recipe' and therefore vary little between batches. May be moist or semi-moist but are most commonly dry foods

Complementary diets

Unsuitable as single source of food as they lack one or more essential dietary components and are not necessarily nutritionally balanced. Commercial packaging usually suggests what is needed to make the diet balance. May be life stage-oriented and should be fed appropriately. Usually intended to be fed with another complementary diet (e.g. tinned food plus mixed biscuit) or as a treat

Moist foods

Usually high water content (70–80%) and meat-based. Most common forms tinned or foil-packed 'pouches'. Preservation achieved by heat sterilization. Tend to be highly digestible, palatable and have reasonable (months to years) shelf life until opened. Often life-stage preparations. Energy contents may be low, with tendency to protein excess

Semi-moist foods

Contain moderate amount of water (15–30%) with shelf life of several months. Preservation achieved by the use of humectants (sugar, salt or glycerol, which bind water), mould inhibitors and low pH. Can be made from a variety of products and have a fairly high nutritional density, digestibility and palatability. Propylene glycol used as a preservative in some semi-moist dog foods can be toxic to cats

Dry foods

Low water content (<10%). Some are preserved by drying (where shelf life is short) but more modern methods of heat treatment and packing can extend shelf life to a year or more. Some are complementary foods (mixer biscuits); others are complete foods. Most complete foods (and some mixers) are life stage-oriented. Nutritional density is high; digestibility and palatability can be lower than with more moist foods. Because of low water content, free access to water must be allowed with these foods. In cats, low water content together with formulation of some dried foods can predispose to urolithiasis (see Chapter 9)

2.8   Diet types and formulations.

Exotic pets

Dietary recommendations for the common exotic pets are given in Figure 2.9. As in dogs and cats, the formulation of homemade diets for these species can lead to dangerous nutritional problems and commercial pelleted feeds are often preferred as at least part of the diet, to ensure that the correct balance of vitamins, minerals, fibre, protein and energy is provided. Pelleted feeds also have the advantage of avoiding selective feeding in small pets, where the pet eats only the bits it likes rather than the whole meal. Selective feeding can also be reduced by feeding small meals that are eaten completely, rather than giving large amounts of food at one time. For more detail on feeding exotic pets consult the *BSAVA Manual of Exotic Pets* and manuals on specific groups.

Pet	Feeding biology	Dietary recommendations
Rats and mice	Herbivorous/ omnivorous	Best fed commercial (ideally pelleted) rodent diet plus fruit and vegetables. Avoid excess sugary treats and foods
Hamsters	Omnivorous	Feed commercial mix plus fruit, vegetables and nuts. Avoid excessively sweet foods and treats
Guinea pigs	Herbivorous	Feed commercial mix formulated for guinea pigs (not for general herbivores or rabbits) plus hay, grass and assorted vegetables. Require vitamin C level >10 mg/kg, increasing to >30 mg/kg in pregnancy, achieved by feeding complete pelleted guinea pig food and fresh vegetables. Water supplementation with vitamin C also possible
Gerbils	Herbivorous, occasional omnivores	Feed commercial food plus vegetables (lettuce, apple, carrot) and seeds. Avoid excessively sweet foods and treats
Rabbits	Herbivorous	Feed commercial mix (ideally pelleted) plus hay, grass and vegetables (roots, kale, cabbage, etc.). Avoid commercial mixes that allow selective feeding. Avoid sugary feeds and treats. Avoid sudden dietary changes
Ferrets	Carnivorous/ omnivorous	Feed commercial ferret food or good quality cat food. Avoid excessive treats. Allow *ad libitum* feeding to accommodate short gut
Birds	Various according to species	Budgerigars, cockatiels, parrots: feed species-specific commercial mix or pellets plus fresh fruit, vegetables and sprouted seeds. Insectivorous (mynah birds, touracos): require additional mealworms or crickets. Raptors: require 'whole carcasses', usually frozen and thawed day-old chicks

2.9   Feeding common exotic pets. (continues)   ▶

Pet	Feeding biology	Dietary recommendations
Tortoises	Herbivorous or omnivorous	Adequate calcium:phosphorus ratio must be achieved in diet. Herbivores: feed on mixture of vegetables only. Omnivores: require additional insects, mealworms, worms, slugs, etc.
Lizards	Herbivorous or carnivorous	Varying diets depending on whether herbivorous or carnivorous. Most are fed on arthropods (crickets, mealworms). Calcium:phosphorus ratio must be balanced; supplements often given to achieve this. Legislation in UK limits feeding of live prey items
Snakes	Carnivorous	In the wild, usually eat variety of prey (eggs, fish, small mammals, earthworms, insects). In captivity, usually fed on frozen and thawed young mice and rats ('pinkies'). Legislation in UK limits feeding of live prey items

2.9   (continued) Feeding common exotic pets.

Dietary deficiencies and excesses

Deficiencies and excesses of nutrients (Figure 2.10) may occur for several reasons:

- Poor feeding by the owner due to:
  - Neglect in attention to feeding or failure to recognize problems in the pet
  - Pet becoming fussy about food and owner allowing the diet to become limited
  - Failure to feed a diet appropriate to the life stage of the pet
  - Poor or incorrect choice of homemade diet ingredients
  - Excessive supplementation of the diet
- Lack of nutritional intake by pet (inappetence, dysphagia)
- Lack of absorption of nutrients (vomiting, diarrhoea, small intestinal disease, pancreatic insufficiency)
- Increased nutritional demand (cachectic states) due to disease (neoplasia, heart disease, endocrine problems)
- Excessive nutrient loss (gut disease, diabetes, renal disease)
- Breed-specific problems resulting in poor absorption or increased loss of nutrients (e.g. zinc deficiency in Alaskan Malamutes, Fanconi syndrome in Basenjis).

Medical reasons are further discussed in Chapter 9.

Nutrient	Causes and consequences of deficiency	Causes and consequences of excess
Protein	Rare, as low protein diets are unpalatable. Most serious in growing animals which are undergrown with poor joint cartilage and bone mineralization. In adult animals, protein malnutrition is reflected in a dull coat, skin lesions, lethargy and hypoproteinaemia	None in healthy animals. There is no evidence to link the feeding of high protein diets to dogs or cats with normal kidney function to the onset of renal disease
Carbohydrate	None as long as energy requirements are met by fats and proteins	Digestive disorders (e.g. lactose intolerance). If the capacity for carbohydrate digestion is exceeded then the excess is fermented by bacteria in the large bowel, producing fatty acids and lactate resulting in an acidic osmotic diarrhoea. Carbohydrates are poorly tolerated in animals needing high energy diets (e.g. lactation, work) and by puppies/kittens who have low amylase activity
Fat	Sufficient energy levels can rarely be provided by a fat-deficient diet, hence the animal will lose weight Essential fatty acid deficiencies include hair loss, fatty liver degeneration, anaemia, infertility	Obesity
Biotin	Excessive feeding of raw eggs where the avidin binds biotin produced by intestinal microorganisms, particularly in combination with oral antibiotics Causes dry scurfy skin, alopecia and dried secretions around the nose, mouth and feet	Not reported

2.10   Common dietary deficiencies and excesses in dogs and cats. (continues)   ▶

Nutrient	Causes and consequences of deficiency	Causes and consequences of excess
Calcium and phosphorus	Highest requirements in young fast-growing dogs. Ratio is as important as absolute amounts and should be between 0.9:1 (cats), 1:1 (dogs) and 2:1 *Nutritional secondary hyperparathyroidism* – usually seen in animals fed all-meat diets (calcium deficient) and results in the reabsorption of bone. Affected animals have problems walking and in severe cases standing; there is pain on palpation. Ghost-like bones and pathological fractures can be seen on radiography *Eclampsia* – occurs at whelping (large breeds) and mid-lactation (small breeds) and is seen as muscle twitching and tremor. Can occur in animals fed too little or too much calcium	Excess is usually only a problem in young rapidly growing dogs and is seen as skeletal abnormalities In adults, particularly cats, there may be an increased risk of calcium oxalate crystalluria or uroliths Eclampsia
Copper	Puppies and kittens fed home-cooked diets based on milk, milk products and eggs Excessive zinc supplementation Causes anaemia, depigmentation of hair and skeletal disorders	Chronic toxicity not reported
Iodine	Animals fed meat or cereals produced in iodine-deficient areas. Cooking also reduces iodine Causes enlargement of thyroid gland (goitre), lethargy, alopecia, disorders of growth and fertility, weight loss and oedema	None reported. Cyclical high and low iodine-containing diets have been suggested as a cause of hyperthyroidism in cats
Iron	Seen in puppies and kittens fed inappropriate milk substitutes. Causes a non-regenerative anaemia	May impair the availability of other elements. Excessive supplementation tends to cause vomiting
Magnesium	Usually occurs in animals fed a poorly formulated 'struvite prevention' diet. Causes depression and muscle weakness	Increased risk of struvite urolithiasis, especially if water turnover is low
Potassium	Seen mainly in cats fed on low-potassium vegetarian diets. Affected cats are initially stiff and have poor hair coat; this progresses to weakness and an inability to raise the head. Renal failure has been reported in cats fed high-protein acidifying diets, which require higher levels of potassium supplementation	None known
Zinc	Poor bioavailability due to high calcium levels or diets based on soybean or cereals Causes parakeratosis (scaly skin) and depigmentation of hair	Rare, secondary to ingestion of zinc-containing coins Causes vomiting, weight loss, anaemia and anorexia
Taurine	CATS ONLY: deficiencies can lead to blindness, dilated cardiomyopathy, reproductive failure and developmental abnormalities in kittens. Deficiency is seen in cats fed dog food or vegetarian food	None known
Vitamin A	Dogs fed cereal or offal-based diets or cats fed vegetarian diets Causes skin and eye lesions, increased susceptibility and poor response to infection, problems with bone development and reproduction	Cats or dogs oversupplemented with cod liver oil or cats fed predominantly liver-based diets Causes weakness, anorexia, pain, lameness and stiffness associated with bony hyperplasia, particularly affecting the neck (in cats) Changes are not reversible if the diet is discontinued, although some improvement in clinical signs occurs with time
Thiamine	As there are poor body reserves, deficiency can occur quickly. Most commonly seen in cats fed high levels of uncooked fish (which contain thiaminase), cats and dogs fed uncooked meat preserved with sulphur dioxide, or poorly formulated cooked diets where the thiamine is destroyed by heating and not replaced In young animals, causes poor growth progressing to weight loss, neurological signs and death. Neurological signs seen in cats include abnormal posture, neck weakness, ataxia and seizures	Not reported

2.10   (continued) Common dietary deficiencies and excesses in dogs and cats. (continues) ▶

Nutrient	Causes and consequences of deficiency	Causes and consequences of excess
Niacin/tryptophan	Dogs fed corn-based diets Causes severe tongue (black tongue) and buccal ulceration, drooling saliva and halitosis	Not reported
Vitamin D	Rarely seen Causes ricketts and osteomalacia	Usually associated with oversupplementation (vitamin D is also used as a rodenticide) Causes calcification of the soft tissues, including the skin, and can lead to organ failure (e.g. of the kidneys)
Vitamin E	Deficiency is usually relative where high fat (dry) diets have become rancid or in cats fed diets based predominantly on fish, particularly tuna Causes steatitis (inflammation of the fat) associated with lethargy, fever, pain and palpable subcutaneous masses	Not reported

2.10   (continued) Common dietary deficiencies and excesses in dogs and cats.

Advice on obese patients

Obesity is the most common nutritional problem in dogs and cats. It is an excess of body fat and is associated with many health problems. About 50% of pet dogs and cats are overweight to some degree. It is most common in older female animals.

Why obesity is dangerous

Overweight animals suffer most from physical ailments and do not live as long as animals of average weight. Obesity often reduces the pet's enjoyment of life, its performance and the owner's enjoyment of the pet. Specific health risks associated with or influenced by obesity include:

- Heart and respiratory disease
- Diabetes
- Increased risk with surgery and anaesthesia
- Joint disease (e.g. arthritis, back or spinal disc problems)
- Ruptured ligaments (e.g. cranial cruciate ligament rupture)
- Liver disease (e.g. hepatic lipidosis in cats)
- Heat intolerance
- Cancers
- Urinary incontinence
- Reduced healing and response to infection.

Reasons for obesity in pets

Most pets become obese as a result of incorrect feeding and exercise. Good advice to the client when the pet is first owned (see 'Advice on buying pets and on pet behaviour', above) can go a long way to preventing the occurrence of obesity problems.

Although an incorrect balance of diet and exercise is the leading cause of obesity, genetic predisposition may play a role. Certain breeds, including Labradors, Beagles, Basset Hounds and Dachshunds, are thought to be more susceptible to obesity than some other working or sporting breeds of dog, for example.

Hormonal imbalances, such as those due to thyroid or pituitary gland dysfunction, may also lead to obesity, and these should be investigated by the veterinary surgeon as appropriate.

Neutered animals may tend to gain weight, due to reduced metabolism. This should be explained clearly to the owner at the time of neutering, so that they can be more aware of possible weight gain and more conscientious when feeding. (See also 'Disadvantages of neutering', below.)

Management of obesity

Many owners will not face up to the fact that their pet is obese or is being overfed. Frequently used excuses for pet obesity include statements such as:

- We don't overfeed her
- He hasn't had much exercise lately
- It's my husband/wife/children – they give him extras
- She only got fat after she was neutered
- He only has one meal a day
- It's not what she eats…

Because control of obesity in pets has as many owner issues as pet issues, it requires time and patience in order to be successful and avoid owner despondency. As in human obesity management, the use of weight clinics allows time for discussion and encouragement. Veterinary nurses are usually responsible for weight clinics within veterinary practices. Such clinics improve the profile of both the veterinary nursing team and the practice.

Running weight clinics

Weight clinics are usually run on an appointment basis. At the first weight consultation a specific target must be arranged, with an estimated time to reach the goal weight (see below). This should be written down for the owner and a chart for subsequent visits and targets of achievement should be made available.

Useful advice to owners might include the following:

- Keep the pet out of the room when preparing and eating food; this will discourage the pet from scrounging extra food
- Make one person in the house responsible for feeding the animal so that the pet does not get overfed and there is no risk of duplication of feeding
- Ensure that everyone in the family knows to stick to the diet – there must be no extra treats or meals from anyone
- Do not feed overweight pets with other pets
- Do not feed anything other than the pet food prescribed
- Ensure that dogs do not steal food from small children's hands
- Set a routine when feeding and exercising that suits the owner and the pet
- Start regular exercise, or increase existing exercise
- Return for regular weigh-ins, at least once every 2 weeks, and record weight loss on a graph.

At each subsequent weight consultation, the pet is weighed (Figure 2.11) and progress is discussed.

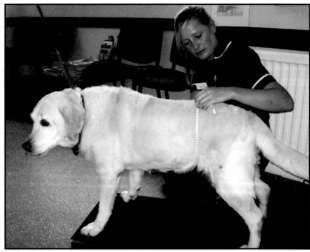

2.11 Regular checks of weight and girth should be made.

Tips for successful weight clinics

- **Weigh the animal every few weeks. This encourages the owner to come into the practice and see how the pet is progressing. Give lots of encouragement (however small or large the weight change might be) and possibly incentives (e.g. vouchers for food, toys, certificates of achievement) to encourage owners to continue to bring their pets to be weighed.**
- **Measure the pet's waist and girth behind the ribs. Sometimes they may not lose any weight, but may have lost several centimetres around the circumference, which can be encouraging.**
- **Discuss the diet and how the animal and owner are finding the changes to feeding. Ask about treats and titbits.**
- **Ask what exercise is being taken by the pet.**
- **Encourage the owner to ask questions.**
- **Changes to diet, exercise and targets may need to be made depending on the progress of pet and owner.**
- **Once the pet has reached the target weight, a new challenge begins in maintaining the weight loss and ideal weight. This means not falling back into bad old habits. The animal's weight must continue to be monitored (though this can be reduced to every few months) together with food intake and exercise.**

Choice of food

As with all diets, the most important points in managing obesity are to reduce the calorie intake, cut out treats and titbits and increase exercise. In many cases simply reducing the amount of food fed and addressing issues regarding treats and exercise are enough to produce successful weight loss. Without these lifestyle changes, pets are unlikely to lose weight regardless of what is fed.

Commercial diets are available through veterinary practices to assist with weight loss and weight control in pets. These diets have the advantage of being able to reduce calorie intake greatly, whilst maintaining the correct balance of nutrients. Veterinary nurses should make themselves aware of the different types of products available and incorporate them into weight clinics as required. A veterinary examination is advisable before significant dietary changes are made.

Two main groups of weight diet are available. The most common types are low in fat and calories and have an increased fibre content. The pet will still have a good portion of food and feel 'full' whilst having a much reduced calorie intake. Due to their fibre content, these diets can have the disadvantage of being much less palatable than the pet's normal food and also result in the pet producing an increased faecal volume, which owners may find undesirable. Different levels of fibre content may be used for initial weight loss and subsequent weight maintenance.

A more recent form of weight management diet is low in carbohydrate but high in protein. These diets rely on similar principles to the 'Atkins diet' used in humans. High protein levels encourage the metabolism of fats stored in the body as a main source of energy and may also have appetite-suppressive effects. Such diets may be fed at 'weight loss' or 'maintenance' levels. There may be some specific medical contraindications for feeding high levels of protein.

In addition to any dietary changes, owners should avoid giving any supplements unless advised to do so by the veterinary surgeon and must be made aware of the importance of fresh drinking water always being available to the pet.

Setting a target

Regardless of how overweight the animal is, an initial target for weight loss of around 15% of current bodyweight should be set. This is usually achievable over a period of 18–20 weeks. For example, a 50 kg Labrador would have an initial target weight of 42.5 kg and an average anticipated weight loss of about 400 g/week.

How much weight loss to expect

A good and safe rate of weight loss is around 1% per week. This means that a 6 kg cat would lose around 60 g/week and the 50 kg Labrador 500 g/week. With smaller pets such as cats, it is such a small amount of weight loss per week that fortnightly rather than weekly weighing might be more appropriate.

Treats

Treats are allowable, and often desirable, as the owner feels less unkind to their pet and is more likely to stick to other dietary restrictions. They should be kept to a sensible level and the calorific content of the treat must be taken into account when calculating the size of the main meal(s). Where possible, if owners insist on giving some form of treat, they should be encouraged to offer low-calorie treats (e.g. raw vegetables or commercial low-calorie treats). Ideally the owner should weigh out the animal's daily amount of food in the morning and keep a few biscuits behind for treats throughout the day if required.

Exercise

Along with changes to the diet, the importance of an increased amount of exercise needs to be explained to the client. This can simply mean regular walks, more frequent walks or more play time; more ideas for increased exercise are given in the box below. If the animal is unable to increase exercise due to a clinical disease, it is essential that veterinary advice is obtained.

Exercise suggestions for dogs (based on physical ability and veterinary advice)

- Fetch a toy
- Jogging with the owner
- Running alongside a cycling owner (special leads are available for this)
- Swimming and hydrotherapy (see Chapter 9)
- Longer walks and brisker walks.

Exercise suggestions for cats

- Playing with toys
- Catch the light or flying toys
- Harness and lead walks
- Obstacle courses (around house or in garden)
- Being encouraged to run up and down stairs
- Boxing games.

Advice on reproduction and care of neonates

In order to be able to advise clients on reproduction in their pets, it is important that veterinary nurses have a good understanding of what might be considered normal, as well as knowing when veterinary attention should be sought.

Drugs used to manipulate the reproductive system and control breeding are described in Chapter 3. Further detail on the biology of reproduction can be found in the *BSAVA Textbook of Veterinary Nursing*.

Female dogs and cats

Oestrous cycle in the bitch

The oestrous cycle is made up of four phases (Figure 2.12). The term 'season' or 'heat' includes pro-oestrus and oestrus, and usually lasts for about 3 weeks. The oestrous cycle in the bitch first occurs at puberty, which is defined as the onset of sexual function. The age of puberty is variable: usually the bitch is 8–9 months old, but the range is between 5 and 24 months. Bitches come into season every 4–12 months and these commonly occur in the spring and autumn. On average most breeds have two seasons a year.

Phase	Duration	Signs
Pro-oestrus [a]	7–10 days (range 4–14 days)	Some vulval swelling; blood-stained discharge. Attracts dogs but repels mating; sometimes behavioural changes
Oestrus [a]	8–12 days (range 5–15 days)	More swollen and flaccid vulva; discharge more mucoid, less blood. Attracts dogs and allows mating; has escapist tendencies
Metoestrus [b] (luteal/post-oestrus phase, also called dioestrus)	Approximately same length of time as pregnancy (55 days)	No external signs. Not attractive to dogs. Vulva is normal size; possible whitish discharge at start. Possible mammary enlargement towards the end
Anoestrus	3–4 months (range 1–9 months)	Period of quiescence following the luteal phase or pregnancy

2.12 Oestrous cycle of the bitch. [a] Pro-oestrus + oestrus = heat/season; lasts about 3 weeks. [b] False pregnancy and pyometra can occur during metoestrus.

Oestrous cycle in the queen

The oestrous cycle in the queen is made up of four phases (Figure 2.13), as in the bitch. Pro-oestrus and oestrus (the 'season' or 'heat') are less distinct than in the bitch and together only last 3–10 days. This time is shortened if mating occurs. Ovulation is usually induced (or 'reflex'), associated with the stimulation of mating. Unless there is spontaneous ovulation (see below), oestrus is usually followed by an interoestrous phase rather than true metoestrus (Figure 2.14).

Phase	Duration	Signs
Pro-oestrus and oestrus	3–10 days, shortened by mating Difficult to separate the two phases except that the male is accepted when female is in oestrus	Behavioural signs (vocalization, rubbing against objects, rolling on floor). Few physical signs
Interoestrus	About 3–14 days Follows oestrus when no mating has occurred or when mating does not result in a pregnancy	Diminishing behavioural signs. No physical signs
Anoestrus	Over the period of winter when there are no hormonal cycles	No physical signs

2.13   Oestrous cycle of the queen.

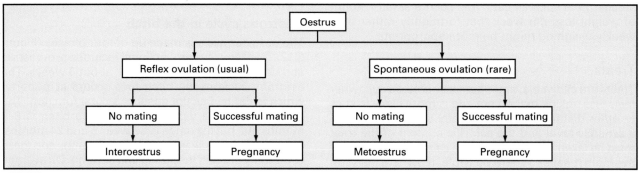

2.14   Ovulation in the queen.

Puberty in cats is dependent on daylength, age and weight. Usually the first oestrus is seen in the first spring in which a bodyweight of 2.5 kg is attained, which is usually at 5–6 months of age. Queens have an oestrous cycle every 2–3 weeks in spring, summer and autumn; this is described as being seasonally polyoestrous. Sometimes indoor cats also cycle in the winter months.

Male dogs and cats

- In male dogs the age of puberty is 6–8 months (up to 1 year in larger breeds). In cats it is 9–12 months (pedigree cats tend to be later than domestic breeds).

- Most male dogs and cats are introduced to stud at about 1 year of age.
- Male animals should be used at stud no more than 2–3 times in their first year. If the owner wishes to increase this, they must first be confident that the stud dog or cat is not siring puppies or kittens with hereditary defects. Overuse may in addition adversely affect the male animal's fertility.

Exotic pets

Details of gestation periods and other reproductive parameters for commonly encountered exotic pets are given in Figure 2.15.

Species	Age at puberty	Gestation (days)	Litter size (average)	Age at weaning (days)
Mice	6–7 weeks	19–21	6–12 (8)	21 [b]
Rats	6–8 weeks	20–22	6–16 (10)	21 [b]
Hamster, Syrian	6–8 weeks	15–18	5–9	21–28
Hamster, Chinese	7–14 weeks	21	4–5	21
Hamster, Russian	6–8 weeks	18	4	16–18
Gerbil	10–12 weeks	24–26 [a]	3–7 (5)	2–26
Guinea pig	M: 9–10 weeks F: 4–6 weeks	59–72 [a]	1–6 (3–4)	21
Chinchilla	M: 6–8 months F: 4–5 months	111	1–6 (2)	42
Rabbit	M: 4–8 months F: 3–4 months	28–32	4–12	42
Ferret	First spring (March) after birth	41–42	8	42–56

2.15   Reproductive parameters of common mammalian exotic pets. [a] Gestation in gerbil is extended to 27–48 days if female also lactating; in guinea pig depends on litter size. [b] Earliest.

Mating

Male animals mate more successfully when they are in a familiar environment; therefore it is preferable to take the female to the male for mating. It is also preferable that either the male or the female has been previously bred from successfully.

The timing for mating is critical, especially in dogs. The most fertile time in female dogs and cats is considered to be from the 10th to 14th day of oestrus. However, the range can be from day 3 or as late as day 18. As cats are induced ovulators, under most circumstances timing is less critical.

Laboratory tests can be carried out in veterinary practices to determine when a bitch is most fertile. These include:

- A microscopic examination of vaginal cells (cytology), to detect numbers and types of cells. This method is reasonably reliable
- Blood sampling for changes in the progesterone levels around ovulation. This will give a good indication of when mating is most likely to be successful.

Mating in the dog

Normal mating behaviour in the dog is described in Figure 2.16. As described above, tests may be carried out in advance to indicate when the bitch is in oestrus and will be most fertile and receptive to the dog. Alternatively, the bitch and dog may be introduced to each other at what is likely to be the most receptive time. Mating should be allowed as soon as the bitch accepts the dog. If the bitch is not fully receptive, either the bitch or the dog can become aggressive. Care should be taken when introducing strange animals to each other. Breeders typically allow two matings with the same dog to occur in the oestrous period.

1. The bitch and dog often exhibit play behaviour, jumping up and chasing each other, as part of the courtship.
2. The bitch will then settle and stand with her tail to one side (flagging).
3. The dog's penis will be partially engorged and extruded from the sheath.
4. The dog mounts the bitch and may ejaculate a small amount of clear fluid.
5. Slow thrusting movements allow the penile tip to enter the vulva.
6. The penis becomes fully erect and enters the vagina (intromission).
7. Thrusting movements become rapid and the second fraction is ejaculated.
8. The dog then dismounts from the bitch and turns through 180° with the penis still in the vagina (the tie).
9. The third fraction is ejaculated into the vagina.
10. The animals remain tied for up to 30 minutes, after which the dog's penis slowly deflates and the pair disengage.
11. Both animals should be allowed to clean and lick themselves.

2.16 Canine mating behaviour.

Mating in the cat

Mating behaviour in the cat is described in Figure 2.17. Multiple matings usually occur in one day.

1. Courtship is variable and often non-existent.
2. Queen adopts the mating position, fore-end crouched and tail up.
3. Male grasps skin on her neck in his teeth and lies over her.
4. Intromission and ejaculation occur quickly.
5. As the penis is withdrawn the queen often howls – coital stimulus.
6. Queen then rolls and licks herself vigorously.
7. She will not allow further mating for about 1 hour.

2.17 Mating behaviour in the cat.

Selection of animals for breeding

Animals selected for breeding should be:

- A good example of the breed
- Of good temperament
- In good health
- Of the correct age for breeding (usually 2–6 years old)
- Free from known contagious diseases (for example, all breeding cats – males and females – should be tested for FeLV and FIV before each breeding)
- Free from known hereditary defects; where screening programmes exist (see below) animals should be screened and shown to be negative.

Schemes to control hereditary defects in dogs

The schemes below, run by the British Veterinary Association (BVA), are those most often encountered for pedigree dogs and routinely offered in veterinary practices. As genetic testing has become more advanced and available, many other tests are being developed (usually DNA blood tests) for specific defects in specific breeds and clients may request these. Often the best advice for clients on what is commonly tested for in a breed can be sought from other reliable breeders.

Further information on the schemes below is available and frequently updated on the BVA website.

BVA/Kennel Club/International Sheepdog Society Eye Scheme

Dogs are tested annually for inherited eye conditions. Conditions of the lens, retina and other internal structures of the eye are included. Some of these conditions are:

- Inherited cataracts
- Primary lens luxation
- Primary glaucoma
- Collie eye anomaly
- Retinal dysplasia
- Central and generalized progressive retinal atrophy (PRA).

Conditions of the eyelids (entropion, ectropion and distichiasis) are not included.

Testing is carried out by BVA-appointed eye panellists who are experienced veterinary ophthalmologists. There are two schedules:

A. Known inherited diseases in specific breeds (these are certifiable)
B. Monitoring of breeds for conditions that may be emerging inherited problems.

BVA/Kennel Club Hip Dysplasia (HD) Scheme

Dogs (male and female) are radiographed on one occasion when the animal is over 1 year old. The radiograph is taken with the dog on its back, so some sedation or general anaesthesia is needed (see Chapter 11).

- Radiographs can be taken in any veterinary practice that has suitable facilities.
- Images are sent to the BVA and a 'score' is given for each hip. High scores (up to 106) represent poor hips; a score of 0 represents 'perfect' hips.
- Hip scores are compared with an average for that breed.
- Animals selected for breeding should have scores *well below* the breed average.

BVA/Kennel Club Elbow Dysplasia (ED) Scheme

Dogs (male and female) are radiographed on one occasion when the animal is over 1 year old. Two views of each elbow are taken (flexed and extended). Some degree of sedation or general anaesthesia is needed to allow good positioning (see Chapter 11).

- Radiographs can be taken in any veterinary practice that has suitable facilities.
- Images are sent to the BVA and a 'grade' is given for each elbow (0–3). If the scores differ, the overall score is the higher of the two grades.
- Grade 0 is normal; grade 3 indicates severe elbow dysplasia.
- Animals selected for breeding should have a grade of 0 or 1.

Pregnancy

Pregnancy, also called the gestation period, ranges from 60 to 67 days in the bitch and from 56 to 70 days in the queen. Most bitches deliver (whelp) between 63 and 65 days after mating. The queen will usually kitten on average between days 65 and 67, but this is commonly difficult to predict accurately due to multiple matings. Gestation periods for exotic species are given in Figure 2.15.

An examination can be carried out by a veterinary surgeon approximately 21 days from the date of mating to detect signs of pregnancy by abdominal palpation or by ultrasound scan.

During the final stages of pregnancy, both the bitch and queen often start to look for a secure safe place for delivery. Prior to the time of delivery, for bitches a whelping box should be made available in a secluded place, ideally somewhere the bitch would normally choose to go. The whelping box should be large enough for the bitch to move around freely, with short sides to enable her to get in and out, but high enough to keep the puppies confined. It should be lined with thick newspaper, which can be used to absorb fluid and can be shredded for nest making, with some additional comfortable bedding such as towels or blankets. Queens should ideally have a kittening box (Figure 2.18) but they usually choose their own space in the house or outbuildings.

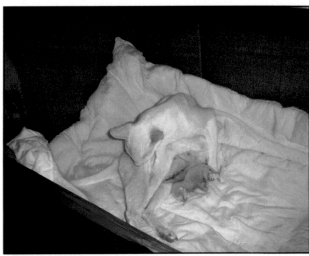

2.18   Kittening box. This queen has had a Caesarean section.

Onset of parturition

The most reliable indicator of impending parturition is the fall in rectal temperature some 8–24 hours earlier. The body temperature fluctuates during the last week of pregnancy and prior to parturition will decrease usually by 1°C in large breeds and 3°C in small breeds. The decrease in body temperature is responsible for shivering, which is recognized at the first stage of parturition. Other signs of impending parturition include:

- Nest making
- Seeking solitude
- Anorexia (not in all cases)
- Enlargement and flaccidity of the vaginal lips
- Obvious mammary development and colostrum production from the teats (this should not be expressed unnecessarily before parturition).

Parturition

For a successful parturition:

- The lower genital tract must permit passage of fetuses
- The cervix must dilate
- The fetuses must be actively propelled from the uterus to the vulva
- The neonate must be capable of survival.

Stages of parturition

Parturition can be divided into five component parts: preparation; first stage; second stage (labour); third stage (including expulsion of placenta); and puerperium.

Stage of preparation

- Colostrum present in the mammary glands.
- Relaxation of the vaginal and perineal tissue.
- Drop in body temperature to around 37°C.
- Dam/queen seeks the nesting site.

This stage may take 1–3 days. Clients should be advised to treat the pet as normally as possible in this period but equally allow the pet some quiet time to settle where they are happy, ideally in the whelping or kittening box.

First stage of parturition

- Restlessness.
- Onset of myometrial contractions.
- Panting.
- Nest making.
- Anorexia, shivering and vomiting may be seen.
- Queens may vocalize and groom themselves.

This stage usually lasts 1–12 hours, but in animals having their first litter (**primiparous**) it may last up to 36 hours. Clients should be advised to observe their pet quietly during this period whilst allowing them to settle reasonably undisturbed. At the end of this stage, cervical dilation should be complete and the first water bag (**allantochorion**) will be passed through the cervix.

Second stage of parturition

- Involuntary myometrial contractions.
- Coordinated voluntary contractions of the abdominal muscles.
- Dam may crouch, stand or lie.
- First allantochorion (see above) seen at vulva, may be broken or bitten by the dam, resulting in release of allantoic fluid.
- Puppy or kitten born, contained in amnion that is usually intact; dam will lick and chew to break the amnion and stimulate the neonate.
- Umbilical cord will be broken during parturition or by actions of dam.
- Body temperature returns to normal.

This stage of labour (which overlaps with third-stage labour in animals producing multiple fetuses) usually lasts 3–12 hours. Clients should be advised to observe their pet quietly during this period, with minimal intervention. If the dam fails to release the neonate from the amnion within a few minutes, this can be done gently by the owner. Umbilical cords not broken by parturition or the dam should be gently tied off with thin cotton approximately 0.5 cm from the umbilicus. All such intervention should be kept to a minimum and neonates handled must be quickly returned to the dam.

Intervention should be actively discouraged in the more exotic pets, where disturbance may result in rejection of the neonates or even in them being eaten by the dam.

It is common for clients to phone for advice during this period. It may be the job of the veterinary nurse to advise clients if all appears to be progressing normally. If unsure, the nurse should seek veterinary advice. Veterinary assistance should be sought if:

- The puppy or kitten is not born within 30 minutes of the production of the allantochorion
- The dam is straining unproductively for more than 1 hour
- The dam becomes weak and straining becomes unproductive
- More than 2 hours elapse between the birth of the fetuses
- A red/green discharge is seen (**uteroverdin**) and no fetuses are being born (this discharge is the product of placental breakdown and may suggest the fetuses are losing their placental blood and oxygen supply through premature separation of placentas)
- The dam is in second-stage labour for a total duration of over 12 hours.

Third stage of parturition

- Myometrial and abdominal contractions continue.
- Expulsion of placentas alternating approximately with birth of fetuses (sometimes a fetus may be born without its placenta as another fetus quickly follows).
- Production of uteroverdin (this is the normal breakdown product of maternal blood trapped between the placenta and fetal membranes).
- Dam/queen may eat placentas.

This stage of pregnancy overlaps with second stage of parturition in species producing more than one fetus.

Puerperium

- Uterine involution takes place, usually rapidly at first, and is completed within 4–6 weeks post partum.
- Uteroverdin production and any bleeding should stop after 1 week.
- The dam's temperature may be slightly elevated for up to 1 week.

During this stage the dam's reproductive tract begins to return to normal. Veterinary advice should be sought if:

- Vaginal discharge is heavy or persists beyond one week
- The dam is unwell in any way
- The neonates are not feeding and thriving normally.

Recognizing parturition-related problems

Dystocia

Dystocia (difficulty giving birth) is a common problem in both the bitch and the queen but less common in smaller mammalian pets. It is defined as the inability to expel the fetus through the birth canal without assistance. There is an increase in frequency of dystocia in pedigree cats and in breeds of dog with larger heads (including brachycephalic breeds).

The causes of dystocia may be maternal or fetal in origin (Figure 2.19).

Cause of dystocia	Comments
Maternal causes	*Account for approximately three quarters of all dystocia cases in the bitch and approximately two thirds of cases in queens*
Primary complete inertia	About two-thirds of maternal dystocia cases
Primary partial inertia	About one third of maternal dystocia cases
Birth canal too narrow	Uncommon, though more common in queen than in bitch
Uterine torsion	Uncommon, bitch
Uterine prolapse	Uncommon, queen
Uterine strangulation	Uncommon, queen
Hydrallantois	Uncommon, bitch
Vaginal septum formation	Uncommon, bitch
Fetal causes	*Account for approximately a quarter of all dystocia cases in the bitch and one third of cases in queens*
Malpresentations	Most common fetal cause
Malformations	More common in queen than in bitch
Fetal oversize	More common in bitch than in queens
Fetal death	Uncommon

2.19   Causes of dystocia in bitches and queens.

Uterine inertia

This is the most common cause of dystocia. It may be primary or secondary.

Primary inertia

This is when the uterus fails to respond to the requirements of parturition and contractions of the myometrium are absent. Primary complete uterine inertia is the failure to initiate labour, whereas primary partial uterine inertia occurs when parturition is initiated but the entire process cannot be completed. Reasons for this may be:

- Insufficient stimulation (small litter or small fetus)
- Over-stretching of the uterine muscles by large litters
- Inherited predisposition
- Older or overweight animals
- Bitch exhibiting excessive anxiety.

Primary inertia may be treated by:

- Calming the nervous or unsettled bitch or queen
- Encouraging the settled bitch to exercise (a walk around the garden is appropriate)
- Gentle manual stimulation of the dorsal vaginal wall.

Secondary inertia

This is always due to exhaustion of the myometrium, usually caused by obstruction of the birth canal. If the condition is diagnosed early enough the animal should still be quite bright; otherwise she will be exhausted and depressed.

In the case of secondary inertia, provided that the birth canal is not obstructed in any way, the veterinary surgeon may prescribe oxytocin, an injectable hormone product (see Chapter 3) that results in contraction of the myometrium. Failure to respond to administration of oxytocin may lead to the addition of intravenous calcium to the medical treatment or a move to elective Caesarean section (see Chapter 13).

Obstruction of the birth canal

The causes of birth canal obstruction may be fetal or maternal in all species.

Fetal obstruction may result from:

- Malpresentation (fetus not in the normal position for delivery)
- Oversized fetuses (often in association with low fetal number)
- Malformations of the fetus
- Fetal death.

Maternal causes include:

- Narrow pelvic canal
- Soft tissue abnormalities (neoplasms, polyps, fibromas)
- Uterine torsion/rupture
- Congenital malformations of the uterus.

If the fetus is in the birth canal, manual manipulation may be attempted to remove the fetus. If this is the case:

- The dam must be gently restrained
- Gentle examination should be used to establish the cause of the dystocia
- Aseptic conditions must be observed (clean hands or surgical gloves)
- Lubrication must be used (obstetrical lubricant)
- Limbs of the fetus must never by pulled – hold only around the shoulders or pelvis
- If the fetus cannot be quickly and safely removed, a Caesarean 'section' must be carried out.

Caesarean operation

Caesarean section (removal of the fetuses from the uterus by surgical intervention) may be a necessary procedure if there are signs of dystocia, trauma or infection. The indications that this procedure might be necessary are:

- Complete/partial uterine inertia that is unresponsive to medical treatment
- Secondary uterine inertia that does not respond to medical treatment
- Fetal malposition
- Fetal oversize
- Fetal death
- Excess/deficiency of fetal fluids

- Maternal birth canal deficiency
- Neglected dystocia
- Toxaemia of pregnancy
- Illness/trauma of dam.

Further information on Caesarean operations is given in Chapter 13.

Management of the neonate

Maternal care of the newborn

Following a normal birth, the mother should tend to her young by:

- Licking off the amniotic membranes, especially around the mouth and nose
- Biting the umbilical cord
- Nuzzling the neonate to stimulate and keep it warm.

In dogs and cats the neonatal period is classed as the first 10 days of life. Neonates are totally dependent on the mother. They have very little subcutaneous fat and no ability to shiver to protect themselves from hypothermia, and cannot regulate their own body temperature. Normal neonatal characteristics are given in Figure 2.20.

Suckling

Under normal circumstances the neonate will find its way to the mother's teats immediately following birth and begin to feed. This is most important, as the neonate requires the first milk (colostrum) within the first few hours of life. Colostrum contains:

- Antibodies to give 'passive immunity' (see vaccination section, below) to the neonate. The importance of this varies between species, some relying on antibodies in colostrum and others to a greater or lesser extent on antibodies passed across the placenta

- Laxatives to help expel meconium (the contents of the digestive tract formed during development in the uterus; if this is not expelled soon after birth it can cause gut obstruction, evidence of which will be a distended abdomen)
- Nutrients to protect against hypoglycaemia and to start growth.

In addition, the temperature of the milk protects against hypothermia.

Ambient temperature

The ambient temperature in which neonates are kept for the first 24 hours should be not less than 30°C; after this the nest temperature can be dropped to 26°C over a few days. It is important that the mother can escape the heat, but the neonates must stay in their enclosure at their ambient temperature (see earlier descriptions of whelping boxes for this purpose).

Elimination

The mother will lick the neonate's perineal area to encourage urination and defecation. After 2–3 weeks of age the young will urinate and defecate voluntarily. Soiled bedding material should be removed from the whelping box or kittening pen at frequent intervals and replaced with clean material.

Hand-rearing puppies and kittens

Wherever possible, neonates should be left with the dam. In some cases (e.g. large litters) supplementary feeding may be necessary but the neonates should still spend most of their time with the dam. Hand-rearing is time-consuming, increases the risk of neonatal infections, and increases future behavioural problems in the offspring. Reasons for hand-rearing puppies and kittens include:

- Orphaned or abandoned young
- Mother unsuitable (aggressive, inexperienced, nervous)

Characteristic	Puppies	Kittens
Birth weight	Very variable	Cross-breed: 110–120 g Small breed: 90–110 g Larger breed: 120–150 g
Temperature	Day 1: 36°C Day 7: 37°C	36°C falling to 30°C and rising to 38°C at 7 days
Heart rate	200/minute	200–250/minute
Respiratory rate	15–35/minute after birth	15–35/minute after birth
Eyelids open	10–14 days	5–12 days
Hearing develops	Around 2 weeks	Around 2 weeks
Shivering reflex	Around 1 week	Around 1 week
Suckles	Every 2 hours for first 2 weeks	Every 1–2 hours for first few days
Weight gain	Doubles weight in 8 days	Loses weight to begin with, then gains 15 g/day
Locomotion	Standing: 14 days Walking: 21 days	

2.20 Normal neonatal development.

- Too large a litter (see above)
- Eclampsia
- Mother unwell or has no milk.

Basic requirements when hand-rearing include warmth, food and good hygiene.

Warmth

This can be attained by use of:

- Incubators
- Hot-water bottles
- Heat lamps
- Heat pads
- Suitable insulated bedding.

Food and feeding

Orphaned young may be fed with a commercial milk replacer or substitute, which should match the composition of the mother's milk. Ideally they should receive the benefit of colostrum for the first 48 hours of life; commercial replacers for this are available.

- Neonates should be fed at approximately 2-hourly intervals for the first 2 weeks of life. A volume of 2–5 ml per feed is usually taken initially, but the manufacturer's guidelines for feeding commercial milk replacers should be followed.
- As the orphan grows, the quantity taken at each feed increases and the frequency of feeds can be reduced.
- Weight gains should be checked and recorded regularly, to ensure that nutrition is adequate.
- After feeding, the neonate's perineal area should be gently rubbed with some warm, damp cotton wool, to stimulate urination and defecation.

Hygiene

Strict cleanliness of environment, equipment and the neonates themselves should be observed.

Sick neonates should be isolated from their litter mates.

Complications of the neonatal period

Neonates should be carefully examined shortly after their birth to detect any defects. Some of the most common defects include:

- Cleft palate or lip
- Overshot or undershot jaw
- Polydactyly (extra digits)
- Umbilical or inguinal hernia
- Cryptorchidism (undescended testes)
- Spina bifida (lack of spinal fusion).

Unless the defect is minimal, easily corrected and unlikely to affect the quality of life, affected neonates should be euthanased on welfare grounds. These defects may have a genetic basis and will therefore affect the decision to breed again from the same sire and dam (see 'Selection of animals for breeding', above).

Fading puppy syndrome

The definition of this syndrome is 'failure to thrive despite a normal birth and ideal weight'. Usually death will occur 3–5 days after birth. The causes of this condition are wide ranging. In order to diagnose the possible cause, a postmortem examination should be carried out. The possible causes of death could include:

- Infection
- Poor mothering
- Congenital abnormalities
- Inadequate management.

Weaning

Puppies and kittens are usually weaned at 3–4 weeks of age. This is achieved by allowing access to soft, moist foods 4–6 times a day. Traditionally, foods such as minced meat, breakfast cereals, baby foods and scrambled eggs have been used for weaning. Commercial moist puppy or kitten foods are perhaps more suitable weaning foods as they are balanced for immediate and longer-term growth and development. They can be mashed or liquidized. Palatability can be an issue with some commercial foods and the short-term mixing of these with more traditional weaning foods can be useful. Inappropriate feeding can lead to developmental problems, including bone disease (see 'Advice on feeding and nutrition', above).

The weaning ages for some common exotic pets are given in Figure 2.15. Most are weaned on to adult food, though commercial foods for juvenile rabbits and guinea pigs are available and to be recommended.

Advice on control of reproduction (neutering)

Neutering removes the sexual urge for both male and female animals and prevents the production of unwanted offspring. It is carried out surgically. For females, removal of the uterus and both ovaries is usual; and for the male, removal of the testicles. These procedures are irreversible. Temporary or semi-permanent control of reproduction can be achieved through the use of certain drugs (see Chapter 3). Further information on neutering is also given in Chapter 13.

Advantages of neutering

If breeding is not intended, neutering has undoubted advantages in both the male and female.

Male animals

- Removes sexual behaviour (for example, if a neutered dog gets the scent of a bitch in oestrus, he is unlikely to show any interest).
- Minimizes male characteristics such as dominance (though additional training may also be required) and aggression because testosterone levels are reduced.

- No straying, looking for a mate.
- Reduces risks of prostatic disease, perineal hernia, perineal adenoma.
- Prevents testicular disease.

Female animals

- Prevents oestrus as well as breeding; therefore prevents oestrus-related behavioural problems.
- Female will not come into heat, therefore will not have to be confined and deprived of the usual exercise and companionship regime.
- Prevents unwanted puppies/kittens.
- Prevents phantom pregnancies.
- Reduces cats calling (can be irritating to owner).
- Reduces risks of uterine diseases, uterine and ovarian tumours, pyometra.
- Reduces risks of mammary disease; prevents mammary tumours, if carried out before the first season.

Disadvantages of neutering

It is a common fallacy that neutered animals will become overweight and lazy following neutering. Neutering does reduce metabolic rate and neutered pets will need less food, which means that dietary choice plays an important role. Owners need to ensure that the animal is fed a suitable diet for its size and amount of exercise. Routinely feeding a scientifically prepared complete food and the correct amount for specific breed and size will be sufficient to control development of obesity after neutering.

Another common question from owners is whether the pet will lose its character. Neutering is sometimes performed to help to control certain behavioural abnormalities and often dogs will become more gentle, but they will not lose their temperament or character.

As there are many more advantages than disadvantages, neutering is usually recommended by most veterinary practices.

When to neuter

Dogs and cats are usually neutered at between 5 and 12 months of age. Suggested neutering ages for other common species are given in Figure 2.21. Many owners will have their own views on age; for example, some owners want their bitch to have one season before being neutered, but there is no advantage in this. Studies have shown that concerns associated with the occurrence of incontinence in bitches spayed before their first season are largely unfounded and greatly outweighed by the benefits of prevention of mammary cancer through early spaying. The actual age that neutering is recommended will be determined by individual practice policy.

Species	Males	Females
Ferret	6–9 months	6–9 months
Rabbit	3–4 months	Around 6 months
Guinea pig	3–4 months	6–9 months

2.21   Suggested neutering ages for commonly neutered small pets.

Vasectomy

It is unusual to vasectomize most companion animal species. The exception to this is in ferrets, where a vasectomized male may be used to prevent continuous oestrus in female animals. Vasectomies are usually carried out in healthy, sexually mature male ferrets.

Advice on infection control and disease prevention

Infection control is an important subject for veterinary nurses and is covered additionally in Chapter 4. Information on specific infectious diseases is given in Chapter 9. The following section deals with the sort of advice that veterinary nurses may be required to give to clients on how they might prevent and control infections in their pets.

Spread of infection

Infectious diseases can be spread by 'horizontal' or 'vertical' transmission (Figure 2.22).

Type of disease transmission	Examples
Horizontal transmission	
Direct contact	
Animal to animal	Feline leukaemia virus, feline immunodeficiency virus
Airborne over short distance	*Bordetella bronchiseptica*, *Chlamydophila felis*
Indirect contact	
Via inanimate objects (fomites)	*Canine parvovirus*, *Toxoplasma gondii*
Airborne over larger distance	Canine parainfluenza virus, canine distemper virus
Via biological vectors: - Mechanical - Definitive host - Intermediate host	- Sandflies transmitting *Leishmania* - Cat carrying *Taenia taeniaeformis* - Flea carrying *Dipylidium caninum*
Vertical transmission	*Toxocara canis*, feline panleucopenia virus, feline leukaemia virus

2.22   Routes of disease transmission, with examples of diseases spread in each way.

Horizontal transmission

Horizontal transmission may occur through direct or indirect contact.

- **Direct contact:** infection is passed directly from animal to animal.
  - Occurs when the body surfaces of two or more animals come into very close contact. This may be as a result of grooming, sleeping in close contact, fighting, or mating.

- Infection may also be spread directly through the air over short distances by coughing or sneezing.
- **Indirect contact:** infection is spread via an intermediary.
  - Infection may be spread via inanimate objects (known as fomites), such as feeding bowls, through contaminated food, or through environmental contamination, for example from poorly cleaned kennels or bedding. This is why owners and kennel staff must pay great attention to hygiene (see below).
  - Airborne spread can also occur and is influenced by the proximity of kennelling and by the appropriate (or inappropriate) use of ventilation units.
  - Alternatively, indirect spread may involve another organism (living or animate carriers) called a biological vector. Vectors may just carry the organism (mechanical vectors) or may be part of the organism's life cycle (e.g. definitive or intermediate hosts of parasites).

Horizontal disease transmission may occur at several stages of the disease process, and clients should be aware of this. There may be:

- Transmission during the incubation period before the animal is unwell
- Transmission during the time that the animal is sick
- Transmission after the animal has partially or fully recovered (see Carrier animals, below).

Vertical transmission

Vertical transmission of infection is when it is passed from a mother to her offspring before birth, as a result of the dam being infected at the time of conception or becoming infected during pregnancy.

Carrier animals

A carrier animal is one that does not show clinical signs of disease but carries the disease-producing organism in its body and may continue to excrete or 'shed' it. Carrier animals may be described as either 'convalescent' or 'healthy':

- **Convalescent carriers** have had the disease, with the usual signs, but do not rid themselves of the organism completely for a long time (sometimes for life) and may show recurring signs of disease
- **Healthy carriers** have been exposed to the disease and possess a degree of immunity sufficient to prevent clinical signs, but not to prevent infection. Vaccinated animals can become carriers in this way.

Carriers may be continuous or intermittent excreters of the microorganism:

- **Continuous excreters** excrete the infectious agent continuously and can infect other animals at any time; they are easier to identify than intermittent excreters

- **Intermittent excreters** only excrete organisms under certain circumstances, usually periods of stress (e.g. parturition, lactation, rehoming, other disease, use of immunosuppressive drugs such as corticosteroids).

Infectious agents may be excreted in:

- Faeces
- Urine
- Nasal and ocular discharges
- Saliva
- Genital discharges
- Fluid from skin lesions
- Blood
- Milk
- Vomit.

They may also be released by dead animals.

Prevention of exposure of other animals, fomites or vectors to these substances can be used as a method of disease control.

Methods of disease control

Methods of controlling the spread of disease from infected to susceptible animals are illustrated in Figure 2.23.

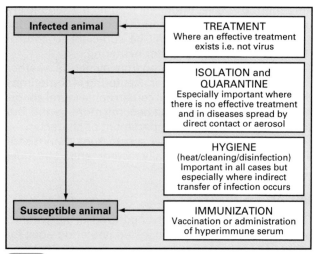

2.23 Methods of prevention of spread of disease.

Treatment of infected animals

Treatment of infected animals can be used as a way of limiting spread of disease, as well as benefiting the individual. There are four potential aims of treatment:

- To kill the pathogenic organism involved – rarely possible in the case of viral disease
- To prevent secondary opportunistic infection (usually bacterial) that can make the situation worse
- To assist the animal's own immune system to eliminate the organism as rapidly as possible, through the provision of nutrition, fluids and other non-specific support
- To modify the immune response directly, making it more effective.

Specific treatments for common diseases of dogs, cats and exotic pets are discussed in more detail below and in Chapters 3 and 9.

Isolation and quarantine of infected animals

Isolation is the segregation and separation of infected or potentially infected animals from uninfected animals, particularly high-risk groups such as neonates, sick animals or unvaccinated animals. Quarantine is the segregation of animals of unknown disease status usually on first entering a premises or country.

Isolation of diseased animals

Potentially infectious animals should be isolated in a specially constructed or designated isolation facility in the veterinary practice (see Chapter 4). Kennels and catteries should have similar facilities. In a client's house, a separate room – ideally with its own airspace – may be used. Basic hygiene, as described in Chapter 4, should be employed.

Routine quarantine for new animals

New animals entering an existing colony (e.g. breeding group) or a multi-animal household should be kept separate for at least 3–4 weeks in case they are incubating an infectious disease. During this time any necessary diagnostic testing (e.g. for FeLV and FIV) and vaccination should be carried out.

Young and other susceptible animals

Young animals have no, or poor, immunity to many diseases and parasites. They are therefore best kept isolated from kennels, airspaces and runs used for older animals. Elderly, immunosupressed or otherwise disease-susceptible animals should ideally be treated in a similar way.

Hygiene

Thorough cleansing of all surfaces will remove many of the viruses, bacteria and parasites that may be present. The efficient cleaning of surfaces with soap or detergent plus water (preferably hot), followed by thorough rinsing, is much more effective than using disinfectants to try to kill organisms. Cleaning in this way removes most organisms so that they are no longer present to produce infection. Many disinfectants can kill infective organisms but none will reliably kill some bacterial spores and parasite eggs. Disinfectants are rendered much less effective by the presence of dirt, blood, pus, faeces or soaps. Disinfection alone should not be relied upon, nor should it be assumed that all infectious agents will be destroyed. This applies to all feeding and bedding materials, as well as all surfaces in kennels, catteries and owners homes. Reducing the weight of infection increases the chances of an animal mounting an effective immune response if it should become infected. Further information on cleaning methods and products is given in Chapter 4; many of these can be easily adapted to the home environment.

Immunity and immunization

Natural acquired (active) immunity

When infection occurs, the body responds by producing antibodies specific to the agent responsible. Once recovery is complete, the animal is resistant to further infection from that agent and is said to be immune. Immunity can last for variable periods, from a few months to the rest of the animal's life, depending on the degree and type of stimulation (immunogenicity) of the microorganism involved. This natural process can be copied by the use of vaccines.

Maternally derived (passive) immunity

Newborn kittens and puppies have little or no acquired immunity at birth. Also, their immune systems are immature and slow to react, and their body reserves are limited. In order to increase survival in the first few weeks of life, passive immunity is gained from the dam. Passive immunity can be transferred from the dam to her offspring in two ways:

- Via the placenta: antibodies pass directly from the mother's blood to that of her fetuses through the placenta (this accounts for <5% of immunity transferred to puppies and kittens)
- Via the colostrum (first milk).

Colostrum is very rich in antibodies; these are not digested by the offspring in the first 24–48 hours of life but are instead absorbed into the bloodstream. By 48 hours after birth, closure of the gut to absorption of these antibodies has occurred and the amount of antibodies in the milk also begins to reduce. In order to gain maximum maternal immunity it is essential that kittens and puppies suckle from their dam in the first few hours of life. Although alternative colostrum supplies may be available, they are unlikely to be of the quality of that provided by the neonates' own dam. The dam will have raised colostral antibodies against pathogens present in her own environment and, provided she is not moved prior to parturition, offspring will gain protection from pathogens in this environment.

The transfer of antibodies from dam to neonate, via both placenta and colostrum, can be maximized by ensuring that the mother's antibody levels are high around the time of parturition. Vaccination prior to mating is advised. In some disease situations it is necessary to vaccinate a pregnant bitch or queen, and this should be performed at least 4 weeks before parturition, according to the manufacturer's recommendations.

Advice on vaccination

Vaccines work by mimicking the body's own natural acquired immunity to disease. The principles of vaccination are described in further detail in other texts, including the BSAVA *Textbook of Veterinary Nursing*.

Types of vaccine

Vaccines do not cause the disease they aim to protect against because the organisms in them have been killed or changed (attenuated) in some way, often through genetic modification. Types of vaccine used to prevent disease in dogs, cats and exotics in the UK and regimes for their use are described in Chapter 3. Veterinary nurses must be familiar with this information in order to be able to give the correct advice to clients. Clients should be made aware that vaccines may be given via several routes (e.g. intramuscular, subcutaneous, intradermal, intranasal (Figure 2.24)) so that they fully understand the procedures involving their pets.

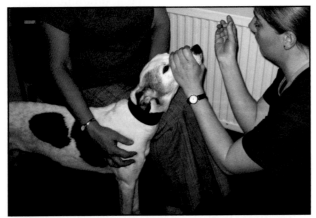

2.24 Some vaccines, for example the kennel cough vaccines, are given via the intranasal route.

Vaccination of puppies, kittens and other young pets (primary vaccines)

Provided the dam was vaccinated and neonates received colostrum correctly (see above), protection against disease for the first few weeks should be achieved in the first 24–48 hours of life. During this period, maternally derived antibodies would work against vaccination, as they would bind to the vaccine antigen themselves. As the young animal gets older, maternal antibody levels decrease until they reach a level at which they no longer interfere with vaccination.

The scheduling of vaccinations for puppies, kittens, young rabbits and ferrets varies between different vaccines and manufacturers. The majority of vaccination schedules begin at 9–10 weeks of age for kittens, and 6–10 weeks for puppies, with a final injection being given at 12 weeks of age in kittens, and 10–12 weeks in puppies. These vaccines are described as 'primary courses'. It is important to inform the client that full immunity is not reached until around 7–10 days after the second injection (depending upon manufacturer's recommendations); hence, puppies and kittens should remain relatively isolated until that time.

Vaccination of puppies, kittens and other pets may be the first contact with the veterinary practice for the pet or owner. This can be an opportunity to bond the client to the practice and advise on general health care. Veterinary nurses should be a key component of this service.

Vaccination of adult animals (booster vaccinations)

The immune response to naturally acquired infection or vaccination lasts for a variable period, depending on how strongly the infection/vaccine has stimulated the immune response (its immunogenicity). As natural immunity is so variable, it is not sensible to rely upon its protection for diseases where vaccination is possible. Equally, the protection given by vaccination does not last forever, and animals who have received primary vaccine courses will therefore require 'booster' vaccinations as adults. The exact frequency of booster vaccinations will depend upon the vaccine type and the manufacturer's recommendations. Typically, pet animal vaccines last 1–3 years, requiring the animal to have booster vaccines for at least some diseases annually (see Chapter 3). Pets that have missed booster vaccines or whose vaccination status is uncertain may be required to re-start their primary vaccine courses as above.

As well as ensuring animals are adequately protected against disease, booster vaccinations offer an opportunity for veterinary staff to carry out an annual general health check on each pet, including a clinical examination by a veterinary surgeon.

Vaccination cards

Each vaccinated dog and cat should be issued with a certificate of vaccination. The vaccine and its batch number should be recorded both on the animal's record card and on the vaccination card. Record cards are supplied by the vaccine manufacturers and usually have the practice's name and address on them. It is very important that ALL details are filled in correctly, especially when groups of puppies or kittens are being vaccinated for a breeder. Certificates must be signed by the veterinary surgeon and stamped with the practice's details. Certificates will have to be produced by owners if their animals are going to stud, shows or boarding kennels.

Client concerns regarding vaccination

Clients typically have two concerns regarding vaccination of their pets. These are that the vaccine may cause some kind of ill health (adverse reaction) or that the vaccine may not work (vaccine failure). Veterinary nurses should be able to advise clients about each of these.

Adverse reactions to vaccines

Minor reactions are relatively common. These are usually a reflection of the immune response to the vaccine or are caused by reaction to a chemical in the vaccine. They include:

- Small swellings at the site of injection (local reaction) that resolve spontaneously
- Lethargy and depression with a poor appetite for 24–48 hours following vaccination (generalized reaction).

Unless the reaction is very mild, veterinary examination should be advised in each of these situations in order to alleviate client concerns.

More serious vaccine reactions include allergic responses to components of the vaccine such as preservatives. The reactions include generalized itching or swelling of the face. These cases should be seen immediately by a veterinary surgeon; medical treatment may occasionally be required.

Vaccine-related sarcomas have been reported in cats, associated in particular with some feline leukaemia virus (FeLV) vaccines. In common with other neoplasms, the cause of these sarcomas is thought to be multifactorial (genetic factors, other tissue irritants at the site of vaccine) rather than being caused just by the vaccine itself. The risks to an individual cat of developing a vaccine-related sarcoma are, however, very low and certainly considerably lower than the risks of developing FeLV infection, and so vaccination is recommended.

There is much current, and often ill-informed, debate about the safety of vaccination, particularly with respect to booster vaccinations and long-term health issues. Whilst vaccination is not guaranteed or 100% safe, the benefits of vaccination outweigh the risks and it is easy to forget the severity of diseases like parvovirus or distemper in areas where, because of vaccination, the conditions are now very rare. The following should be considered when giving advice to clients:

- Vaccination should be carried out according to the manufacturer's data sheet instructions
- Vaccination of elderly animals should be encouraged as their immune system is less effective and, should they become infected, less able to mount an effective immune response
- Whilst dogs or cats living in more isolated areas are less likely to meet infectious disease, their immunity is likely to wane more rapidly than animals in more highly populated areas who are continually being exposed to low levels of infectious diseases that serve to stimulate their immune systems repeatedly. Hence, should an individual from an isolated area happen to meet an infectious disease they may be fully susceptible
- Over-vaccination and repeatedly restarting a primary vaccination course should be avoided
- Suspected adverse reactions to vaccination should be reported to the Veterinary Medicines Directorate (VMD) on a special form for this use.

Failure to respond to vaccine

Vaccination can appear to fail for a variety of reasons (listed below) but in most cases it is not the vaccine that is at fault.

- Out-of-date vaccine.
- Incorrect storage resulting in the vaccine becoming inactive (see Chapter 3).
- Incorrect administration (e.g. needle passing all the way through the skin, resulting in vaccination of the fur).
- Persistence of maternal antibodies for longer than anticipated (the exact age should always be determined before first vaccination).
- Animal is already incubating the disease. Most animals are presented for first vaccination at the time that maternal antibodies have waned and they are susceptible to disease; in some cases they have already become infected but are asymptomatic. Disease tends to develop very shortly after vaccination (within 2–3 days). Vaccination is unlikely to be harmful but is too late to provide protection.
- Sick animals. Administration of vaccine to a sick animal is unlikely to be harmful but the animal may be unable to produce a normal antibody response to the vaccine. A thorough examination should always be performed by a veterinary surgeon on animals presented for vaccination.
- Corticosteroid treatment. These and other immunosuppressive agents will interfere with the immune response. Animals known to be on such treatment should not be vaccinated.
- Stress (e.g. rehoming) can have a similar effect by increasing endogenous corticosteroid production.
- Overwhelming infection. The incubation period of a disease is dependent on the virulence and infectious dose. If a vaccinated animal encounters high levels of virulent pathogen, it may not be able to raise a strong enough immune response within the incubation period. In such cases clinical signs will generally be less severe than those in unvaccinated animals.
- Strain variation. Most viruses have several strains and although vaccines tend to cover the most common ones some strains are not fully covered and new strains may develop; hence a vaccinated animal will appear unprotected if it should meet a strain where there is no cross-protection from the vaccine strains.
- Individual immune deficiency.

Advice on overseas travel

Pet Passports and the EU Pet Travel Scheme

A European 'Pet Passport' allows movement of dogs, cats and ferrets within the European Union (EU) and also between other approved countries. Under the Pet Travel Scheme (PETS) a passport permits the re-entry of animals into the UK without quarantine, via approved routes, provided that blood tests show adequate rabies antibody titres following vaccination (see below). The actual countries and routes covered by PETS are subject to change; for the most up-to-date information the Department for the Environment, Food and Rural Affairs (Defra) website should be consulted.

Although there has been an increased interest in owners taking their pets on holiday with them due to relaxation in quarantine requirements, quarantine still remains the most efficient barrier to rabies and exotic diseases (see 'Risks of exotic diseases', below) that are not seen in the UK. Many of these diseases are transmitted by biting insects and ticks and can pose significant health risks to travelling pets, their owners and the UK disease status as a whole.

An EU Pet Passport can be issued for any animal (dogs, cats, ferrets) that has been microchipped (Figure 2.25) or is tattooed (to give unique identity) and is vaccinated against rabies. Vaccination must take place after the microchip has been implanted (or, if already microchipped, after scanning).

The EU passport allows entry into most EU countries, and other approved countries, currently 21 days after rabies vaccination. If the animal is required to return to the UK, a blood test will be required, usually

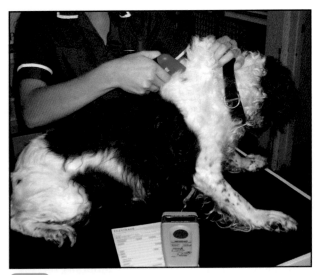

2.25 Microchipping.

between 20 and 30 days after vaccination (depending on the vaccine manufacturer's recommendation). The blood test will confirm that post-vaccination anti-rabies antibody levels are adequate to give protection against the disease. Re-entry to the UK is not permitted until 6 months after the blood test was carried out (the maximum recorded incubation period of the rabies virus). At the time of writing the re-entry requirements to the UK are under review and the Defra website should be consulted for the most up-to-date recommendations.

For entry into countries outside the EU, it is recommended that owners contact Defra or the embassy of the country or countries being visited for advice on their current requirements.

Booster vaccinations against rabies

In order to maintain the EU passport and prevent the need for additional blood tests, a rabies booster is required within the manufacturer's recommended interval. For booster requirements for specific EU countries it is advisable to check with Defra or the embassies of the countries being visited.

Issuing the PETS Passport

Depending upon the practice's policy, it is likely that a routine appointment can be made at the practice for all the components of the Pet Passport described above. The pet should be fasted for 4–6 hours prior to blood sampling. Reports of the rabies antibody results should be received within 2–4 weeks. When confirmation of adequate blood results (titre >0.5 IU/ml) are obtained a passport can be issued. The passport (Figure 2.26) must be signed and stamped by a veterinary official, usually a veterinary surgeon in the practice who is also a Local Veterinary Inspector for Defra.

Treatment against parasites

Due to the risks of parasitic diseases in some of the EU countries, it is recommended that pets are treated appropriately prior to and during their travels, depending on local risks (see 'Risks of exotic diseases', below). Before re-entry into the UK, it is a Defra requirement that all animals *must* be treated against external and internal parasites in order to prevent bringing these diseases into the UK. The pet must visit a veterinary practice no less than 24 hours and no more than 48 hours prior to returning to the UK. Approved treatments must be given and certified by a suitably qualified veterinarian.

Risks of exotic diseases

Rabies vaccination and parasitic treatment before re-entry to the UK are required by the government as part of the PETS scheme to protect public health. Additionally, depending on the countries visited, pets travelling overseas can be at risk of diseases not commonly seen in the UK, many of which are potentially fatal.

Heartworm

Heartworm is a parasitic worm (*Dirofilaria immitis*), primarily causing disease in dogs but cats are also at risk. It is transmitted and carried by mosquitoes. Once transmitted to the pet, it migrates to the blood vessels of the heart and lungs, causing disease which, if untreated, results in death.

- Diagnosis can be confirmed by blood samples.
- It is commonly found in Southern Europe, the USA and many tropical countries.
- Prevention is through the use of insect-repellent collars or spot-on products, or regular preventive treatment with appropriate anthelmintics.

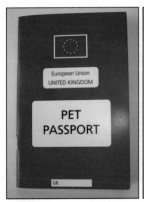
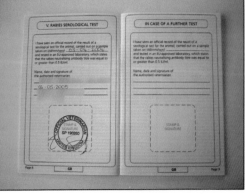
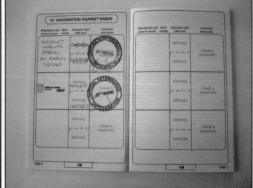

2.26 EU Pet Passport.

Leishmaniasis

Leishmaniasis is caused by the protozoal parasite *Leishmania infantum*. It is primarily a disease of dogs, but also cats, and is zoonotic; the parasite is transmitted by sandflies. Once transmitted to the pet, it affects the cells of the immune system and causes skin infections, weight loss, and eye, liver and kidney damage. If untreated, infection is fatal.

- Diagnosis can be confirmed by blood samples and microscopic examination of tissue samples.
- It is commonly found throughout the tropics and especially the Mediterranean coastal areas of Southern Europe.
- Prevention is through fly-repellent collars or spot-on products.

Babesiosis

Babesiosis is caused by the protozoal parasite *Babesia canis* or *B. gibsoni*. It is primarily a disease of dogs, but cats are also at risk. The parasite is transmitted by ticks. Once transmitted to the pet, the parasites destroy the red blood cells, usually causing anaemia. Other clinical signs are jaundice, anorexia, red urine, lethargy and development of fever. Infection can be fatal.

- Diagnosis can be confirmed by blood samples.
- It is relatively common on the continent of Europe and in other countries outside it.
- Prevention is by killing, removing or repelling ticks. Pets should be checked twice daily for ticks and suitable tick-repellent products used.

Hepatozoonosis

Hepatozoonosis is caused by the protozoal parasite *Hepatozoon*. It is primarily a disease of dogs and cats and is transmitted by blood-sucking insects, mites or, most commonly, ticks. Two main species affect dogs:

- **H. canis**
  Can cause lethargy, anaemia, weight loss and secondary liver, lung and kidney disease
  - Found in Europe, Africa, Asia and South America
  - Diagnosis by blood sampling
- **H. americanum**
  Can cause severe pain, lameness and paralysis, abscesses of the muscles
  - Commonly found in southern states of the USA
  - Diagnosis by muscle biopsy.

Prevention for both species is by killing, removing or repelling ticks. Pets should be checked twice daily for ticks and suitable tick-repellent products used.

Ehrlichiosis

Ehrlichiosis is a rickettsial infection (*Ehrlichia canis*) that primarily affects dogs and cats and is transmitted by ticks. Once transmitted to the pet, the infection affects the cells of the immune system and can cause destruction of the bone marrow. If untreated, it can be fatal. Clinical signs include depression, fever, swollen glands and haemorrhage under the skin.

- Diagnosis is by blood sampling.
- It is widely distributed throughout the world.
- Prevention is through killing, removing or repelling ticks. Pets should be checked twice daily for ticks and suitable tick-repellent products used.

Advice on parasitic infections

Although under current prescribing legislation (see Chapter 3) veterinary nurses are not able to prescribe all types of antiparasitic medication to clients for use in their pets, they will still be called upon to give general advice on the types of parasites encountered, the impact of parasite life cycles on their control, and the common methods of prevention that are available. Antiparasitic drugs are used to kill parasites or stop them from breeding (see also Chapter 3).

Parasites are organisms that exist for the whole or part of their life cycle living on or in another organism. There are two types:

- **Endoparasites** live inside the host organism
- **Ectoparasites** live on the surface of the host organism.

Endoparasites

The most common endoparasites in dogs and cats are tapeworms (cestodes) and roundworms (nematodes).

It is uncommon for dogs and cats in the UK to suffer from true disease due to worm infestation, unless they have very heavy worm burdens. Regular routine parasitic control is essential to rid the animal of any possible infestations and additionally (and importantly) to prevent any risk of zoonosis (transmission to humans). The choice of antiparasitic products to control endoparasites (anthelmintics) will depend on both the lifestyle of the pet and the type of owner it has; this will be discussed later. It should be remembered than anthelmintics kill only the worms present in the pet at the time of treatment and convey no residual protection.

Protozoal parasites are discussed above in the section on exotic diseases.

Roundworms

Toxocara canis and *Toxocara cati*

The most common roundworms are *Toxocara canis* in the dog and *Toxocara cati* in the cat. The life cycle of *T. canis* is described in Figure 2.27. These parasites are most common in young puppies and kittens and are the most important aspect of ownership to be discussed at first consultation. Heavy infections of *Toxocara* may cause vomiting, diarrhoea, gut obstruction and coughing in heavily infected animals. *Toxocara* eggs, passed in the faeces of the pet, can cause blindness or illness in humans if ingested. Children are most likely to be at risk, as they may play in an environment contaminated by faeces, such as grassy playgrounds and sandpits.

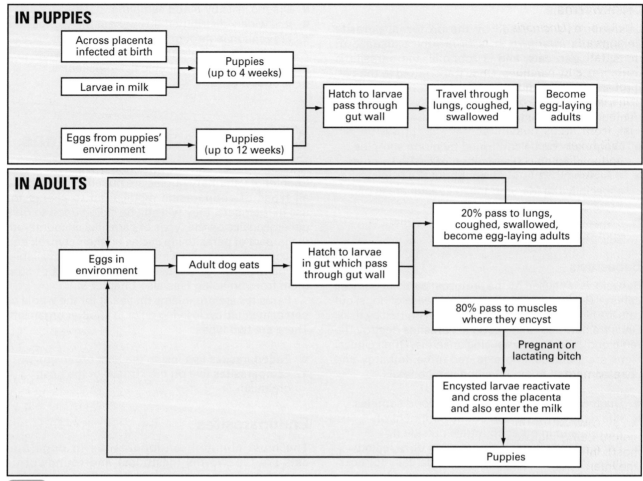

IN PUPPIES

Across placenta infected at birth → Puppies (up to 4 weeks)

Larvae in milk → Puppies (up to 4 weeks)

Eggs from puppies' environment → Puppies (up to 12 weeks)

Puppies → Hatch to larvae pass through gut wall → Travel through lungs, coughed, swallowed → Become egg-laying adults

IN ADULTS

Eggs in environment → Adult dog eats → Hatch to larvae in gut which pass through gut wall → 20% pass to lungs, coughed, swallowed, become egg-laying adults

80% pass to muscles where they encyst

Pregnant or lactating bitch

Encysted larvae reactivate and cross the placenta and also enter the milk

Puppies

2.27   *Toxocara canis* life cycle.

Essential information for dog owners regarding *Toxocara canis*

- Puppies can be born with *T. canis*, passed to them from their mother in the womb.
- Further infections can occur in puppies through milk.
- The worms move into the lungs. They are then coughed up and swallowed, and produce egg-laying adults until the puppy is approximately 14–16 weeks old.
- Puppies should be wormed twice after weaning (for example at 4 and 6 weeks old) with an appropriate roundworm treatment according to the manufacturer's recommendations.
- After 16 weeks of age, all dogs should be routinely wormed 3–4 times a year, according to the manufacturer's recommendation and risk factors for pet and owner.
- More frequent worming is required in the pregnant bitch, to help prevent or reduce levels in her offspring. Roundworm products should be used from mid-pregnancy through lactation, according to the manufacturer's recommendations.
- *T. canis* is zoonotic and a particular risk to young children.

The life cycle of *Toxocara cati* is essentially the same as for *T. canis*, but there is no transplacental transmission.

Essential information for cat owners regarding *Toxocara cati*

- Kittens become infected through their mother's milk.
- Kittens should be wormed twice from weaning (for example at 4 and 6 weeks old) with an appropriate roundworm treatment according to the manufacturer's recommendations.
- After 13 weeks of age, all cats should be routinely wormed 3–4 times a year, according to the manufacturer's recommendations and risk factors for pet and owner.
- Pregnant queens should be wormed in late pregnancy and lactation with a suitable roundworm product, according to the manufacturer's recommendations.
- *T. cati* is zoonotic and presents a risk to children through cat faeces being buried in sandpits; for this reason sandpits for children should be covered when not in use.

Hookworms

Hookworm (*Uncinaria stenocephala*) infection occurs in dogs after ingestion of infected larvae, or by larvae penetrating the skin. It can cause mild anaemia or skin irritation and reaction. Hookworm is traditionally a problem in dogs housed in poorly cleaned kennels or runs, where a build-up of contamination has occurred. As the disease also occurs in foxes, there is an added risk from areas heavily contaminated by (usually urban) foxes. Faecal sampling is recommended for a definitive diagnosis of hookworm infection, allowing a suitable anthelmintic product to be selected.

Whipworms

Trichuris vulpis infection is through ingestion of infected larvae, which attach to and feed from the gut lining, causing diarrhoea and eventual debilitation.

As in the case of hookworms, some anthelmintics may not be effective against whipworms. When either species is suspected, faecal sampling can be undertaken to confirm a diagnosis of infection (see Chapter 10). This ensures that a correct and effective anthelmintic treatment can be given.

Tapeworms

Tapeworms are segmented parasites, flat in cross-section. They require an intermediate host (Figure 2.28) in which to undergo a stage of development before being ingested by the dog or cat (definitive host). Infection is through ingestion of all or part of the intermediate host.

Dog and cat tapeworm

Dipylidium caninum is the most common type of tapeworm found in dogs and cats. Its intermediate host is the flea. The life cycle of *Dipylidium caninum* is described in Figure 2.29. Flea larvae eat tapeworm eggs and gravid segments passed by infected dogs and cats. Adult fleas are then ingested by the dog or cat whilst grooming and release the immature stage of the tapeworm (metacestode) into the gut of the pet. The adult tapeworm develops in the gut and the life cycle is completed as tapeworm eggs and gravid segments are passed in the faeces. The tapeworm life cycle can be completed in as little as 3 weeks, which means that infection can recur very quickly if fleas (as well as the tapeworms) are not controlled.

Segments of *D. caninum* may be seen around the anus of dogs and cats, where they can cause irritation. The adult worms cause few clinical signs unless burdens are very heavy in young or debilitated pets.

Taenia species

The intermediate hosts of several *Taenia* species (see Figure 2.28) are either ruminants (sheep and cattle) or small rodents. Infections are therefore more common in farm dogs fed raw meat and in feral or hunting cats that catch rodents. These tapeworm species have minimal effects on the infected dogs and cats, but are important in livestock species both clinically (where the intermediate stages may occur in gut, liver or brain) and at meat inspection (where they can result in rejection of affected areas of the carcass).

Tapeworm species	Intermediate host	Definitive host
Dipylidium caninum	Flea (*Ctenocephalides felis*)	Dog or cat
Taenia multiceps	Cattle, sheep	Dog
Taenia ovis	Sheep	Dog
Taenia pisiformis	Rabbit	Dog
Taenia taeniaeformis	Rodents	Cat
Echinococcus spp.	Sheep, cattle, humans	Dog

2.28 Some common dog and cat tapeworms and their intermediate hosts.

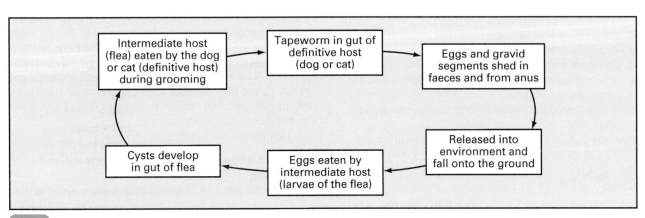

2.29 Life cycle of *Dipylidium caninum*.

Echinococcus granulosus

This infection occurs in certain parts of the UK, including areas of Wales and some parts of Scotland. The usual intermediate host is the sheep, but humans can also be infected by ingestion of eggs. The definitive host is the dog. In humans, hydatid cysts can cause severe disease depending on where in the body they are situated and they require surgical removal. Control methods include correct disposal of sheep carcasses and appropriate regular worming of dogs. In areas where *Echinococcus* is a risk, local government eradication programmes are in place to ensure that disposal and worming are carried out efficiently and human risk is minimized.

Endoparasites in exotic species

The small mammals, birds and reptiles seen in veterinary practices all have their own specific endoparasites that include not only roundworms and tapeworms but also protozoal parasites (coccidians, amoebae, flagellates and ciliates). Since most exotic pets are kept in relative isolation, little 'routine' treatment is necessary. In cases of weight loss, diarrhoea or general ill thrift, endoparasitic infections may be considered and diagnostic tests on fresh faecal samples carried out. In cases where clients keep large groups of such species, routine screening of faecal samples from representative animals may also be considered. Treatment is usually based on diagnosis and specific requirements. For more information refer to the *BSAVA Manual of Exotic Pets* and to those manuals that cover specific groups.

Ectoparasites

Fleas

Ctenocephalides felis, whose common name is the cat flea, is a major ectoparasite of the dog as well as the cat and may also affect ferrets. The dog flea *Ctenocephalides canis*, rabbit flea *Spillopsyllus cuniculi* and hedgehog flea *Archaeopsylla erinacei* may also occasionally be encountered in pet dogs and cats. Fleas are not fully host-specific and are zoonotic. They cause irritation and disease in affected animals and people.

Problems in humans include:

- Bites and irritation
- Fleas acting as vectors of disease (cat-scratch fever).

Problems in animals include:

- Scratching and irritation
- Pruritus, with possible self-trauma
- Development of an allergic dermatitis
- Intermediate host of tapeworm *Dipylidium caninum* (see above)
- Transmission of disease (e.g. feline infectious anaemia)
- Anaemia in heavily infested animals (often the young or debilitated).

Control of fleas in pets

In order to advise clients on the control of fleas in pets, it is important to understand the flea's life cycle (Figure 2.30). Important features are as follows.

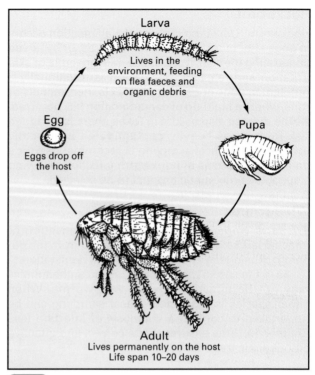

2.30 Flea life cycle.

- Adult fleas are only 5% of the problem. The majority of the infestation is made up of eggs, larvae and pupae, the immature stages that usually live in the house.
- The immature stages may remain in the house for up to a year before hatching.
- Many non-veterinary products bought from the supermarket or pet store may not be fully effective when trying to control the infestation.
- The choice of product should relate to level of infestation, the pets affected and type of problem.
- All pets in the house must be treated (see Chapter 3 for current treatments for pets).
- The environment (house, kennel, hutch, bedding) must also be treated, usually with a household spray. In cases of severe infestation it may be necessary to seek help from the local council or professional pest eradication companies in order to carry this out efficiently.

Ticks

The most common tick acquired by dogs and cats is the sheep tick (*Ixodes ricinus*), both the nymph and the adult forms of which can be found on pets. The animals pick these up whilst walking in fields that are or have been grazed by sheep and cattle or are populated with wildlife. The nymphs and adults attach themselves firmly to the host animal, take a blood meal until fully engorged, and then drop off. The tick will attach itself to any host, including humans.

Tick problems in animals include:

- Direct irritation at the site of attachment and feeding
- Transmission of diseases (e.g. Lyme disease, tick pyaemia, ehrlichiosis) (see also 'Overseas travel' section in this chapter)
- Difficulty in removal.

Ticks are treated by removal of individual parasites (special tick removers are available: it is important that the tick's head is not left in the animal as this can be the source of further irritation, infection and abscess formation) and the use of tick-repellent products, most of which are also licensed to kill fleas.

Lice

These insect parasites spend their whole life cycle on the host. They are not zoonotic and are host-specific. Transmission is directly from dog to dog or cat to cat. Environmental hygiene is important in controlling and preventing louse infestation.

The common species of lice found on domestic pets are given in Figure 2.31. They are just visible to the naked eye but differentiation of species requires microscopic examination.

Species of louse	Type of louse	Species affected (host)
Trichodectes canis	Biting	Dog
Linognathus setosus	Sucking	Dog
Felicola subrostratus	Biting	Cat
Gliricola porcelli	Biting	Guinea pig
Gryopus ovalis	Biting	Guinea pig
Polyplax serrata	Sucking	Mice, rats
Haemodipsus ventricosus	Sucking	Rabbit

2.31 Common louse species.

Clinical signs include:

- Excessive scratching, secondary skin infection
- Anaemia in severe cases in young or debilitated animals.

Lice are relatively easy parasites to kill using most of the licensed products available for fleas.

Mites

Cheyletiellosis

Cheyletiella mites are referred to as 'walking dandruff'. They are surface mites and permanent parasites, their whole life cycle taking place on the host. The life cycle occurs over about 3 weeks from egg to adult. *Cheyletiella* spp. are not host-specific and can be transmitted from animal to human. Pruritus is seen in some animals.

Rabbits are the most commonly affected pet (the species responsible being *Cheyletiella parasitovorax*) and usually present with scaling of the skin on the neck and back. Various products are available for the treatment of *Cheyletiella* (see Chapter 3).

Demodectic mange

Demodex canis is a subsurface mite and parasite of dogs. It can be found in small numbers in normal healthy animals, but can become a more significant infection if an animal's immune system is compromised in any way. Clinical disease is usually seen in juvenile animals (under 18 months old) or as adult-onset disease in immunocompromised individuals. The mite is host-specific and not zoonotic. It should be identified by skin scraping and microscopic examination (see Chapter 10). Clinical signs are usually alopecia and scaling. Lesions usually start off as localized to the head and feet, but may become more generalized to extensive areas of the body. Secondary bacterial infections and self-trauma make the signs more severe.

Demodex cati is a relatively uncommon parasite that causes similar clinical signs in cats. *Demodex* species are also found in some of the smaller mammalian pets such as hamsters (*D. criceti* and *D. aurati*).

Demodectic mange can be difficult to treat due to its relationship with the animal's own immune status. Repeat treatments with licensed products in dogs and cats and use of these products off-licence in small mammals can be successful.

Canine scabies (fox mange)

Sarcoptes scabiei is a subsurface burrowing mite that is a permanent resident on the host. The mites can be transmitted by close or indirect contact between dogs or between dogs and foxes. Clinical signs include intense pruritus and localized areas of alopecia, scaling, erythema and crusting. The ears, muzzle, hocks and elbows are common areas for the first visible lesions to develop. Eventually generalization of the infection results in severe hair loss, self-trauma and secondary bacterial infection. Untreated, the infection is highly debilitating and can result in death.

Scabies is a zoonotic disease, so careful handling and treatment are essential. The infection can be easily diagnosed by skin scraping and analysis (see Chapter 10). Treatment is now relatively easy using licensed products (see Chapter 3).

Ear mites

The most common ear mite, *Otodectes cynotis*, can affect dogs, cats and ferrets. Ear mites cause irritation and thick black wax in the ear canal. They are just visible to the naked eye and can be seen on otoscopic examination. Various ear products are suitable for treating ear mites (see Chapter 3) and may be dispensed following examination by a veterinary surgeon.

Other mite infections

Many species of mite affect exotic pets. One of the most common of these is *Trixacarus caviae*, which causes scaling and irritation on the dorsum of guinea pigs. Rats and mice are not uncommonly affected by fur mites (*Myobia musculi*, *Radfordia affinis* and *Mycoptes musculinus*), resulting in irritation and hair loss. *Notoedres* species may cause irritation around the head area of hamsters. Feather mites in birds, in particular pigeons (affected by *Falculifer rostratis*), and snake mites (*Ophionyssus natricis*) in snakes and lizards are also common causes of irritation in affected individuals. In all cases clients with pets showing signs of such infestations should seek veterinary advice. This usually involves examination, laboratory diagnosis of the problem and treatment, which is often ivermectin administered by the veterinary surgeon.

Fly larvae (maggots)

Larvae of the bot fly and of dipterids (in particular *Lucilia sericata*) may affect all types of pet. The flies are attracted to tissue that is damaged or contaminated with faeces and urine. Large numbers of fly eggs (usually white or yellow) are laid on the pet and hatch into larvae (maggots) that can cause tissue damage. Such damage is called myiasis or 'fly strike'. Fly strike may rarely affect debilitated or disabled dogs and cats, but rabbits and other small mammalian pets are most susceptible. Fly strike is most commonly seen in rabbits in the summer months, when flies are around and weather conditions are warm. If rabbit and guinea pig hutches are not cleaned out regularly and efficiently, they become an attractive place for the flies to lay their eggs. Rabbits with a history of urine or faecal soiling that are not checked daily are particularly susceptible. Fly eggs take as little as 12 hours to hatch (this is temperature-dependent), which means that strike can happen very quickly and may not be recognized early if pets are not frequently checked.

Parasiticides are available that prevent fly strike by arresting the development of the fly larvae, and owners of rabbits should be encouraged to use such products. Once a rabbit (or other pet) has been exposed to fully developed maggots the tissue damage can become extensive very rapidly. Intensive care, including removal of the maggots, fluid therapy and wound treatment, must be implemented immediately. Often euthanasia is necessary if the wounding is extensive or if body cavities have been penetrated.

Advice on antiparasitic treatments

Dogs and cats

There are many different preparations on the market today for prevention and control of parasites and these are discussed in detail in Chapter 3. The recommendation of a specific product will depend upon the lifestyle of both the pet and the people in contact with it (Figure 2.32). In order to assist with product choice, routine questions that should be asked of the client are outlined in Figure 2.33.

Type of pet	Lifestyle	Additional risks	Suggested treatments
House cat	Less exposed to parasites than most cats. Does not hunt	None	6-month multi-wormer. Flea treatment in summer months
Hunting cat	Outdoor cat. Catches mice	High risk of ecto- and endoparasites	3-month multi-wormer. Regular flea treatment
Kitten	Indoors. Increased roundworm risk due to age	Zoonotic risk for people, especially children, handling the kitten	Regular roundworm treatment. Tapeworm and flea treatment
Outdoor dog	Risk of both endo- and ectoparasites	Increased risks if in the countryside	3–6-month multi-wormer. Regular flea treatment. Tick treatment as required
Travelling dog	Goes overseas with owners	Risk of 'exotic' diseases	Appropriate parasite treatments for areas of travel (see 'Advice on overseas travel')
Puppy	Mostly indoors. Increased roundworm risk due to age	Zoonotic risk for people, especially children, handling the puppy	Regular roundworm treatment. Tapeworm and flea treatment

2.32   Choice of antiparasitic treatments for dogs and cats.

Question	Reason for question
Have you treated the pet with other parasitic controls?	May be contraindications to mixing products
Have parasites been found on the pet?	May indicate a large burden or determine product choice
Is prevention of infestation required?	Should always be suggested/discussed
How old is the pet?	Determines choice of product and roundworm risk
How is the pet housed?	Affects type of environmental control
Does the pet have a mostly indoor or outdoor lifestyle?	Affects level of risk of infection with most parasites
Does the pet have access to farmland or hill land?	Affects tick and tapeworm risk especially
Has the pet travelled or is it about to travel overseas?	Affects range of parasitic risk (see 'Advice to clients on pet passports, the pet travel scheme and overseas travel')
Are there any other pets in the house that also need treating?	Affects choice of product
Are there young children in the household or visiting?	Affects roundworm risk especially
Are there temperament issues with the pet (feral, difficult to handle) or owner disabilities?	Affects selection of a suitable product

2.33   Choosing a suitable antiparasitic: questions for owners.

It is also essential to make a correct diagnosis of the problem. This is relatively easy with fleas, ticks and tapeworms but more difficult with burrowing mites and some roundworms. If it is not obvious which parasite is causing the problem, microscopic examination (see Chapter 10) is essential in order to ensure that the correct parasiticide is selected for treatment and, importantly, that any necessary prevention of reinfestation is instituted. It must be remembered that anthelmintic preparations only kill the parasite present in the animal at the time of administration, and so ongoing prevention (or regular repeat treatment according to the manufacturer's recommendations) will be necessary to prevent reinfestation.

As well as choosing an effective product based on the questions in Figure 2.33, owners are likely to be influenced by:

- Frequency of application
- Ease of application
- Cost (per month).

Exotic pets

Because many small pets live enclosed in relatively solitary conditions, their risks of parasitic infections are lower than in more free-roaming dogs and cats. There may, however, be problems encountered when pets are purchased from large or already infected colonies. Additionally there is a need to protect against certain specific problems such as fly strike in rabbits.

Very few products are licensed for the treatment of parasitic infections in species other than dogs and cats, but licensed products do exist for the treatment and prevention of fleas, *Cheyletiella* and blowfly strike in rabbits. Similar questions to those outlined in Figure 2.33 for owners of dogs and cats can be asked when assisting clients in making a choice between these products. As blowfly strike is such a serious condition, preventive treatment should be recommended to all rabbit owners.

As products used for the treatment and prevention of parasitic problems in other exotic pets may have to be used 'off licence', it is essential that:

- A correct diagnosis of the problem has been made using appropriate laboratory techniques
- The owner is made aware if a product is being used 'off licence' and gives signed consent to this
- The pet is carefully monitored during treatment by a veterinary surgeon.

Euthanasia and bereavement

The human/pet relationship is very strong for many clients. Pets enrich our lives in numerous ways: they provide companionship and comfort, give us something to care for and love, keep us active and often enable us to meet other people with similar interests. Pets are family members and when they die their owners will often feel that it is 'like having a death in the family'. Many owners experience real grief upon the death of their pet and need help and support to cope with their loss.

Although the loss of a pet is a significant life event, in many circumstances euthanasia is vital to relieve the suffering of a dying animal and most owners appreciate the humanity of the euthanasia process. 'Put to sleep' is a term often used when an animal is to be euthanased. Great care must be taken if and when this term is used so that all concerned are absolutely clear that it actually means euthanasia; for example, a client might interpret being 'put to sleep' as being given an anaesthetic that puts their animal to sleep for a while, not for ever.

Around 2% of patient contacts at the veterinary surgery will result in euthanasia. This means that in a busy multi-vet practice several euthanasias occur each day and it can be easy to forget that, although routine for the practice staff, this is a rare and often highly emotional event for the owner.

No two euthanasia events will be exactly the same; every client and situation will be different. Euthanasia of a pet can profoundly affect the owner, the veterinary surgeon and the nurse, especially if the pet has spent a lot of time at the practice being treated before the decision for euthanasia is made.

Much of what is described below is time-consuming and difficult to organize in a busy practice, but it is an important part of veterinary care. The care provided at this time has a profound influence on the way a client will view the practice in the future and on the way that the public views the veterinary profession in general.

Euthanasia carried out in the veterinary practice is the cause of death of around 75% of animals and is therefore the most likely way in which a pet is going to die. However, 'convenience euthanasia' should be strongly discouraged.

No matter what nurses may think or feel about whether or not a pet should be euthanased, they must not appear judgmental. There are often many complex issues involved in the decision that may not be obvious at the time. This can be particularly difficult when euthanasia is requested for a young healthy animal for what appears to be a fairly trivial matter. Under these circumstances, nurses should ask to speak to the veterinary surgeon concerned to find out whether it is appropriate to offer to rehome the pet – a gesture for which some clients will be immensely relieved.

Many owners have difficulty making a decision for euthanasia and will ask the nurse, 'What would you do if it was your pet?'

- The nurse should never make an off-the-cuff answer to this question. Many clients are extremely vulnerable at this time and will take the advice literally. It can also sound as if the nurse is disinterested.
- A nurse unfamiliar with the case should say so and advise the client to talk with the veterinary surgeon concerned.
- Under no circumstances should a client be told what they ought to do.
- In virtually all cases the client will have already made their decision and is simply looking for support. The nurse should try to find out what that decision is and support it.
- In general, the nurse should try to make the client understand that this is an individual and personal decision and that there are no right or wrong choices. The client knows their pet best and so they are in the best position to make the decision.

Arranging the environment

Many clients have great difficulty in going back to a veterinary practice after euthanasia of their pet. The professionalism and care of the practice at the time has a great influence on the way the client feels about their pet's treatment and their use of the practice in the future.

- The client should have to wait as short a time as possible. In most instances an appointment shortly before the beginning of a surgery should be given, as appointments at the end of a surgery can sometimes mean a long wait if the veterinary surgeon is running late.
- If waiting is unavoidable, somewhere outside the main waiting area should be provided.
- It can be helpful to arrange for a nurse or receptionist to wait with the client, allowing them to talk about their pet. Nurses should always appear sincere and interested in what the client is telling them. Talking about their pet will often help the client's grieving process.
- When euthanasia has been performed, the client should be able to leave the surgery without walking through a waiting room full of people
- Removal of the body should not involve carrying it through any client areas.

Arrangements for disposal of the body

The method of disposal of the body can be a big decision for the client and they need to be able to make an informed decision as to what they would like done. A client may wish to bury their pet at home; alternatively, they have the option of mass cremation and disposal of ashes, or individual cremation and return of their pet's ashes in either a casket for retention or a box from which they can scatter the ashes if they wish (Figure 2.34). The difference between mass cremation and individual cremation must be explained fully and carefully, as should the costs of the different options. Individual cremation is significantly more expensive than mass cremation and the cost of a casket a lot more than a 'box for scattering'.

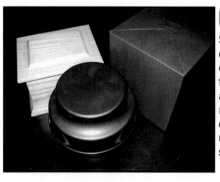

2.34 Some examples of options for the return of ashes. Left to right: wooden casket; metal urn; box for scattering.

It is essential that:

- The client's instructions regarding postmortem examination, disposal of the body or return of ashes are clearly understood, preferably in writing (see Figure 2.35)
- Great care is taken to identify and label bodies correctly for individual cremation

- The disposal service is supervised when bodies are collected and the correct paperwork completed and exchanged.

Dead animals are treated as clinical waste and disposed of only to licensed organizations unless the client wishes to take the body home for burial.

Paperwork

Signing the euthanasia form

Many owners find signing the euthanasia form upsetting, but it is a legal document and owners have been known to deny having given permission, particularly during the grieving process. A signed consent form (Figure 2.35) is particularly important when the client is not well known to the practice, if there are differing family opinions on the desirability of euthanasia, or if the person bringing the pet is not the owner. A consent form cannot be signed by a person under 16 years of age and should usually be signed by a person over 18.

NAME OF VETERINARY SURGERY
(Address ....)

EUTHANASIA CONSENT FORM

Euthanasia consent form for (Pet name) on (date)

(Client Name)   (Pet species)
(Client address)   (Pet breed)
                                                 (Pet age)

I hereby give my consent for the euthanasia of the above animal.

Please complete the rest of the form by ticking the box(es) as appropriate.

☐   I give my authorization for a postmortem examination of (pet's name)'s body to be carried out

☐   I wish to have (pet's name)'s body cremated

☐   I DO NOT want the ashes to be returned to me

☐   I would like the ashes returned to me:
    ☐ In a box for scattering
    ☐ In a metal urn
    ☐ In a wooden casket

Quoted price: (amount)

Signed ....

Name in block capitals ....

2.35 Example of a euthanasia consent form. The form must be signed by the owner, or their representative, who must be over 18 years of age.

Settling the account

This can add great stress to the situation, particularly if the bill is large for what eventually has been unsuccessful treatment. Some clients prefer to pay the bill before the euthanasia, which is possible as long as all the paperwork is complete and the euthanasia attracts a standard charge. Other clients will settle their bill after the euthanasia is complete, while others will be too upset and prefer to have the bill sent to them. There should be a clear practice policy as to how accounts are settled following euthanasia and nurses should know what this policy is and follow it. If there are problems the nurse should refer the matter to the Practice Manager or owner.

Practice records

Following euthanasia, practice records for the pet must be updated **immediately**. On no account should an owner receive a reminder about a booster vaccination a few weeks after losing their pet. If a reminder has already gone out, the owner should be informed that it will be arriving and apologies should be made accordingly.

Sympathy cards

Personalized sympathy cards can be much appreciated by owners and show that the practice cares about the owner and their pet. They can also give the client an excuse to telephone the practice, ostensibly in thanks for the card but in reality to discuss other issues regarding their pet's death that may have been bothering them.

The euthanasia process

Different owners react in different ways and their wishes should be accommodated if possible. For example, some will arrive, hand over their animal and leave immediately; usually their reason for not staying is that they are afraid of expressing their emotion in public. If it is appropriate, the nurse should reassure them that crying is understandable and natural.

Preparing the owner

It helps the owner if they are warned what to expect during euthanasia, as it will be easier for them to keep calm when some of the following occur:

- The pet's hair might be clipped
- The veterinary surgeon will inject anaesthetic
- The pet will 'go to sleep' as it would if given an anaesthetic, but the high dosage of the drug stops the heart
- The majority of animals lose urinary continence and some also defecate
- There may be reflex gasping movements even after the animal is dead
- Dead animals do not close their eyes.

Problems during euthanasia

Euthanasia of hard-to-handle, nervous or aggressive pets can be particularly stressful. The key is to remain calm. Some of the following measures may help to alleviate potential problems:

- Sedation of the patient may help but many sedatives reduce blood pressure, making finding the vein more difficult
- An intravenous catheter may be inserted (away from the owner if necessary)

- Before starting the procedure, all equipment should be to hand (e.g. scissors, clippers, swabs, drugs, needles, syringes)
- If a dog needs to be muzzled, tape should be avoided
- If the nurse feels that the needle is not in the vein or that the injection appears to be perivascular, the veterinary surgeon should be alerted immediately because:
  - The animal will not die
  - Perivascular injection is painful
  - The animal may become hyperexcitable if only a small amount of barbiturate has been given intravenously before the injection becomes perivascular.

After euthanasia

Some owners like to stay for a few minutes with their pet after it has died and some time alone with their pet should always be offered. To give them that time the consultation room should not be booked immediately following a euthanasia appointment, or a 'special' consulting room should be used for the procedure so that normal consulting is not affected.

If the nurse does not know what to say to the client at this stage, it is often better to say nothing and simply remain quietly with the client or leave if requested, returning a short time later. No matter how busy the practice is, it is important not to appear to be rushing the client.

Placing the animal in a plastic sack in front of the client should be avoided – this should be done after the owner has left. Even though the animal is dead, the client will be very sensitive about how it is handled. Owners taking pets home should be given incontinence pads and blankets for the pet to be wrapped in or the offer of a cardboard coffin.

Client reaction to euthanasia

Clients react in many different ways to the euthanasia of a loved pet and it is important to be able to recognize and deal with the emotions that they may exhibit.

'Shock'

'Shock' is usually exhibited by a refusal to accept that euthanasia is the only option. Shock and disbelief most frequently occur following a traumatic accident in a young animal, or where the owner believes that the problem is trivial and is told that their animal has serious advanced and terminal disease. Often owners will request a second opinion and this should be provided, wherever possible from within the practice.

Shocked people tend to become pale, weak and confused and may have difficulty grasping simple information. A cup of sweet tea is a traditional but effective measure. It is important that initial explanations are given slowly and as simply as possible. Any decisions that are made should be recorded in writing.

Shock tends to be a brief phase, lasting a few hours and rarely more than a day.

Dealing with shocked owners

- If clients are expressing disbelief, they should not be contradicted directly. Sympathize with their situation.
- If a second opinion is requested, try to provide one from within the practice. Shocked owners with dying pets travelling distances by car are a danger to themselves and other road users. If it is unavoidable, persuade the client to rest for a short while, make them a drink and stay with them if possible.
- If an animal is brought in following a road traffic accident:
  - It may have died en route and it may be necessary to call in a veterinary surgeon to confirm death
  - If the owner is convinced that the animal has been recently breathing, resuscitation should be attempted (see Chapter 7) until help arrives – even if the situation appears hopeless.

Anger

This is a common emotion and is often directed at the practice or at a neighbouring practice that has previously treated the pet. In many cases owners feel guilty (see below) and are seeking to blame someone for their pet's death. The type and quality of treatment are often questioned and such complaints, however unjustified, can sometimes lead to more serious actions such as litigation.

Dealing with angry owners

- Verbal attacks may be directed against the practice or the staff. They can be hurtful, particularly when the practice has put considerable time and effort into a case.
- It is important to stay calm and courteous and not become too defensive. Any failings on the part of the owner, such as time taken to seek veterinary advice, should not be raised.
- If the client refuses to be placated:
  - Try to find a quiet place for them to sit
  - Locate someone more senior to talk to them, preferably the veterinary surgeon who has dealt with the case, even if this is the person with whom the client appears unhappy
  - If it is impossible to find this particular veterinary surgeon make sure that the person who does talk to the client has full case notes and as much other detail as possible, including the nurse's impression as to why the client is upset
  - If no-one else is available, either book an appointment for the client to come back or arrange for the veterinary surgeon involved to telephone them to discuss the case. In

the latter situation it is essential that the veterinary surgeon makes the call when promised. If they cannot, the nurse must phone the client to rearrange contact.
- Avoid making statements that could be interpreted as an admission of carelessness, neglect or error.
- In many cases sincere expressions of sympathy and understanding at their loss may be all that the client requires. For many clients it is not so much whether the practice was right or wrong, but more that its staff cared and tried.
- If an error has been made, it is the responsibility of the veterinary surgeon, not the nurse, to explain the circumstances to the client.

Guilt

Most pet deaths are surrounded by a degree of guilt on behalf of the owners, who may feel that if the pet became ill prematurely it was due to a failing on their part.

Common areas of guilt are:

- Not spotting how unwell their pet had become
- Seeking veterinary advice too late
- Being unable or unwilling to afford more extensive investigations and treatments
- Failing to bring the pet back when requested or when its condition deteriorated
- Not requesting euthanasia at an earlier time
- Being responsible for a traumatic injury.

Dealing with owners who feel guilty

- It is important not to intensify feelings of guilt, as this can lead to aggression, blame or depression.
- Reassure the owner that it is not their fault, for example, if the pet has developed cancer. It is also helpful to sympathize with the owner and reassure them that it is always easier to see what would have been best after the outcome is known, or that accidents do happen and they are by no means alone in leaving a gate open leading to the pet being run over.

Depression

Sadness following the loss of a pet is natural. In some cases, especially where there is a single pet belonging to a person living on their own, clinical depression can occur. Such cases are rarely just about the pet and usually involve other personal experiences, particularly the loss of a relative. Guilt can also play a part in the onset of depression.

Depressed people can become physically ill, not eating or sleeping properly and losing interest in their daily responsibilities and appearance. Such owners are prone to break down in tears for no apparent reason.

Depression usually occurs within a few days of the loss, reaches a peak in about 2 weeks and then subsides.

Dealing with depressed owners

- **Sometimes the client will telephone the surgery with an apparently trivial enquiry, or become a frequent visitor with other pets with minor problems.**
- **Care must be taken to make sure that the client does not become emotionally dependent on the nurse or the practice, as neither has the time or training to be of long-term help.**
- **In many cases the client wants to talk to someone who understands their loss. They may have questions or want to have situations explained again that they were unable to take in at the time. The nurse should find time to answer these enquiries in a quiet place where there will be no interruption. If the case has been complicated, ask a veterinary surgeon to speak to the client.**
- **Clients should be assured that their feelings are normal and to be expected. Where appropriate, they should be reassured that they have done everything they could for their pet.**
- **The grieving process can be helped by encouraging a client to make a memorial gesture – for example, sponsoring a rescue animal.**
- **On rare occasions professional help may be necessary. The practice should be aware of any local support group so that it can be recommended.**
- **In extreme cases of profound depression, continuing for more than 3 weeks and where there may be a risk of self-harm, professional medical help should be sought. It is the responsibility of the veterinary surgeon dealing with the case to make the initial contact with the client's doctor or social services.**

Nurses should speak to someone more senior in the practice if clients are showing excessive dependency on the nurse, or if the nurse is concerned about a client's wellbeing. Details of conversations should be recorded on the client record, or someone else should be made aware of all the conversations.

Acceptance

This is essentially the recovery phase, when the client can rationalize their loss and view the circumstances of their pet's death objectively. The client is then able to talk about their pet more rationally and without excessive emotion.

During the acceptance phase:

- No action may be required
- This may be the time when suggesting a new pet is sensible, unless the previous pet died of an infectious disease that may still be present in the owner's home
- The practice should advise the client on how to find a new pet, what will be most suitable and what to look for (see 'Advice on buying pets' section, above). The client should be encouraged to bring the new pet to the practice for a check-up, preferably 4–5 days after they have brought it home
- Many owners are keen to adopt rescue pets at this stage. Having gone through the emotional turmoil of a sick pet, taking on a new animal with problems may not be the best solution. A young healthy pet may be more suitable.

Assessing the client's needs

Assessing the client's needs is often a matter of experience, helped by previous contact with the client. For newly qualified nurses or those who have recently joined the practice, help from senior nursing colleagues can be invaluable.

Situations that tend to suggest that an owner will have problems coping with the death of their pet include the following:

- There has been a lack of time to prepare for, or come to terms with, the loss (e.g. traumatic episodes or rapidly advancing disease)
- The owner has suffered problems following the death of a pet in the past
- The owner lives alone and it was their only pet
- The pet has been nursed through a period of intense care and dependency
- The pet has helped an owner through a personal crisis, such as divorce or loss of a close relative
- The pet belonged to someone close to the owner who has now died – the last living link
- The owner is forced to opt for euthanasia for financial reasons, or because they are unable to provide the necessary support at home.

Such clients should be contacted, where appropriate, a few days after their pet's death or encouraged to phone the practice 'if they have any questions or just want a chat'. When contact is made the conversation need not be prolonged but should appear sincere, concerned and unhurried. Asking how the client is feeling can allow them to express their grief or give clues to their state of depression. Reassurance is the key, particularly if it is necessary to suggest that they contact a support agency. The nurse should always end the conversation by saying that they can contact the surgery again for a chat.

Grief within the practice

Grief at the loss of an animal may not be confined to the owner but may profoundly affect members of the practice staff, particularly when an animal has been hospitalized for a long period and has undergone intensive treatment. Support should be provided where possible, particularly to trainees and less experienced staff. Older staff may appear less affected but this is usually due to the necessity of developing coping strategies; it does not mean that they do not care about the pet's death. Nurses should be prepared to talk about and share grief with their colleagues, recognize grief in others and offer support.

Advice when admitting and discharging patients

Admission of patients

Patients often have to be admitted to the veterinary practice in order for tests to be carried out and operations to take place. The admission procedure is often carried out by a veterinary nurse under the direction of a veterinary surgeon responsible for the case.

The importance of consent

When admitting patients for procedures or operations, informed signed consent for the procedure must be obtained from the owner. It is important that the owner reads and fully understands everything that is involved before signing the consent form.

Consent forms are legal documents and must only be signed by an informed adult (over 18 years old). Ideally the person signing the form will be the owner. In certain circumstances it may be necessary for another adult to sign on behalf of the owner, with the owner's consent, and in this instance this person takes on the legal responsibilities of consent.

Obtaining consent and admission of patients

The exact process of admitting animals and obtaining consent for procedures will vary between veterinary practices, but the admission process usually includes some or all of the following:

- Produce a consent form (photocopied or computer-generated). An example is shown in Figure 2.36
- Confirm client and pet details (name, address; breed, sex, age)
- Confirm and explain the procedures that will take place
- Clarify if the pet is to be sedated or anaesthetized in any way
- Explain any risks involved
- Confirm that the pet's condition has not changed in any way since last seen by the veterinary surgeon
- Confirm any medication being given to the pet and when the last dose was given
- Confirm any known allergies or previous adverse reaction the pet may have
- Confirm when the pet was last fed (important if the pet is to be sedated or anaesthetized, or if blood samples are to be collected)
- Confirm any additional client requests (e.g. clip nails, groom, check ears)
- Confirm and record any possessions left (leads, blankets, toys, etc.)
- Check additional information on the consent form

Anyplace Veterinary Hospital
Consent form

Owner: *Mrs Smith*   **Date of admission:** *01/01/06*

Address: *1, Brown Street*   **Contact phone No:** *01234 56789*
Anytown
Somewhere

Consent for: *Daisy*   **Species:** *Canine*
                                 Breed: *Dobermann*

Last meal: *Last night 8 pm*

Medication today: *None*

Allergies/reaction: *None*

Possessions left: *Red collar and chain lead*

Procedure: *General anaesthetic and spay*

Extra requests: *Clip nails, check anal glands*

Estimated price: *£200–250*

I hereby give permission for the performance of the procedures listed on the above named animal. I understand that this includes:

* Administration of an anaesthetic/sedation as necessary
* Surgical operations and associated procedures as necessary
* Other procedures as necessary, including those described above

I understand that all anaesthetic and surgical procedures involve some risk to the animal, and in the case of emergency I consent to such procedures as might be necessary.

I agree to the estimated costs and will be responsible for payment. I agree to pay full fees on collection of my pet.

2.36   Example of a consent form.

- Confirm client contact details for the day (mobile and 'landline' phone numbers)
- Explain the estimated costs involved (see 'Estimates and quotes', below) and the method of payment expected according to practice policy
- Give owner an opportunity to read the form and ask any questions
- Obtain owner's or agent's signature on the consent form
- Admit the pet to the practice in a secure way (on a lead or in a basket) without any risk of escape.

Ideally the admission procedure will take place somewhere quiet (for example, a consulting room) where there are no distractions and the owner feels able to ask questions. Specific appointment times for admissions ease congestion and allow adequate time for the process to be carried out properly and for the client to avoid feeling at all rushed. The nurse should try to use language that the owner will fully understand and avoid abbreviations – for example, use 'general anaesthetic' rather than 'GA' when talking to the client and on the consent form. The owner may be upset at leaving the pet or worried about its condition and the procedures that are to take place. It is the nurse's job to support and reassure the client if they are in any way distressed. Other clients may be in a hurry to go to work if the admission is in the morning; this again is helped by specific appointment times. The admitting nurse must act quickly and efficiently if the client is in a hurry but must ensure that this does not in any way compromise the admission. In all cases, fully informed signed consent for the correct procedures must be obtained.

If the nurse feels unsure in any way about explaining the procedures involved they must seek veterinary advice. If the client is unhappy about giving consent for any reason, the assistance of a senior member of staff should be sought.

The ability of the practice to be able to contact the client throughout the day is essential. Equally the owner should be informed of how and when contact with the practice to discuss the progress of the animal will be made. This will depend upon the practice's policy and the type of case. The owner might be asked to telephone the practice at a specific time, or the nurse may need to confirm that the practice will contact the owner when the procedure is finished. Owners are likely to be concerned about the pet and having contact with the practice as soon as is practical after the procedure will help to alleviate their concerns.

Additional procedures at admission

After admission it may be necessary for the nurse to:

- Place the animal in a safe and secure kennel or cage (see Chapter 5)
- Weigh the pet
- Record the admission in an operations diary
- Liaise with the veterinary surgeon regarding administration of premedication (see Chapter 12).

Discharging patients

It is often the job of the veterinary nurse to discharge patients from the veterinary practice to their owners. This is especially the case after routine procedures such as neutering, and nurses must be especially familiar with these procedures. The actual protocol for discharging patients will vary between practices but will usually involve some or all of the following:

- Identify the owner and animal that they have come to collect
- Confirm that the animal is ready for collection
- Confirm who is to discharge the animal
- Gather together any medications for the pet
- Gather together any items belonging to the pet (leads, beds, etc.)
- Explain the procedures that have been carried out
- Explain the aftercare that the animal requires at home

- Check that the owner understands what is required and feels able to carry it out at home
- Check that the owner understands how and when any medication should be given
- Check that the owner knows when to report progress or return for follow-up appointments
- Perform any follow-up activities as necessary (take payments, make appointments)
- Hand over the animal in a professional manner, safely restrained.

The discharge procedure should take place somewhere quiet and private, such as a consultation room, where the owner is able to concentrate on what is being said and feels able to ask questions. As with admissions, a specific appointment time helps to avoid unnecessary congestion and the client or nurse feeling rushed.

As the owner may concentrate on the pet rather than on what is being said, it is often better to speak to the owner first and then bring the pet to the owner. Written instructions are also beneficial so that the owner is not expected to remember every detail of what is said. Clients may be unsure as to how to administer medications and it is the job of the veterinary nurse to explain this and demonstrate as necessary.

An example discharge sheet is shown in Figure 2.37.

**Anyplace Veterinary Hospital
Discharge form for Daisy Smith**

Daisy has been spayed today under general anaesthetic. She has been given pain-killing injections and antibiotics today and has some additional medication to start tomorrow. This medication should be given once daily with food as directed.

A small area of hair has been clipped from Daisy's leg to allow the veterinary surgeon to give an injection into the vein, producing a smooth anaesthetic. Hair has also been clipped from her abdomen to allow the surgery to take place. The hair will regrow over a few weeks.

Daisy should sleep indoors this evening and only be taken for short walks on a lead until next seen by the veterinary nurse. A light meal as provided should be given this evening.

Daisy has skin sutures (stitches). These should be checked daily and any swelling or discharge reported. If Daisy licks and chews at the sutures you must contact the practice and a preventive collar will be provided.

We would like to see Daisy again in 5 days for a check up and in 10 days to remove the sutures. Please make appointments at reception to see the veterinary nurse.

If you have any queries or concerns please do not hesitate to contact the Hospital.

At all times telephone 01246 81012

2.37   Example of a discharge form.

Processing client payments

Practice payment policy

All veterinary practices expect non-account clients to pay at the time their pet is treated, except perhaps in the case of euthanasia (see above). Where animals are hospitalized, payment is often requested on an ongoing basis. Farm animal and equine clients, as well as dog and cat breeders where large and regular amounts of work are carried out, are usually sent monthly accounts. It is very important that the nurse is fully aware of, and adheres to, the practice payment policy when requesting and taking payment from clients.

The cost of treatment

The nurse should be aware of the cost of the common and regular procedures, drugs and materials (e.g. consultations, neutering, vaccination, microchipping, flea and worm products, food) and be able to explain these costs to the client. It is useful to be able to break down the cost of treatments such as flea and worm control or food products into cost per day or per week as examples for the client. This may help to show the client that, on a daily or weekly basis, costs are relatively low and the products are good value for money.

Estimates and quotes

Estimates should be given to all clients for operations, dental treatments and any other non-routine procedures.

- An **estimate** is the price that the practice expects the treatment to cost the client; this price may vary to some degree depending upon the circumstances of the operation and if extra work needs to be carried out. The estimate should give the client a very good idea of cost, but the final price may be a little more or a little less.
- A **quote** is a firm price given for a procedure and is not changed, whatever change in circumstance there may be.

In some practices only the veterinary surgeon is able to give estimates. The estimate should always be recorded on the client's record and they should be given a paper copy of the estimate so that there is no misunderstanding at a later date. An estimate gives an expected cost of treatment for the client's animal and it is important that this is clearly explained to the client so that they understand that the final bill may be more or less than the estimate given. If the cost of treatment is likely to be much greater than the estimate (for example, an operation is more complicated or time consuming than anticipated) the client should be contacted as soon as possible to discuss the change in cost. The estimate should always be put on the consent form for any operation (see Figure 2.36) and the nurse should check that the client is aware of this.

Methods of payment

Clients can pay their bills by a variety of methods.

Cash

- Always check the amount of cash handed over and do not put notes into the till until the change has been given.
- Ensure that the cash and notes are valid currency. Banks often provide information on how to check paper money for the following characteristics:
  - Watermarks
  - Paper quality
  - Metal strips
  - Printed shapes at the bottom of each note enclosing the letters ER.

Cheques

- Always watch as the client signs a cheque and make sure that the signature matches the one on the guarantee card and that the written amount matches the numbered amount.
- Record the cheque card number, expiry date and type of card (e.g. Mastercard, Visa) on the back of the cheque.
- Never accept a postdated cheque, i.e. a cheque dated in the future.
- If the client makes an error when writing the cheque, the mistake can be crossed out and rectified but the correction must be initialled by the client.
- A cheque that is more than 6 months old will not be honoured by the bank when it is presented.
- A cheque may be returned to the practice by the bank stamped 'refer to drawer'. This usually means that there are insufficient funds in the client's bank account to cover the amount written on the cheque. Occasionally it will be because the cheque has not been signed, or words do not agree with figures. In these cases the client should be contacted and asked to pay by another method.
- A cheque takes 3 working days to clear, i.e. for the money to pass into the payee's account.

Debit cards and credit cards

Credit cards

When a credit card is used, the cardholder is in effect borrowing a sum of money from the credit card company. This will be recorded on their credit card account. At the end of each month they will receive the account, which they can pay in full or in part. If they pay in part, interest will be charged on the outstanding amount.

Debit cards

When a debit card is used, the sum of money is immediately debited from the cardholder's bank account. The cardholder cannot use a debit card for a sum of money greater than they have in their bank account. Debit cards also act as cheque guarantee cards.

Chip and pin

Debit and credit cards are now protected by 'chip and pin' technology. The **chip** is a small microchip embedded into the card and it holds the card owner's unique details. The **pin** is a four-digit personal identification number assigned to the cardholder. When the card is placed in the practice's electronic card terminal (Figure 2.38) and the cardholder keys in their pin number, online authorization is given and a receipt is printed. Signatures are now only accepted if a client has special difficulties or is disabled in some way.

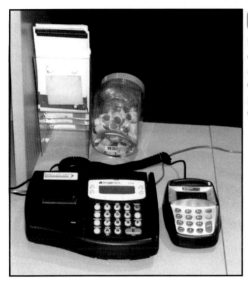

2.38 Examples of debit and credit card payment equipment.

Standing orders

A standing order is a fixed amount paid into the veterinary practice's bank account from a client's account on a fixed date. A standing order can be altered by the client but not by the practice. A small number of clients use this method of payment to keep their account in credit.

Direct debits

A direct debit differs from a standing order in that the amount paid into the practice's bank account from the client's account can be altered by the practice, depending on how much the client owes. As with the standing order, a few clients use this method to pay their veterinary bills.

Value added tax (VAT)

All veterinary practices are registered for VAT. If a business is VAT-registered it must charge 17.5% VAT on the services and products it sells to its customers. This amount is then paid by the business to HM Customs and Excise. There are some products, such as food for human consumption, that do not attract VAT and there are some services, such as the provision of gas and electricity, that attract a lower rate of VAT.

The veterinary practice must charge the full rate of 17.5% on all its services and product sales, the only exception being for charities, where VAT is not charged on drugs purchased. VAT must be added to the client's bill after all the items on the bill have been calculated.

Examples of VAT calculations

Example 1

Consultation	£20.00
Drugs	£ 6.00
Total	£26.00
VAT at 17.5% = (£26.00 x 17.5)/100 =	£ 4.55
Total payment due	£30.55

Example 2

Total payment incl. VAT	£30.55
Bill before VAT charge = (£30.55	
x 100)/117.5 =	£26.00
VAT element of bill = £30.55 – £26.00 =	£ 4.55

Processing payments

However the client has paid their bill, the payment must be recorded on the client's record so that they are not charged again for their animal's treatment. Most veterinary practices now have computerized client records. If this is the case, the payment should be entered into the client's financial record and the nurse should check that the correct payment has been credited to the client's account. If written records cards are being used, the amount paid should be recorded by hand and deducted from the outstanding amount on the client's record.

Itemized billing

It is good practice, and will soon be a legal requirement, to produce an itemized bill for the treatment of a client's animal. An itemized bill should be given to each client; it should include details of all services and products supplied and it must be possible to distinguish prescription-only medicines (POMs) from other veterinary products.

Itemized billing

Consultation	£18.00
Drugs *(specify drugs)*	£ 9.50
Wormer *(specify wormer)*	£ 6.00
Food *(specify food type)*	£15.00
Total goods and services	£48.50
VAT	£ 8.49
Total payment due	£56.99

The itemized bill is a very useful communication aid. It shows the client how the costs of their animal's treatment are broken down and it can be used to explain what treatment the animal has been given. In addition, the nurse can use the itemized bill to explain to the client what good value they have received.

Receipts

A receipt should always be offered to clients and should include details of the amount received from the client. The receipt can either be produced by the computer or handwritten. In some cases the bill can be used. The nurse should write on the bill:

- The date
- The nurse's name or initials
- The amount received
- 'Received with thanks'.

Insurance claims

Some pet owners have their pet insured. If this is the case, they may only be liable to pay the 'excess' on their veterinary bill. If a client says that they are insured, it is important to check their records and make certain that their insurance is up to date and that they are covered for the condition for which the pet is being treated. Depending upon the company with which the client is insured and the practice's policy, the practice will either bill the insurance company direct for the treatment minus the 'excess', or the client may have to pay the whole bill to the veterinary practice and then claim back the costs from the insurance company.

Since January 2005 veterinary practices have had to be authorized by the Financial Services Authority (FSA) before appointed representatives in the practice are allowed to recommend individual pet insurance companies, explain policy details, help clients to complete proposal forms and assist in the completion of claim forms. If a practice is not authorized by the FSA in regard to specific policies, they can only provide general information on the advantages of pet insurance and supply but cannot give advice on insurance material.

Disagreement over the cost of treatment

There may be instances where a client becomes upset about their bill and challenges the cost of the treatment. This may be because the cost is higher than the estimate given, or because the amount is higher than expected. Much disagreement can be avoided if carefully calculated estimates are given (see 'Estimates and quotes', above). If the bill is higher than the estimate, the nurse should explain why this is so. For example, it might be that more teeth were extracted during a dental procedure, or an extra lump was removed, or ears were cleaned. The next step is to go through the itemized bill with the client to explain the costs and the treatment given or drugs dispensed. If the client is still not satisfied, the nurse should suggest that they speak to the veterinary surgeon concerned or to the Practice Manager.

Inability to pay

There will always be some genuine clients who find it difficult to pay their veterinary bills. In such cases the nurse should provide the client with information and contact details about local and national charitable organizations that may be able to help. It may also be appropriate to discuss pet insurance as a future option to help with the payment of veterinary bills. Another suggestion might be that the client should set up a direct debit or standing order account with the practice to spread the cost of bills, if it is felt that the client might be receptive to such an arrangement. In a very few cases practices allow payment of veterinary bills by instalments. The nurse needs to know what the practice's policy is regarding this and, if it might be an option, should suggest that the client speaks to someone with more authority about their bill payment.

Ideally, any discussions about costs and payment should always take place *before* treatment is carried out, except in the case of life-saving acute emergency treatment.

Further reading and useful websites

British Veterinary Association website: www.bva.co.uk

Corsan J and Mackay AR (2001) *The Veterinary Receptionist: Essential Skills for Client Care*. Butterworth-Heinemann, Oxford

Department for Environment, Food and Rural Affairs website: www.defra.gov.uk

Horwitz D, Mills D and Heath S (2002) *BSAVA Manual of Canine and Feline Behavioural Medicine*. BSAVA Publications, Gloucester

Lane DR, Cooper B and Turner L (2007) *BSAVA Textbook of Veterinary Nursing, 4th edition*. BSAVA Publications, Gloucester

Meredith A and Redrobe S (2001) *BSAVA Manual of Exotic Pets, 4th edition*. BSAVA Publications, Gloucester

Ramsey I and Tennant B (2001) *BSAVA Manual of Canine and Feline Infectious Diseases*. BSAVA Publications, Gloucester

Shilcock M (2001) *The Veterinary Support Team*. Threshold Press, Newbury

Shilcock M and Stutchfield G (2003) *Veterinary Practice Management – A Practical Guide*. Saunders, Edinburgh

Acknowledgement

The authors and editors would like to acknowledge the contributions to the *BSAVA Manual of Veterinary Nursing* by Kit Sturgess and Janet Parker.

3

Practical pharmacy for veterinary nurses

Heather Roberts and Sally Anne Argyle

> ## *This chapter is designed to give information on:*
>
> - The different types of drugs used in veterinary practice
> - Commonly used abbreviations associated with drug dosing
> - The different formulations and routes of drug administration
> - Calculation of drug doses and infusion rates
> - The legal categories of drugs and legislation affecting their use
> - Safe handling, record keeping and storage of drugs
> - Labelling and dispensing of drugs in a safe, responsible manner

Introduction

Two terms commonly encountered in the discussion of medicines are pharmacology and pharmacy.

Pharmacology can be defined as the study of the way in which living organisms are affected by chemical agents. It encompasses pharmacodynamics and pharmacokinetics.

- **Pharmacodynamics** can be seen as the effect that the drug has on the body.
- **Pharmacokinetics**, in contrast, can be seen as the way in which the body handles the drug. Pharmacokinetics therefore covers the absorption, distribution, metabolism and excretion of the drug. (For definitions of these terms, refer to 'Administration and formulation of drugs' later in this chapter.)

Pharmacy focuses on the drugs themselves and encompasses the preparation, formulation and dispensing of drugs.

Figure 3.1 shows how drugs may be categorized by:

- Mode of action
- The body system on which they act.

Drugs categorized by mode of action
Antimicrobial agents
Antineoplastic drugs
Immunosuppressive agents
Antiparasitic agents
Anti-inflammatory agents
Antiepileptics
Diuretics
Vaccines
Analgesics
Sedatives/tranquillizers
Anaesthetic agents
Nutraceuticals

Drugs categorized by system on which they act
Cardiovascular system
Respiratory system
Gastrointestinal system
Urinary system
Endocrine system
Reproductive system
The eye
The integument
Musculoskeletal system
Nervous system

3.1 Drugs may be categorized by mode of action or by the system on which they act.

> ⚠️ **WARNING**
> It should be noted that on occasions it will be necessary to use drugs not licensed for a given species. 'Off-label' use is discussed later in this chapter. Veterinary nurses in practice should be mindful of this, especially when involved with medicating exotics and small pets, where the likelihood of encountering off-label use is increased.

Drugs categorized by mode of action

Chemotherapeutic agents

These are drugs used to treat either invading microorganisms or aberrant host tissue growth (neoplasia). Drugs in this category therefore include antimicrobial and antineoplastic agents. An important characteristic of these agents is that they should by some means be able, selectively, to affect the invasive agent or tissue without damaging healthy host tissue.

For example, the antibiotic benzyl penicillin prevents cross-linking of peptidoglycan, an important constituent of bacterial cell walls. This antibiotic will therefore disrupt the cell walls of susceptible bacteria, thereby killing the organisms. Animal cells do not have cell walls and are therefore unaffected by the antibiotic.

Antimicrobial agents

Drugs within this group may be divided as follows:

- Antibacterial agents
- Antifungal agents
- Antiprotozoal agents
- Antiviral agents.

Antibacterial agents

By strict definition, **antibiotics** are the products of other microorganisms and are therefore naturally occurring agents, while **antibacterial** drugs include not only naturally occurring agents but also synthetic or semi-synthetic agents, such as the sulphonamides. However, the terms antibiotic and antibacterial are often used interchangeably, since many of the traditional antibiotics (e.g. those within the penicillin group) have been modified so that they too are synthetic or semi-synthetic and therefore the distinction is no longer relevant.

Antibacterials can be described as either bacteriostatic or bactericidal.

- **Bacteriostatic** implies that the drug slows down the growth of the bacteria, allowing the host's own defence system to overcome the infection.
- **Bactericidal** agents kill the invading bacteria.

Figure 3.2 lists the main groups of antibacterial agents, together with examples and modes of action.

Antifungal agents

These are used to treat fungal infections and may be described as either fungistatic or fungicidal.

- **Fungistatic** agents slow or inhibit the growth of the fungal organism, thereby allowing the host's own defence system to overcome the infection.
- **Fungicidal** agents kill the fungus.

Class	Examples	Bactericidal or bacteriostatic	Mode of action
Penicillins [a]	Ampicillin, amoxicillin	Bactericidal	Disrupt bacterial cell wall
Cephalosporins [a]	Cefalexin	Bactericidal	Disrupt bacterial cell wall
Sulphonamides [b]	Sulfadiazine, sulfasalazine	Bacteriostatic	Block bacterial folate synthesis
Diaminopyrimidines [b]	Trimethoprim	Bacteriostatic	Block bacterial folate synthesis
Aminoglycosides	Gentamicin, neomycin	Bactericidal	Inhibit bacterial protein synthesis
Tetracyclines	Doxycycline, oxytetracycline	Bacteriostatic	Inhibit bacterial protein synthesis
Macrolides	Erythromycin, tylosin	Bacteriostatic/bactericidal	Inhibit protein synthesis
Quinolones	Enrofloxacin, marbofloxacin	Bactericidal	Inhibit DNA gyrase (interfere with DNA processing and protein synthesis)
Chloramphenicol	Chloramphenicol	Bacteriostatic	Inhibits protein synthesis
Nitroimidazoles	Metronidazole	Bactericidal	Prevent DNA synthesis
Lincosamides	Clindamycin, lincomycin	Bacteriostatic/bactericidal	Inhibit protein synthesis

3.2 Classification and mode of action of commonly used antibacterial drugs. [a] The penicillins and the cephalosporins are collectively known as the β-lactams. [b] The sulphonamides and the diaminopyrimidines are often combined; for example, trimethoprim and sulfadiazine may be combined in a single preparation.

They may be applied topically or given systemically. Figure 3.3 summarizes the main antifungal agents used in small animal practice and gives examples of some of their uses.

Route of administration	Examples of drugs	Uses
Topical	Miconazole	Treatment of *Malassezia pachydermatis* skin infection. Also effective against ringworm, including treatment of lesions in rabbits
	Enilconazole	May be used for irrigation of nasal *Aspergillus fumigatus* infection
	Amphotericin B	Useful in birds for oral *Candida* lesions
Systemic	Griseofulvin, ketoconazole, itraconazole	Main use is in treatment of ringworm. Ketoconazole and itraconazole are also used to treat a variety of fungal infections in dogs, cats and exotic pets

 Examples of antifungal agents used in companion animal practice.

Antiprotozoal agents

These are discussed later in the section on Antiparasitic agents.

Antiviral agents

Treatment of viral infections generally involves supportive therapy and the use of agents, such as antibacterial agents, to control secondary infections. A number of antiviral drugs (such as aciclovir, zidovudine and trifluorothymidine) are available but are not licensed for animal use. Until recently they have been used primarily for ocular manifestations of herpesvirus infection in horses and cats. Interferon omega can be used systemically to enhance the body's natural defence system in cases of enteric parvovirus in dogs, and may be used topically in cases of ocular herpes keratitis.

> ⚠ **WARNING**
> **Antiviral agents are highly toxic, with a narrow safety margin, and should therefore be used with extreme care.**

Antineoplastic and immunosuppressive agents

Drugs are frequently used in the treatment of neoplastic diseases in companion animals. They are of particular importance in systemic neoplastic diseases

that are not amenable to surgical management (e.g. lymphosarcomas and leukaemias). They may also be used as an adjunct to surgery, to reduce tumour size prior to surgery or as an additional treatment following surgery. Drugs used to destroy tumour cells are termed **cytotoxic** drugs. Examples include prednisolone, which is licensed for animal use, along with vincristine, doxorubicin and cyclophosphamide, which may also be used.

> **WARNING**
> **Many of these agents are highly toxic. Safety precautions should be strictly adhered to in the handling, dispensing and administration of these drugs (see later).**

Many cytotoxic drugs are also immunosuppressants, and drugs such as prednisolone and cyclophosphamide are used in the treatment of conditions such as immune-mediated haemolytic anaemia and thrombocytopenia.

Antiparasitic agents

Antiparasitic agents encompass anthelmintics, ectoparasiticides and antiprotozoal agents.

■ **Anthelmintics** are drugs that can be used to prevent or remove a parasitic worm infection from an animal. Most internal parasites (**endoparasites**) are worms (helminths).
■ **Ectoparasites** live on the surface of the animal and include fleas, ticks, mites and lice. Drugs used to kill ectoparasites are termed **ectoparasiticides**.
■ **Antiprotozoal** agents are used in the treatment of protozoal infections such as toxoplasmosis and giardiasis. Clindamycin may be used to reduce oocyst shedding in cats infected with *Toxoplasma gondii* as well as in the treatment of clinical signs due to this protozoan in both dogs and cats. A combination of a sulphonamide antibacterial and pyrimethamine has also been used in the treatment of toxoplasmosis. Metronidazole is effective in the treatment of giardiasis in cats; fenbendazole is used to treat giardiasis in cats and dogs. Giardiasis may also affect chinchillas, in which fenbendazole and to a lesser extent metronidazole may be used. The microsporidium protozoan *Encephalitozoon cuniculi* is often associated with neurological disease in rabbits, and control with a benzimidazole anthelmintic, such as fenbendazole, is indicated.

Anthelmintics

Figure 3.4 lists some of the anthelmintics commonly used to treat endoparasitic infections and provides information on their spectrum of activity.

Many anthelmintics have a broad spectrum of activity, with drugs such as fenbendazole being effective against all stages of the parasitic life cycle. Other drugs, such as piperazine, have little effect on the larval stages of the parasite and therefore have a much shorter duration of effect.

Anthelmintic	Tapeworms			Roundworms		
	Echinococcus	*Taenia*	*Dipylidium*	*Toxocara*	*Uncinaria*	*Trichuris*
Fenbendazole [a]		✓		✓	✓	✓
Pyrantel (not cats)				✓	✓	
Febantel (not cats)				✓	✓	✓
Piperazine				✓	✓	
Praziquantel	✓	✓	✓			
Nitroscanate (not cats)		✓	✓	✓	✓	
Milbemycin				✓		✓
Moxidectin				✓	✓	✓ dogs only
Selamectin				✓		
Emodepside				✓		

3.4 Anthelmintics commonly used to treat endoparasites (adult nematodes and cestodes) in the dog and cat (for full details relating to efficacy against larvae, refer to current data sheet information at www.noahcompendium.co.uk). For combination products that have effect on both ecto- and endoparasites, see Figure 3.6. [a] Fenbendazole is also used for the prevention or treatment of *Encephalitozoon cuniculi* infection in rabbits.

The control of certain endoparasitic infections is of importance from a public health point of view. Parasites such as *Echinococcus* and *Toxocara* can cause disease in humans (zoonoses) and in order to prevent this type of infection, anthelmintics are often used routinely to prevent infection in pets, thus reducing human exposure to these parasites. Tapeworms have an indirect life cycle with only the adult inhabiting the intestine of the dog or cat. This means that part of the development (larval stages) occurs in an intermediate host. In the case of *Dipylidium caninum*, the flea is the intermediate host. Therefore to control this parasite adequately, flea control should also be implemented. See Chapter 2 for further details on advice for clients.

Rabbits are commonly infected with the nematode *Passalurus ambiguus*, although its presence is often non-pathogenic, even with a significant worm burden. Fenbendazole may be used in the control of the pinworm in rabbits; piperazine is also effective. Praziquantel may also be used for cestode treatment in rabbits.

Ectoparasiticides

Control of ectoparasitic infestations is also of importance in domestic animals. These parasites not only produce discomfort and skin disease in the host animal, but they may also be responsible for the transmission of other diseases or parasites. For example, fleas act as an intermediate host for the tapeworm *Dipylidium*, which infests dogs and cats; lice, fleas and ticks are involved in the transmission of *Mycoplasma haemofelis*, an organism that causes haemolytic anaemia in cats.

Parasites may also infest and be responsible for skin lesions affecting in-contact humans. Along with UK-derived zoonoses, it is worth noting the increased vector risks associated with overseas travel, particularly pertinent since the introduction of Defra's Pet Travel Scheme (see Chapter 2). For example, dogs have the potential to carry leishmaniasis, carried by sandflies that are endemic to the Mediterranean region.

There is now a vast array of veterinary ecto-parasiticides. They can be broadly divided into those that act systemically and those that act topically. Figure 3.5 summarizes the main groups of drugs within these two categories. Imidacloprid is licensed for use in rabbits to control flea infestation, and lufenuron has also been used.

In the case of flea infestations, it is important not only to treat the animal, but also to treat the bedding and the environment. Some of the more novel preparations, such as fipronil, (s)-methoprene and lufenuron, contribute towards environmental control of the parasite by affecting egg laying and larval development. In addition there are separate products specifically designed to treat the environment, e.g. permethrin combined with cyromazine or pyriproxyfen.

Group	Example	Uses
Systemic (oral administration)		
Neonicotinoids	Nitenpyram	Fleas (adult)
Benzoyl urea derivatives	Lufenuron	Fleas (larval)

3.5 Ectoparasiticides commonly used in small animals. Many of these products have age restrictions regarding use in young animals. Also, there are species restrictions for different products. Always refer to data sheet prior to administration (see www.noahcompendium.co.uk for recent advances). (continues) ▶

Group	Example	Uses
Topical		
Amidines	Amitraz	*Sarcoptes, Demodex* in dogs (and *Cheyletiella* unlicensed use)
Phenylpyrazones	Fipronil	Fleas, ticks, *Trichodectes canis* and *Felicola subrostratus*. Fipronil may aid control of *Cheyletiella* and *Sarcoptes*, along with *Neotrombicula autumnalis*, which may affect ferrets as well (unlicensed)
Chloronictinyl nitroguanides	Imidacloprid	Fleas (dogs, cats and rabbits). When combined with permethrin, also effective against ticks and will repel sandflies and mosquitoes
Avermectins	Selamectin	Fleas, ear mites and heartworm prevention in dogs and cats. In addition, dogs benefit from protection against *Toxocara canis*, *Sarcoptes* and *Trichodectes canis*. Cats are covered for *Toxocara cati*, *Ancylostoma tubaeformae* and *Felicola subrostratus*
	Moxidectin	Ear mites and heartworm prevention in dogs and cats. In addition, dogs benefit from protection against *Demodex* and *Sarcoptes*, along with *Toxocara canis*, *Ancylostoma caninum*, *Uncinaria stenocephala*, *Toxascaris leonina* and *Trichuris vulpis*. Cats are covered against *Toxocara cati* and *Ancylostoma tubaeformae*
Pyriproxyfen	Pyriproxyfen	Fleas (eggs and larvae only)
Pyrethrins and synthetic pyrethroids	Permethrin	Fleas and ticks. When combined with imidacloprid, will repel sandflies and mosquitoes. Cats are very susceptible to permethrin toxicity; avoid accidental exposure by keeping cats away from treated dogs until the product is dry

3.5 (continued) Ectoparasiticides commonly used in small animals. Many of these products have age restrictions regarding use in young animals. Also, there are species restrictions for different products. Always refer to data sheet prior to administration (see www.noahcompendium.co.uk for recent advances).

Myiasis (fly strike) is a significant seasonal concern for rabbits and some other small pets. Infection by the bot fly or dipterids can escalate rapidly and the seriousness of such infestation should not be underestimated. Ivermectin may be used with care to kill the larvae, with antibiotics to treat secondary infection. Cyromazine does not repel flies but is an insect growth inhibitor which will prevent development of the *Lucilia sericata* larvae. It is licensed for use in rabbits.

Figure 3.6 shows commonly used combination products currently available for control of endoparasites and ectoparasites.

Anti-inflammatory agents

These are drugs that inhibit or reduce the formation of some of the mediators of inflammation and pain. The two main groups are:

- Corticosteroids
- Non-steroidal anti-inflammatory drugs (NSAIDs).

Both groups of agents are anti-inflammatory, **analgesic** (reduce pain) and **antipyretic** (reduce fever). For further information on analgesia, see Chapter 12. Use of these drugs in exotic and small pets such as rabbits is likely to be unlicensed. Meloxicam and carprofen are widely documented for 'off-label' use in rabbits.

There is also a group of nutraceuticals used as an adjunct to traditional therapy for musculoskeletal diseases, such as osteoarthritis. These include combinations of glucosamine and chondroitin supplements. Glucosamine is a sugar that helps production of new cartilage and is essential for joint maintenance. Chondroitin nourishes the joint, enabling it to remain spongy, which is essential to absorb shock and cushion the joint. Another nutraceutical worth noting is the extract from the green-lipped mussel *Perna canaliculis*, which provides a natural anti-inflammatory agent, in some cases at a potency equivalent to NSAIDs such as aspirin.

Trade name	Active ingredients	Uses
Drontal Plus	Praziquantel, pyrantel, febantel	Roundworms and tapeworms in dogs
Drontal Cat	Praziquantel, pyrantel	Roundworms and tapeworms in cats
Advocate	Imidacloprid, moxidectin	Fleas, ear mites, heartworm and intestinal nematodes in cats and dogs. *Sarcoptes* and *Demodex* in dogs
Profender	Emodepside, praziquantel	Roundworms and tapeworms in cats
Milbemax	Milbemycin, praziquantel	Roundworm, tapeworm and heartworm in dogs and cats
Advantix	Imidacloprid, permethrin	Fleas, ticks, sandflies and mosquitoes in dogs

3.6 Commonly used combination products for ecto- and endoparasites.

Corticosteroids

Corticosteroids are frequently used for the management of inflammatory disease, such as arthritis or chronic bronchitis. An example is prednisolone. They also have an important role as antineoplastic and immunosuppressive drugs, because in addition to reducing the formation of inflammatory mediators, they reduce the cellular and (to a lesser extent) the antibody responses, which often play an important role in these diseases. A corticosteroid such as prednisolone is often used as part of a drug protocol for the medical management of neoplasia, or of immune-mediated disease, such as autoimmune-mediated thrombocytopenia.

Associated side effects of corticosteroid use include prolonged recovery from illness and delayed wound healing. Systemic use is broadly contraindicated in patients with diabetes insipidus or renal disease; in such cases alternatives should be sought. On occasions, corticosteroids remain of use in treatment of musculo-skeletal diseases, particularly pain with acute onset.

NSAIDs

NSAIDs are also used for the management of acute and chronic inflammatory conditions. Examples of NSAIDs include carprofen, meloxicam, ketoprofen and tepoxalin. Like the corticosteroids, these drugs reduce the formation of inflammatory mediators. The most common side effect involves gastrointestinal ulceration. Other side effects include renal toxicity, hepatotoxicity and blood dyscrasias.

Cats are particularly susceptible to the toxic effects of paracetamol, due to a reduced ability to metabolize the drug. Its use should therefore be avoided in this species. Considering the number of licensed alternative products available for use in dogs, paracetamol is probably best avoided, as is ibuprofen.

Aspirin can also cause toxicity in cats, since the excretion of the drug is slow. Aspirin may still be used in cats for treatment of iliac thrombosis, provided dosing is closely monitored.

Antiepileptics

These drugs are used to control epileptic seizures (Figure 3.7).

Key points relating to the use of antiepileptic drugs are as follows.

- Start treatment if the seizures are more frequent than once every 6 weeks, or if they occur in clusters, or if status epilepticus occurs (i.e. repeated seizures with no conscious interval).
- Monitor for hepatotoxicity.
- Sudden withdrawal of antiepileptic drugs can lead to seizures or status epilepticus.
- Monitor plasma levels of the drug.
- Avoid the administration of drugs that lower the threshold for seizures to occur. For example, the sedative acepromazine will have this effect and should be avoided in animals with epilepsy.

Diuretics

This class of drugs acts to remove excess water from the body, through increased total urine output (diuresis). They are principally employed for use in patients with hypertension, or fluid retention associated with cardiac or renal disease.

There are several different types:

- Loop diuretics (e.g. furosemide), which inhibit reabsorption of chloride and sodium in the ascending loop of Henle
- Potassium-sparing diuretics (e.g. spironolactone), which are particularly useful where other diuretics have resulted in hypokalaemia
- Thiazide diuretics (e.g. hydrochlorothiazide)
- Osmotic diuretics (e.g. mannitol), which may be used in the treatment of glaucoma or cerebral oedema.

Vaccines and immunological preparations

Immunity can be active or passive. Further details on the different types of immunity can be found in Chapters 2 and 9.

Vaccines comprise antigenic material that is given to an animal in order to induce an immune response, usually against bacteria or viruses.

'**Live**' vaccines contain organisms that have been modified so as not to cause disease. They replicate in the body and stimulate the production of antibodies specific to the organism. These vaccines may be given systemically, or topically to generate immunity at the site. For example, 'kennel cough' vaccinations are administered intranasally, where they act on the

Use	Name of drug	Comments
Seizure control	Phenobarbital	Commonly used in canine epilepsy and can be used in cats
	Primidone	Used in dogs; start at low doses and gradually increase. Metabolized to phenobarbital
	Phenytoin	Contraindicated in cats; rapidly metabolized in dogs. Less commonly used
	Potassium bromide	Can be used as adjunct to therapy with phenobarbital where seizures are not controlled with phenobarbital alone
Treatment of status epilepticus	Diazepam	One of drugs of choice if given intravenously
	Propofol	Given under intravenous infusion, preferably with endotracheal tube placement, with constant monitoring

3.7   Examples of drugs used in control of epilepsy.

mucosa of the respiratory tract. However, it is possible that the organism may mutate after administration, reacquiring its pathogenicity.

'Killed' or 'inactivated' vaccines contain antigenic organisms to stimulate antigen production without replication. These types of vaccinations are generally safer in use, particularly if required during pregnancy. Genetic modification may be employed during manufacture of these types of vaccines. As an example: with inactivated rabies vaccines, strains of the virus are grown on cells originating from embryonic cells from hamsters. The virus is then inactivated by a chemical process and absorbed into an adjuvant. (**Adjuvants** are agents that, when added to a vaccine, enhance the immune response. Examples are aluminium hydroxide and aluminium phosphate.)

Other types of vaccine include **toxoids**, which are toxins, obtained from microorganisms, that have been modified so that they will still induce an immune response but are no longer harmful. Tetanus toxoid is the main example.

Figure 3.8 summarizes the vaccines routinely used in companion animals in the UK. All diseases listed are endemic in the UK apart from rabies.

Anaesthetics, sedatives and analgesics

These are described in Chapter 12.

Nutraceuticals

The term nutraceutical is a combination of 'nutritional' and 'pharmaceutical' and refers to foods that act as medicines, either alone or as an adjunct to traditional therapy. Those commonly encountered are glucosamine and chondroitin, and the green-lipped mussel extract (see Anti-inflammatory agents, above, and Figure 3.20).

Drugs categorized by the system on which they act

Cardiovascular system

Cardiac disease is very common in dogs and cats. Figures 3.9 and 3.10 summarize the drugs used in the management of cardiac disease.

Agent/disease	Species	Type of vaccine	Suggested regimen
Canine distemper virus	Dog (and ferret)	Live	Initial vaccine at 6 weeks of age; repeat 2–4 weeks later (at least 10 weeks of age)
Canine parvovirus	Dog	Live	Depends on vaccine used. Usually first dose at 10 weeks of age; then 2–4 weeks later
Infectious canine hepatitis	Dog	Live; inactivated also available	Initial as early as 8 weeks of age; repeat at 10–12 weeks
'Kennel cough'	Dog	*Bordetella bronchiseptica* live intranasal	From 3 weeks of age. Immunity lasts 6–12 months, depending on the brand used
		Parainfluenza virus live	Two vaccinations, 3–4 weeks apart; second at 10–12 weeks of age
Leptospirosis	Dog	Inactivated	From 8 weeks of age, two doses 2–6 weeks apart
Rabies	Dog and cat	Inactivated	May give first dose at 4 weeks of age; second dose must be given at 12 weeks. Antibody titres recommended to confirm sufficient immunity
Chlamydophila	Cat	Live	From 9 weeks of age, two doses 3–4 weeks apart. More often incorporated into flu and enteritis combinations
Feline panleucopenia (feline infectious enteritis)	Cat	Live or inactivated	From 9 weeks of age, two doses 2–4 weeks apart
Feline viral respiratory disease	Cat	Herpesvirus and calicivirus live or inactivated	From 9 weeks of age; second dose 2–4 weeks later
		Bordetella bronchiseptica live intranasal	One dose (from 8 weeks of age) at least 72 hours prior to risk of exposure (e.g. cattery). Immunity lasts up to 1 year
Feline leukaemia	Cat	Inactivated	From 9 weeks of age; second dose 2–3 weeks later
Myxomatosis	Rabbit	Live	From 6 weeks of age. Repeat every 6 months
Viral haemorrhagic disease	Rabbit	Inactivated	From 10–12 weeks of age (repeat dose after 1 month if <10 weeks at initial vaccination). Revaccinate every 12 months

3.8 Vaccines commonly used in small companion animals within the UK. Note: The regimens suggested here may vary depending on the particular vaccine used. Longevity of immunity with individual vaccinations (and manufacturers) is regularly under review; therefore it is pertinent to consult the relevant data sheets (see also www.noahcompendium.co.uk).

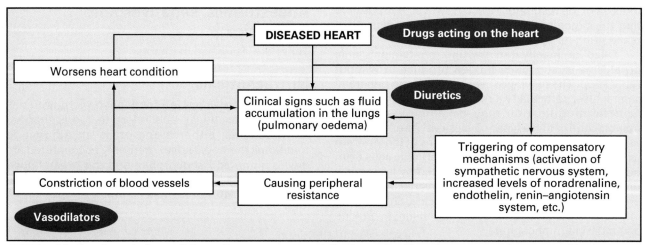

3.9 Mechanisms in heart failure. Drugs may: target the heart itself; reduce congestion caused by heart failure; or act directly on blood vessels. See also Figure 3.10.

Category	Drugs	Example	Effect
Acting on the heart	Cardiac glycoside	Digoxin	Increases force of the contraction and slows heart rate
	Antiarrhythmic	Lidocaine, mexiletine	Reduces or abolishes abnormal rhythms
	Calcium channel blockers	Diltiazem, amlodipine	Diltiazem is used in hypertrophic cardiomyopathy. Amlodipine is used to control hypertension in cats
	Calcium sensitizing drugs	Pimobendan	Indicated for management of congestive heart failure and myocardial contractility deficits
To reduce congestion and oedema formation	Diuretic	Furosemide, spironolactone	Increases water loss through kidneys
To dilate blood vessels	Arteriodilators	Hydralazine	Dilate the arteries
	Venodilators	Glyceryl trinitrate	Dilate the veins
	ACE inhibitors [a]	Enalapril, benazepril, imidapril, ramipril	Dilate both arteries and veins

3.10 Summary of main types of drugs used in the management of cardiac disease. The categories are not absolute; for example, venodilators will also help to reduce congestion and oedema formation. [a] Angiotensin-converting enzyme inhibitors block the formation of angiotensin in the kidney. This results in vasodilation, which promotes excretion of salts and water from the body and this reduces hypertension.

Respiratory system

Groups of drugs such as antibacterials, anti-inflammatories and antihistamines are used in the management of respiratory disease. In addition, certain groups of drugs are used specifically for their effects on the respiratory system and three of these may require definition.

■ In the presence of respiratory disease, the respiratory tract often becomes quite dry, with a reduction in volume and an increase in the viscosity of the secretions produced. This leads to a harsh dry non-productive cough. An **expectorant** increases the production of secretions, thus helping to alleviate the condition.

■ A **mucolytic** is a drug that breaks down the secretions, making them less viscous.
■ An **antitussive** is a cough suppressant.

Figure 3.11 lists the main categories of drugs used in the management of respiratory disease. A couple of additional points are worth making.

■ Antitussives should only be used when the coughing is such that it is causing discomfort and distress to the animal. These drugs should certainly be avoided in conditions such as bronchopneumonia, where inflammatory secretions are being produced.
■ The main indication for respiratory stimulants is to stimulate respiration in newborn animals.

Drug type	Examples	Action
Bronchodilators	Etamiphylline, theophylline	Dilate the airways
Expectorants	Ipecacuanha	Increase volume of secretions
Mucolytics	Bromohexine	Make secretions less viscous
Antitussives	Butorphanol	Suppress coughing
Stimulants	Doxopram	Act as central nervous system stimulant
Antibacterials	Cephalosporins	Against respiratory disease due to bacterial infection
Nasal decongestants	Pseudoephedrine	Constrict vessels in nose and help reduce congestion

3.11 Types of drugs used in conditions affecting the respiratory system.

Gastrointestinal system

Many of the drugs used in the management of gastrointestinal disease, such as antimicrobial agents and corticosteroids, may also be used for other conditions. Figure 3.12 lists a number of groups of therapeutic agents that are used more specifically for the management of gastrointestinal diseases.

Urinary system

Figure 3.13 summarizes some of the common conditions affecting the urinary bladder, together with examples of therapeutic strategies used to control or treat the conditions listed. A combination of drugs is often required to address both primary and secondary problems.

Drug category	Type	Example	Action
Emetics		Xylazine i.v., i.m. (may cause sedation) Apomorphine i.v., s.c. (works best subcutaneously) Washing soda orally Ipecacuanha orally	Induction of vomiting
Antiemetics		Metoclopramide, ondansetron, maropitant	Prevention of vomiting
Antidiarrhoeal agents	Adsorbent	Kaolin, charcoal, montmorillonite	Adsorbs toxins and coats the gut wall
	Agent that decreases gastrointestinal motility[a]	Loperamide, diphenoxylate	Reduces propulsive motility and increases segmental motility
Agents used in chronic diarrhoea	Anti-inflammatory	Prednisolone, sulfasalazine	
	Antibacterial	Metronidazole	Used for bacterial overgrowth and treatment of specific infections
Laxatives	Lubricant laxative	Liquid paraffin, linseed oil	Softens and lubricates faecal mass
	Bulk-forming laxative	Bran, sterculia	Increases faecal bulk and promotes peristalsis
	Osmotic laxative	Lactulose, magnesium sulphate	Increases water in bowel and induces peristalsis
	Stimulant laxative	Bisacodyl	Promotes colonic peristalsis
Antacids		Aluminium hydroxide	Neutralizes gastric acid
	H$_2$ receptor antagonist	Cimetidine, ranitidine	Blocks gastric acid secretion
	Proton pump inhibitor	Omeprazole	Blocks gastric acid secretion
	Prostaglandin E1 analogue	Misoprostil	Inhibits gastric acid secretion
Gastroprotectants	Sucralfate	Sucralfate	Protects ulcer site
Prokinetics		Metoclopramide	Promotes gastric emptying and gut motility Useful in rabbits

3.12 Drugs used in the management of gastrointestinal disease. [a] Drugs that reduce motility are sometimes contraindicated in diarrhoea, since hypomotility rather than hypermotility may be a feature in some cases. Also, if invasive organisms are involved, reducing motility will only further decrease the rate of expulsion of the pathogens.

Condition	Treatment	
	Drug	**Action/comments**
Cystitis	Antibacterials, e.g. amoxicillin, cefalexin Acidifiers, e.g. ammonium chloride, methionine Alkalinizers, e.g. sodium bicarbonate, allopurinol	Acidification or alkalinization may improve the action of certain antibiotics. For example, penicillin is more efficacious in an acidic environment, while sulfadiazine is more efficacious in an alkaline environment
	Glycosaminoglycosan	Lines bladder wall so that it is less likely to become irritated Used for maintenance after crystalluria
Urinary retention due to paralysis of detrusor muscle	Phenoxybenzamine	Blocks receptors on the bladder neck and sphincter, allowing it to relax for urination
Urinary retention due to excessive urethral sphincter tone	Bethanecol	A parasympathomimetic drug; stimulates receptors in the detrusor muscle causing it to contract
Urinary incontinence due to detrusor muscle instability (not common)	Propantheline	A parasympatholytic drug; blocks receptors in the detrusor muscle reducing contraction
Urinary incontinence due to lack of urethral sphincter tone	Phenylpropanolamine	Stimulates receptors of the sphincter, increasing tone and reducing urine leakage
	Estriol	Short-acting synthetic oestrogen; increases tone in lower urinary tract and is indicated for urinary incompetence in spayed bitches

3.13 Common conditions affecting the urinary bladder and examples of therapeutic strategies.

Chronic renal failure

Benazepril is the primary treatment of choice for management of chronic renal insufficiency in cats. Benazepril is an ACE inhibitor, preventing the conversion of angiotensin I to angiotensin II. It therefore serves to alleviate hypertension, along with reducing protein loss in the urine.

Additional treatment is largely palliative and is aimed at reducing the associated secondary changes. It includes:

■ Fluid therapy
■ Diet low in protein of high biological value

■ Treatment such as aluminium hydroxide to lower blood phosphate levels
■ Use of recombinant human erythropoietin to treat anaemia.

Endocrine system

Endocrine disorders are generally characterized by under- or over-production of a variety of hormones. Figure 3.14 summarizes the more frequently encountered endocrine disorders of the dog and cat, listing some of the drugs commonly used in the medical management of these conditions. Periodic

Gland	Endocrine disorder	Medical treatment / management
Thyroid	Hypothyroidism – most common endocrine disorder in dog; due to underactivity of thyroid gland	Liothyronine, levothyroxine
	Hyperthyroidism – mainly elderly cats, due to overproduction of thyroid hormones	Methimazole, carbimazole, radioactive iodine
Adrenal gland	Cushing's disease (hyperadrenocorticism) – overproduction of adrenal glucocorticoids	Trilostane, mitotane
	Addison's disease (hypoadrenocorticism) – underproduction of mineralocorticoids and glucocorticoids	Fludrocortisone acetate. Prednisolone required initially or desoxycorticosterone pivalate (DOCP)
Pancreas	Insulin-dependent diabetes mellitus – reduced insulin production	Insulin: types include bovine, porcine and human
	Type 2 non-insulin-dependent diabetes	Glipizide
Pituitary gland	Central diabetes insipidus – underproduction of antidiuretic hormone (ADH) by the pituitary gland (ADH increases reabsorption of water by the kidney)	Desmopressin
	Nephrogenic diabetes insipidus – kidney is resistant to effects of ADH	Hydrochlorothiazide

3.14 Most frequently encountered endocrine disorders of the dog and cat, with examples of drugs used in medical management.

monitoring of drug levels in the blood is necessary to allow accurate dosing and adjustments to be made accordingly.

Reproductive system

Examples of drugs used to manipulate the reproductive system are listed in Figure 3.15. Reasons for use in females may include:

- Prevention or suppression of oestrus
- Prevention of pregnancy following mating
- Abolition of pseudopregnancy and milk production
- Stimulation or suppression of parturition.

In males, reasons for use may include:

- Management of male behavioural traits
- Management of conditions such as prostatic hypertrophy.

> **WARNING**
> Care should be exercised at all times in the handling of hormonal substances. Gloves should be worn. Some hormonal preparations should not be handled by pregnant women or by asthmatics.

The eye

A wide range of conditions may affect the eye, either primarily or as part of a more generalized disease. Many of the drugs are applied directly on to the surface of the eye in formulations designed specifically for this purpose. In addition, drugs may be injected into the subconjunctival region or administered systemically. Figure 3.16 lists some of the more frequently used ocular preparations, together with their actions and some of the situations in which they may be employed.

Drugs	Action/classification	Uses
Cabergoline	Stimulates dopamine receptors in anterior pituitary, which inhibits release of prolactin. Prolactin controls milk production and maintains pregnancy from day 35	Pseudopregnancy in the bitch
Estradiol benzoate	Oestrogenic effect, prevents implantation	Misalliance: used to prevent pregnancy in the bitch. Administered on 3rd and 5th days following mating. A third injection may be given on the 7th day. **Do not use in cats**
Medroxyprogesterone acetate Megestrol acetate Progesterone Proligestone	Progesterone-like activity	Prevention or suppression of oestrus in the bitch. Prevention of oestrus in the queen. Proligestone is used to prevent prolonged oestrus in the jill ferret
Methyltestosterone Testosterone esters	Androgens	Suppression of oestrus and pseudopregnancy in the bitch. Also used in male dogs and cats for deficient libido
Aglepristone	Antiprogestogenic	Misalliance and termination of pregnancy up to day 45. Given twice, 48 hours apart
Delmadinone acetate	Progesterone-like activity, acts as antiandrogen	Prostatic hypertrophy, prostatic carcinoma and perianal gland tumours in male dogs. Management of male aggression and hypersexuality in male cats and dogs
Oxytocin	Normally secreted by the posterior pituitary; causes uterine contraction and stimulates milk letdown	Promotion of milk letdown after parturition in the bitch and queen. Treatment of uterine inertia (lack of uterine contraction) in the bitch and queen
Vetrabutine	Inhibits oxytocin-induced contraction of the uterus	Used to delay parturition in the bitch. **Do not use in cats**

3.15 Examples of drugs that have an effect on the reproductive system, with some indications.

Type of drug	Examples	Uses
Antimicrobial	Chloramphenicol, chlortetracycline, gentamicin, fusidic acid	Bacterial infections
Anti-inflammatory	Corticosteroids, e.g. betamethasone	Inflammatory conditions such as uveitis. Do not use where there is corneal ulceration

3.16 Drugs used for treatment of conditions affecting the eye. (continues) ▶

Type of drug	Examples	Uses
Immune-modulating	Ciclosporin	Immune-mediated disease such as plasmacytic conjunctivitis of the third eyelid and keratoconjunctivitis sicca
Mydriatics (dilate pupil) Cycloplegics (reduce spasm of ciliary muscle)	Atropine sulphate, cyclopentolate, phenylephrine, tropicamide	Anterior uveitis Pupillary dilation for examination or ocular surgery
Miotics (constrict pupil)	Pilocarpine	Glaucoma
Drugs that decrease formation of aqueous humour	Acetazolamide, timolol maleate	Glaucoma
Tear replacement preparations	Hypromellose, polyvinyl alcohol	Keratoconjunctivitis sicca
Diagnostic stains	Fluorescein, Rose Bengal	Diagnosis of corneal ulcers
Local anaesthetics	Proxymetacaine, tetracaine	Minor surgical procedures

3.16 (continued) Drugs used for treatment of conditions affecting the eye.

The integument

Figure 3.17 summarizes the types of agent used in the treatment and control of skin disease.

Treatment of skin disease may be achieved by either systemic or topical administration of drugs.

- **Topical** application allows direct delivery of the drug to the affected site with minimal systemic effects. Topical treatment may be formulated as shampoos, sprays, powders, ointments, lotions, gels or creams. The formulation is important as it may aid in the penetration of the active ingredient to the skin.
- A **systemic** approach may be more appropriate if the condition is affecting the deeper layers of the skin or if the disease is widespread.

Treatment should aim to:

- Alleviate clinical signs
- Treat the underlying cause.

While the symptomatic approach is quite straightforward, the aetiology of the skin disease is often difficult to ascertain, or it may not be possible to prevent exposure of the animal even if the cause is identified. For example, many dogs suffer from allergic skin disease associated with allergens such as housedust mite and fleas. Flea control may be relatively straightforward to implement but exposure to housedust mite is unavoidable, though vacuuming may reduce levels of the mite.

Type of drug	Route of administration	Examples	Uses
Corticosteroids	Systemic	Prednisolone, methylprednisolone	Control of immune-mediated and inflammatory skin disease
	Topical	Betamethasone	
Antihistamines	Systemic	Diphenhydramine, promethazine, chlorpheniramine	Allergic skin disease
Antibacterials	Topical	Neomycin	Pyoderma
	Systemic	Cefalexin	
Sunscreens	Topical	Titanium dioxide, butyl methoxydibenzoylmethane	Prevention of sunburn and sun exposure, which can be associated with squamous cell carcinoma (white cats' ear tips)
Essential fatty acids	Systemic	Evening primrose oil	Coat condition and allergic skin disease
Antifungal agents	Systemic	Griseofulvin, itraconazole	Treatment of ringworm and *Malassezia pachydermatis* infection
	Topical	Clotrimazole, miconazole	
Ectoparasiticides	Systemic	Lufenuron	Flea control
	Topical	Fipronil, selamectin	Flea control (and other parasites; see above)

3.17 Drugs used in the treatment and control of conditions affecting the skin. (continues) ▶

Type of drug	Route of administration	Examples	Uses
Keratolytic agents (promote loosening of the horny layer of the epidermis)	Topical	Benzoyl peroxide	Pyoderma, seborrhoea
Hormonal agents	Systemic	Melatonin	Available as subcutaneous implant and may be used to manage recurrent flank alopecia, pattern alopecia and alopecia X in dogs
Immune-modulating	Systemic	Ciclosporin	Chronic atopic dermatitis in dogs

3.17 (continued) Drugs used in the treatment and control of conditions affecting the skin.

Ears

The different types of drug used in the treatment of otitis (inflammation of the ear) are summarized in Figure 3.18. Ear disease may occur as part of a generalized skin condition, or may be present in isolation. In addition to topical treatment of otitis, systemic administration of drugs such as corticosteroids and antibacterials may be necessary.

> **WARNING**
> Many of the agents used topically can penetrate the skin of the operator as well as that of the animal. In particular, care should be taken with the application of topical corticosteroids. Disposable gloves should always be worn when applying these agents. Gloves (preferably latex-free) should be dispensed to owners, along with the drug.

Musculoskeletal system

There are three main categories of drugs employed in managing diseases of the musculoskeletal system.

- **Non-steroidal anti-inflammatory drugs (NSAIDs)** (Figure 3.19) are widely incorporated into treatment regimens for alleviation of pain associated with muscular and joint disease, both chronic and acute.
- **Corticosteroids** (Figure 3.19) have long been used in the management of pain, though their use in practice has somewhat declined in favour of NSAIDs.
- **Nutraceuticals** are a more recent and holistic approach to pain management in musculoskeletal disease. These natural supplements can aid conventional therapy and help to alleviate symptoms. Figure 3.20 lists the commonly used derivatives. Nutraceuticals are often used as an adjunct to prescribed medicines.

Condition	Type of agent	Examples
Otodectes (ear mites)	Ectoparasiticide	Selamectin, moxidectin
Bacterial infection	Antibacterial	Neomycin, gentamicin, framycetin
Fungal infection	Antifungal	Miconazole, nystatin
Inflammation	Anti-inflammatory	Prednisolone, betamethasone

3.18 Examples of drugs used to treat otitis externa. Some ear preparations contain no identified ectoparasiticide but are still effective against ear mites. Many ear preparations contain a combination of drugs, e.g. they may contain an ectoparasiticide, an antibacterial, an antifungal and an anti-inflammatory drug.

Drug	Action and indications
Non-steroidal anti-inflammatory agents	
Carprofen	Preferentially inhibits COX-2 pathway, leading to limited production of inflammatory prostaglandins. Limited COX-1 inhibition. Indicated for mild to moderate pain
Meloxicam	Preferentially inhibits COX-2 pathway, leading to limited production of inflammatory prostaglandins. Limited COX-1 inhibition. Indicated for mild to moderate pain. Effect is improved by pre-emptive administration
Ketoprofen	Dual inhibitor of COX-1 and LOX. For control of mild to moderate pain
Tepoxalin	Inhibits COX and LOX. Indicated for control of pain and inflammation associated with canine osteoarthritis

3.19 Anti-inflammatory agents commonly used in musculoskeletal disease. COX = cyclooxygenase; LOX = lipoxygenase. Both are enzymes in inflammatory pathways, and their inhibition can result in a reduction in pain and inflammation. Selective inhibition is preferable since it limits negative effects on organs such as the gastrointestinal tract and kidney. (continues) ▶

Drug	Action and indications
Corticosteroids	
Prednisolone	A synthetic corticosteroid used for its anti-inflammatory properties. Can be used for treatment of osteoarthritis when combined with cinchophen
Dexamethasone	Strong anti-inflammatory properties, far greater than those of prednisolone

3.19 (continued) Anti-inflammatory agents commonly used in musculoskeletal disease.

Supplement	Nature and action
Glucosamine	A sugar substance synthesized in the body that is a component of proteoglycan, which forms cartilage. Helps to produce and maintain healthy cartilage
Chondroitin	Nourishes the joint, enabling it to remain spongy, enabling effective shock absorption and cushioning. Commonly used in combination products with glucosamine
Green-lipped mussel extract (*Perna canaliculus*)	A natural anti-inflammatory which some claim may have potency equivalent to some prescribed NSAIDs

3.20 Nutraceuticals used in musculoskeletal disease.

For further details, see the relevant section of 'Drugs classified by mode of action', above. For up-to-date information on licensing, refer to www.noahcompendium.co.uk

Nervous system

A number of groups of drugs affect the nervous system, including:

- Antiepileptics
- Steroids
- NSAIDs
- Antiparasiticides
- Antibiotics (cell-wall penetrating).

These drugs are discussed earlier in the chapter.

Administration and formulation of drugs

In order for a drug to have the desired effect, several criteria must be fulfilled:

- The drug must reach the site at which it is to act
- It must be present at the appropriate concentration
- The appropriate concentration must be present for a sufficient length of time.

In order to understand how this may be achieved, it is important to have some concept of the fate of a drug after it has been administered to the animal. Figure 3.21 illustrates the main steps involved in the disposition of drugs after administration.

- **Absorption** involves the movement of the drug from the site of administration into the plasma. By definition, drugs administered intravenously

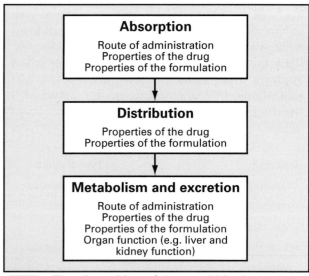

3.21 The disposition of drugs within the body. Above are the three main steps in drug disposition. Listed under each are some of the most important factors that influence drug disposition. Both metabolic rate and environmental temperature may also affect the disposition of drugs in the body. This is an important consideration, especially in ectotherms, e.g. reptiles.

bypass the absorption stage. Local blood flow at the site of administration can have an important effect on the rate of absorption. Some drugs can be formulated as 'depot' preparations. This means that there is a more prolonged release of drug from the site, decreasing the frequency of administration required. A good example of this would be a depot preparation of procaine penicillin, which is slowly released. Some drugs may be enteric-coated to prevent premature digestion by gastric acid.

- **Distribution** is important, as it determines whether the drug reaches the target tissue or not. Some drugs are distributed widely throughout the body and will enter most tissues, while others have a more limited pattern of distribution.
- **Metabolism** involves alteration of the drug in some way. It is generally associated with inactivation of the drug but there are exceptions to this. The liver is the main organ involved in drug metabolism and liver dysfunction can reduce the body's ability to deal with certain drugs. The metabolic rate or ambient temperature of some exotic pets may result in a change in rate of metabolism of the drug and thus a need to alter dosage or frequency of administration accordingly.
- **Excretion** can occur through a variety of routes, such as the kidney, the gastrointestinal tract and the respiratory system. The presence of renal disease, for example, may reduce the ability of the body to excrete certain drugs. In birds and reptiles the presence of a renal portal system means that drugs injected into the caudal part of the body may be rapidly excreted or may reach the kidneys at potentially nephrotoxic concentrations (e.g. aminoglycosides such as gentamicin).

> **WARNING**
> **Administration of medicines to exotic and common small pets needs careful consideration. Many drugs are not licensed for use in these species. Further caution should be exercised in dosing, as very small quantities may be required for clinical effect.**

As shown in Figure 3.21, two important factors that influence the fate of the drug within the body are:

- The site or route of administration
- The formulation of the drug.

These two factors go hand in hand, in that in general drugs are formulated in a specific way in order to facilitate their administration by a particular route.

Routes of administration

Techniques of drug administration are illustrated in Chapter 5.

Oral administration

This route is commonly used in veterinary practice. Factors that can influence gastrointestinal absorption include gastrointestinal motility, splanchnic blood flow, and particle size and formulation of the drug.

There are several potential problems with the oral route.

- The drug may be inactivated by gastric acid or gastrointestinal enzymes. In such cases an enteric-coated preparation should be used, or an alternative route should be considered. For example, S-adenosylmethionine (SAMe), a stabilized salt, is enteric-coated. This prevents gastric acid digesting SAMe, thus enabling effective absorption through the duodenum.
- The drug may not be absorbed from the gastrointestinal tract. In some instances this may be desirable. For example, some of the sulphonamide antibacterials are designed to remain in the gastrointestinal tract so that they have a local effect in the gut.
- Drugs may be absorbed and undergo rapid metabolism and hence inactivation by the liver (known as first-pass metabolism). This can preclude the oral administration of certain drugs. An example is glyceryl trinitrate, which is administered transdermally to avoid this effect.
- The drug may interact with certain food components. For example, the tetracycline antibiotics bind to calcium-rich foods, hindering absorption. Some drugs should specifically be given with food (e.g. griseofulvin) or after fasting (e.g. ampicillin).

Formulation of oral preparations

Drugs for oral use are given as tablets, capsules or liquids (either solutions or suspensions).

Tablets may or may not be coated. Reasons for enteric-coating a tablet may include:

- Improving the palatability
- Protection from the atmosphere
- Protection from gastric acidity
- Reducing the rate of disintegration of the tablet in the gastrointestinal tract.

Capsules comprise a hard gelatin case (generally two halves slotted together) containing the drug in granules or powder form. The capsule may contain a mixture of fast- and slow-release particles to produce a more sustained release of the drug and hence decrease the frequency of dosing required. Capsules should be given whole to the animal, unless specified otherwise by the manufacturer.

Liquids may contain the drug either in solution (the drug is dissolved in the liquid) or in suspension (the drug particles are suspended in the liquid, and often settle to the bottom if left standing). Prior to use, suspensions must always be well shaken to re-suspend the drug particles.

More recently, rapidly dissolving oral tablets have been developed, whereby contact with the mucosal surface of the mouth melts the tablet. Their intention is to improve ease of administration, and subsequently adherence to the prescriptive regimen for clients at home. An example would be tepoxalin, an NSAID indicated for musculoskeletal pain in dogs.

Oral administration in small pets

Oral administration in rabbits and other small pets may pose difficulties. Tablets are difficult to administer and thus suspensions are preferable. It has been suggested that some rodents (e.g. chinchillas) may voluntarily eat tablets hidden in raisins.

If the drug is only available in tablet form, as is often the case for exotics, it may be necessary to prepare a suspension, mixing the drug with water or another substance (e.g. baby cereal) to ease administration. Orogastric tubes may also be employed in this circumstance and are of particular use in tortoises and other reptiles.

Parenteral administration

Parenteral (or non-enteral, i.e. not via the gastrointestinal tract) administration implies injection of the drug. Examples of reasons why drugs may be injected rather than given orally include the following:

- The drug may not be well absorbed by the oral route
- The drug may be inactivated by gastric secretions
- Injection may achieve more rapid and reliable therapeutic levels of the drug.

WARNINGS
- **All solutions, needles and syringes used for injection must be sterile and pathogen-free.**
- **Aseptic precautions should be observed at all times.**
- **Drugs should not be mixed in the same syringe as they may react with one another, having a detrimental effect.**

Drugs may be injected into the following sites:

- Subcutaneous (s.c.)
- Intramuscular (i.m.)
- Intravenous (i.v.)
- Intradermal
- Intrathecal
- Subconjunctival
- Intraperitoneal (i.p.).

Subcutaneous and intramuscular injection

The main determinant of absorption of drugs administered subcutaneously or intramuscularly is local blood flow. Subcutaneous injections are administered in areas where the skin is loose (mainly the scruff of the neck). The plunger of the syringe should always be drawn back before injecting, to ensure that the needle is not located within a blood vessel.

Intramuscular injections are generally more painful. The main site for intramuscular injection is the muscle mass of the hindlimb. Care should be taken to avoid the sciatic nerve in this region.

When using either of these routes, due consideration should be paid to the volume being administered at one site, particularly in small pets. Where there is a choice it is preferable to use smaller volumes over several sites, to reduce the incidence of discomfort.

Intravenous injection

This is the fastest route for drug distribution, bypassing absorption. Intravenous administration requires the drug to be in solution, as particles in suspension may obstruct small vessels. Intravenous injection should be carried out slowly. Rapid injection of a drug bolus may cause adverse reactions, such as collapse. Drugs administered intravenously include some antimicrobials, diuretics and intravenous anaesthetics.

The cephalic vein in the forelimb, the saphenous vein in the hindlimb and the jugular vein in the neck are examples of vessels used for intravenous injection of drugs. In rabbits, the marginal ear veins may be employed, and the use of topical anaesthetic will minimize the jerk reaction often demonstrated on insertion of the needle or cannula.

Some drugs are so irritant that they may *only* be administered intravenously, such as the antitumour antibiotic doxorubicin and the intravenous anaesthetic thiopental. Extravascular injection of these substances can lead to severe tissue necrosis and sloughing of the skin overlying the site of injection.

Intradermal injection

This is used for intradermal skin testing: a panel of allergens is injected intradermally to determine the cause of allergic skin disease. More commonly encountered, the vaccine to guard against myxomatosis in rabbits is in part administered intradermally, usually in the skin on the dorsal aspect of the ear base.

Intrathecal injection

This is injection of a drug into the subarachnoid space. It is rarely used in veterinary practice.

Epidural injection

An epidural injection is used to administer drugs into the epidural space around the spinal cord. In practice this may be a route of administration for anaesthetic and analgesic drugs (see Chapter 12).

Intraperitoneal injection

This may be useful in small animals (e.g. rodents and feline neonates) for the administration of fluids or anaesthetic agents. The peritoneum provides a large surface in the abdominal cavity for the absorption of the drug, where generous blood supply facilitates rapid absorption. It is possible to administer up to 10 ml i.p. to rats and up to 4 ml i.p. to hamsters.

Rectal administration

Rectal administration of drugs is not frequently used, although rectal diazepam may be employed in immediate treatment of epileptic seizures in dogs.

Inhalation of drugs

This is the route of administration of volatile and gaseous anaesthetics such as isoflurane and nitrous oxide (see Chapter 12). Drugs used in the treatment of respiratory conditions may also be administered by this route. For example, the antimicrobial gentamicin may be administered by nebulization to dogs with bronchopneumonia, in addition to the administration of systemic antimicrobials. Whilst inhalation is intended to provide action of the drug in the respiratory tract proper, intranasal drugs (e.g. the kennel cough vaccines) aim to act on the nasal mucosa.

Transdermal administration

Drugs may be applied to the skin in order to produce a systemic effect. This can be useful to avoid first-pass metabolism by the liver (seen with some drugs on oral administration). The vasodilator glyceryl trinitrate is administered this way. Fentanyl (an opioid agonist) is also available in patches for treatment of prolonged pain associated with surgery or neoplasia.

Topical administration

In this case the drug is applied directly to the area where it is required. This is suitable for administration of drugs to a number of sites, such as the skin, the ear and the eye. Topical administration of a drug may avoid undesirable systemic effects, though in some cases drugs applied topically can be absorbed to give significant systemic levels. This tends to be the case with drugs that have good lipid solubility (fat solubility), which enables them to cross the barriers of the skin and conjunctiva (e.g. the topical administration of corticosteroids to the eye or ear). Figure 3.22 lists the different types of formulation used for topically administered drugs.

Formulation	Description
Creams	Water-miscible, non-greasy and easily removed by washing and licking
Ointments	Greasy, insoluble in water and generally anhydrous; more difficult to remove than creams
Dusting powders	Finely divided powders (care should be taken not to inhale these)
Lotions	Aqueous solutions or suspension; evaporate to leave thin film of drug at the site
Gels	Aqueous solutions that are semi-solid; easy to apply and remove
Sprays	Liquid solutions that may be applied by pressurized or pump-action means, resulting in fine mist (care should be taken not to inhale)
Shampoos	Liquid solutions used to clean hair and underlying skin

3.22 Drug formulations used for topical administration.

Calculation of drug doses

> **WARNING**
> Currently the ultimate responsibility for the calculation of doses lies with the veterinary surgeon. Nurses given the responsibility for calculation of doses should always check with the veterinary surgeon responsible for the case.

Most doses are described in terms of weight, and the recommended dose for an animal is generally expressed in terms of the weight of drug per unit of bodyweight of the animal (e.g. mg/kg). Alternatively, the dose may be expressed in terms of weight of drug per unit of body surface area (usually per square metre, e.g. mg/m^2). This is the case for digoxin and some of the drugs used in the chemotherapy of malignant disease. Conversion charts are available allowing the conversion of bodyweight into body surface area (see the *BSAVA Small Animal Formulary*).

Units of weight

The main units of weight are: kilogram (kg); gram (g); milligram (mg); and microgram. Microgram can be abbreviated to mcg or µg but in longhand it may be difficult to distinguish mg and µg. Therefore it is wiser not to abbreviate in this instance.

1 kg = 1000 g
1 g = 1000 mg
1 mg = 1000 micrograms

- Drugs in **tablet** and **capsule** form state the weight of the active drug contained in each tablet or capsule. A particular drug may come in a variety of different strengths.
- Drugs in **liquid** form contain the weight of drug per unit volume of liquid, e.g. the number of milligrams per millilitre (mg/ml), where 1 litre (1 l) = 1000 ml.
- The concentration of drugs in liquid form may also be expressed as percentage solutions. For example, a 1% solution means that there is 1 g of drug in 100 ml of the solution.
- There are some exceptions to these formats. For example, insulin is expressed in international units/ml (IU/ml). Insulin is administered in dedicated syringes that are graduated in international units rather than millilitres. They are available in 100 IU, 50 IU and 40 IU sizes, for human and animal use.

>
> **WARNING**
> Care should be taken when dosing with insulin. For animal use only, 'Caninsulin' doses are to be administered solely from 40 IU/ml syringes, rather than the standard 100 IU/ml.

Examples of how to calculate drug doses are given below. For further information on the calculation of infusion rates, see Chapter 8.

Drug dose calculation: Example 1

A 27 kg Labrador requires treatment with clindamycin for 7 days. The recommended dose rate is 5.5 mg/kg twice daily. The capsules come in strengths of 25 mg, 75 mg and 150 mg. Calculate the daily dose of clindamycin for this dog.

5.5 mg/kg (dose rate) x 27 kg (bodyweight of dog) = 148.5 mg twice daily ▶

Which strength capsule would you use?

The 150 mg size. The dog would require one capsule twice a day.

How many capsules should be dispensed to the owner?

1 capsule twice daily = 2 capsules per day x 7 days = 14 capsules required in total.

Drug dose calculation: Example 2

A 4 kg cat requires treatment with ketoprofen. The recommended dose for injection is 2 mg/kg daily. There is a 1% solution of ketoprofen for injection. Calculate a dose for this animal.

A 1% solution contains 1 g/100 ml, or 10 mg/ml. The dose required by the cat will be:

2 mg/kg (dose rate) x 4 kg (body weight) = 8 mg

The volume for injection will be the total required dose divided by the concentration:

8 mg (dose) ÷ 10 mg/ml (concentration) = 0.8 ml of the 1% solution

Drug dose calculation: Example 3

A 10 kg Lhasa Apso has developed a heart rhythm abnormality after abdominal surgery. A bolus injection of lidocaine intravenously has abolished the rhythm but the dog now needs to be maintained on a constant-rate infusion of the drug at a rate of 50 micrograms/kg/minute given in intravenous fluids. The fluids in a 1 litre bag are to be given at a rate of 10 ml/kg/hour. How much lidocaine needs to be added to the bag to give the drug at a rate of 50 micrograms/kg/minute?

As both the rate of fluid administration and the rate of drug administration required are known, it is easier to express them both in the same units of time:

Drug administration:

50 micrograms x 10 kg (weight of dog) = 500 micrograms/minute

This equals 500 x 60 = 30,000 micrograms/hour = 30 mg of lidocaine per hour.

Fluid administration:

At a rate of 10 ml/kg/hour = 100 ml per hour for a 10 kg dog. ▶

Therefore there needs to be 30 mg of lidocaine in every 100 ml of fluid. In a 1 litre bag there is 10 x 100 ml, so it needs 10 x 30 mg of lidocaine. The 300 mg of lidocaine is added to the 1 litre bag of fluids, which will give an infusion rate of 50 micrograms/kg/minute if the fluids are administered at a rate of 10 ml/kg/hour.

Legislation

In veterinary practice, legislation governs the handling, usage, storage, prescribing and administration of veterinary medicines. Veterinary surgeons and nurses working within veterinary practice must be aware of the legislation: it has been set in place to protect the animal, the practitioner, the nurse and the client.

Legislation is constantly changing; indeed, at the time of writing this chapter, significant changes were taking place in the legislation governing veterinary medicines in the UK. The Medicines Act 1968 and the Medicines (Restrictions on the Administration of Veterinary Medicinal Products) Regulations 1994 were superseded by the Veterinary Medicines Regulations 2005, from 30 October 2005. At this time, therefore, the relevant legislation governing these areas includes the following:

- Veterinary Medicines Regulations 2005
- Health and Safety at Work etc. Act 1974
- Control of Substances Hazardous to Health Regulations 2002 (enacted under the Health and Safety at Work etc. Act 1974)
- Misuse of Drugs Act 1971 (Modification) Order 2001

The Veterinary Medicines Directorate website is a useful source of information on current drug legislation and provides excellent links to other informative and relevant sites. The address is www.vmd.gov.uk

Classification of veterinary medicines

A 'veterinary medicine' can be defined as any substance or combination of substances presented as having properties for treating or preventing disease in animals, or any substance or combination of substances that may be used in or administered to animals with a view either to restoring, correcting or modifying physiological functions by exerting a pharmacological, immunological or metabolic action or to making a medical diagnosis.

Under the recent legislation there are some changes to the way in which veterinary medicines are classified. The current categories are as follows:

- Prescription Only Medicine – Veterinarian (POM–V)
- Prescription Only Medicine – Veterinarian, Pharmacist, Suitably Qualified Person (POM–VPS)
- Non-Food Animal – Veterinarian, Pharmacist, Suitably Qualified Person (NFA–VPS)
- Authorised Veterinary Medicine – General Sales List (AVM–GSL).

POM–V

POM–Vs can only be prescribed by veterinary surgeons for administration to animals under their care, i.e. following clinical assessment. They may also be supplied by a pharmacist or another registered veterinary surgeon, but only on production of a written prescription from the animal's own veterinary surgeon. This category corresponds closely with the former POM category (Prescription Only Medicine).

POM–VPS

A clinical assessment is not necessarily required prior to prescription of a POM–VPS. This category corresponds closely to the former PML (Pharmacy Merchants List) group of medicines.

Medicines in this category can only be prescribed by a registered qualified person (RQP). An RQP is defined as a:

- Registered Veterinary Surgeon
- Registered Pharmacist
- Registered Suitably Qualified Person (SQP). Veterinary nurses can become SQPs. SQP training modules are being incorporated into some nurse training modules. Established nurses, or nurses whose training did not include this module, may complete an additional training module to achieve SQP status.

The client may request a written prescription from the RQP and this prescription may be issued by any other RQP.

NFA–VPS

This category corresponds to medicinal products on the former PML list, for non-food producing animals. As with POM–VPM, a clinical assessment is not a prerequisite but only a registered qualified person may prescribe medicines in this category. This would be a:

- Registered Veterinary Surgeon
- Registered Pharmacist
- Registered Suitably Qualified Person.

AVM–GSL

Medicinal products under this category may be supplied by any retailer (including supermarkets and pet shops) with no restrictions on supply. Moreover, they may be supplied by personnel other than veterinary surgeons.

This category corresponds closely to the former GSL (General Sales List). Products in this category have a wide safety margin, and tend to be used to alleviate or prevent clinical signs of common ailments, such as diarrhoea or worm burden.

Controlled drugs (CD)

These are drugs that might be abused, and they are controlled under the Misuse of Drugs Act 1971 (modification) order 2001. Controlled drugs are divided into five Schedules, in decreasing order of severity.

- **Schedule 1.** Veterinary surgeons have no reason or authority to possess or prescribe these drugs. This category includes LSD and cannabis. Essentially, they are not used medicinally.
- **Schedule 2.** Examples in this group include fentanyl and morphine. All purchases must be recorded, and individual use must be recorded in a Controlled Drugs Register within 24 hours (see below). Drugs must be stored in a locked secure cabinet. Drugs must not be destroyed or disposed of unless under supervision of an appointee of the Secretary of State.
- **Schedule 3.** This group includes buprenorphine and phenobarbital. Buprenorphine must be kept in a locked secure cabinet, though it is advisable to store all Schedule 3 drugs in a locked receptacle. Purchase invoices should be kept for 2 years. *Under RCVS guidelines, it is recommended that ketamine be stored under Schedule 3 guidelines and kept in a locked cabinet due to risk of abuse. An informal register of use is also suggested.*
- **Schedule 4.** This includes butorphanol and androgenic steroids. These are exempted from control when used in veterinary practice.
- **Schedule 5.** This includes preparations containing codeine at muted strengths, making them exempt from the controlled drug requirements except that purchase invoices must be kept for a period of 2 years.

Entries made on obtaining the drug			
Date supply received	Name and address of supplier	Amount obtained	Form in which the drug was obtained

Entries made when supplying the drug					
Date transaction occurred	Name and address of person supplied	Licence or authority of person supplied to be in possession	Amount supplied	Form in which supplied	Amount of drug remaining

3.23 Recommended layout of Controlled Drugs Register for Schedule 2 drugs. (This is intended as an example only; there are several variations on the format.)

Controlled Drugs Register

Records are required for Schedule 2 drugs. This must be in a bound book with sections designated for each drug. An entry must be made within 24 hours of receipt of the drug and every time the drug is used. Entries must be written legibly in indelible ink and must not be amended. The Register must be kept for 2 years from the last entry. Figure 3.23 shows the recommended layout of the Register, but purpose-made published versions are preferable.

Requisition of controlled drugs

A requisition, written in longhand and signed by the veterinary surgeon, must be obtained by the supplier before delivery of Schedule 2 and 3 drugs. It must state the name and address of the veterinary practice, the purpose for which the drug will be used and the amount of the drug required, in both words and numbers.

Prescribing and the 'cascade'

Legislation governs which medicines may be prescribed for a particular condition in a particular species:

A veterinary medicine may only be administered to an animal if that medicine has a product licence for the treatment of that particular condition in that particular species.

The exceptions to this (referring only to non-food-producing animals) are defined in the Veterinary Medicines Regulations 2005 as the **cascade method of prescribing**, as numbered below.

If, and only if, no drug is licensed for that condition in that species, then:

1. A veterinary medicine licensed in another species or for another condition in the same species may be used. This is considered to be **'off-label'** use, which is defined as use of the medicine outside the purpose for which it has market authorization.
2. If no product as in (1) exists, then a licensed human product may be used or a veterinary product licensed in another EU member state may be used (see Importing veterinary medicines, below).

3. If no product as in (2) exists, then a product can be prepared on a one-off basis by an authorized person in accordance with a veterinary prescription.

When it is necessary to prescribe 'off-label', the owner or guardian of the animal should be made aware of the potential hazards and **signed consent** should subsequently be obtained. The reason determined for 'off-label' use should be recorded in the patient's clinical notes.

Importing veterinary medicines

Veterinary surgeons may apply for importation of drugs using special certification:

- *Special Import Certificate* (SIC) – may be used to import a product licenced in another EU member state if no suitable product is available in the UK
- *Special Treatment Certificate* (STC) – may be used to import a product licensed in a non-EU country if no appropriate product exists in the UK or other member state.

For both SICs and STCs application for certification is made through the Veterinary Medicines Directorate and a fee is charged.

Prescriptions

A veterinary prescription may be required under several different circumstances. In the case of POM–V and POM–VPS medicines, a client may elect to be supplied with the medicine elsewhere. In this case a veterinary surgeon may write a prescription so that another RQP may supply the medicine to the client. Veterinary prescriptions are also required for controlled drugs and these prescriptions have different legal requirements.

Requirements for a POM–V prescription

The points shown here in bold are legal requirements. An example prescription is shown in the box below. The prescription:

- **Must be written legibly in indelible ink or other indelible format**
- **Must state the name and address of the prescriber and substantiate that the prescriber is a veterinary surgeon, e.g. MRCVS**

- Must state the date of issue
- Must state the name and address of the person to whom the product is supplied
- Must give a description of the animal (e.g. name)
- Should state the name and the strength of the drugs to be dispensed, using either the generic name or a proprietary (trade) name (avoiding abbreviations)
- Should state precise directions for use, including route, dose and formulation
- Must declare that the prescription is issued in respect of an animal under the veterinary surgeon's care
- Must be signed by the prescribing veterinary surgeon
- Should state 'For animal treatment only' and 'Keep out of reach of children'
- If applicable, should also state 'For topical use only'
- Should contain directions for repeat prescriptions.

A prescription must be dispensed within 6 months of the prescription being written.

Example prescription

The Veterinary Centre, Any Street, Any Town, Postal code

Please supply the following drug to Mr Owner of Another Street, Any Town, Postal code for treatment of 'Pet', an animal currently under my care.

Clindamycin 150 mg x 14 (fourteen)
Give one tablet by mouth, twice a day, for seven days.
No repeats.
For animal treatment only. Keep out of reach of children.

Signed: .... Mrs I.M.A. Vet MRCVS
28/1/07

Requirements for Schedule 2 and Schedule 3 controlled drugs

Additional legal requirements for prescriptions of Schedules 2 and 3 controlled drugs are as follows.

- The prescription must be written in the prescribing veterinary surgeon's own handwriting (exceptions to this are phenobarbital and pentobarbital).
- The form and strength of the drug to be dispensed must be included. The quantity to be dispensed must be written in both numbers and figures. Abbreviations should not be used.
- The drug may only be dispensed within 13 weeks of issue of the prescription.
- Prescriptions for controlled drugs may not be repeated.

Abbreviations

Abbreviations may be used when writing prescriptions or within medical notes. Common abbreviations include:

- od (*omni die*), sid (*semel in die*) or q24h – once daily
- bd (*bis die*), bid (*bis in die*) or q12h – twice daily
- tid (*ter in die*) or q8h – three times daily
- qid (*quarter in die*) or q6h – four times daily

Storage of veterinary medicines

Most of the requirements for the storage of veterinary medicines are based on common sense. The important points are as follows.

- Store in accordance with the manufacturer's instructions.
- Refrigeration must be available and maintained between 2°C and 8°C. Refrigerators should be fitted with a maximum/minimum thermometer to allow monitoring of the temperature. Insulin and vaccines are examples of products that must be kept refrigerated.
- The designated storage area should not be accessible to the public.
- Storage areas should be kept clean and should be well ventilated. Eating or drinking should be forbidden in this area.
- Flammable products should be stored in appropriate cabinets.
- Dates of delivery should be logged and marked on products. For multi-use products, the date of first use should be marked on the product.
- Products returned by clients should not be reused as they may have been inappropriately stored.
- An effective stock control system should be implemented allowing routine checking and detection of products requiring reordering or approaching their expiry date. In addition, new legislation under the Veterinary Medicines Regulations 2005 requires more data to be kept relating to purchase and usage of drug stock. Records need to include information regarding expiry date and batch number. A detailed audit will be legally required at least once yearly and records kept for a five-year period.
- Controlled drugs in Schedule 2 and some in Schedule 3 should be stored in a locked cabinet. Keys for this cabinet should only be available to the veterinary surgeon and/or an authorized person designated by the veterinary surgeon. Other drugs such as ketamine are liable to abuse and it is recommended that they also should be stored in a locked cabinet. Under RCVS recommendations, it is suggested that usage be recorded in an informal register.
- Drugs in consulting rooms and in vehicles should be kept to a minimum and should not include controlled drugs.

■ POM–VPS, AVM–GSL and NFA–VPS drugs may be displayed to the public but only 'dummy' packs may be used. POM–V drugs may not be displayed to the public, though posters advertising them may be displayed within the veterinary practice since this is advertising only to clients and not to the general public. Under the new legislation, advertisement of POM–V drugs to veterinary nurses and veterinary students is also not allowed, which has implications for veterinary education. Up-to-date information on this topic is available at www.vmd.gov.uk

Handling, labelling and dispensing of medicines

The important legislation involves:

■ Health and Safety at Work etc. Act 1974
■ Control of Substances Hazardous to Health Regulations 2002 (enacted under the Health and Safety at Work etc. Act 1974).

Currently, the veterinary surgeon is responsible for ensuring that the requirements of the relevant legislation are fulfilled. A practice manual should be available that provides the staff with details of the practice's policy, including handling and dispensing of medicines.

> ⚠ **WARNING**
> **Anyone involved in the handling or dispensing of veterinary medicines should be adequately trained.**

COSHH Regulations

These regulations relate to work involving substances that are deemed to be hazardous to health, including certain veterinary medicines and animal products. It is the employer's responsibility to perform a risk assessment of each of these substances used. Manufacturers of veterinary products now provide a product safety data sheet to aid this risk assessment. The employer must aim to prevent or control exposure of employees to these substances by information, instruction and training.

Practical points for handling and dispensing of medicines

■ Direct contact between the skin of the person dispensing the drug and the drug itself should be avoided. This can be achieved through wearing protective clothing, such as disposable gloves, or by using pill counters.
■ Notify the veterinary surgeon of skin abrasions and avoid dispensing drugs under these circumstances.
■ Particular care should be taken with drugs marked as teratogenic or carcinogenic.
■ The data sheet should always be consulted, especially if the dispenser is not familiar with the particular drug in question.

■ Drugs should be appropriately labelled and should be dispensed in an appropriate container (see separate section below).
■ COSHH regulations extend to a responsibility to the client. The client should be given clear instructions with regard to the safe handling, storage and disposal of the medicine. For example, disposable gloves (preferably latex-free) may need to be given to the client for the application of certain products for external application, or the client should be advised that some products should be kept refrigerated.

> ⚠ **WARNING**
> *Cytotoxic drugs,* **such as cyclophosphamide, require extreme care in handling and administration as many are highly toxic and irritant. Appropriate protective clothing should be worn and the drugs should be prepared in a designated area. Tablets must never be divided or crushed. These drugs should not be handled by pregnant women.**

Labelling

All drugs that are dispensed must be appropriately labelled. Figure 3.24 gives an example of a drug label.

> Date
>
> Ms A Vet MRCVS
> The Veterinary Clinic
> Any Street, Any Town, Postal code
>
> Antirobe 25 mg x 14
> One capsule to be given twice a day
>
> For 'Pet'
> Mr Owner
> Another Street, Any Town, Postal code
>
> Keep out of reach of children.
> For animal use only.

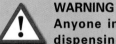 Example of information required on labels of dispensed medicines described under the Veterinary Medicines Regulations 2005. This information should be written in an indelible manner on the container of the medicine or, if this is not possible, on the package of the medicine. The label should not obscure the manufacturer's information. If the product is for topical application then '**For external use only**' should be included on the label. The omission of the recommended information could be considered professionally irresponsible and negligent if the product were used in an unsafe way.

Essential information that **legally must be provided** on the label includes:

■ **The statement 'For animal treatment only'**
■ **The name and address of the owner and the identity of the animal (i.e. the animal's name)**
■ **The date**

- **The statement 'Keep out of the reach of children'**
- **The name and address of the veterinary practice and prescribing practitioner.**

Additional information that it is *recommended* as good practice includes:

- Details of the drug (name, strength and amount)
- Instructions for administration
- Instructions for storage.

Containers

Many veterinary medicines may be dispensed from bulk containers and should therefore be packaged in suitable containers when dispensed to the public.

- Reclosable child-resistant containers made of light-resistant glass, rigid plastic or aluminium should be used. Elderly or infirm clients may require more easily opened containers and discretion may be operated in these circumstances.
- Blister-packed medicines may be dispensed in paper board cartons or wallets. Paper envelopes and plastic bags are not acceptable as sole containers of products.
- Creams, dusting powders, ointments, powders and pessaries should be supplied in wide-mouthed jars made of glass or plastic.
- Light-sensitive medicines should be in opaque or dark-coloured containers.
- Certain liquids for external use, as specified under the Medicines (Fluted Bottles) Regulations 1978, should be dispensed in fluted (vertical-ridged) bottles so that they are discernible by touch. These bottles are no longer in production and so may be difficult to obtain at present. If possible these liquids should therefore be dispensed in the manufacturer's own container.

Disposal of veterinary medicines

Tablets, capsules, creams, ointments, injections, etc. are classed as pharmaceutical waste and should not be included with clinical waste.

- Disposal is complex and local authorities can provide information on companies dealing with effective disposal.
- Schedule 2 controlled drugs may only be destroyed in the presence of a person authorized by the Secretary of State, such as a police officer.
- Once the product reaches the final user (i.e. the client) the legislation affecting disposal no longer applies, but advice should be given with regard to safe disposal of medicines.

Further reading

Bishop Y (ed.) (2004) *British Veterinary Association Code of Practice on Medicines*. BVA Publications, London

Bishop Y (ed.) (2004) *The Veterinary Formulary, 6th edn*. Pharmaceutical Press, London

Gorman N (ed.) (1998) *Canine Medicine and Therapeutics, 4th edn*. Blackwell Science, Oxford

Elliott J and Rock A (2007) Medicines: pharmacology, therapeutics and dispensing. In: *BSAVA Textbook of Veterinary Nursing, 4th edn*, ed. DR Lane *et al*. pp. 153–174. BSAVA Publications, Gloucester

Meredith A and Redrobe S (eds) (2002) *BSAVA Manual of Exotic Pets, 4th edn*. BSAVA Publications, Gloucester

Moore M (2001) *Calculations for Veterinary Nurses*. Blackwell Science, Oxford

Orpet H and Welsh P (2002) *Handbook of Veterinary Nursing*. Blackwell Science, Oxford

Tennant B (ed.) (2005) *BSAVA Small Animal Formulary, 5th edn*. BSAVA Publications, Gloucester

4

Managing clinical environments, equipment and materials

Sue Dallas, Marie Jones and Elizabeth Mullineaux

This chapter is designed to give information on:

- Environmental conditions that should be maintained in each clinical area
- Methods of prevention of spread of infection, including methods of cleaning
- Methods of waste disposal
- Isolation and barrier nursing
- The management of stock in the veterinary practice

The inpatient environment

Animals are hospitalized in order to:

- Be observed
- Have surgical procedures carried out
- Have medical procedures carried out
- Be nursed
- Have samples collected from them.

In order for veterinary staff to do this, the environment must be correct. To ensure a high standard of care, there must be adequate facilities, equipment and human resources.

Locations within the practice for the care of patients include:

- Consultation rooms
- Operating theatre
- Preparation/triage rooms
- Recovery area
- Kennels
- Grooming area
- Exercise areas
- Kitchen/food preparation room.

General considerations for the inpatient include:

- Environmental temperature
- Hygiene and cleaning
- Light, heat, ventilation, noise and security.

Environmental temperature

In most mammals and birds, body temperature is regulated within the ideal thermoneutral zone. This varies between species to allow for the working of the internal body environment of each, and the balance attained is known as **homeostasis**.

Reptiles and amphibians interact with their environmental temperature to maintain a body temperature that is optimal for the particular species, given the opportunity to do so. Thus, monitoring of their body temperature is not always necessary.

However, all species, whatever means they use to control their own body temperature, sometimes need help. When an animal is conscious and healthy, its internal mechanisms are functioning; but when it is ill or injured, it may need assistance from the nursing environment.

In most clinical situations, it is usually desirable to maintain an animal's normal or optimal body temperature. Patients in the veterinary clinic that are unable, for a variety of reasons, to maintain their own body temperature within normal limits will benefit (often dramatically) when the environmental temperature is either raised or lowered to suit their special needs.

Methods of assisting patients to raise their body temperature include:

- Heat pads
- Bubblewrap
- Water-circulating pads

- Incubators
- Hot-water bottles (well wrapped)
- Ceramic heat lamps (especially for reptiles)
- Lightweight blankets
- Space blankets
- Synthetic fleece
- Beanbags.

Methods used to lower body temperature include:

- Cool pads
- Fans
- Air conditioning.

In each clinical area of the veterinary practice temperatures should be maintained appropriately; temperature fluctuations should be monitored and recorded using maximum–minimum thermometers. The ideal range is 18–21°C, and the temperature should not fall below 15.5°C.

Prevention of the spread of infection

How disease spreads

Disease is spread from one animal to another by various methods (see also Chapter 2). Microbes leave the body in or on:

- Oral, nasal and ocular discharges (e.g. rabies via the saliva; feline respiratory diseases and distemper via ocular and nasal discharge)
- Urine (e.g. leptospirosis and hepatitis)
- Vomit (e.g. canine parvovirus)
- Blood (e.g. microorganisms transmitted by fleas to another animal)
- Skin surface (e.g. surface bacteria and fungi such as ringworm)
- Milk from mother to offspring (e.g. some worms, some viruses).

The microbes are passed on from one animal to another, sometimes by a carrier animal. These animals do not show clinical signs of disease but are individuals that:

- Have had the disease and recovered (**convalescent carriers**)
- Never show clinical signs of the disease (**healthy carriers**).

Both types will shed the disease-carrying microbes into the environment, putting other animals at risk. Microbes are passed from one animal to another by means of:

- Direct *contact* – parts of the bodies of two animals come into contact (e.g. nose to nose or nose to anus)
- Indirect *contact* – the contact is with an inanimate object (e.g. bedding, water bowl or lamp post)
- Aerosol transmission – through the air, in the form of droplets from sneezing, coughing or using air currents

- Contaminated food or water – contaminated by urine and faeces of passing rodents or other animals (due to incorrect storage of dried foods)
- Carrier animals – shedding microbes in discharges, urine or faeces yet unaffected themselves (e.g. canine hepatitis).

Development of disease

Entry into a new host

Routes of entry include the following.

- Eating:
  - Infected food or water
  - Contact with contaminated food/water bowls
  - Eating faeces (coprophagia)
  - Eating the disease carrier (e.g. flea, while grooming).
- Inhalation:
  - Breathing in airborne microbes, or sniffing contaminated surfaces.
- Through the skin:
  - Wound
  - Scratch
  - Insect bite
  - Subsurface mite (e.g. *Sarcoptes*).
- Via damaged mucous membranes:
  - Mouth
  - Nose
  - Eye.

Infection

If the microorganism has entered the host animal and overcome its resistance, infection may ensue. Some infections are confined to a restricted area (e.g. abscesses); others are called **systemic** because they spread through the whole body via the bloodstream.

Resistance to infection

Individual resistance will depend on:

- Age
- Nutritional state (too thin or overweight)
- Skin being intact
- Vaccination status
- Immune response and white blood cell activity.

Incubation

Incubation refers to the time between the animal receiving the microbe and showing clinical signs of disease.

Methods used to control disease

- Avoid direct contact with infected animals (use of isolation, see later).
- Maintain high levels of hygiene/disinfection in the animal's environment.
- Reduce the number of animals kept within the same air space, or improve the efficiency of air movement to reduce aerosol transmission.
- Provide early and effective treatment of infected animals to prevent others becoming infected.
- Control parasites to prevent passing of disease from one animal to another.
- Maintain vaccination status of animals and staff.

Cleaning and maintaining clinical environments

The practice hospital environment may house high concentrations of microorganisms that are potentially pathogenic (i.e. can cause disease). When patients are injured or diseased, they are even more at risk because of a decreased resistance to infection. Every effort must be made to decrease the microbe population in order to safeguard patients.

The aims are to:

- Eliminate or control sources of disease
- Prevent transmission of disease
- Increase host resistance to disease.

Methods of achieving these aims include:

- Isolation and quarantine
- Vaccination
- Improved diet
- Hygiene
- Chemotherapeutic agents
- Euthanasia of animals with uncontrollable infections.

Sources and transmission of disease can be controlled by:

- Improved ventilation
- Physical cleaning
- Chemical disinfectants and antiseptics
- The use of protective clothing (plastic disposable aprons and gloves; see Figure 4.12).

Standards will be adjusted according to the area within the hospital practice.

General cleaning

In the case of general cleaning equipment (to include commercial cleaners), the level of care is standard.

Mopping

If mops are used for washing floors, the following rules apply.

- Mop heads should be washed daily in the washing machine (>40°C) and dried.
- If used more than once daily, they should be soaked for 30 minutes in a bucket of disinfectant.

- They should never be left standing in soaking solution for any longer than 30 minutes.
- They should be wrung out thoroughly before use on the floors.

Cleaning a floor with a mop

- **Move the mop from left to right across the body; never push it back and forth in front of you.**
- **The mop head should be agitated in the disinfectant solution and wrung out before proceeding to clean.**
- **Start with the area of floor furthest from the door.**
- **When the area immediately around you has been cleaned, move and repeat the mop rinsing for a new area.**
- **No one should be allowed to walk on the floor until it is dry.**
- **Change the disinfectant solution between rooms, or more frequently if the floor is heavily soiled.**
- **A separate mop or other cleaning equipment should be used in areas where high standards of clinical cleanliness are important (e.g. theatre).**

Cleaning surfaces

Checks should be made throughout the day on:

- Doors
- Cabinet/cupboard doors
- Walls
- Lighting
- Monitor/keyboards, if present.

Spot-cleaning should be carried out as required, using the appropriate solutions. Cleaning between each patient must be carried out on:

- Tables
- Surfaces
- Equipment used.

To prevent spread of disease, the appropriate disinfectant (Figure 4.1) or antiseptic solution on a disposable cloth or wipe is used and protective clothing is worn to protect staff and other patients.

Type/active ingredient	Examples of commercial products	Formulation and recommended use	Advantages	Disadvantages
Phenol compound	Jeyes	Liquid – environment	Good activity against a range of bacteria; inexpensive	Variable activity against viruses; poor activity against spores. **Toxic to cats**
Chloroxylenol	Dettol	Liquid – environment and skin	Good activity against Gram-positive bacteria	Inactivated by hard water/ organic matter; poor activity against Gram-negative bacteria

4.1 Disinfectants and antiseptics. (continues)   ▶

Type/active ingredient	Examples of commercial products	Formulation and recommended use	Advantages	Disadvantages
Hypochlorites (bleach)	Domestos	Liquid – environment	Effective against bacteria, fungi, viruses and spores; inexpensive	Corrosive; strong smell; inactivated by organic matter; can give off gas if mixed with urine
Halogenated tertiary amines (contain quaternary ammonium compounds)	Trigene, Vetaclean	Liquid – environment	Good activity against bacteria, fungi and viruses; low toxicity; low corrosion	Inactivated by hard water
Iodine / Iodophors	Pevidine	Liquid – topical skin application	Good activity against spores; wide range of activity	May stain; allergic reactions
Peroxygen compounds	Virkon	Powder – environment	Active against a wide range of microorganisms; fast acting	Activity reduced by organic matter; corrosive to metal; irritant
Aldehydes (glutaraldehyde)	Cidex, Parvocide	Liquid – environment	Active against a wide range of organisms	Slow acting; high irritancy/sensitivity
Alcohol	Surgical spirit	Liquid – skin and environment	Good activity against bacteria and fungi; fast acting	Flammable; not sporicidal; inactivated by organic matter; can be irritant
Biguanides	Chlorhexidine, Hibiscrub	Liquid – skin	Good activity against most bacteria and fungi; low toxicity/irritancy	Not active against spores; limited activity against viruses

4.1   (continued) Disinfectants and antiseptics.

Different inpatient areas

Consultation rooms

These are the outpatient, examination and consultation zones (Figure 4.2). They are normally decorated in similar warm tones to the clinic reception area.

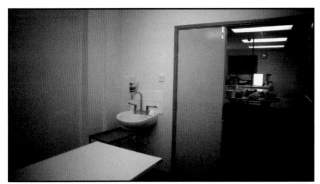

4.2   Consultation room, with a wide door leading to the treatment area.

It is important to maintain a high standard of repair and hygiene here because this is where the client will spend the greatest amount of time. Excessive fittings are normally avoided; those that are in place are necessary for the purposes of examination of patients.

Fixtures might include:

- Examination table (either floor-mounted or cantilevered from the wall)
- Wall-mounted shelf (with drawers for equipment)
- Hand washbasin
- Wall-mounted antiseptic solution dispenser
- Paper towel dispenser
- Appropriate bins or containers for clinical and non-clinical waste (see later)
- X-ray viewer
- Wall-mounted ophthalmoscope/auriscope.

It is in the consultation room that the client and veterinary surgeon meet, often for the first time. It is important that everything required for a thorough examination is to hand and has been cleaned and disinfected between patients. For this reason, the ideal design allows the veterinary surgeon to use two consultation rooms, with a separate dispensary (Figure 4.3). This type of layout enables each soiled room in turn to be thoroughly cleaned between clients (Figure 4.4) without hindering consultations.

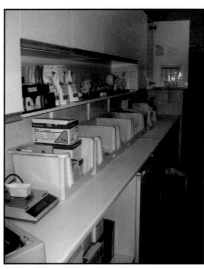

4.3   Dispensary area between two consultation rooms.

Between clients
Clean and disinfect the surface of the examination table
Spot-clean other surfaces if soiled
Check and clean soiled instruments
Collect up and remove soiled dressings or bandage materials

Between consultation surgeries
Clean and disinfect all surfaces (morning, afternoon and evening)
Collect used instruments and sterilize or clean them
Dispose of all waste in the appropriate containers, bins or bags (see Figure 4.11)
Empty and disinfect bins
Restock (as required):

- Selection of curved and straight scissors
- Dressings and bandages
- Cotton wool
- Antiseptic solutions
- Stethoscope
- Thermometer
- Selection of forceps
- Stitch cutters
- Paper towels

4.4   Cleaning routines for consultation rooms.

Preparation and triage area

This central area is one of the most important rooms in a modern veterinary clinic. It is a non-sterile area, but because of the variety of patients passing through the room it is essential to maintain a high level of hygiene.

Triage (examination and rapid classification of a case) may also take place here (Figure 4.5). It is a multipurpose room in which patients from the ward, kennels and consultation rooms will:

- Receive medication and treatment
- Have samples collected for diagnostic procedures
- Be examined
- Have bandages, splints or casts removed or changed
- Be prepared for surgical procedures.

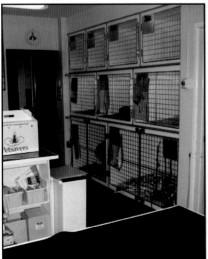

4.5   Preparation and triage room.

It is important that this is a secure area, ideally with a double self-closing door system to be passed through before escape is possible. Instructions to all staff about the opening and closing of these doors are usually displayed on a nearby wall.

- Surfaces in the preparation/triage area must be of a high standard, allowing easy disinfection and excellent hygiene.
- The walls should be covered with durable low-maintenance material, allowing regular wiping down.
- Floors have to withstand constant traffic (staff and patients) and frequent cleaning.
- Considerable storage space is required for both large equipment and disposable materials.
- Due to the many functions of this area, it is frequently up to four times the size of the clinic's operating theatre.
- Preparation for surgical procedures (anaesthetic induction and clipping up) requires a gas scavenging system, an oxygen supply, an anaesthetic machine and a vacuum facility to collect hair.
- Good lighting is essential:
  - Fluorescent lights inset into the ceiling with diffuser panels for general room light are an alternative to normal daylight
  - Spotlights (with a dimmer facility) over the treatment tables ensure good light levels in the key work areas of the room.
- Ventilation systems, via air conditioning using forced intake and extraction of atmosphere, should be installed; they will also provide constant temperature and humidity.
- Windows should not be present, unless escape-proof and with blinds.
- In order to reduce noise levels, high-set windows should be double-glazed; purpose-lagged wall panels and fire doors should be kept shut to prevent the transfer of sound through the clinic or outside the clinic.

Cleaning routines for the preparation/triage area are shown in Figure 4.6.

The preparation/triage room is always sited near the theatre suite for easy movement of patients. Also nearby are:

- Surgical team's scrub-up area
- Sterilizers
- Instrument cleaning and packing facility.

Due to the many roles that this area plays in the work of the clinic, it is essential that order and organization of equipment and disposable materials are well established. Systems include:

- Good shelving
- Cupboards and cabinets with obvious labels concerning equipment and use
- Sterilizing dates and equipment named on all packs
- Stock lists required, with quantities.

Between patient preparations or treatments
Dispose of waste materials and body fluids as clinical waste (see Figure 4.11)
Clean the clipper blades and clippers
Check the walls, surfaces, worktops and treatment table and spot-clean with dilute disinfectant (see Figure 4.1)
Check the vacuum collection bag or container and empty it if necessary
Spot-clean the floor
Check levels of disposables

After preparation/treatment sessions
Dispose of all waste material; disinfect bins and fit new liners
Wipe down all surfaces with dilute disinfectant
Restock cupboards
Check equipment (e.g. clippers and blades)
Refill dispensers for hand-cleaners and antiseptics
Clean all sinks
Replace towels and paper towel rolls

4.6 Cleaning routines for the preparation/triage area.

Recovery area

On completion of surgical procedures, patients recover consciousness in an area where staff are able to monitor and observe them (Figure 4.7).

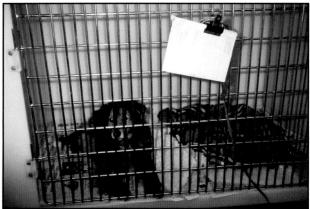

4.7 Recovery kennel, allowing good patient observation.

These animals should not be disturbed by unnecessary cleaning routines, but it is essential to allow thorough cleaning to take place at some point in each day, when patients have been moved to the ward kennels.

Patients in the recovery stage may vomit, defecate, urinate or salivate. These body fluids must be removed immediately, and disposed of in the correct manner by staff wearing protective clothing.

Cleaning should include the following routines:

- Dispose of waste; disinfect bins and replace plastic liners
- Wipe down all surfaces and equipment such as drip stands
- Clean and disinfect recovery areas
- Check supplies of disposable materials and restock
- Clean the floor.

Kennels and wards

Patients are moved from the recovery area to an inpatient ward (Figure 4.8). These wards are normally situated as far as possible from the consulting and reception areas of the clinic.

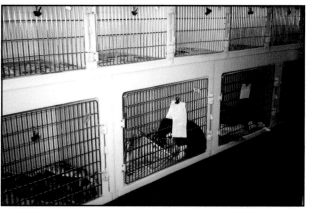

4.8 Tiered hospital kennels in an inpatient ward.

- Kennel wards must:
  - Be durable
  - Be secure
  - Be easy to clean
  - Retain heat
  - Allow good observation of the patient.
- Kennels must be of the correct size for the type of patient housed and should be made of a material that is non-permeable and is easy to clean and disinfect.
- Heating and ventilation are important to assist in maintaining a patient's body temperature, while providing good oxygen levels in the room atmosphere.
- For further improvement of the atmosphere, a combination of air conditioning and scavenging systems may be used.
- Noise from inpatients is controlled by good soundproofing. Materials used to isolate the noise in the animal ward area include:
  - Acoustic tiles fitted to ceiling and floor
  - Walls well insulated and lagged
  - Double-glazing fitted to any window
  - Self-closing internal doors.

The daily cleaning routine for kennels and wards is shown in Figure 4.9.

- Remove waste from all bins; replace the plastic liner
- Clean and disinfect walls
- Spot-clean surfaces, doors, cupboard doors, light fixtures, drip stands and any other items routinely kept in this area
- Check and restock any disposable materials
- Clean and disinfect the sink (if any)
- Clean and disinfect the floor
- Disinfect and store cleaning equipment
- Launder all used bedding on high temperature setting (minimum 40°C)

4.9 Daily cleaning routine for kennels and wards.

Sick and recovering animals often cannot control urination and defecation; therefore, more frequent attention and cleaning of a soiled kennel is required (for details on bedding materials, see the *BSAVA Manual of Practical Animal Care*).

Before disposal of urine and faeces, it is important to check whether a sample is required. If a sample has been requested by the attending veterinary surgeon, it should be collected in an appropriate container, sealed, labelled and refrigerated. There should be a note on the case card that collection has taken place.

Exercise run

For reasons of security, exercise areas should be adjacent to the kennel wards with escape-proof fences or walls between the two (Figure 4.10). The run area is often located within an insulated area of the clinic for control of environmental temperature and noise levels.

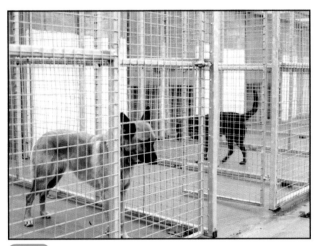

4.10 Individual run areas for long-stay patients.

Grooming facilities

Grooming facilities may be attached to the clinic as an additional customer service and to enable patients to be groomed as a part of essential routine care before discharge. A bath tub, grooming table and dryers are required. The grooming clippers, combs and brushes are stored and cared for here. (For details on grooming, see the *BSAVA Manual of Practical Animal Care*.)

Kitchen/food preparation area

The kitchen is where food is stored and prepared for inpatients.

- With a variety of species being catered for, a range of tinned, dry and fresh foods needs to be stored:
  - The dry foods must be stored in dry rodent-proof containers and labelled for content
  - A storage area is needed for the various types of tinned food, with easy viewing for stock control
  - A refrigerator should be available for the storage of part-used tinned foods, perishables and fresh foods.
- The work/preparation surfaces must be durable and easy to clean and disinfect.
- There should be a good-sized sink unit, with drainer, for the preparation and washing of fresh leafy foods.
- There needs to be a sufficient area of work surfaces to accommodate the washing up, drying and storage of bowls and containers.

Waste disposal

All waste materials must be disposed of safely and in accordance with legal requirements (Figure 4.11).

Type of waste	Things included	Type of disposal
General waste	Paper; cardboard; kitchen waste	Recycle if possible. Otherwise dispose of via local council usually in blue or black bags
Non-hazardous veterinary healthcare waste	Blood-stained theatre waste; kennel waste; consulting room waste	Yellow and black striped ('wasp' or 'tiger') bags
Hazardous veterinary healthcare waste	Blood-stained, faecal contaminated or body fluid-contaminated waste from animals with diseases infectious to other animals or humans	Orange clinical waste bags OR Yellow clinical waste bags or bins
'Sharps'	Needles; blades; broken contaminated glass	'Sharps' bin, usually yellow with a white or red lid
Chemotherapeutic waste	Contaminated needles, vials, giving sets	'Chemotherapeutic' bin, with a purple or black lid
Pharmaceutical waste	Used and empty medicines containers and used syringes	'Pharmy' bin, usually a green or yellow container
	Part used or expired drugs; empty bottles; vials; other pharmaceutical waste	'DOOP' containers (Destruction Of Old Pharmaceuticals), usually green with a red lid
	Cytotoxic medicines	Yellow 'pharmy' bin with a black or purple top (or use 'sharps' bin, as above)

4.11 Classification of waste, according to Control of Hazardous Waste (England and Wales) Regulations (HWR) 2005. (continues) ▶

Type of waste	Things included	Type of disposal
Cadavers	Deceased pets and wildlife	Release for home burial or to pet crematorium. May change in the future if infectious and classified as 'hazardous waste'
Radiography chemicals	Used or expired developer and fixer; contaminated water	Special containers and contractors needed. Regarded as 'hazardous healthcare waste'
Other 'special' waste	Aerosols; computer monitors and TVs; fridges; freezers; fluorescent light tubes	Local council disposal sites specified for this type of waste. Classified as 'hazardous waste'

4.11 (continued) Classification of waste, according to Control of Hazardous Waste (England and Wales) Regulations (HWR) 2005.

Isolation and barrier nursing

If an animal in the practice hospital shows signs of ill health that could be transmitted to other patients, it should be moved immediately to the isolation unit so that other patients are not exposed and put at risk. For various reasons (disease, stress, injury or not yet vaccinated) these other patients are considered to be susceptible hosts.

The methods used to control the transmission of microorganisms shed by a patient will vary.

- Good ventilation of the isolation area is essential in the control of airborne disease; therefore isolation units need to have a separate air-handling system from the rest of the clinic.
- A range of environmental disinfectants is kept in the isolation unit, providing choice in the elimination of specific microbes.
- Antiseptic hand-cleaners for use between patients and the wearing of disposable gloves when handling patients are essential.
- Although a surgical mask may not be needed routinely, wearing it as well as goggles or eye visor is recommended when nursing animals with airborne zoonoses (e.g. birds with psittacosis).
- Use of disposable paper towels for hand-drying and cleaning will further reduce transmission of infection.
- No visitors should be allowed in the isolation unit, only key nursing staff.
- The presence of all disease vectors such as flies, fleas and lice should be actively investigated and eliminated.
- Any reusable materials or equipment should be autoclaved within the isolation area before being used on other patients.

Isolation unit

- **The unit must be totally self-contained, with all its own equipment for feeding, nursing and cleaning.**
- **One nurse should be allocated to this area and should have no other duties in the animal areas.**
- **A footbath should be used and clothing changed on entering and leaving the unit.**
- **There should be a supply of disposable protective clothing.**
- **Effective and appropriate disinfectants should be used.**
- **Personal and environmental hygiene should be strict.**
- **All waste from the unit should be disposed of safely.**
- **The patient should have no contact with other animals.**
- **Cages, kennels and runs should be contained within the unit.**
- **The unit should have its own sink/kitchen area (with hot and cold water).**
- **There should be a treatment table and medical supplies.**
- **There must be a good ventilation system (to deal with airborne microbes).**

If the unit is well designed, its entrance will be separate from that of the main hospital. This enables patients with suspected contagious diseases to be taken directly to isolation.

All soiled cage papers and bedding, also other body discharges such as blood, saliva, urine, faeces and eye and nasal discharges, should be disposed of in the normal way (i.e. as clinical waste).

Apart from possible transfer of microorganisms to other patients, there may also be a risk of the transfer of zoonoses to the nursing staff; therefore it is vital that protective clothing is used (Figure 4.12).

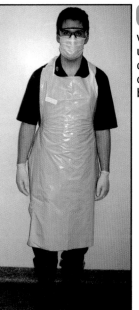

4.12 Suitable protective clothing for working in an isolation unit: disposable gloves; disposable plastic apron; disposable plastic over boots; goggles; and mask.

In certain cases, the owners of a patient discharged from isolation should be informed that their pet may shed the infectious microorganism responsible for its disease for some time. Therefore they should limit contact with other animals during that period and be aware of hygiene issues in the case of diseases transmissible to humans (e.g. leptospirosis).

Stock control

The purpose of stock management and control is to have every drug, vaccine, or supply item always available when needed, yet not waste money acquiring and storing surplus supplies. This is a delicate balance, because the amount and trends of use of drugs and supplies can change rapidly.

If too much stock is stored, extra money and storage space are required and the stock will be paid for long before the last is used. If too little stock is kept, needed items will sometimes not be available to provide the preferred treatment for the patient, or an opportunity for the sale of a product will be missed. Close attention to stock levels of surgical supplies, pet food, pharmaceuticals, vaccines, X-ray film and other items will ensure that an adequate stock is maintained. An effective stock control system is needed to reorder and replenish items before they run out.

Most practices use one large wholesaler but may also order from other smaller suppliers (e.g. chemists, laboratories, stationery companies) and this will mean that stock control needs to be cross-referenced between several companies. Nurses need to be aware of who are the official suppliers for the practice.

Responsibility for stock control

Practice managers, veterinary nurses and occasionally reception staff may be assigned responsibility for stock control. Sometimes the responsibilities will be divided between several staff, each being responsible for a specific area. One person should be the primary person placing orders, making sure that what is received is what was ordered and invoiced.

Once a delivery of stock arrives, it should be dealt with immediately and checked thoroughly prior to being stored. The order should be checked for:

- Damage – broken glass, open boxes, wet boxes, vaccines etc. not stored at correct temperature
- Expiry dates – ensure that all are in date
- Presence of all items on the invoice or delivery note
- Price increases on the invoice
- Items requiring special storage (e.g. vaccines or controlled drugs) – ensure that these are dealt with appropriately.

Storage

Good stock control not only involves ordering and maintaining of stock; it also requires the correct storage of goods to ensure that they reach the client in good condition and that they do not perish due to incorrect storage. As a general rule the majority of stock is stored away from client access in a clean and dry environment, such as a pharmacy/dispensary area. There are exceptions to this: certain products have special requirements. For example, vaccines require refrigeration on arrival, and controlled drugs must be correctly recorded and stored in a locked cupboard. For more details of storage of medicines, see Chapter 3; for the storage of radiographic material, see Chapter 11.

Stock control systems

Considerable money is involved in stock purchases. Much can be lost through inadequate stock control procedures. This loss may occur because the practice was billed for materials that were never received, or the practice was double-billed for an order, billed for damaged goods, or billed for more or different items than were actually received. Losses also occur because of ordering too many months' supply of perishable goods that deteriorate or go beyond the expiry date on the container and are no longer effective or legally safe to use.

Stock rotation is important to ensure that older stock is used first, thereby reducing the chance of items going out of date. All new stock should be placed under or behind existing stock, ensuring that the oldest products are at the front so that they are used first.

There are many computerized and manual stock control systems available for use within a veterinary practice, including:

- Handheld computers
- Bar coding
- Direct computer link to wholesaler
- Paper-based checklists.

In order to be accurate, computerized systems require the input of everything that is sold and used. As a result of human error or inconsistencies they are only moderately successful in providing all the stock control information needed. Manual procedures, such as taking frequent stock counts of all supplies, can go a long way to helping the computerized stock control process to be successful.

An effective stock control system should:

- Be easy to use
- Ensure that all medications and supplies are available when needed
- Reduce expenses by achieving a good turnover rate
- Provide a signal when each item needs to be ordered
- Track seasonal variations
- Track past usage
- Provide purchase cost information to keep the pricing and supply of products current
- Ensure that ordered items are actually received and back-ordered items are tracked so that over-ordering does not occur
- Make it easy to account for when and where items are used so cost can be allocated to various areas within the practice

- Provide a procedure for checking invoices to make sure that they are accurate for amounts ordered and prices quoted
- Allow the practice to obtain the best prices available, identify expired or outdated items and return to suppliers for credit as required.

Definitions of terms used in stock control are given in Figure 4.13.

Delivery note	Arrives with the goods ordered and can be used to check goods received
Invoice	Gives details of goods received with a breakdown of costs and balance owed
Invoice number	The invoicing company's reference number
Order number	The practice's reference number
Unit price	Price per individual item
Recommended retail price	Price at which products should be sold
Terms of delivery	Supplier's delivery terms (e.g. 'balance payable on delivery of goods')
Terms of payment	Supplier's payment terms (e.g. 'within 30 days of receipt of invoice')
Credit note	Issued to allow products up to that value to be purchased without charge

4.13   Terms used in stock control.

As with all business documents, records should be stored in a logical manner so that they can be easily found if required and only the appropriate staff (e.g. person responsible for ordering, practice manager and practice principal) should have access to the information.

Rules of good stock control

- **Check all goods against the delivery note.**
- **Check delivery note against original order.**
- **Unpack all stock immediately upon receipt.**
- **Dispose of all packing immediately and correctly (e.g. clinical waste in yellow bags).**
- **Sort out special storage products (e.g. vaccines, insulin, controlled drugs).**
- **Keep minimum stock level records and reorder when stock reaches this.**
- **Rotate all stock.**
- **Carry out regular stock audits.**
- **Maintain auditable records and security of these.**

Further reading

Platten D (2007) Management of an animal ward. In: *BSAVA Manual of Practical Animal Care*, ed. P Hotston Moore and A Hughes, pp. 88–107. BSAVA Publications, Gloucester
Monsey L (2007) Maintaining animal accommodation. In: *BSAVA Textbook of Veterinary Nursing, 4th edn*, ed. DR Lane *et al.*, pp. 210–227. BSAVA Publications, Gloucester

An introduction to care and monitoring of the inpatient

Sue Dallas

This chapter is designed to give information on:

- Provision of basic nursing care for the hospitalized patient
- Monitoring of standard parameters
- Practical approaches to restraint for routine procedures

Introduction

Nursing care is one of the most important duties of the veterinary nurse. Attending to patients' wellbeing and monitoring vital signs are paramount in providing good nursing care. Nursing care for specific groups of patients is discussed in more detail in the relevant chapters.

It is important to consider the individual patient. Quite often in a busy veterinary establishment, where there may be an urgency to get the job done, it is easy to forget the simple approaches to caring for the patient. A nursing plan is a useful method of ensuring total individual patient care takes place (see Chapter 6). It is important to monitor standard parameters of hospitalized patients on a regular basis and to record the findings. Early detection of abnormalities permits rapid intervention, preventing deterioration of the individual patient.

Normal parameters

Temperature

Normal values for body temperature	
Dog	38.3–38.7°C
Cat	38.0–38.5°C
Rabbit	38.5–40.0°C

When taking a temperature:

- Take the temperature at the very least twice a day (it is always lower after sleep)
- Leave the thermometer in position for at least 1 minute; in the case of a subnormal temperature, leave in position for at least 2 minutes
- After insertion into the rectum, tilt the thermometer to contact the epithelial wall lining the tract. This ensures that the thermometer is not placed into faeces in the rectum, which would give a false reading.

Equipment required to take a temperature includes:

- Thermometer (ideally digital for use in the ear or per rectum)
- Lubricant such as K–Y Jelly or medicinal liquid paraffin
- Small amount of cotton wool
- Propyl alcohol
- A watch with a second hand.

Taking a rectal temperature

1. Collect and prepare all required equipment.
2. Correctly restrain the patient.
3. Shake down the thermometer (if using a mercury thermometer) and check the reading.
4. Apply lubricant to the thermometer tip.
5. Insert into the rectum for the correct length of time. Never be tempted to reduce this time (1 minute for mercury, or until the timer bleeps for digital).

▶

6. **Remove, wipe with the cotton wool and read.**
7. **Wipe clean using antiseptic solution.**

The reading should always be written down, so that a record can be built up of any changes to the patient's condition and the time of day that the recording took place.

Abnormalities in body temperature are defined in Figure 5.1.

Term	Definition	Causes include
Hyperthermia	High body temperature above normal range	Heatstroke; exercise; seizures; incorrect use of heat pads
Fever (pyrexia)	Increase in body temperature	Bacterial or viral infection; pain
Hypothermia	Reduction of body temperature below normal range	Hypovolaemic shock; general anaesthesia; can commonly occur in neonatal, geriatric or compromised patients and impending parturition
Diphasic	Fluctuating temperature	Canine distemper and other infections

5.1 Abnormalities in body temperature.

Storage of thermometers

Thermometers should be stored in the correct manner, depending on their type.

- Always wipe clean of faecal material before placing in the jar or container.
- Protect the bulb end of the thermometer by placing a layer of cotton wool at the bottom of the container.
- Never store or clean in a hot solution as this could damage the thermometer.
- Before use, wipe clean of the antiseptic solution, which could irritate the rectal lining.

Pulse

Blood pumped into the aorta during ventricular contraction creates a wave that travels from the heart to the peripheral arteries. This wave is referred to as a pulse.

Normal values for pulse rate

Dog	**60–100 beats per minute**
Cat	**160–200 beats per minute**
Rabbit	**180–300 beats per minute**

The pulse is palpated by lightly placing the index and middle fingers on a part of the body where an artery crosses bone or firm tissue.

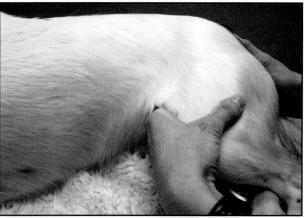

5.2 Taking a femoral pulse. (Reproduced from *BSAVA Textbook of Veterinary Nursing*.)

Sites used include:

- Femoral artery – located in the groin region on the medial aspect of the femur (Figure 5.2)
- Digital artery – located on the cranial surface of the hock
- Coccygeal artery – located on the ventral aspect of the base of the tail
- Lingual artery – located on the ventral aspect of the tongue (used only in unconscious or anaesthetized patients).

Taking a pulse

1. **Correctly restrain the patient.**
2. **Place fingers over the chosen artery.**
3. **Using a watch with a second hand, count the pulse for a minute.**
4. **Record the result.**

Pulse abnormalities are given in Figure 5.3.

Abnormality	Causes include
Raised rate	Pain Fever or high temperature Early shock Exercise Excitement or stress
Lowered rate	Unconsciousness Debilitating disease Sleep Anaesthesia
Weak pulse	Poor peripheral perfusion Hypovolaemia
Irregular pulse	Cardiac arrhythmias

5.3 Pulse abnormalities.

Mucous membrane colour

Non-pigmented mucous membranes should be pink. The colour depends upon blood haemoglobin concentration, tissue oxygen levels and peripheral capillary blood flow. Mucous membrane colour is most commonly assessed in the gums (Figure 5.4) but the conjunctiva of the eye or unpigmented membranes of the vulva or penis can also be used.

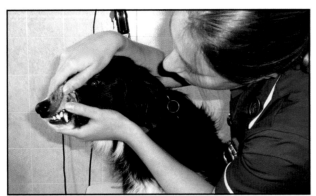

5.4	Assessing the colour of the mucous membranes of the gums.

Abnormalities in mucous membrane colour are listed in Figure 5.5.

Colour	Indication of
Pale	Shock Serious haemorrhage
Blue (cyanotic)	Lack of oxygen to tissues (hypoxia)
Red (congested)	Over-oxygenation of tissues, seen after exercise, sepsis, fever
Yellow (icteric, jaundiced)	Excess of bile pigment in the circulation, seen in hepatobiliary disorders
Red spots/blisters (petechiae)	Small haemorrhages into surface tissues caused by clotting disorder or warfarin poisoning

5.5	Abnormalities in mucous membrane colour.

Capillary refill time

Capillary refill time (CRT) is a measure of blood flow to the capillary beds of the membranes. This flow depends on cardiac output.

To determine capillary refill time, pressure is applied by the index finger to a non-pigmented area of the mucous membranes (over the root of the upper canine tooth) and then released (see Figure 7.14). The time required for colour to return to the blanched area is recorded as the capillary refill time. The normal value is 1–2 seconds. Abnormalities are given in Figure 5.6.

Abnormality	Causes include
Prolonged time (>2 seconds) – poor peripheral perfusion	Later stages of shock Heart failure
Rapid time (<1 second)	Anxiety Compensatory shock Fever Pain

5.6	Abnormalities in capillary refill time.

Respiration

Respiration is the exchange of oxygen and carbon dioxide between the air and body tissues. The rate and pattern of breathing and the effort required to breathe are controlled by the brain and respiratory muscles.

Normal respiration values	
Dog	10–30 breaths per minute
Cat	20–30 breaths per minute
Rabbit	30–60 breaths per minute

To monitor respiration requires observation of movements of the thoracic wall, or placing the hands lightly on either side of the ribs. The respiratory rate is assessed by recording the patient either breathing in or breathing out. This is ideally recorded when the patient is not panting and is awake.

Abnormalities in respiration are listed in Figure 5.7.

Abnormality	Causes include
Increased rate (tachypnoea)	Pain; fever; trauma to the central nervous system or thorax; anxiety; heat; exercise
Decreased rate (bradypnoea)	Trauma to the central nervous system; low blood carbon dioxide levels; drugs (e.g. sedative); sleep
Noisy loud breathing (stridor or stertor) may be observed with the following:	
Difficulty breathing in (inspiratory dyspnoea)	Diseases of the nasal passages, larynx, pharynx or trachea (e.g. elongated soft palate, laryngeal paralysis, tumours)
Difficulty breathing out (expiratory dyspnoea)	Collapsing intrathoracic trachea
Rapid shallow breathing	Disease of the pleural space (air or fluid accumulation, e.g. pneumothorax, pneumonia)
Laboured breathing on inspiration and expiration	Pulmonary oedema; contusions
Coughing: harsh and dry, or fluid and productive, or blood (haemoptysis)	Congestive heart failure; kennel cough; bronchitis; pneumonia

5.7	Abnormalities in respiration.

Demeanour

The demeanour (behaviour) of inpatients should always be monitored carefully. The hospital environment is not a normal one for any animal and often gives rise to fear, stress or aggression towards any subsequent handling and restraint for a veterinary procedure.

It is important to become familiar with each individual inpatient to assess behaviour and body language. Points to bear in mind in the initial approach to any inpatient include the following:

- Be quiet but confident in approaching the animal
- Be reassuring in manner and voice
- Never corner an animal: always leave perceived choices
- Stroke the animal and accustom it to voice and scent
- Only lift the animal if the approach has been accepted.

Figure 5.8 describes typical behaviour seen when animals are unwilling to be handled. Body language is further illustrated in the *BSAVA Manual of Practical Animal Care*.

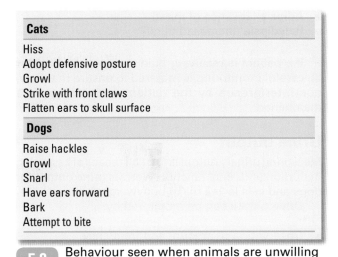

Cats
Hiss
Adopt defensive posture
Growl
Strike with front claws
Flatten ears to skull surface

Dogs
Raise hackles
Growl
Snarl
Have ears forward
Bark
Attempt to bite

5.8   Behaviour seen when animals are unwilling to be handled.

For any long-stay patients, allowing visits from the owner and familiar-smelling bedding or toys may be beneficial. Walking a patient outdoors may improve demeanour. General assessment is often easier away from the hospital environment. Figure 5.9 describes normal and abnormal patient demeanour.

Normal	Abnormal
Alert	Depressed
Responsive to contact and voice	Unresponsive to contact and voice
Relaxed	Tense
Settles into accommodation	Restless and unable to settle into accommodation

5.9   Patient demeanour.

Posture

The posture or position of the patient may indicate an abnormality, pain, or distress that may be the cause of stress or aggression when approached by hospital staff.

- Curled-up position – may indicate that the animal is cold.
- Spread-out position – may indicate high temperature, or environment too hot.

- Praying position (sternal recumbency with the forelimbs extended and slight elevation of the abdomen) – often indicates abdominal pain.
- Reluctance to lie down – seen in animals with dyspnoea, muscular or sketetal pain, stress or anxiety.

Limb problems that require assessment include:

- Lameness – scored from 1 (slight lameness) to 10 (non-use of limb)
- Pain, heat or swelling
- Paraplegia (loss of use of two limbs, generally hind limbs)
- Quadriplegia (loss of use of all four limbs – causes include spinal cord disease or injury).

Appetite

Appetite is a significant parameter when caring for the hospitalized patient. Careful observation, measurement and recording of the amount and type of food consumed are important. Recording the bodyweight daily, or even twice daily, will indicate the efficiency of nutritional support. Good nutritional support is essential for the recovering or ill animal, to provide energy and additional support for the demands of the immune system, for wound healing and for cell division and growth.

Changes in environment and diet may affect the patient's willingness to eat and it may be necessary to encourage free-choice eating. In animals reluctant to eat, free-choice intake can be improved through good nursing techniques such as hand-feeding, petting and positive reinforcement while the animal is eating, and through improving palatability and aroma by warming the food.

Loss of appetite is an early parameter indicating that the animal is unwell and it should be investigated immediately, before the condition of the animal deteriorates. There are many causes for loss of appetite, such as pain anywhere in the body, dental infection, pharyngitis, nasal congestion and pyrexia.

Feeding for life stage requirements

To aid recovery of inpatients, it is essential to provide the most appropriate diet and correct level of nutrients. However, the best diet is useless unless it is eaten by the patient. Nursing staff face a balance between adequate provision of nutrients that aid recovery and ensuring that the smell and taste of the food are attractive enough for the patient to want to eat it.

Life-stage requirements for inpatients require variation in nutrients, biological values and feeding intervals (see Chapter 2 and *BSAVA Manual of Practical Animal Care*). Special diets for specific clinical conditions are discussed in Chapter 9.

Neonates

It is essential that neonates are fed by their mother as soon as possible after birth in order to get maximum benefit from the maternal colostrum. If for any reason the mother is not available, the neonate will need bottle feeding. A proprietary milk formula should be used, fed from a bottle feeder of appropriate size (various sizes are available), to provide the correct protein and fat levels. The formula is fed at body temperature or just above, initially every 2 hours, with frequency of feeding decreasing as the quantity taken increases.

Growth phase

The energy demands of growing young animals are high and are met by using an energy-dense highly digestible diet with a suitable amount and balance of vitamins and minerals, particularly calcium and phosphorus. Inpatients can either be fed continuously or approximately 4–5 times daily to ensure that adequate energy uptake via food takes place.

Maintenance (adult)

To avoid loss of appetite or the development of stress or diarrhoea in a patient, a familiar diet should be provided (in consultation with the owner). The diet must be balanced and the daily nutrients should be divided into 2–3 feeds per day, which will allow continuous monitoring and will be more comfortable for the patient than one large meal.

Pregnancy

Depending on the stage of pregnancy and the species of inpatient, dietary requirements may be unchanged from normal maintenance (bitches only require an increase in dietary intake in the last 3 weeks of pregnancy) or may need to be increased from the time of mating (during pregnancy, cats require dietary increases to approximately 30% above maintenance amounts). Feeding may be continuous or via small feeds throughout the day.

In the lactation phase, energy requirements depend on litter size, with the greatest demands occurring 4 weeks after parturition. Small meals should be fed to supply the correct quantities of nutrients, often using a proprietary diet for lactating animals that will provide the necessary increased energy density.

Activity

Diets for working animals (e.g. sheepdogs, police dogs and racing Greyhounds) should meet the needs for muscular work and stress. Diets that have increased energy and fat levels are often referred to as 'active diets', but in recovering inpatients from this group it is important to provide a familiar diet that is palatable, digestible and balanced.

Old age

Aged inpatients will vary considerably in condition and health status. They should be fed a familiar diet, given in small frequent meals and warmed to increase palatability. Older patients may require special diets in order to help deal with specific medical problems (see Chapter 9). Elderly patients may have sensory loss as well as a poor appetite. Many also have reduced mobility and will need assistance to take up the required daily nutrients.

Fluid intake

Water is one of the non-energy-producing nutrients that animals require in the largest amounts. Fresh drinking water (in a container appropriate to the species) should always be available to patients, unless contraindicated.

Water forms 60–70% of bodyweight. Water (as fluid) is involved with nearly every body process and is essential for maintaining balance and health. It cannot be stored in the body and is lost daily via the lungs and in urine, faeces and sweat.

Average water requirements for healthy dogs and cats are 50–60 ml water/kg bodyweight/day, though there is variation. Animals may drink significantly more, depending on diet, exercise and environmental factors. Abnormalities in fluid intake include:

- **Adipsia** (absence of thirst)
- **Polydipsia** (increased thirst).

If a patient is receiving fluid therapy (see Chapter 8), careful monitoring is required to ensure that flow, non-interference by the patient and delivery are maintained.

Urine output

Measuring urinary output is a useful means of assessing hydration and renal function. Normal urine output for dogs and cats is 1–2 ml/kg bodyweight/hour.

Urine output can be monitored by:

- Observation of amount and frequency
- Indwelling urinary catheterization.

The act of urination (**micturition**) should be carefully observed and any difficulty recorded. Assessment of colour, smell and clarity should be recorded.

Hospitalized patients should be given regular opportunities to urinate and defecate and, if at all possible, a range of surfaces (grass, concrete or gravel) should be offered, to provide familiar ground. The majority of dogs will not soil indoors and may become distressed and uncomfortable if unable to go outside. Cats should be provided with clean litter trays. For the requirements of exotic pets, see the *BSAVA Manual of Practical Animal Care*.

Abnormalities in urine output and urination include:

- **Anuria** (absence of urination)
- **Dysuria** (difficult or painful urination)
- **Haematuria** (presence of blood in passed urine)
- **Polyuria** (increased urine production).

Defecation

The amount and frequency of faecal material passed should be monitored and recorded. The faeces should be assessed for texture/consistency, colour, smell, and presence of blood or mucus.

Abnormalities in defecation are described in Figure 5.10.

Record keeping

Standard parameters of hospitalized patients are monitored and recorded on a regular basis. Figure 5.11 shows an example of a record sheet from a kennel.

Abnormality	Description	Causes include
Constipation	Passing small amounts of hard faeces	Obstructions of the colon or rectum (tumours, foreign bodies); dehydration; environmental factors, such as kennel confinement, soiled litter trays; prostatic enlargement; ingested bones
Diarrhoea	Frequent passage of abnormally soft or liquid faeces	Unsuitable diet or changes in diet; bacterial infection; canine parvovirus; colitis
Dyschezia/tenesmus	Pain on defecation	Rectal/anal disease; back pain

5.10   Abnormal defecation.

5.11   Example of a kennel sheet.

Basic care of the neonate

Neonate refers to an animal during the first 10 days of life. Newborn puppies and kittens are completely dependent and helpless. Essential care includes the following.

▪ Stimulate urination and defecation after feeding by rubbing the perineum area gently with moistened cotton wool (this simulates the mother's licking). The neonate should sleep after feeds and not cry. Daily checks on weight gain should be made.

■ Warmth is essential to orphaned neonates and is supplied by careful use of an incubator, heat lamp or heated pads.
■ Hygiene and cleanliness ensure that the neonate is not overexposed to microbes in its environment. Wash hands before handling the neonate and keep any utensils and equipment sterilized if possible. Remove any milk, urine and faeces from the neonate and from its bedding.
■ Remove any eye or nose discharges using dampened cotton wool, using a separate piece for each eye.

Further information on the care of neonates is given in Chapter 2.

Basic handling and restraint procedures

Reasons for restraint include:

■ Physical examination
■ Blood sampling
■ Administering treatment or medicines
■ Application of dressings and bandages
■ Clinical examination
■ Grooming.

Patients require restraint to prevent injury both to themselves and to handlers. The majority of patients can be restrained with the minimum of force; heavy handling can often exacerbate the situation. Time taken to become familiar with each animal can assist in the restraint procedure.

Aggressive patients

Some patients may require additional methods of restraint due to their aggressive behaviour. Depending on species, there is a range of equipment available.

■ Dogs:
  – Commercially available muzzles (Figure 5.12)
  – Tape muzzles (made from 5 or 7.5 cm white open-weave bandage: a loop is placed over the dog's muzzle, crossed under the jaw and tied securely at the back of the neck).
■ Cats:
  – Commercial cat-calming muzzle (similar to the dog muzzle but also covers the whole of the cat's face, including the eyes) (Figure 5.12)
  – Crush cage (useful for administering intramuscular injections)
  – Towel, rolled around the cat and covering head, body and limbs (a limb can be excluded to access a vein)
  – Commercial cat bag: the cat is placed in the bag for restraint (exclusion of a limb allows access to a vein).

General restraint

Dogs

■ Use a suitable slip lead or collar and lead.
■ Have the patient in a standing position.

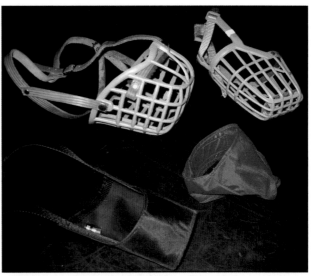

5.12   A selection of muzzles. From bottom left, clockwise: fabric dog muzzle; basket-type dog muzzle suitable for brachycephalic breed; basket-type dog muzzle; cat muzzle.

■ Hold the head gently but firmly on either side of the neck. Alternatively, place an arm under the neck, encircling and gently drawing the patient's head towards the handler's body (Figure 5.13). The latter technique is more suited to large dogs, or medium-sized to large dogs being restrained on an examination table.

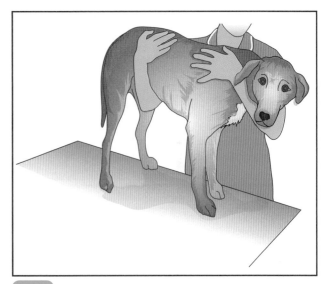

5.13   General restraint of a large dog.

Cats

■ Always transport cats in a cage.
■ Check that doors and windows are closed.
■ Take time to speak to and stroke the cat in the cage before lifting it out.
■ If the cat responds in a friendly manner it can be lifted out of the cage: place a hand under the thorax and hold the two front legs between the fingers, with the other hand supporting the hindquarters (Figure 5.14).

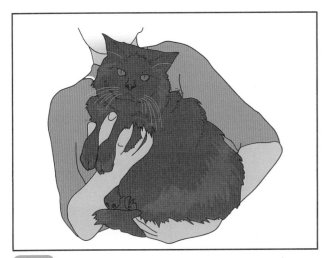

5.14   Lifting a cat.

To carry a cat (Figure 5.15):

1. Place one hand over the back of the head.
2. Place the other hand under the thorax and grasp the forelimbs between the fingers.
3. Lift into the handler's body, positioning the cat's hindquarters under the handler's elbow.
4. The cat is supported in sternal recumbency along the handler's forearm.

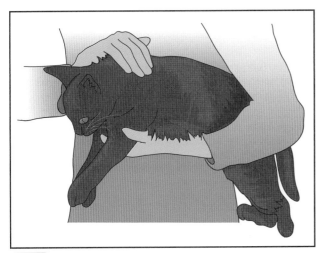

5.15   Carrying a cat.

The majority of cats do not like to be scruffed and so gentle but firm handling should be exercised. Light restraint by placing the hand over the top of the neck may be all that is required for a physical examination.

Aggressive cats require more forceful restraint, and scruffing may be necessary: the scruffed cat should be held in lateral recumbency with the hindlimbs drawn away from the body and firmly held between the fingers.

Exotic pets

For restraint of exotic pets, see the *BSAVA Manual of Practical Animal Care* and the *BSAVA Manual of Exotic Pets*.

Restraint for common procedures
Jugular venepuncture
Dogs

1. The dog should be placed in a sitting position.
   a. Small and medium-sized dogs are easily restrained on a non-slip examination table (Figure 5.16).
   b. Larger breeds are better restrained on the floor with their backs against a solid surface.
2. Place a hand under the dog's chin and extend the head upwards.
3. Take the other arm over the dog's shoulders, pulling the dog's body into the handler's body; place the fingers between the forelimbs and hold firmly (this technique is not always possible in larger breeds: the hand can be placed around the front of the forelimbs).
4. A second handler may be required to support the hindquarters of a larger dog to prevent reversing.

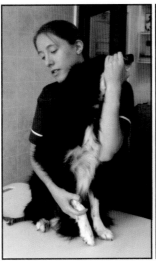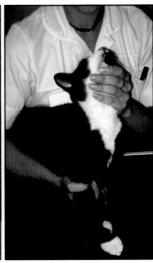

5.16   Positioning and restraint for jugular venepuncture.

Cats
It is possible to restrain cats in the same manner as small dogs (Figure 5.16). If a towel is used to cover the cat's body and limbs, the handler has better control and is less likely to get scratched.

Another method of control and restraint for jugular venepuncture is to position the cat with all four limbs and body wrapped in a towel or in a cat bag, upside down on the handler's lap, extending the head and neck away from the handler.

Cephalic venepuncture
Dogs

1. Place the dog in a sitting position or in sternal recumbency.
2. Place an arm under the dog's neck and gently draw the dog's head towards the handler's body; restrain firmly.
3. The other arm is taken over the dog's shoulder to hold the dog's elbow in the palm of the hand.

Place the thumb over the radius to compress the vein (Figure 5.17).
4. A second handler may be required to support the hindquarters of a larger dog to prevent reversing.

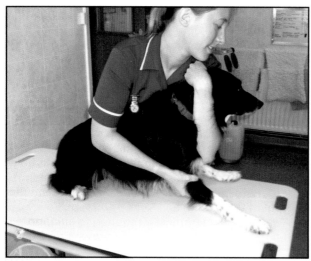

5.17 Positioning and restraint for cephalic venepuncture.

Cats

Cats can be restrained for cephalic venepuncture in a similar manner to small dogs, but instead of placing the arm around the neck, it is placed over the top of the neck, turning the head into the handler's body.

Scruffing should only be instituted if the cat becomes difficult to handle.

Injections

For subcutaneous and intramuscular injections the patient should be restrained in a manner that protects the handler and administrator from being bitten or scratched.

■ The animal's head should always be firmly held in any of the positions described above.
■ Dogs can be positioned either sitting or standing.
■ Cats should always be restrained on a non-slip examination table, placed in sternal recumbency with restraint at the head and hindquarters. The person administering the injection can assist by restraining the front or back (depending upon the injection site).

For information on the restraint of exotic pets for injections see the *BSAVA Manual of Practical Animal Care* and the *BSAVA Manual of Exotic Pets*.

Oral medicine administration
Dogs

1. Place the patient in a sitting position.
2. Support the head by firmly holding either side of the neck.

3. The person administering the oral medicine should approach from behind, or from one side of the patient, and take a firm hold of the upper jaw with one hand, gently pulling upwards and slightly backwards. This causes the lower jaw to drop, enabling the medicine to be placed into the mouth (Figure 5.18).
4. Try to place the medicine at the back of the tongue.
5. Close the mouth, keeping the nose elevated.
6. Gently massage the pharyngeal area to encourage swallowing.

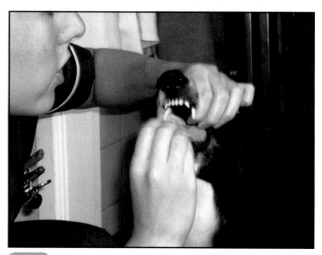

5.18 Administration of oral medicine to a dog.

Cats

Cats can be restrained in the same manner as described above, with additional restraint of the forelimbs.

The head is drawn back by placing a hand around the back of the neck and holding below the ears. This encourages the bottom jaw to drop, enabling oral treatment to be administered in the same manner as described above. A pill giver may also be used.

Further reading

Hotston Moore P and Hughes A (eds) (2007) *BSAVA Manual of Practical Animal Care*. BSAVA Publications, Gloucester

Houlton JE and Taylor PM (1987) *Trauma Management in the Dog and Cat*. Wright, Bath

Seymour J (2007) Observation and assessment of the patient. In: *BSAVA Textbook of Veterinary Nursing, 4th edn*, ed. DR Lane *et al.*, pp. 228–234. BSAVA Publications, Gloucester

McCurnin DM (1994) *Clinical Text for Veterinary Technicians*. WB Saunders, Philadelphia

Meredith A and Redrobe S (2002) *BSAVA Manual of Exotic Pets, 4th edn*. BSAVA Publications, Gloucester

Pratt PW (1996) *Medical Nursing for Animal Health Technicians*. American Veterinary Publications, Goleta, California

6

The nursing process and nursing models

Carole Davis

> ### This chapter is designed to give information on:
>
> - The importance and relevance of the nursing process in patient care
> - The veterinary nurse's role in assessing, diagnosing, planning, implementing and evaluating care
> - What is meant by the term 'nursing model'
> - How nursing models can be adapted to good effect by veterinary nurses
> - Documentation that enables veterinary nurses to plan and record care using the nursing process and a nursing model

Introduction

There need be no great mystery about frameworks or models for day-to-day practice; they are simply a way of organizing knowledge and understanding for the benefit of the patients entrusted to the nurse's care. We use theory in everyday practice whether we are aware of it or not, and the challenge now is for veterinary nurses to use it more consciously and formally.

Veterinary nurses are beginning to think seriously about the development of veterinary nursing theory and knowledge. This approach is well established amongst their human nursing colleagues and there is every reason to be confident that veterinary nursing, a much more recently established profession, will adopt this approach to care and most importantly adapt it to the context in which they practice with great effect.

Importantly, through the use of the nursing process and nursing models, veterinary nurses will be better able to articulate and demonstrate the nature of their role and the unique skills and knowledge they bring to their practice.

The nursing process

The nursing process was first introduced in the USA in the early 1980s as a reaction to dissatisfaction with a task-centred disease-oriented approach to care which failed to take into account the needs of the individual patient. In its early stages it was born out of a desire to show nursing as a distinct yet complementary discipline to medicine. Parallels may be seen with veterinary nurses currently striving to illustrate how their set of skills and knowledge, although complementary, differs from that of veterinary surgeons.

The introduction of new ways of working tends to be deemed most effective when these are seen less as something imposed on nurses delivering the care at grass roots level, without due preparation and consultation, than as an exercise in partnership, involving other veterinary and hospital assistants from the onset in how change is implemented.

What is the nursing process?

The nursing process:

- Is a problem-solving framework that enables the nurse to plan care for a patient on an individual basis
- Is a dynamic interactive fluid process, which is cyclical rather than linear
- Is not undertaken once only, for example on admission; a patient's needs change frequently and the veterinary nurse must respond appropriately
- Consists of five steps:
  - Assessment
  - Diagnosis
  - Planning
  - Implementation
  - Evaluation.

The nurse uses these five stages in every interaction with a patient, no matter how brief. Expert veterinary nurses will have mastered this process to such a sophisticated degree that they are often unaware of using the different stages, doing so instinctively. Less experienced veterinary nurses are likely to be more methodical.

The main outcome of the nursing process is a comprehensive plan of care for the patient which is carried out by all nursing staff involved with the patient.

Characteristics of the nursing process

The nursing process is:

- **Systematic** – it encompasses an ordered sequence of stages which are deliberate and purposeful in nature, i.e. seeking to maximize efficiency and attain long-term beneficial results
- **Dynamic** – it recognizes that there is overlap between the stages and that nurses frequently experience moving backwards and forwards between them
- **Interpersonal** – it recognizes the uniqueness of individual animals and thus is less likely to make generalizations and assumptions and overly focus on the task in hand
- **Outcome-focused** – the stages are designed to enable nurses to focus on achieving the best and most efficient results through the most appropriate and effective nursing actions
- **Universally applicable** – it will allow veterinary nurses to practice nursing with a wide and inclusive range of animals, healthy or unwell, young or old, in any environment.

How veterinary nurses can benefit from the nursing process

- It offers the possibility of individualized care of animals.
- It provides a systematic way of thinking about patients or clients.
- It creates nursing care plans.
- It records that nursing care has been carried out.
- It evaluates the effectiveness of nursing care.

As will be shown later in the chapter, the nursing process works well with nursing models. It provides an excellent framework for education and practice, in particular for inexperienced veterinary nurses and those new to the profession. Already, veterinary nurses are beginning to see its potential as a tool with which to generate new theories specific to veterinary nursing practice through research.

Assessment

Data collection is a key nursing skill and the first stage of the nursing process. The importance of this stage cannot be overemphasized. A nursing care plan will only be as good as the quality and accuracy of the information that goes into it, and the shift from assessment to diagnosis is a crucial one. Animals are complex and each is unique, so it is important not to rush this stage or allow oneself to be rushed by others. This will save time overall, not to mention possibly save lives.

Recently, approaches to healthcare have witnessed a departure from an approach to assessment which focuses exclusively on 'diagnose and treat', rather akin to the medical model approach, to one which aims to 'predict, prevent and manage' as well.

The assessment stage encourages the veterinary nurse to identify the patient's potential and actual health problems. Some of these problems may be linked to specific medical conditions; others will be specific to individual animals, any behavioural and psychological problems, the patient's social situation, and relationships with their owners.

Assessment is when initial ideas and impressions are formulated about existing health problems. Good observational and interviewing skills are critical here.

The main data collection methods for small animals include:

- Observation
- Interviewing the owner
- Conducting a physical assessment
- Discussion with the veterinary surgeon.

Data can be:

- **Objective:** from physical examination, e.g. temperature, respiration, condition of skin or hair, pain or tenderness on touch
- **Subjective:** statements and feelings made by the owner, e.g. 'He's not been himself lately'.

Sources of assessment data are:

- The patient
- Owners
- Current and previous nursing records
- The records of other professionals such as veterinary surgeons
- Statements and information from RSPCA officers, police, witnesses to an accident, and others.

Effective assessment depends on:

- Identifying problem areas for the patient
- Prioritizing the patient's care needs to ensure their safety and comfort

- Good social skills – used to establish rapport and a relationship with the owner that may develop over a period of care
- Interviewing skills – used to gather and give information and to clarify the purpose and intention of the procedure, admission, etc.
- A problem-solving approach and decision-making skills – applied to the available information
- Observing non-verbal cues
- Recording what is factual and observable
- Handling and care of the animal.

It is very important for the veterinary nurse to be aware of his/her own limitations and to know when to request help or to ask for a second opinion. This is a strength not a weakness and frequently an excellent way of learning.

Nursing 'diagnosis'

This stage did not appear in the first nursing process but latterly has been seen as a critical step in the nursing process. It is the culmination of assessment and is seen to be synonymous with problem identification.

As a term it can cause confusion, and it is important to make clear that veterinary nursing diagnosis is different from the diagnosis made by a veterinary surgeon. The latter aims to provide a causal explanation for the patient's presenting signs and symptoms, e.g. heart failure, diabetes. The former is essentially a nursing judgement about matters which are within the scope of nursing practice, e.g. assisting with restoring fluid balance, pain management and mobility. Nursing diagnoses are amenable to nursing actions for which the veterinary nurse is then accountable.

Planning care

Considered and informed planning will facilitate improved or optimal levels of functioning for patients, based on problem areas identified in the nursing diagnoses. It will also enable the nurse to establish realistic outcomes within realistic time frames.

There are three types of planning:

- Initial planning
- Ongoing planning
- Discharge planning.

There are four stages of the planning process:

1. Setting priorities amongst the identified problems.
2. Establishing goals that are achievable and realistic.
3. Selecting nursing interventions.
4. Developing nursing care plans.

Goals may be short term, intermediate or long term in nature. They should clearly state what the criteria for success are and when they should be reviewed, e.g. 4-hourly, daily, twice weekly. Action plans should set the nursing interventions required to enable patients to achieve these goals.

The planning and recording of care are a great means of communicating effectively with other nurses and others involved in the patient's care. They provide purpose, meaning and guidance to care, while providing a sound basis for the continuity of care.

Implementing care

Having set the goals, the veterinary nurse should now be in a position to carry out the plan of care through a series of nursing interventions. All the steps of the nursing process are inter-related and successful implementation is wholly dependent on the quality of the assessment, diagnosis and planning stages.

The best nursing actions:

- Base their care on evidence-based practice, nursing research and professional standards of care
- Understand the rationale for the nursing actions to be implemented, and question any that are not readily understood
- Adapt care to the individual patient
- Are safe and take account of risk
- Respect the dignity of the patient and owner
- Adopt a holistic approach, i.e. take account of physical, psychological and social needs
- Continue to assess the patient.

Nursing intervention should be communicated effectively to relevant others and accurate records made following the intervention.

Evaluation of care

The purpose of the evaluation stage is to enable nurses to measure the extent to which the patient care goals have been met. It enables assessment of both the standard of nursing care and its quality. Importantly, evaluation enables the nurse to discover which nursing actions are most consistently effective in solving a particular patient problem. Through evaluation, feedback is obtained on the effectiveness of the care plan and any need for adaptation.

Types of evaluation:

- **Ongoing:** evaluation carried out during or after implementing a nursing intervention to demonstrate a patient's need for, and response to, that particular nursing intervention
- **Intermittent:** evaluation performed at specific intervals to demonstrate the extent of a patient's progress towards achieving goals
- **Summative:** evaluation performed at the time of discharging the patient to demonstrate its condition at that time.

Possible outcomes following evaluation are:

- Attainment of the goal, e.g. patient is now fully mobile
- Progress being made towards the goal, e.g. patient is now partially mobile
- No progress made towards the goal, e.g. patient's mobility has not improved
- Movement away from the goal, e.g. patient's mobility has deteriorated.

The following actions may be taken when a goal has not been reached:

- Adaptation of goals
- Alteration of nursing actions
- Revision of evaluation dates.

Time spent on evaluation is crucial and to neglect it is to undermine all the other stages of the nursing process. Conversely, because there is overlap between all stages, the effectiveness of the evaluation is dependent on the degree of attention and thoroughness given to assessment, diagnosis, planning and implementation.

Evaluation provides veterinary nurses with a way of demonstrating accountability, thus implying responsibility for their own actions and advancing their professional status.

Integrated care pathways

The nursing process as a formal tool for care planning has been well established in human nursing for some time. When something has been around for a long time there is a danger of it becoming stale and jaded, hence a need to modernise and develop it as a useful clinical process rather than a paper exercise.

One successful way of doing this in human nursing has been by using it as a springboard for integrated care pathways. These are an increasingly common approach to defining the patient's journey through the healthcare system. They have been used to standardize treatment for diagnostic-related groups, thus reducing variation in treatment for patients with similar conditions.

Integrated care pathways specify the contributions of the different professionals involved in delivering care for an individual (e.g. the integration of physiotherapy, hydrotherapy, behavioural therapy, etc.) to provide a complete picture of the patient's care episode.

Nursing models

If the nursing process provides a framework for care, nursing models provide the vehicle for the delivery of that care. In short, nursing models enable the nursing process to 'come to life' by providing a further set of ideas about patients and the factors that can cause health-related problems to arise.

The medical model

Before introducing nursing models, it is useful to give a brief account of the 'medical model' as for many years this has provided the basis for nurse training. The medical model is not a model in the same sense that nurses apply the term. Essentially it describes the approach by which doctors examine, diagnose and treat patients. It is an approach that is viewed as systematic, reductionist and scientific.

According to the medical model, the person or animal is a complex set of anatomical parts and physiological systems. Within the medical model, the individual's social behaviour and psychological problems may be explained and thus oversimplified in terms of biological processes. The emphasis on anatomical, physiological

and biochemical malfunctions as the causes of ill health causes a disease-oriented approach to care, rather than an individualized holistic approach to care that takes into account the whole patient – not just physical factors but psychological, social, environmental and spiritual aspects as well.

The nature of assessment within the medical model focuses on signs and symptoms. Following a medical diagnosis, interventions are introduced to bring about change in particular body systems or parts. Goal setting will rarely be patient-centred and the focus is on 'putting things right'.

It is important to state that in recent times this approach has come in for increasing scrutiny and criticism, particularly by nurses, who through the introduction of their own 'models' have sought to develop a set of beliefs that enables them to understand and respond effectively to all health-related needs.

The change from a medical model to a nursing model is seen as one of the most profound in the history of human nursing.

What is a nursing model?

A nursing model is generally described as a collection of ideas, beliefs and values about the nature and purpose of nursing, which influence the way in which nurses work with their patients.

The nursing process describes how care will be organized, whereas a nursing model describes what the nursing care will be like. A wide range of nursing models have been introduced and developed over the years, with some being more popular and widely used than others. As with the nursing process, most models originated in the USA.

The key ideas or concepts which should be made explicit in any nursing model are:

- The nature of the individual person or animal
- The nature of health and illness
- The role of nursing in health and illness
- The nature of the environment.

Nurses hold views about all of these, and their own personal philosophy, beliefs and values underpin the care they give. Thus, the philosophy underlying a nursing model must be made explicit, not purely for theoretical reasons, but to enable the nurse to give the required care. The description of the Roper, Logan and Tierney Model (later) will make this clear.

In working with veterinary nurses in the classroom and in practice it is seen that some human nursing models are more readily adaptable and relevant to the care of animals than others. However, it is important that veterinary nurses make up their own minds.

It is possible to classify nursing models into four broad categories, according to their theoretical origins.

- **Developmental** models concentrate on human development and maintain that nursing care is required when the process of development is affected by illness or accident. They emphasize the processes of growth, development and maturation. The major thrust is change. Example: Orem.

■ **Systems** models see the body as a system made up of several inter-related subsystems, and focus on these physiological systems in addition to the psychological and social systems within the person as a whole. Systems models operate on the assumption that nursing interventions are required when parts of the human system are not interacting effectively or when stress occurs to disrupt equilibrium. Example: Neuman.

■ **Interaction** models focus on the interaction between the nurse and the patient, emphasizing social acts and relationships between people. These models believe that nursing interventions are necessary when a person cannot perform a role that supports or sustains health. Example: King.

■ **Energy fields** models are epitomized by the incorporation of the concept of energy, and claim that human patients are best understood not as systems or discrete parts but as unified fields of energy that interact with their environment. Example: Rogers.

Later in the chapter, one particular model will be discussed in detail to offer insight into the usefulness and potential of nursing models for veterinary practice.

Orem's Self-Care Model

Orem, a well respected nursing theorist, based her model on the concept of 'self-care' thus reducing dependency and paternalism within healthcare settings. Orem maintains that all individuals have self-care needs and have the right to meet those needs unless it is impossible for them to do so. The following offers a brief overview of the model's framework.

Universal needs with regard to self-care

■ Maintenance of sufficient intake of air.
■ Maintenance of sufficient intake of water.
■ Maintenance of sufficient intake of food.
■ Balance between activity and rest.
■ Balance between solitude and social interaction.
■ Prevention of hazards to human life, human functioning and human wellbeing.
■ Promotion of human functioning and development within social groups in accordance with human potential.
■ Known human limitations and the human desire to be 'normal'.

It seems that all apart from the last two could potentially be applied to the care of animals.

Developmental self-care requisites

These include:

■ Infancy
■ Childhood
■ Adolescence
■ Pregnancy.

Human deviation with regard to self-care requisites

■ Ill health, illness or disability result in a demand for changes in self-care behaviour.
■ The emphasis is on self-care *versus* self-care deficit.

Categories of nursing systems

■ Total compensatory nursing systems – the nurse takes full responsibility, e.g. unconscious patient, acutely ill patient.
■ Partially compensatory nursing systems – activities shared between nurse and patient, e.g. the elderly.
■ Educative/supportive nursing systems – it is acknowledged that the patient is potentially capable.

The overall goal of care planning with Orem is the elimination of self-care deficits expressed in the form of problem and goal statements. Initially, when veterinary nurses are introduced to the Orem model they may be unconvinced by its relevance and usefulness to their practice. Frequently, on closer investigation it is possible to see some potential here for adapting and revising it for their particular purpose.

The Roper, Logan and Tierney Model

One of the very few models for nursing developed in the UK and originally created as an education tool, the Roper, Logan and Tierney (RLT) Model has been widely used in veterinary practice in this country. It seems to offer veterinary nurses a framework they feel is relevant to their work and one they can more readily identify with. Educationalists have found that it provides a valuable guide to caring for animals, and as a means of enhancing student learning.

Its origins lay in Roper's study carried out in 1976 of the experience of student nurses in clinical practice and developing a conceptual framework which would enable a progression away from a disease-oriented approach to care, with medical labels attached to patients, to seeing the person as a whole. For Roper, activities of daily living were an important way of identifying the common nursing requirements shared by all patients.

An overview of the model will now be given for use by veterinary nurses; the recommended Further reading at the end of this chapter should be consulted for more detail and to gain a deeper understanding.

The model is divided into two parts: the model for living and the model for nursing.

The model for living

There are five components to the model (Figure 6.1):

■ Activities of Living (ALs)
■ Progression of a person along a lifespan that indicates movement of an individual from life to death, linked to age: infancy; childhood; adolescence; adulthood; old age

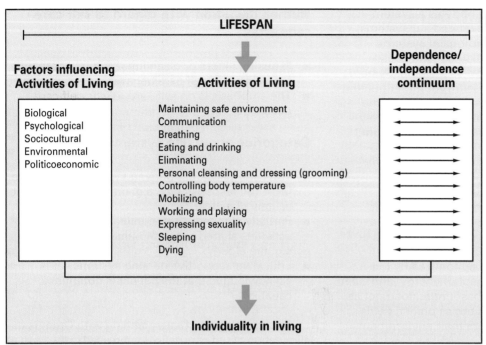

6.1 The Roper, Logan and Tierney Model for living.

- Dependence/independence continuum, which acknowledges that there are stages of a person's life when an individual cannot yet, or can no longer, perform certain ALs independently
- Factors influencing ALs:
  - Biological – the body's anatomical and physiological performance
  - Psychological – intellectual, e.g. cognitive development and emotional aspects
  - Sociocultural – societal and cultural norms, along with religious and spiritual beliefs
  - Environmental – including atmospheric components, household environment, vegetation, buildings
  - Politicoeconomic – encompasses the role of the state, the law and the economy
- Individuality in living, which stresses that each individual is unique and therefore will carry out the ALs differently.

The model for nursing

The model for nursing is the same as the model for living in all but one component, that of individualized nursing (Figure 6.2), which covers the components of the nursing process.

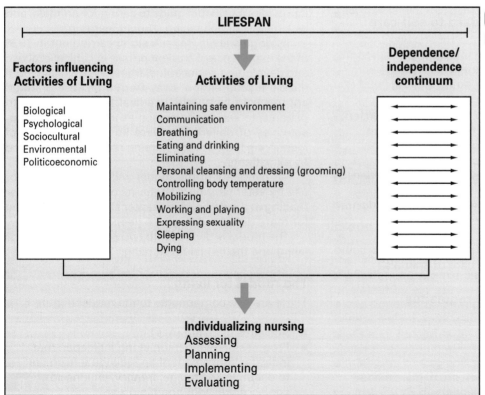

6.2 The Roper, Logan and Tierney Model for nursing.

Nurses working in the field of veterinary practice and using the RLT Model need to acknowledge how the ALs are influenced by:

- The position of the patient in the lifespan
- The levels of dependence and independence, and the methods the patient uses to cope with dependence
- The factors (biological, psychological, sociocultural, environmental, politicoeconomic) that have influenced or are influencing the patient's individual lifestyle and quality of life.

Individualized nursing care and the nursing process

An example of a form that can be used for documentation is given in Figure 6.3. These will be useful in helping veterinary nurses to plan care, using the RLT Model, for patients with a range of commonly encountered conditions such as diabetes, heart failure, renal failure, mobility issues and pain. An example of a specific condition is given in Figure 6.4; while details may vary the key principles remain the same.

PATIENT ASSESSMENT

Activities of living	Actual problems	Potential problems
Maintaining safe environment		
Expressing normal behaviour for species and age		
Breathing		
Eating and drinking		
Urinating and defecating		
Grooming		
Controlling body temperature		
Mobilizing		
Playing and going for walks		
Sleeping		
Dying/Euthanasia		
Date: Time: Signature:		

6.3   Example of a form that can be used during the assessment phase.

Patient's nursing records

OWNER'S NAME: *Mr Bloggs*
PATIENT'S NAME: *Snarf*
ADDRESS: *10 Imaginary Lane Maidupville*
POSTCODE: *MA8 4UR*
TEL NO: *01234 567890*
AGE: *Approx. 2 wks*

HOSPITAL: *ABC Vets*
WARD: *Isolation ward*
ADMISSION STATUS: *Healthy*
ADMITTED FROM: *Owner*
DATE: *3 January 2007*
TIME: *13.10*
CONSULTANT: *A. Vet*

REASON FOR ADMISSION: *Orphan kitten*
PREVIOUS MEDICAL HISTORY: *None*
CURRENT MEDICATIONS: *None*
ALLERGIES: *Unknown*

PRIMARY/NAMED NURSE: *FRED*
ADMITTING NURSE: *PHYLLIS*
INFORMATION OBTAINED FROM: *Mr Bloggs*

ADMISSION DEPENDENCY SCORE: *High*
PRESSURE ULCER RISK SCORE: *Low*
MOVING & HANDLING RISK SCORE: *Low*

VALUABLES: Retained/Sent home *Cat box*

6.4   Example of a nursing care plan for an orphaned kitten. (Template adapted from Holland *et al.*, 2003) (continues) ▶

Actual (A) and potential (P) problems

Maintaining a safe environment *Limited awareness of surroundings*	*A – Cannot maintain safe environment* *P – Injury caused to patient*
Communication *Limited ability to communicate needs*	*A – Not able to indicate needs* *P – Needs not met by nurse*
Breathing *Achieved independently*	*A – None* *P – Inhale milk while feeding*
Eating & drinking *Dependent on nurse*	*A – Cannot feed self* *P – May not receive adequate food and water*
Urinating and defecating *Dependent on nurse*	*A – Needs stimulation to eliminate* *P – Waste products may build up and cause illness*
Grooming *Dependent on nurse*	*A – Not able to clean food/urine/faeces off self* *P – Sores may develop*
Controlling body temperature *Dependent on nurse*	*A – Loses body heat rapidly* *P – Develop hypothermia*
Mobilizing *Limited ability to mobilize*	*A – Cannot move away from danger or soiling* *P – Injury occurs or sores develop*
Playing *Limited ability, dependent on nurse*	*A – Absent mother/no companion* *P – Mental boredom/separation anxiety*
Expressing sexuality *N/A – Sexually immature*	*N/A*
Sleeping *Independent* *– environmental changes needed by nurse*	*A – Requires more sleep* *P – Noise may cause lack of sleep*

6.4 (continued) Example of a nursing care plan for an orphaned kitten. (Template adapted from Holland *et al.*, 2003) (continues) ▶

Dying/Euthanasia	N/A
N/A	

Date:................................. Time:................................. Signature:.................................

PROBLEM

The patient *is neonatal with immature development of all activities of living. Requires nursing interventions to achieve maintaining safe environment, eating and drinking, eliminating, cleansing and controlling body temperature*

GOAL

The patient *needs to be provided with sufficient nursing care to increase his body weight by 15g per day, and maintain his body temperature within normal ranges. The patient should commence weaning within two weeks of admittance*

To be achieved by *(date)*

NURSING INTERVENTION

1) Maintain safe clean environment	Clean kennel daily and when soiled. Wash hands before and after handling. Isolate as unvaccinated. Make sure cannot fall through bars
2) Provide adequate nutrition	Syringe feed milk replacer, 5ml every 3 hours. Ensure milk is not inhaled. Weigh daily
3) Ensure regular elimination	Wipe perineum to encourage elimination after each feed
4) Maintain patient's hygiene	Clean patient after each feed and if necessary
5) Maintain body temperature	Supply warming blanket. Monitor body temperature daily
6) Provide mental stimulation to patient	Provide opportunities for play, e.g. provision of toys. Provide TLC at least 8x daily
7) Limit noise, light and activity during periods of sleep	Notify other staff of quiet times, dim lights to allow sleep

Signature:.................................

6.4 (continued) Example of a nursing care plan for an orphaned kitten. (Template adapted from Holland *et al.*, 2003) (continues)

▶

EVALUATION

The patient *has continued to gain weight on a daily basis. Syringe feeding should continue until 4 weeks old when weaning should commence.*

Date:................................... Signature:...

Daily evaluation/communication/progress

PATIENT'S NAME:.....*Snarf*...................................... WARD:....*Isolation*...........

A.L...

Date/Time	Remarks	Designation & Signature
8am	Snarf sleeping. Woken to change bedding and clean kennel	ME
8.10	Snarf syringe fed 5 ml Cimicat. Took slowly but finished all	FRED
	Cleaned Snarf's face and paws	
	Stimulated perineum to encourage elimination	
	Good quantity of urine and faeces passed	
	Cleaned Snarf's perineum	
9am	Weight 112g	SAM
	Temperature (rectal) 38.5°C	
	Snarf vocalizing and alert	

6.4 (continued) Example of a nursing care plan for an orphaned kitten. (Template adapted from Holland *et al.*, 2003)

Conclusion

This chapter has sought to provide an introduction to the huge topic of the nursing process and nursing models. It is hoped that the veterinary nursing profession will embrace these concepts and use them as a way of taking practice forward.

The really important thing, especially with nursing models, is to remember that they should never be used in a rigid or inflexible manner. All approaches to care should be kept 'alive' by regular questioning and testing.

Further reading

Aggleton P and Chalmers H (2000) *Nursing Models and Nursing Practice, 2nd edn.* Palgrave Macmillan, Basingstoke

Cherry M (2000) Care pathways for urinary continence problems. *Nursing Times* **96** (19), suppl. pp. 7–10

Davis S (2006) *Roper's Model for Vet Nurses. VN Times* July 2006

Holland K, Jenkins K, Solomon S and Whittam S (2003) *Applying the Roper–Logan–Tierney Model in Practice.* Churchill Livingstone, Edinburgh

Jeffery A (2007) The nursing process; Models of nursing. In: *BSAVA Textbook of Veterinary Nursing, 4th edn,* ed. DR Lane *et al.*, pp. 271–279. BSAVA Publications, Gloucester

Johnson S and Keating M (2000) Use of integrated care pathways to manage unpredictable situations. *Professional Nurse* **16,** 956–958

McGee P (1998) *Models of Nursing in Practice: A Pattern for Practical Care.* Stanley Thorne, Cheltenham

Roper N, Logan W and Tierney A (2000) *The Roper, Logan and Tierney Model of Nursing.* Churchill Livingstone, Edinburgh

7

Triage and emergency nursing

Belinda Andrews-Jones and Amanda Boag

> **This chapter is designed to give information on:**
>
> - Setting up and running an emergency room/treatment area
> - Planning for emergencies
> - Evaluation of the emergency patient (triage; primary survey; major body systems assessment)
> - Immediate treatment of life-threatening emergencies
> - Nursing and monitoring the emergency patient

Introduction

This chapter provides information for student and qualified veterinary nurses on assessing and dealing with emergency patients quickly and with confidence and competence. When presented with an emergency patient, the first aim is to recognize the severity of the problem and to take urgent action to preserve life. Especially in busy emergency practices, it is important that the nursing staff can evaluate patients accurately as they are presented, and work with the veterinary surgeon, so that patients are prioritized, and treated in the order that will maximize benefit to all patients. It is also vital that further suffering is prevented and that the emergency patient is monitored, so that any deterioration can be identified and acted upon quickly.

The term 'first aid' is often used by the general public to describe the emergency treatment administered to an injured or sick patient before professional care is available. *The best tool an emergency veterinary clinician can have is a good veterinary nurse.*

Setting up an emergency room/treatment area

All practices, including general practices and those that do predominantly emergency or out-of-hours work, should have a designated area for dealing with emergency patients. This emergency area or room should be easily accessible from as many other areas of the building as possible, including the client entry area, consulting rooms, areas with diagnostic equipment such as radiology, and any laboratory areas. Anaesthetic equipment (including oxygen) should be readily available in the emergency area. In most practices, the preparation area or induction room is most suitable, as this room is usually fitted with most of the emergency equipment needed.

All staff (including all veterinary surgeons, veterinary nurses and reception staff) should know that any emergencies should be brought to this area. The area should be well lit, spacious and tidy, and items and equipment should be placed in an orderly and methodical fashion. There should be a mobile crash box or trolley (Figure 7.1) that is well stocked and ready for use at all times. It should be the responsibility of one person in the practice (commonly a veterinary nurse) to ensure that it is checked at least once a week, as well as after every use.

Planning for emergencies

The key to treating emergency patients successfully is careful and thorough planning. This includes thinking about different emergencies that could come into the practice and how they could be assessed and helped quickly. For example:

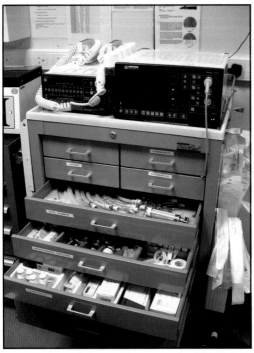

7.1
A well stocked mobile crash trolley.

■ Are the anaesthetic circuits and oxygen easily accessible?
■ Are the endotracheal tubes in order of size and are all cuffs working?
■ Are intravenous catheters of varying sizes readily available?
■ Are emergency drugs easily accessible and in date?

It is useful to have a chart of emergency drug doses for different patient weights displayed in the designated emergency area, or in the crash box or trolley itself. During an arrest situation it is essential that the correct drug dosages can be drawn up and administered rapidly without the need for prolonged or complex calculations. An example of an emergency drug dosage chart is given in Figure 7.2.

Staffing for the 'crash' situation

Successful cardiopulmonary–cerebral resuscitation (CPCR) requires a team approach and the key is planning and practice. The more people in the practice who are trained and able to help, the better it will be for the patient. The minimum number of people for CPCR is three but more (four to six) would be ideal.

Crash alarms

Large veterinary hospitals should be equipped with a commercial crash alarm that can be used to alert all staff in the building that a patient has undergone cardiorespiratory arrest and to summon all available staff to the designated emergency area. In smaller practices this may not be feasible, but a system should still be in place to alert all staff members.

Resuscitation and emergency equipment

The equipment that should be readily available in the designated emergency area is listed in Figure 7.3. All equipment should be checked regularly. An oxygen supply should be made available at all times. This is typically via an anaesthetic machine attached to a cylinder or piped oxygen supply.

Drug	Concentration	Dose	Patient bodyweight								
			3 kg	*5 kg*	*10 kg*	*15 kg*	*20 kg*	*30 kg*	*40 kg*	*50 kg*	*60 kg*
Adrenaline	1 mg/ml	0.02–0.2 mg/kg	0.6 ml	1 ml	2 ml	3 ml	4 ml	6 ml	8 ml	10 ml	12 ml
Atropine	0.6 mg/ml	0.02–0.04 mg/kg	0.1 ml	0.2 ml	0.3 ml	0.5 ml	0.7 ml	1 ml	1.3 ml	1.6 ml	2 ml
Lidocaine	20 mg/ml	2–4 mg/kg	0.3 ml	0.5 ml	1 ml	1.5 ml	2 ml	3 ml	4 ml	5 ml	6 ml
Diazepam	5 mg/ml	0.5 mg/kg	0.3 ml	0.5 ml	1 ml	1.5 ml	2 ml	3 ml	4 ml	5 ml	6 ml
Mannitol	200 mg/ml	0.5–1 g/kg over 20 min	15 ml	25 ml	50 ml	75 ml	100 ml	150 ml	200 ml	250 ml	300 ml
Furosemide	50 mg/ml	2–4 mg/kg	0.12 ml	0.2 ml	0.4 ml	0.6 ml	0.8 ml	1.2 ml	1.6 ml	2 ml	2.4 ml
Dexamethasone	2 mg/ml	0.25–1 mg/kg	0.38 ml	0.6 ml	1.3 ml	1.9 ml	2.5 ml	3.8 ml	5 ml	6.3 ml	7.5 ml

7.2 Emergency drugs chart, with examples of intravenous dosage based on the patient's bodyweight. *It is essential to check that the concentrations of drugs stocked in the practice are the same as those in the table, in order for the volumes to be correct.* Dose rates from *Plumb's Veterinary Drug Handbook* (Blackwell Publishing, 2005). If intravenous access is not immediately available, the intratracheal route can be used for most drugs (including adrenaline and atropine). In this situation the drug is usually delivered through a urinary catheter placed down the endotracheal tube. In that case, the dosage of the medication should be doubled and a deep patient breath given just after the drug is delivered. The catheter must be flushed with 5 ml sterile saline to ensure that drug is not left in catheter. **Drugs should only be administered under the direct instruction of a veterinary surgeon.**

Oxygen supply (piped or cylinder)	Anaesthetic circuits, ideally: modified T-piece for patients <10 kg; Bain for patients >10 kg 'Ambu' bag
Airway	Cuffed endotracheal tubes of varying sizes (all cuffs checked regularly) Stylet to facilitate intubation (e.g. proprietary stylet, rigid plastic male urinary catheter) Syringe for inflation of endotracheal tube cuff White open-weave tape for securing (tying-in) of the tube Laryngoscope with blades of varying size Large-bore over-the-needle catheter for tracheal oxygen delivery Tracheostomy kit with tubes of varying size Artery forceps Suction equipment; syringe with urinary catheter attached; hand-held suction; suction pump
Drugs (see Figure 7.2 for doses)	Adrenaline (epinephrine)[a] Atropine[a] Lidocaine[a] Calcium gluconate (10%) Dextrose (glucose) (50%) Dobutamine Dexamethasone Doxopram Diazepam Furosemide Glyceryl trinitrate (2%) paste Sodium bicarbonate Mannitol Multiple syringes of heparinized saline should be available Emergency drug dosages chart should be readily available
Catheters	Over-the-needle catheters of varying sizes for intravenous access Intraosseous needles Tape to secure catheters Butterfly catheters for thoracocentesis Equipment for placement of intravenous catheters (see Chapter 8)
Fluid therapy	Isotonic replacement crystalloid (e.g. Hartmann's solution, 0.9% saline) Colloid
Equipment	Scalpel blades Syringes (multiple sizes) Electrocardiograph Electrode gel Defibrillator with external and internal paddles Defibrillator dosage chart Stopwatch/clock Pen and paper for recording information
Asepsis	Surgical scrub and surgical spirit Sterile surgical gloves of appropriate sizes

7.3   Resuscitation equipment. [a] These can be preloaded and labelled so that they are ready to use in an emergency, saving valuable seconds.

Triage of the emergency patient

Triage (meaning 'sorting out') is the process of determining rapidly the urgency of the problem in an emergency patient. This is an extremely important role for the nurse working in emergency practice. All emergency patients should be assessed ('triaged') by a trained nurse as soon as they arrive. The information collected by the nurse can greatly affect the treatment and thus outcome for that patient.

The nurse should assess the severity of the problem and then decide whether the patient must be seen by the veterinary surgeon immediately. This may involve calling the veterinary surgeon away from another consultation or operation. Ideally, the nurse and veterinary surgeon work as a team to make sure that patients are prioritized and treated in the most appropriate order.

When the veterinary surgeon is unavoidably busy, the triage nurse should deliver patient information accurately and should note, for example, whether the patient is unconscious or conscious and whether there are any breathing problems, circulation problems, wounds, bleeding, or bone, joint or soft tissue injuries. This triage does not replace a full clinical examination, which should always be performed by a veterinary surgeon, but it does provide an initial assessment of the severity of the patient's problem, allowing prompt, appropriate and potentially life-saving action.

Telephone triage

The veterinary team commonly becomes aware of veterinary emergencies when an owner telephones. A form of triage is also used on the telephone, with the nurse gaining information about the pet and its problem that can help to determine the urgency of the problem. It also enables the nurse to give appropriate advice regarding whether the pet needs to be seen and any advice regarding transportation. The information obtained during the telephone call will be useful when preparing the emergency room for the patient's arrival.

Caution should be used concerning the owner's interpretation of the patient's condition, as most owners are not medically trained and may be quite distressed by the situation.

If an owner reports any of the following problems, they should be advised that their pet needs to be evaluated by a veterinary surgeon as soon as possible:

- **Respiratory distress or difficulty with breathing**
- **Pale mucous membranes**
- **Collapse**
- **Sudden weakness**
- **Rapidly distending abdomen**
- **Inability to urinate**
- **Ingestion of toxins**
- **Traumatic injuries**
- **Severe vomiting**
- **Blood in vomit**
- **Unproductive retching**
- **Neurological problem or seizures**
- **Difficulty with giving birth**
- **Large wounds**
- **Bleeding**

Any patient that has, or could have, suffered a traumatic injury should be seen with urgency, even if the owner reports that the pet looks well.

A lot of information can be obtained in a short time and important questions for traumatic and medical emergencies are summarized below. This information is very valuable both in preparing for the arrival of the patient and in considering what urgent treatment might be needed. It will also help the veterinary surgeon to start to form an idea of what the underlying nature of the patient's problem might be.

Questions to ask in trauma cases:

- **How did the trauma happen?**
- **When did it happen?**
- **How is the animal breathing?**
- **Carefully lift up the animal's lip: what is the colour of the gums?**
- **Is there any bleeding?**
- **Is the animal conscious?**
- **Is the animal walking/moving?**
- **Can you see any injuries or wounds?**
- **Species and breed?**

Questions to ask in non-trauma emergencies:

- **Species, breed and sex?**
- **Can you explain the problem?**
- **How is the animal breathing?**
- **Carefully lift up the animal's lip: what is the colour of the gums?**
- **Is the animal conscious?**
- **Is there any vomiting or diarrhoea? If so: how often and what colour?**
- **Has the animal had this problem before?**
- **Is the animal on any medication?**

Capsule history

A 'capsule history' should be obtained from owners of all emergency patients. This form of history focuses on obtaining important information that could alter the early management of the patient. It may be necessary for either the nurse or the veterinary surgeon to return to the owner for a more detailed history once the patient is more stable. Important questions to ask in a capsule history include:

- Age, sex and neutering status of the animal?
- If an entire female, when was her last season or litter?
- Is the animal on any medication?
- Has the animal been diagnosed with any long-term medical problems?
- Does the animal have any known allergies?
- Has the animal had access to any toxins?
- When was the last time the animal ate and drank?
- When was the last time the animal passed faeces and urine and were these normal?

Triage action on arrival of an emergency patient

- **When dealing with a emergency patient the triage nurse should be brisk, calm and controlled.**
- **The priority is to ensure that any risks are identified for the nurse, the patient and anyone else (e.g. the owner).**
- **When evaluating an emergency patient, especially if they may be in pain, caution should be used and the triage nurse should always ask themselves whether they are about to put themselves in any physical danger. If they are in any doubt, further help should be called for. *Never put yourself at risk!***
- **A logical approach to the emergency patient ensures that important problems are not missed. The triage nurse should follow a clear plan of action that will allow the prioritization of patient problems and stabilization and treatment strategies.**

Primary survey

The first procedure that the triage nurse should perform is called the primary survey, which should only take about 60 seconds to perform. Essentially the primary survey involves checking that the patient is still alive and that it does not seem likely to undergo imminent cardiorespiratory arrest. The mnemonic ABC should be followed:

- **A**irway – does the patient have a patent airway?
- **B**reathing – is the patient making useful breathing efforts?
- **C**irculation – does the patient have evidence of spontaneous circulation (heartbeat, pulses)?

It should also be determined whether the patient is conscious.

Once this assessment has been carried out, and as long as the triage nurse is satisfied that the patient is not likely to undergo cardiorespiratory arrest, the next step is to carry out a secondary survey, i.e. a major body systems assessment (see later). However, if the nurse has any concerns at all that the patient's airway, breathing or circulation is not adequate, the patient should be taken immediately to the designated emergency area and the veterinary surgeon called for.

Recognition of cardiopulmonary arrest

Early recognition of actual or impending cardiopulmonary arrest is vital to a successful outcome. Signs of impending or actual arrest include:

- Agonal (gasping, laboured) breathing pattern, *or* absence of useful respiratory movements
- Weak and rapid pulses that will usually slow rapidly and dramatically shortly before arrest, *or* absence of a heartbeat and pulse
- Loss of consciousness
- Fixed dilated pupils and lack of a palpebral and corneal reflex.

Mucous membrane colour and capillary refill time may remain normal for many minutes after cessation of effective circulation. If the patient is being monitored by electrocardiography, the electrocardiogram trace (ECG) may also remain relatively normal for several minutes after death. Presence of an ECG should not be taken to mean that the patient is alive.

Cardiorespiratory arrest will result if oxygen supply to the heart and brain are disrupted, as oxygen is essential to sustain cellular respiration. Oxygen is taken in to the body through the lungs and transferred to the red blood cells in the bloodstream. The heart then pumps the red cells, and hence oxygen, around the body, where it is transferred to cells. When cells are deprived of oxygen, they can die rapidly. The brain tissue is particularly sensitive to lack of oxygen and when brain cells are deprived of oxygen death rapidly follows. The longer the brain is starved of oxygen, the more likely it is that permanent brain damage will occur, even if the animal survives. For a successful outcome, cardiorespiratory arrest must be recognized and treated quickly.

Definitions

- **Respiratory arrest** – cessation of effective respiration
- **Cardiorespiratory arrest** – cessation of effective cardiac output and respiration
- **Basic life support** – chest compressions and artificial ventilation
- **Advanced life support (ALS)** – basic life support plus medical intervention

The term **cardiopulmonary–cerebral resuscitation (CPCR) emphasizes the importance of neurological outcome.**

Importance of an open airway

In an unconscious patient the airway may become blocked or narrowed due to the position of the neck and the tongue. The patient's muscles will tend to relax and could occlude the pharyngeal region, especially in breeds with a large amount of soft tissue in this area such as Bulldogs. It is vital that the airway is clear and open to allow adequate ventilation and oxygen delivery to the lungs.

An unconscious patient should be placed in lateral recumbency (preferably right lateral to aid chest compression if necessary) with its head tilted up (dorsally), its mouth held gently open and the tongue gently pulled out. The airway should be examined to ensure that it is clear, but caution should be exercised and the safety of the staff working with the animal must not be compromised.

WARNING
- **Watch your fingers!**
- **Never place fingers in a conscious patient's mouth!**

Cardiopulmonary–cerebral resuscitation procedure

All members of staff – including student veterinary nurses, animal nursing assistants, receptionists and any lay staff – can and should be trained in basic CPCR. They can all be trained to carry out one or more tasks.

All practices should have regular CPCR training sessions, where all can rehearse their responsibilities.

Various veterinary CPCR models are available but stuffed toys of various sizes can also be used to imitate patients. Different scenarios should be considered. After the practice session, or after a real CPCR, there should be a review/self-evaluation to encourage and facilitate ongoing improvements.

Following recognition that a patient has undergone cardiopulmonary arrest, the following tasks should be carried out as quickly and smoothly as possible:

- Placement and securing (tying-in) of an endotracheal tube
- Provision of oxygen and ventilation

- Placement and securing of an intravenous catheter (listed veterinary nurses must be under the direction of a veterinary surgeon; student veterinary nurses must be under the direct supervision of a listed veterinary nurse or veterinary surgeon)
- Placement of an ECG to help the veterinary surgeon decide on appropriate medications
- Provision of external cardiac compressions if indicated.

The precise order in which these tasks are carried out may vary slightly depending on the patient and the number and experience of staff. The patient is typically placed in right lateral recumbency.

It is also vital that a person is nominated to 'run the crash' as soon as possible. This person would usually be a veterinary surgeon but an experienced nurse may need to take this role until a veterinary surgeon arrives. It is this person's responsibility to direct the other members of the team and ensure that all tasks are being carried out.

Depending on the number and training of staff present, the following roles are usually assigned:

- One person to provide adequate ventilation
- One person to undertake chest compressions
- One person to monitor the patient, including feeling for pulses
- One person to draw up drugs as requested by the veterinary surgeon and to record all medications given as well as any other interventions.

Chest compressions

The aim of chest compressions is to cause pressure changes in the heart itself and in the chest cavity, which force blood forwards through the circulatory system. If successful, an assistant should be able to palpate a femoral pulse that is being created with the compressions.

Abdominal counterpressure

If there are more than four people available, it may be helpful for someone to perform abdominal counterpressure. This involves pressing down firmly on the abdomen between chest compressions. It acts to increase venous return to the chest and improves blood pressure and cerebral and myocardial perfusion.

Advanced life support drugs

Once an ECG has been obtained, the veterinary surgeon may want to administer drugs to return the heart to a normal rhythm. Although a veterinary nurse does not need to understand fully the mechanism of action of each drug, having an understanding of what drug is appropriate and why can make both the nurse's and the veterinary surgeon's jobs quicker and easier. An experienced nurse can start to prepare drugs that are likely to be necessary so that they can be administered as soon as they are asked for.

The three drugs used most commonly during resuscitation are adrenaline, atropine and lidocaine.

Adrenaline (epinephrine)

This is a peripheral vasoconstrictor that acts to increase essential blood flow to the heart and brain. It is used in asystole (flat line on ECG) and pulse-less electrical activity (normal appearance to ECG but no pulse produced), which are the two commonest arrest rhythms in dogs and cats.

Atropine

This anticholinergic drug reduces vagal tone. It is used to control severe bradycardia which may lead to asystole or pulse-less electrical activity.

Lidocaine

This is an antiarrhythmic drug. It is used as a chemical defibrillator and for the treatment of ventricular arrhythmias such as fast ventricular tachycardia.

Electrical defibrillation

The purpose of electrical defibrillation is to shock the heart from a chaotic non-pulse-producing electrical activity (commonly ventricular fibrillation) to a normal sinus rhythm. It does this by passing a large electrical charge through the heart, with the hope of causing the cardiac cells to depolarize and then repolarize.

Defibrillation is only useful in cases where arrest has been caused by ventricular fibrillation or rapid ventricular tachycardia. It is not useful for the treatment of asystole (flat line ECG). Ventricular fibrillation is the most common arrest rhythm in humans, which means that defibrillators are commonly used in human medicine. It is only a rare cause of arrest in dogs and cats but, if a patient does present with fibrillation, a rapid response is required as the chance of successful defibrillation is highest when the heart is defibrillated immediately after onset of the rhythm. Excessive energy levels and repeated defibrillation can cause myocardial damage; therefore it is best to start at the lower energy levels and increase as needed.

Extreme caution must be exercised whenever a defibrillator is being used. One person who is trained to operate the machine should be in charge and should instruct all other personnel to 'Clear!' (stand clear) before discharging the defibrillator. Before the defibrillator is discharged, all personnel must be clear of the patient and of the table the patient is on or there is a risk of serious injury. Defibrillators should never be used by untrained personnel. Alcohol-based solvents should never be used in the proximity of the defibrillator.

Precordial thump

This has been advocated as a method of converting ventricular fibrillation to sinus rhythm if an electrical defibrillator is not available. Firm blunt pressure should be applied to the ribs directly overlying the heart with the aim of temporarily stopping and then resynchronizing cardiac rhythm. The success rate of a precordial thump is poor.

Figure 7.4 summarizes the steps to follow when presented with an emergency patient.

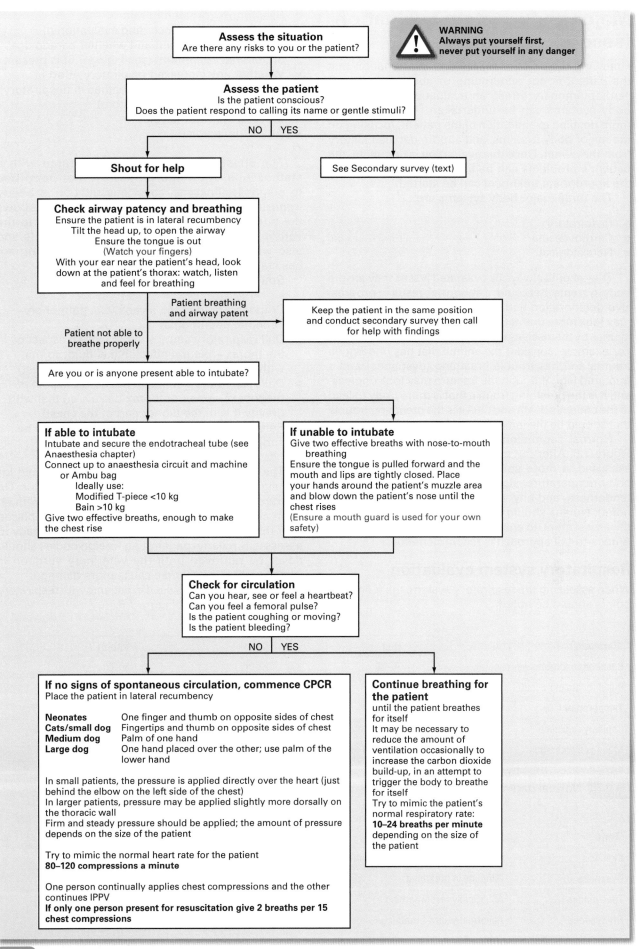

Assess the situation
Are there any risks to you or the patient?

WARNING
Always put yourself first, never put yourself in any danger

Assess the patient
Is the patient conscious?
Does the patient respond to calling its name or gentle stimuli?

NO | YES

Shout for help

See Secondary survey (text)

Check airway patency and breathing
Ensure the patient is in lateral recumbency
Tilt the head up, to open the airway
Ensure the tongue is out
(Watch your fingers)
With your ear near the patient's head, look down at the patient's thorax: watch, listen and feel for breathing

Patient breathing and airway patent

Keep the patient in the same position and conduct secondary survey then call for help with findings

Patient not able to breathe properly

Are you or is anyone present able to intubate?

If able to intubate
Intubate and secure the endotracheal tube (see Anaesthesia chapter)
Connect up to anaesthesia circuit and machine or Ambu bag
Ideally use:
Modified T-piece <10 kg
Bain >10 kg
Give two effective breaths, enough to make the chest rise

If unable to intubate
Give two effective breaths with nose-to-mouth breathing
Ensure the tongue is pulled forward and the mouth and lips are tightly closed. Place your hands around the patient's muzzle area and blow down the patient's nose until the chest rises
(Ensure a mouth guard is used for your own safety)

Check for circulation
Can you hear, see or feel a heartbeat?
Can you feel a femoral pulse?
Is the patient coughing or moving?
Is the patient bleeding?

NO | YES

If no signs of spontaneous circulation, commence CPCR
Place the patient in lateral recumbency

Neonates	One finger and thumb on opposite sides of chest
Cats/small dog	Fingertips and thumb on opposite sides of chest
Medium dog	Palm of one hand
Large dog	One hand placed over the other; use palm of the lower hand

In small patients, the pressure is applied directly over the heart (just behind the elbow on the left side of the chest)
In larger patients, pressure may be applied slightly more dorsally on the thoracic wall
Firm and steady pressure should be applied; the amount of pressure depends on the size of the patient

Try to mimic the normal heart rate for the patient
80–120 compressions a minute

One person continually applies chest compressions and the other continues IPPV
If only one person present for resuscitation give 2 breaths per 15 chest compressions

Continue breathing for the patient
until the patient breathes for itself
It may be necessary to reduce the amount of ventilation occasionally to increase the carbon dioxide build-up, in an attempt to trigger the body to breathe for itself
Try to mimic the patient's normal respiratory rate:
10–24 breaths per minute
depending on the size of the patient

7.4 Steps to be followed when presented with an emergency patient.

Major body system evaluation (secondary survey)

Following the primary survey and confirmation that the patient is not undergoing or about to undergo cardiopulmonary arrest, an evaluation of the major body systems can be undertaken. This involves a more detailed examination of the patient, focusing on the major body systems, and a more detailed history from the owner. Once this evaluation is complete, the patient's problems can be listed and prioritized and the appropriate treatment can be started.

The three major body systems are:

- Respiratory
- Cardiovascular
- Neurological.

They should always be evaluated first as they are the body systems that could, if abnormal, result in progressive deterioration and death. Although other injuries may look more dramatic (e.g. wounds, fractures) these injuries by themselves will not cause the animal's death. For example, consider the animal that has undergone trauma and has trouble breathing (dyspnoea) and a fractured leg. Although the fracture may look unpleasant, it is the breathing trouble that is more likely to lead to the patient's death and thus it is the breathing trouble that should be the initial focus of treatment.

Normal parameters for vital signs are set out in Figure 7.5. After the major body systems have been assessed, a more complete examination including body temperature, signs of abdominal swelling and tenderness, and any wounds or fractures should be noted. Nurses should have a routine for performing the assessment, to ensure that all areas are evaluated. A nose-to-tail approach is recommended.

Respiratory system evaluation

When assessing the respiratory system, the following points should be noted:

- Respiratory (breathing) rate
- Respiratory effort, including evaluation of abdominal movement and whether paradoxical abdominal movement (see Figure 7.6) is present
- Whether any increased respiratory effort is principally as the animal breathes in (inspiratory) or as it breathes out (expiratory)
- Mucous membrane colour
- Any audible noise.

The chest should also be auscultated with a stethoscope. Although nurses are not permitted to diagnose illnesses, chest auscultation is a very important skill to practise and develop. It allows the nurse to provide important information to the veterinary surgeon when the animal presents and also when monitoring the animal after treatment has started.

Sounds that may be heard include:

- Crackles – fluid in the alveoli (e.g. pulmonary oedema, pneumonia)
- Dull respiratory sounds in the ventral aspect of the thorax – pleural effusion (i.e. fluid, so that with gravity it is in the lower part of the chest)
- Dull respiratory sounds in the dorsal aspect of the thorax – pneumothorax (i.e. air, so that with gravity it is in the higher part of the chest)
- Referred upper airway sounds (should also be audible externally without stethoscope).

The external thorax should also be examined for any signs of injury or penetrating foreign bodies. On the rare occasion where the animal presents with an open chest wound, a sterile cover should be placed over this area until the veterinary surgeon is ready to assess it. Similarly, penetrating foreign bodies should never be removed until the veterinary surgeon is ready; early removal may cause more damage.

Definitions of terms used in patients with respiratory distress are shown in Figure 7.6.

Parameter	Dog	Cat	Rabbit
Respiration (breaths per minute)	10–30	20–30	30–60
Pulse (beats per minute)	60–100	160–200	180–300
Temperature (°C)	38.3–38.7	38.0–38.5	38.5–40.0
Capillary refill time	1–2 seconds	1–2 seconds	1–2 seconds
Mucous membranes	Pink and moist	Pale pink and moist	Pale pink and moist

7.5   Normal parameters for vital signs.

Term	Definition
Cyanosis	Blue–purple coloration of the mucous membranes associated with a lack of oxygen
Dyspnoea	Difficulty in breathing
Tachypnoea	Abnormally fast breathing
Bradypnoea	Abnormally slow breathing

7.6   Terms used to describe respiratory distress. (continues)   ▶

Term	Definition
Orthopnoea	Ability to breathe in upright position only; characteristically animals extend their necks and hold their forelimbs with elbows abducted (pointing outwards)
Pneumothorax	Air in the pleural space
Open pneumothorax	Air in the pleural space where there is a direct communication between the pleural space and the outside, often from a traumatic injury
Tension pneumothorax	Large air accumulation in the pleural space where a piece of tissue acts as a ball valve, meaning that air enters but then cannot escape from the pleural space. The pleural pressure increases with every breath and high pressures can be generated. This has negative effects on cardiovascular as well as respiratory function as the heart, great vessels and lungs are compressed. Although very rare, this is life-threatening
Haemothorax	Blood in the pleural space
Pyothorax	Pus/bacterial infection in the pleural space
Pulmonary contusions	Bleeding into the alveoli (equivalent to bruising of the lung)
Haemoptysis	Coughing up blood
Paradoxical breathing	A sign of marked inspiratory effort. When an animal breathes in normally, the chest and abdomen move out together (diaphragm flattens). With paradoxical breathing, as the animal breathes in the chest moves out but the diaphragm gets sucked forward and the abdomen moves in
Hypoxia	Low levels of oxygen in blood and/or tissues
Hypercapnia	Raised levels of carbon dioxide in blood (poor ventilation)
Hypocapnia	Decreased levels of carbon dioxide in blood (increased ventilation)

7.6   (continued) Terms used to describe respiratory distress.

Common causes of tachypnoea or dyspnoea in small animal patients include:

- Upper airway obstruction
- Pleural effusion/disease
- Parenchymal disease
  - Cardiogenic oedema (heart failure)
  - Pneumonia
- Feline asthma
- Pulmonary thromboembolism
- Diaphragmatic/chest wall rupture
- Respiratory fatigue/paralysis
- Severe (acute) anaemia.

Dyspnoea

The most important nursing aims for dyspnoeic patients are to:

- minimize stress
- administer oxygen
- keep the patient cool.

All dyspnoeic patients (especially cats) should be handled very cautiously. Excessive handling and stress can make their breathing worse and may even precipitate respiratory arrest. Struggling against restraint is particularly harmful, as it uses up large amounts of oxygen in the muscles, meaning that this oxygen is not available for more vital organs.

Following arrival at the practice, patients should be placed in a stress-free oxygen-enriched environment to allow them to calm down before any procedures are attempted. Procedures such as placing an intravenous catheter should be done with as little restraint as possible. Plenty of time should be left between different procedures (e.g. catheter placement and drawing blood) to allow the patient to recover. If the patient becomes more dyspnoeic whilst a procedure is being undertaken, the procedure should be stopped and the animal allowed to recover before it is tried again.

Often dyspnoeic patients (especially those whose dyspnoea is caused by an upper airway problem) have increased body temperature. This is associated both with an inability to cool themselves via the respiratory tract (i.e. panting) and with the increased heat generated by the increased effort of breathing. Active cooling measures may be needed (see Hyperthermia).

Ideally, an intravenous catheter should be placed in dyspnoeic patients. This allows administration of drugs on the veterinary surgeon's advice. Drugs used to treat different kinds of dyspnoea that may be administered intravenously include: sedatives such as acepromazine for upper airway dyspnoea; furosemide, for pulmonary oedema; and corticosteroids, for feline asthma and sometimes upper airway dyspnoea. If an intravenous catheter cannot be placed safely due to patient stress, the intramuscular route can often be used.

Oxygen supplementation

Oxygen supplementation is always indicated in the dyspnoeic patient and allows better oxygenation with less respiratory effort from the patient. The methods of oxygen supplementation (Figure 7.7) will depend on what facilities are available. It should be remembered that the administration of oxygen should be done in the least stressful way possible for that patient.

Method	Advantages	Disadvantages
Oxygen cage (commercial)	Well tolerated by the patient. Able to supply oxygen without any restraint. Patient can relax. Some have built-in temperature and humidity controls that allow cooling of hyperthermic patients and prevent the cage becoming too warm or moist. Some have openings of differing size to allow some monitoring and procedures but still maintain required oxygen content	Expensive to buy and to run. Uses a lot of oxygen, but some have built-in circle systems with soda lime, so oxygen can be re-used and carbon dioxide removed. Have to remove patient from oxygen for most procedures. As soon as large cage door is opened all supplementary oxygen is lost
Paediatric incubator	Similar to above. Good visibility. Some have built-in humidifiers	Unlikely to have humidity control. Can be expensive but may be purchased second-hand from human hospitals
Homemade oxygen cage, plastic-covered cage front	Inexpensive to make	Large amount of oxygen needed, and this usually only makes small difference to inspired oxygen content. Humidity can increase to excess. Carbon dioxide has no way of escaping and can build up. Patients often become overheated. As soon as cage door is opened, supplementary oxygen is lost
Elizabethan collar with clingfilm partially covering front	Inexpensive	Not well tolerated by most patients. Humidity levels increase rapidly. Oxygen levels cannot be increased to very high levels due to leakage
Flow-by oxygen (oxygen supply tube held in front of patient's nose and mouth)	Useful on admission of dyspnoeic patients	Acceptable for only very short periods. Some patients dislike sound/presence of tube and air
Mask (clear masks are better than black masks)	Inexpensive	Not well tolerated by most patients; most dislike presence of mask. Only suitable for very short time
Nasal oxygen prongs (Figure 7.8)	Relatively non-invasive and allow easy patient assessment. Inexpensive	Prongs can irritate patient's nares. Can dry nasal mucosa unless humidified oxygen is used. Not as useful if patient is mouth breathing/panting
Nasal oxygen cannula (Figures 7.9 and 7.10)	Can be used even if patient is mouth breathing/panting, as the oxygen is supplied to the caudal nasal chamber. Inexpensive. Good patient cooperation	Can be difficult to place in conscious patients. Very drying to nasal mucosa/oropharynx unless humidified oxygen used. Not tolerated by some patients
Intubation and ventilation	Can provide 100% oxygen. Can be life saving in some diseases where other methods of oxygen supplementation fail	Requires 24-hour facility with intensive nursing facilities. Requires patient be anaesthetized or sedated. Complications may develop if used long term

7.7   Oxygen administration methods: advantages and disadvantages.

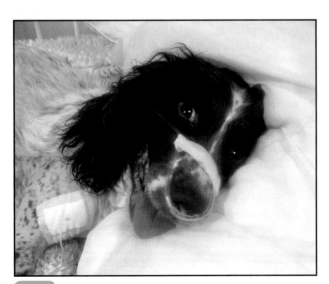

7.8   Dog with nasal oxygen prongs in place.

Nasal cannulation

A very effective and inexpensive method of supplying oxygen therapy is by means of a nasal cannula, the placement of which is described and illustrated in Figures 7.9 and 7.10. Commercial nasal cannulae can be bought but a soft rubber feeding tube can be used instead and is very effective. Inspired oxygen concentrations up to 50% can be achieved.

Humidified oxygen

Humidification of oxygen is important when long-term (more than 2–4 hours) oxygen supplementation is needed. Oxygen supplied from a tank contains no moisture, whereas the air that is normally breathed contains some water vapour. Air also undergoes further humidification in the nasal passages before entering the lower respiratory tract. If dry air is breathed into the lower airways, they can become dry, irritated and damaged.

Materials required
6–10 FG infant feeding tube
Local anaesthetic (ophthalmic local anaesthetic drops work well)
Sterile lubricant
2 x zinc oxide tape strips, 1 cm x 2 cm
Non-absorbable monofilament suture material with needle OR 'superglue'

Method
1. Apply local anaesthetic drops to one or both nares. Wait 5 minutes for the drops to work.
2. Measure the feeding tube against the animal, from the tip of the nares to the medial canthus of the eye. Make a mark with a pen on the feeding tube at the required length.
3. An assistant may be required to hold the patient's head.
4. Apply sterile lubricant to the feeding tube and insert the tube into one of the nares, passing it in a medioventral direction, until the marker is reached. Hold on to the tube until it is secured in place, as the patient may sneeze it out.
5. Secure the tube to the patient using tape and either sutures or glue. Place a piece of tape over the tube at the level of the nares (just lateral to the alar fold). This tape can be glued or sutured to the skin at that point. A second piece of tape should be attached to the tube and then to the skin on either the medial dorsal aspect of the nose or the side of the face.
    Using tape applied to the tube to secure it to the patient prevents occlusion of the tube by sutures and allows a larger surface area if glue is to be used. Glue is painless to apply and easier and quicker to use, but has the disadvantage of being slightly more difficult to remove and may not be as aesthetically pleasing to owners. Sutures can be more painful and take longer to place and are marginally more invasive to the patient but are easier to remove.
6. Attach oxygen tubing with an adapter to the feeding tube and deliver oxygen at 2–3 litres per minute. The oxygen must be humidified.
7. If the patient appears to be irritated by the tube, reduce the oxygen flow and instil local anaesthetic drops into the nares.

7.9 Placement of a nasal cannula for oxygen delivery.

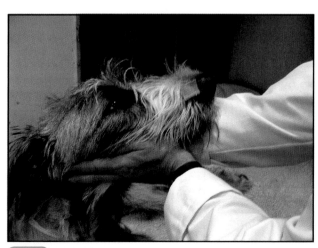

7.10 Patient with nasal cannula in place.

Commercial humidifiers (Figure 7.11) can be attached to the oxygen supply; the oxygen bubbles through the sterile saline in the humidifying bottle, collects tiny droplets of saline and delivers them to the patient's airway.

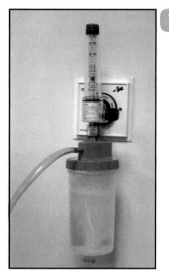

7.11 Humidifier.

Oxygen toxicity

Theoretically, if oxygen is breathed at high concentrations (>80%) for prolonged periods of time (over 24 hours), it can be toxic to the lungs. This situation is very unlikely to arise in veterinary medicine.

Ways of assessing and monitoring oxygen needs

Other than the degree of dyspnoea (as assessed by physical examination), there are a number of techniques that can be used to evaluate the severity of hypoxia and monitor the response to therapy.

Arterial blood gases

This is the 'gold standard' technique for measuring respiratory dysfunction. It involves taking a blood sample from an artery (commonly the dorsal metatarsal artery) and processing it through a blood gas analyser. Although these analysers were traditionally very expensive, cheaper machines can now be bought and an increasing number are now found in veterinary practices, especially those with high emergency caseloads. The analyser allows accurate monitoring not only of blood oxygen levels but also of blood carbon dioxide, pH, bicarbonate and acid–base content.

Carbon dioxide is important, as it is the waste product of tissue respiration. It is carried in the blood to the lungs, then moves into the alveoli and is exhaled. When a patient reduces the amount or rate at which they breathe (or stops breathing), the carbon dioxide within the bloodstream increases rapidly and this can cause further problems.

Pulse oximetry

Pulse oximeters measure the percentage oxygen saturation of haemoglobin (the molecule that carries oxygen) in the blood. They work by passing light through the skin and capillaries, which is differentially absorbed depending on the proportion of oxyhaemoglobin present. The machine gives a reading that reflects the percentage of haemoglobin that is saturated with oxygen. It should be remembered that, due to the shape of the oxyhaemoglobin dissociation curve, pulse oximetry is insensitive to early hypoxia and values of 90–93% should be a cause for serious concern.

A good pulse wave in the peripheral circulation is needed for a pulse oximeter to function correctly and this can be a problem in emergency patients. Other factors that may compromise the accuracy of the pulse oximeter include patient movement and pigmented skin.

Thoracic radiography

Chest radiographs can be very useful in the assessment of the dyspnoeic emergency patient and can help the veterinary surgeon to reach a diagnosis as to the cause of the dyspnoea. Radiography is, however, often very stressful for the patient; supplemental oxygen should be provided and the patient should be monitored very closely for worsening respiratory distress. If this occurs, radiography may have to be delayed until the patient is more stable. **Dyspnoeic patients should never be put on their backs (dorsal recumbency) for radiography.**

Specific causes of dyspnoea and emergency treatment

Upper airway obstruction (including choking)

Patients with upper airway obstruction commonly present with loud breathing sounds audible without a stethoscope, extreme distress, and cyanotic mucous membranes. Rarely, the breathing sounds can be quiet due to very little air movement. Upper airway obstructions are most commonly due to anatomical problems, such as laryngeal paralysis or elongated soft palate, but occasionally airway foreign bodies are seen. A veterinary surgeon's help should be sought as soon as possible.

Key actions with patients with upper airway obstruction are to:

- Calm the patient or sedate it (on the advice of a veterinary surgeon)
- Keep the patient cool
- Administer supplemental oxygen.

Occasionally these patients cannot be treated successfully in this way. In this situation, the nurse should anticipate that the patient might undergo respiratory arrest and should prepare for general anaesthesia and endotracheal intubation or tracheostomy. As these patients often have abnormal airways, a range of different-sized endotracheal tubes should be provided, including some much smaller than would normally be used. A male dog urinary catheter may also be useful. Equipment for tracheal catheterization and tracheostomy should also be made ready.

Pleural space disease

This is a common cause of dyspnoea in dogs and cats. Although a veterinary surgeon would usually make the diagnosis, the nurse may be suspicious if the animal has rapid shallow breaths and dull lung sounds on auscultation. Treatment involves thoracocentesis (i.e. using a needle to drain the pleural space of either fluid or air).

Thoracocentesis

Equipment for thoracocentesis may be urgently required and includes:

- **Butterfly catheter (cats and small dogs) or over-the-needle catheter (large dogs)**
- **Three-way stopcock**
- **Extension tubing if catheter used**
- **Syringe (20 ml for cats and small dogs; 60 ml for large dogs)**
- **Sterile scrub**
- **Plain and EDTA tubes for collection of samples for further analysis.**

The chest wall is clipped and scrubbed prior to the veterinary surgeon inserting the needle. Typically the area clipped should be large and should include rib spaces 7–10 on both sides of the chest.

Diaphragmatic rupture

Diaphragmatic rupture (a tear in the diaphragm) may be seen following blunt trauma to the chest or abdomen (e.g. road traffic accident). Abdominal organs (commonly the liver but sometimes the stomach or intestines) can penetrate through the diaphragm into the chest cavity and cause a space-occupying lesion that reduces the ability of the lungs to expand. Although these patients may show severe respiratory compromise if a large rupture is present, this is very rare. Most diaphragmatic ruptures produce only mild clinical signs. These patients should receive oxygen supplementation and should be encouraged to sit in sternal recumbency to maximize oxygenation.

Cardiovascular system evaluation

When assessing the cardiovascular system the following points should be noted:

- Heart rate
- Heart rhythm (regular, irregular)
- Pulse rate
- Pulse quality
- Synchronicity of pulse rate and heart rate (pulse deficits)
- Mucous membrane colour
- Capillary refill time.

Heart rate and pulses

Heart rate should be between 60 and 100 beats per minute (bpm) in a normal dog at rest, though up to 120 bpm is acceptable in a veterinary consulting room. Contrary to popular belief, this varies very little with the size of the dog. Most normal cats will have heart rates in the range of 160–200 bpm when arriving at a veterinary practice.

The rhythm should be regular and there should be a pulse for every heartbeat. The presence of pulse deficits (a heartbeat heard without feeling a pulse) is indicative of a arrhythmia and suggests that it would be beneficial to record an ECG. The pulse quality should also be described and may range from a tall narrow (or bounding) pulse in early shock, through to a barely palpable weak or thready pulse in late shock (Figure 7.12).

The capillary refill time (CRT) should be assessed by pressing the thumb firmly on the gingival mucosa (usually just above the canine tooth) until it blanches and then noting the time it takes for the colour to return (Figure 7.14). In a normal animal this should be about 1.5 seconds. Both slow and fast CRTs may be seen.

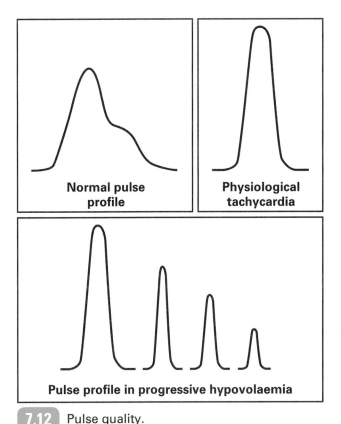

7.12 Pulse quality.

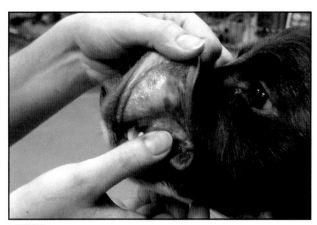

7.14 Assessing capillary refill time.

Mucous membrane colour and capillary refill time

Mucous membranes should normally be pink (slightly paler in cats). Changes in mucous membrane colour may suggest a number of different conditions (Figure 7.13).

Shock

The main purpose of a cardiovascular system examination in an emergency patient is to detect the presence of shock. In the veterinary field, shock is defined as a lack of oxygen delivery to the tissues. This occurs most commonly secondary to a problem with the circulatory system and hypoperfusion. Decreased perfusion, and thus decreased oxygen delivery to the tissues, will have significant effects on the organs, especially the heart, brain and kidneys. If prolonged, it will lead to organ failure and death. Four major types of shock are recognized (Figure 7.15).

- **Hypovolaemic shock** is the most common form and is characterized by:
  - Tachycardia
  - Prolonged capillary refill time
  - Pale mucous membranes
  - Low blood pressure (if severe).
- In **cardiogenic** and **obstructive shock** the findings are very similar to those in hypovolaemic shock, but arrhythmias may also be present.

Colour	Description	Significance
Pink (slightly paler for cats)	Normal	Normal
Red	Congested	Toxins; severe inflammatory response syndrome (SIRS); hyperthermia/pyrexia, sepsis. If only around teeth, may be gingivitis
Cherry red		Carbon monoxide poisoning
Pale/white	Pallor	Anaemia, shock
Blue/purple	Cyanotic	Lack of oxygen – marked dyspnoea
Yellow	Jaundiced/icteric	Acute hepatic failure, biliary obstruction
Orange	Haemoglobin pigment	Treatment with Oxyglobin
Chocolate brown	Methaemoglobin pigment	Methaemoglobinaemia (e.g. paracetamol and onion toxicity)

7.13 Mucous membrane colour chart.

Type of shock	Description	Common causes
Hypovolaemic shock	Decreased circulating blood volume	Haemorrhage; severe vomiting and diarrhoea; third-space fluid loss (loss of fluid into the body cavities)
Distributive shock (includes anaphylactic, toxic and septic shock)	Abnormal distribution of body fluids secondary to body-wide dilation of all blood vessels	Sepsis; systemic inflammatory response syndrome (e.g. severe pancreatitis); severe allergic reaction
Cardiogenic shock	Failure of heart to act as effective pump	Dilated cardiomyopathy; severe arrhythmias
Obstructive shock	Physical obstruction to blood flow within vascular system	Pulmonary thromboembolism; pericardial effusion

7.15 Four major types of shock.

- In **distributive shock**, of whatever cause, there is one important difference: as the body is unable to constrict its blood vessels normally, the mucous membranes appear abnormally red.

A drop in blood pressure is a late change during shock, as the body has a number of mechanisms that try to maintain blood pressure. A mean arterial blood pressure <60 mmHg is of considerable concern, as there may be damage to vital organs such as the brain, heart and kidneys.

When monitoring a patient in shock, measurement of urine output (ml/kg per hour) and urine specific gravity is very useful as it forms a non-invasive way of evaluating perfusion of the kidneys. To put it simply: if the animal is making plenty of urine (>2 ml/kg/hour) the kidneys must be well perfused. Serial measurements of urine output are a useful and cheap monitoring tool that can be used in most practice situations.

Shock should not be confused with dehydration.

- **Shock** implies a loss of fluid from the vascular system and has profound and potentially life-threatening effects.
- **Dehydration** implies a loss of fluid from the interstitial and intracellular spaces. Signs of dehydration include increased skin tenting and dry mucous membranes. Dehydration is very rarely life-threatening.

Treatment of shock

The treatment of shock varies depending on the cause. Most patients with hypovolaemic or distributive shock will require some form of intravenous fluid therapy, often at quite fast rates in the initial stages (see Chapter 8).

If bleeding is an obvious cause of shock, efforts should be made to arrest the haemorrhage. Methods of arresting haemorrhage include:

- Direct digital pressure: ensure that gloves are worn and apply pressure for at least 5 minutes
- Artery forceps (haemostats): if the bleeding vessel can be visualized it may be possible to clamp it directly with artery forceps
- Pressure dressing: apply direct pressure over the bleeding area using an absorbent pad and cohesive bandage
- Cold compress: constricts the blood vessels, reducing the haemorrhage.

Patients with shock are also likely to benefit from oxygen supplementation and being kept in a stress-free, comfortable environment. They may have a reduced body temperature but should be re-warmed slowly and only after fluid therapy has been started. Patients with shock require careful and close monitoring, especially in the first few hours after presentation.

Neurological evaluation

Initial evaluation of the animal's nervous system should include an assessment of gait and also of mentation. It should be interpreted alongside knowledge of the animal's other problems. For example, in an animal known to have suffered major haemorrhage, mental depression may be expected whereas the same degree of depression in another animal may be much greater cause for concern.

In recording an assessment of gait, the following terms should be used:

- **Paresis** – weakness
- **Plegia** – paralysis (unable to move)
- **Quadriplegia** – paralysis of all four limbs
- **Paraplegia** – paralysis of any two limbs
- **Hemiplegia** – paralysis of one side of the body.

In a paralysed animal it is also very important to note whether the animal can feel its limbs (e.g. turns towards the handler when its toes are squeezed even though it cannot move them).

Lameness may be also be identified at this point of the patient's evaluation and should be recorded.

Mentation can be classified as

- **Alert**
- **Obtunded** (mentally dull)
- **Stuporous** (semi-conscious but able to be roused by a painful stimulus)
- **Coma** (unconscious and unable to be aroused).

Other neurological features that should be noted include:

- Pupil size and symmetry
- Presence of pupillary light reflexes
- Facial asymmetry and any head tilt
- Nystagmus (abnormal flicking eye movements)
- Presence of gag reflex (in stuporous or comatose patients only)
- Anal tone (may be assessed when taking temperature).

Seizures

Seizures occur due to a brain disorder in which clusters of nerve cells (neurons) in the brain signal abnormally. The pattern of neuronal activity becomes disturbed, causing some combination of strange sensations, abnormal behaviour, muscle spasms and loss of consciousness. During a seizure, neurons may fire as many as 500 times per second, which is much faster than the normal rate of about 80 times per second.

Common causes of seizures in veterinary patients include:

- Idiopathic epilepsy
- Central nervous system neoplasia
- Inflammation
- Trauma
- Cerebral haemorrhage
- Hepatic disease (hepatoencephalopathy)
- Hypoglycaemia
- Hypocalcaemia
- Toxins/poisons.

When nursing a patient that is having a seizure ('fit'), take the following steps:

1. Note the time.
2. Ensure that the airway is open and clear – do not place anything in the patient's mouth (and do not get bitten).
3. As far as possible, ensure that the animal cannot injure itself.
4. Call a veterinary surgeon.
5. The veterinary surgeon may request the nurse to administer diazepam by the intravenous route if a catheter is present, or by the rectal route if not.
6. Depending on the patient, an intravenous catheter should be placed once the seizure is over so that further medications can be easily given intravenously should the animal have another seizure.
7. Monitor the patient's temperature. Seizuring patients often become hyperthermic due to muscle activity and may need to be cooled (see 'Hyperthermia', below).

HANDY HINT
Diazepam, when drawn up into a syringe, will attach to the plastic within about 15 minutes.

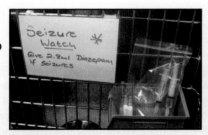

Diazepam should therefore never be drawn up in advance. In patients known to be at risk of seizures, the best solution is to place a card on the patient's kennel saying 'Seizure watch' with a note of the prescribed dose of diazepam required, the vial of diazepam, a sterile syringe and a needle, so that the drug can be drawn up and administered quickly, easily and accurately when required.

After the seizure has stopped:

- Remember that the patient may be disoriented or even blind and care should be taken when handling it
- The kennel may need to be padded
- Keep intravenous access patent
- Closely observe for the first signs of any further seizure activity and record them
- Administer medication as requested by the veterinary surgeon
- Observe and monitor respiratory and cardiovascular systems
- Report any findings to the veterinary surgeon.

Fractured or luxated spine

A fractured or luxated (dislocated) spine is a serious injury in which the neurological condition of the patient can deteriorate, especially as the animal moves. This injury is most commonly seen following road traffic accidents, running into solid objects (e.g. doors) at speed, or falling from a height.

The patient should be kept as still as possible. This may involve a combination of sedative/analgesic drugs and physical restraint, such as strapping to a board (Figure 7.16).

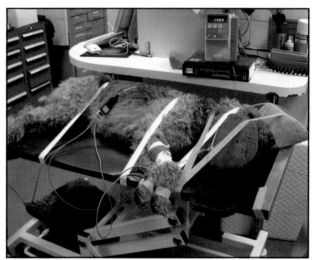

7.16 Strapping a patient with a spinal injury to a tabletop trolley helps to keep the patient immobile.

When the patient needs to be moved (e.g. for radiography) this should be done very carefully and with plenty of people present to help to restrain the patient.

Nursing considerations for the spinal patient

- Ensure that the patient has comfortable and appropriate bedding (e.g. plastic-covered mattress, with clinical bedding covering). Do not use blankets, as body fluids will not be drawn away from the patient. ▶

- **Many spinal patients have lost the ability to urinate. The bladder should be palpated at least every 4 hours and expressed if necessary. Alternatively, a urinary catheter can be placed and drained as required. It is important not to confuse urine overflow with conscious urination: the bladder should be checked for size immediately after urine is passed and if the bladder is still full this implies that overflow may be occurring.**
- **The patient should be turned at least every 4 hours to prevent hypostatic congestion and decubitus ulcers. A note should be made on the monitoring sheet to indicate the time and the position the patient was turned into.**
- **Ensure that the patient is clean and dry at all times to prevent urine and faecal scalding. Clipping the fur and applying a barrier cream (e.g. petroleum jelly) can be useful.**
- **If the patient is able to eat and drink on its own, ensure that the bowls are within easy reach.**

Abdominal assessment

Following evaluation of the three major body systems as described above, the examination should move on to the abdominal cavity, body temperature and any other wounds or injuries.

In the abdominal assessment, the following should be noted:

- Is the abdomen enlarged/distended?
- Are there any external wounds or injuries?
- Does the animal seem to have abdominal pain, either from the way it is standing or when its abdomen is touched?
- Is the animal showing any signs of straining to urinate?
- Is there any evidence of haematemesis (vomiting of blood), haematochezia (passing bright red blood with faeces) or melaena (passing digested or black blood with faeces)?

It is much harder to make an accurate assessment of the function of the intra-abdominal organs from an examination alone. It is also very important to obtain a full history from the owner about any problems relating to the abdomen, including questions about appetite, vomiting and diarrhoea and urination.

Body temperature

Body temperature is controlled by the hypothalamus in the brain. While both hyperthermia and pyrexia present with an elevated body temperature, they should be approached in different ways.

Pyrexia

In pyrexic animals, body temperature is above the normal range but this is an *appropriate* response to the disease process in that patient. Substances (known as pyrogens) produced by white blood cells act on the thermoregulatory centre of the brain and cause it to increase the body temperature. It does this by using heat-conserving measures (e.g. peripheral vasoconstriction) and heat-producing measures (e.g. shivering).

Pyrexia may be caused by any process that can activate white blood cells, such as:

- Infection (bacterial, viral, parasitic)
- Inflammation
- Neoplasia.

Treatment of pyrexia is aimed at dealing with the primary cause (e.g. antibiotics for infections; surgery or other treatment for tumours). Non-steroidal anti-inflammatory drugs (NSAIDs) will reverse the effect of pyrogens on the brain and therefore will tend to lower body temperature. As pyrexia makes the animal feel unwell, NSAIDs may help the animal to feel better but the primary cause must still be found and treated. Intravenous fluid therapy can also be helpful.

Pyrexic animals should not be externally cooled unless their body temperature is so high that it might cause damage to their cells (>42°C). Cooling a pyrexic animal is working against the measures that the brain has put in place and may increase the metabolic stress on the animal.

Hyperthermia

In hyperthermic animals, the body temperature is above the normal range despite the thermoregulatory centre of the brain wanting to maintain a temperature within the normal range. As the body is heated up by external factors, the brain initiates cooling/heat-losing measures (e.g. peripheral vasodilation, panting, lying stretched out). However, if the body continues to be heated (e.g. the animal is trapped in a car on a hot day), or if these heat-cooling mechanisms are not able to work (e.g. upper airway obstruction meaning that the animal cannot pant effectively), there comes a point when these endogenous cooling measures can no longer keep up, and so the body temperature rises above the normal range, i.e. hyperthermia occurs.

Common causes of hyperthermia are:

- Heatstroke
- Severe seizure activity
- Upper airway obstruction.

During hyperthermia the brain wants the body temperature to be within the normal range but cannot make this happen; therefore it is logical that treatment should involve helping the brain and body to achieve this. Active cooling measures are thus appropriate, including:

- Wetting the animal with cool (not cold) water and then applying a fan (most effective)
- Applying alcohol to the pads, pinnae, inguinal areas
- Cool-water enemas
- Intravenous fluid therapy with fluids at room temperature or slightly cooled (not cold).

WARNING
- It is NOT advisable to cover the patient with wet towels/blankets as these can insulate the animal and prevent heat loss.
- Hyperthermic animals should *NOT* be treated with NSAIDs.

It is very important that body temperature is monitored regularly (e.g. every 15 minutes). Cooling measures should be discontinued when body temperature reaches 39.4°C, to try to avoid the development of hypothermia.

Hypothermia

Hypothermia is an abnormally low body temperature and may be seen in patients with shock and in those who have been exposed to low environmental temperatures for prolonged periods.

Treatment revolves around passive or active re-warming. Care should be taken not to re-warm the animal too quickly. The following are tips for treating hypothermia.

- Monitor rectal temperature every 15 minutes until normothermic.
- Maintain a warm ambient temperature (this is the most appropriate way of warming a patient slowly).
- Use warm blankets.
- Use warm continuous-movement waterbeds.
- Warm air blankets (e.g. Bair-Hugger blankets) are excellent for warming patients but in some situations can warm the patient too quickly.
- Any intravenous fluids used should be warmed to 38°C.
- If the patient is anaesthetized, a heat moisture exchange connector can be used on the end of the endotracheal tube.
- Bubblewrap can be wrapped around the limbs (but note that this is more effective at preventing further heat loss than warming).
- Direct heat such as heat pads or hot-water bottles should be avoided. These can cause localized peripheral vasodilation of the heated area which, if the patient is in shock, can make its condition worse. They can also cause burns, especially if the patient is collapsed or immobile and cannot move away easily.

Wounds, bleeding and burns

Following evaluation and initial stabilization of the major body systems, other wounds and injuries can be assessed. It must be remembered that, however dramatic these wounds look, any more life-threatening abnormalities of the patient's major body systems should be addressed first.

Treatment of wounds

Treatment of wounds should only start once the patient is stable. Until that time the wound should be covered with a sterile dressing to prevent further contamination. Any penetrating foreign bodies should be covered and left in place until the patient is stable for definitive treatment.

Any haemorrhage should be controlled using one of the techniques discussed earlier in this chapter. Arterial haemorrhage (bright red blood that is pumping or spurting from the wound) will need addressing more urgently than venous or capillary haemorrhage. Analgesia should be provided after discussion with the veterinary surgeon.

Once the patient is stable, and after discussion with the veterinary surgeon, the wounds should be extensively clipped, cleaned, potentially sutured and dressed. For further information on wound management, see Chapter 14.

Burns

Burns result when intense heat (or, rarely, cold) damages the skin and subcutaneous tissues. Serum leaking from the damaged areas may lead to blister formation.

Burns can be classified by the way in which the burn was caused:

- **Dry burn** – contact with hot objects, flames or friction
- **Scald** – contact with a hot liquid or steam, including splashes
- **Electrical burn** – contact with live electricity (most commonly seen following chewing on live electrical cables; may rarely be seen following lightning strike)
- **Cold burn** – contact with very cold objects, such as freezing metal
- **Chemical burn** – contact with some chemicals, such as caustic soda or paint stripper
- **Radiation burn** – following prolonged exposure to strong sunlight (rarely seen in the UK).

Burns can also be classified by their depth, with a full-thickness burn (especially if covering a large body area) carrying a worse prognosis than a superficial burn:

- **Superficial** – affecting only the outermost surface of the skin; causes redness, swelling, and pain
- **Partial thickness** – affecting slightly deeper layers of the skin, causing the skin to become raw and red with blistering and more severe pain
- **Full thickness** – affecting all layers of the skin; may appear charred or 'leathery'. As the nervous supply to the skin is also destroyed, these burns are not as painful but take much longer to heal.

General advice on treatment of burns

- **Prevent further burning:**
  - **Remove source of problem, or move patient away from source**
  - **Douse area in cold water for minimum of 10 minutes (care should be taken not to overcool the patient and cause hypothermia)** ▶

- **Prevent infection:**
  - **Very gently clip fur over and around burn (include a large area as burns can be much larger than first thought)**
  - **Once cooled, cover area with sterile non-adherent dressing or clingfilm**
- **Relieve pain:**
  - **Discuss with veterinary clinician what analgesia they wish to prescribe**
- **Prevent further damage:**
  - **Elizabethan collar may be needed**
- **Treat shock:**
  - **Extensive burns are often associated with shock, which will need to be treated as a matter of urgency.**

Bones, joints and muscle injuries

Patients that have suffered trauma may have evidence of fractures, or of muscle or joint injury.

As with wounds, treatment of a fracture should be delayed until the major body systems have been evaluated and stabilized. Several general points to consider when dealing with emergencies with fractures or other limb injuries are as follows.

- Prevent/reduce haemorrhage:
  - If there is an open fracture, dress the wound appropriately until definitive treatment can be started.
- Prevent the patient from doing any more damage to itself:
  - Prevent movement – confine patient to small kennel
  - Prevent patient licking or interfering with injury – Elizabethan collar may be necessary
  - Dress any wounds to prevent further contamination.
- Immobilize the fracture (see Chapter 14).
- Analgesia:
  - Fractures cause considerable pain not only from fractured ends of bone but from haemorrhage (causing contusions) and tissue/muscle damage
  - Ask the veterinary clinician what analgesia they wish to prescribe
  - An unstable fracture will cause severe pain; the pain will not be fully controlled until the fracture is stabilized.
- Ensure that other patient comforts are met (e.g. use padded bed and make sure patient is kept warm).

Ophthalmological emergencies

Ophthalmological emergencies can look very dramatic. To avoid further distress to the owner it is generally best to remove the pet from them as soon as possible, even if the patient is stable.

Clinical signs of ocular injury or pain include:

- Proptosed globe
- Misshapen globe
- Foreign object seen in orbit
- Redness or oedema of the conjunctiva or eyelids
- Photophobia (aversion to light)

- Excessive tear production or other ocular discharge
- Blepharospasm
- Self-trauma or rubbing at the eye.

Ophthalmological emergencies may be associated with specific incidents such as trauma or scratches, but some patients with ophthalmological problems (e.g. lens luxation, glaucoma) may appear to develop clinical signs very suddenly with no inciting cause.

Nursing considerations for ophthalmic problems include the following:

- Inform the veterinary surgeon of the problem immediately – some ophthalmic problems require urgent treatment if sight is going to be saved in the eye
- Keep the patient in a quiet dimly lit kennel
- Keep the eye moist with 'artificial tears' solution
- Use an Elizabethan collar to prevent patient interference
- Discuss analgesic requirements with the veterinary surgeon – ocular problems can be very painful.

Rarely, patients are seen with proptosed globes – usually following trauma. Proptosis is commonest in brachycephalic breeds with shallow orbits, such as the Pekingese. It is vitally important that the globe is replaced quickly to prevent permanent loss of sight in that eye. A veterinary surgeon should be called immediately. The eyeball should be kept moist by placing a sterile saline-soaked swab directly over it until the veterinary surgeon arrives. The saline can be cooled to just below body temperature to try to reduce the swelling around the eye. The swab should be kept moist at all times.

 WARNING
Never attempt to replace a proptosed eye. Call for a veterinary surgeon immediately.

Poisoning

A large number of substances may be associated with poisonings in animals. In some cases, owners may witness their pets ingesting something toxic whereas in others the toxin ingestion may only be suspected. It should be remembered that prescribed medications can act as toxins, either if the animal has been given an excessive dose or if the animal has an unusual reaction to the drug. Owners should be questioned carefully, but gently, to check that any prescribed drugs have been given as directed.

Common clinical signs of poisoning include:

- Gastrointestinal signs:
  - Profuse salivation
  - Vomiting
  - Diarrhoea
- Neurological signs:
  - Behavioural change
  - Ataxia
  - Seizures
  - Collapse and coma
- Bleeding
- Unconsciousness and death.

Common poisons

Most poisons are ingested, but some can also be absorbed through the skin or inhaled. The list of potential toxins is very long but common ingested poisons include:

- Rat bait (e.g. brodifacoum, diphacinone), leading to bleeding
- Antifreeze (ethylene glycol), leading to renal failure
- Some insecticides (e.g. organophosphates), leading to neurological signs
- Human non-steroidal anti-inflammatory drugs (e.g. ibuprofen), leading to gastrointestinal signs or renal failure
- Lily plants in cats, leading to renal failure
- Slug bait (metaldehyde), leading to seizures
- Human recreational drugs (e.g. cannabis), leading to neurological signs
- Weedkiller (paraquat), leading to respiratory distress
- Chocolate (theobromine) in dogs, leading to gastrointestinal and cardiac signs.

Treatment

The key aims in initial stabilization of any poisoned patient are to:

- Identify the poison and the amount ingested as accurately as possible
- Prevent further absorption of the poison
- Treat any signs that develop symptomatically
- Administer any antidote or specific treatment (under the direction of a veterinary surgeon)
- Seek expert information. The Veterinary Poisons Information Service (VPIS) (tel. 0207 635 9195 or 0113 245 0530) is a useful source of information but requires that the practice is registered.

If an owner suspects that their animal has been poisoned, they should be asked to bring the pet and the suspect poison with container (if available) to the practice immediately. Some owners may want to try to induce vomiting in their pet at home but this is not recommended. Most of the substances present in the home that can be used to induce vomiting are either ineffective or have the potential for severe side effects (e.g. salt, leading to hypernatraemia). Vomiting can be induced using a number of different emetics (e.g. apomorphine, xylazine, washing soda crystals) under the direction of a veterinary surgeon. Vomiting should *not* be induced if:

- The toxin was a caustic or acidic substance that could cause further damage when it is brought back up
- The patient is depressed or seizuring, where there is a high risk of aspiration.

Some patients may need to be anaesthetized and intubated and gastric lavage performed as a safer option.

Activated charcoal is administered in many patients following induction of emesis, as it binds many toxins within the gastrointestinal tract and prevents further absorption of any remaining toxin. Some dogs will willingly eat activated charcoal mixed with food; in other patients the activated charcoal needs to be delivered by stomach tube.

Although some toxins have known antidotes or specific treatments (e.g. vitamin K for rodenticide intoxication) this is the exception rather than the rule. In most poisoned patients treatment is symptomatic. The patient's cardiovascular, respiratory and neurological status and body temperature should be carefully monitored and abnormalities treated symptomatically as described above.

Skin contamination

In patients where the toxin is on the skin (e.g. some flea products, paint, creosote), the following steps should be followed:

- Inform the veterinary surgeon (drug treatments may be available for some flea products)
- Use an Elizabethan collar to prevent the patient grooming and potentially ingesting the toxin
- Treat any systemic signs symptomatically under the direction of a veterinary surgeon
- Wearing gloves (nurses should not expose themselves to risk), remove the contamination with a combination of grooming, clipping and bathing. Be careful not to cool the patient too much during bathing. Rinse the patient with copious amounts of warmed water.

Inhaled toxins

Occasionally animals inhale toxins such as smoke or carbon monoxide. These patients often show signs of respiratory distress and should be treated symptomatically as described in the section on respiratory emergencies.

Neonatal and paediatric emergencies

Young puppies and kittens may present in a collapsed state with few other clinical signs. There are a number of infectious and non-infectious potential causes, but diagnosis is difficult and treatment is principally supportive. The two most significant contributors to neonatal mortality are hypothermia and hypoglycaemia.

When nursing these patients it is very important that they are kept in a warm non-draughty environment (at least 22°C) and that they receive adequate nutrition. If they present in a collapsed state, a blood glucose measurement should be obtained as early as possible and then glucose supplemented as necessary. In a hypoglycaemic patient, intravenous supplementation is ideal but obtaining intravenous access in these patients can be challenging. Glucose and fluids can also be given by the intraosseous route.

Once they are warmed, artificial feeding can be started. A well formulated canine or feline milk replacer should be used and can be administered by bottle, if the animal is sucking, or via stomach tube. Feeds should take place every 2–4 hours during the first 5 days of life but can be reduced to every 4 hours after day 5. Up to 3 weeks of age, urination and defecation are stimulated by the dam licking the perineal region. If puppies and kittens are hospitalized before this age, nursing staff should provide this stimulation by gently stroking the perineal region with a cotton bud shortly after feeding.

Congenital abnormalities should also be considered in any young animal that is failing to thrive.

Neonatal resuscitation

Resuscitation may sometimes be required in neonatal puppies and kittens delivered by either Caesarean section or vaginal delivery. Equipment that should be prepared prior to delivery includes:

- A warm environment (incubator) or box with heat lamp
- Plenty of soft, dry, warm towels
- Haemostats for clamping the umbilical cord
- Suture material
- Suction bulb syringe for clearing oral secretions
- Emergency drugs (adrenaline, naloxone).

As each puppy is delivered and given to the nurse, the umbilical cord should be clamped about 1–2 cm from the umbilicus. The puppy should be briskly rubbed with a clean, dry towel and the fetal fluids and amnion removed. The oral cavity may be suctioned with a bulb syringe. In most cases, vigorous rubbing is enough to simulate respiration. The old practice of 'swinging' puppies is no longer recommended, due to the potential for damage. If the puppy does not start to breathe on its own, oxygen can be supplied with a tight-fitting facemask or an endotracheal tube. Cardiac massage may be necessary if a heartbeat cannot be felt once the puppy has been warmed and ventilation has been started. Adrenaline can also be administered in this situation. Doxapram is often used in neonates to stimulate respiration but there is no evidence that it is effective; also the therapeutic dose range is very narrow, meaning that an overdose is an easy mistake and can be fatal.

Obstetric emergencies

Bitches may present during parturition if they are having trouble delivering their puppies. There are many causes of dystocia but some of the commoner ones are:

- Primary uterine inertia
- Secondary uterine inertia after prolonged straining
- Fetal malpresentation
- Maternal–fetal disproportion (common in breeds such as Bulldogs)
- Maternal pelvic abnormalities (e.g. previous fractured pelvis)
- Fetal death.

It should be strongly recommended that the bitch be examined by a veterinary surgeon if:

- She has been straining unproductively for more than 1 hour from the onset of stage II labour without producing a puppy
- She has been straining unproductively for more than 30 minutes without producing subsequent puppies
- She has a green–brown vaginal discharge
- She rests for more than 2 hours without straining between puppies
- She appears unwell or depressed herself
- A puppy can be seen stuck in the birth canal.

For queens, the interval between kittens may be longer and the entire parturition process may occasionally last longer than 24 hours, but veterinary advice should still be sought based on the canine guidelines above.

Any bitch with dystocia should be kept in a warm and comfortable environment and examined by a veterinary surgeon as soon as possible so that a decision can be made as to whether to attempt medical therapy (e.g. oxytocin) or whether to proceed to a Caesarean section.

Nutrition

Good nutrition is a vital part of the recovery of many critically ill patients, though it is rarely the focus when initially examining the emergency patient. There are various methods of providing supplemental nutrition (Figure 7.17). It should be remembered that supplementing fluids with glucose only is not a form of nutrition. Further information can be found in Chapter 9 and in the BSAVA *Manual of Advanced Veterinary Nursing*.

Method of feeding	Advantages	Disadvantages
Syringe feeding	Inexpensive. Does not require any special equipment	Time-consuming. Difficult to ensure animal gets correct amount. Often unpleasant for animal. Risk of aspiration
Naso-oesophageal tube	Inexpensive. Can be placed with patient conscious	Tube may be irritating. Only narrow-bore tubes can be used, so feeding may be time-consuming
Oesophagostomy tube	Inexpensive. Easy to place. Can stay in place for weeks. Well tolerated	Requires short period of anaesthesia for placement
Gastrostomy tube	Well tolerated. Can stay in place for weeks to months. Can be large bore, allowing feeds to be given quickly and easily	Requires special equipment (endoscope) or surgery for placement
Jejunostomy tube	Bypasses stomach (useful in some patients with gastric or pancreatic disease)	Requires exploratory laparotomy to place. Ideally requires special food be used as food is delivered to gastrointestinal tract beyond the stomach. Diarrhoea is common complication
Parenteral (intravenous) nutrition	Can be used in patients with non-functional gastrointestinal tract	Expensive. Requires facility with 24-hour care. Nutrition has to be specially compounded for each patient. Total parenteral nutrition requires placement of central catheter. Risk of sepsis or vascular complications

7.17 Supplemental nutrition.

Calculating resting energy requirement

The resting energy requirement (RER) is the energy required by a sick hospitalized patient. This term is preferred to basal energy requirement (BER) when calculating requirements for feeding (see Chapter 9). RER is measured in kilocalories (kcal) and is calculated according to the bodyweight (BW), measured in kilograms (kg), as follows:

- Dog: 30 BW + 70
- Cat: 60 BW

It is recommended that 50% of the calculated resting energy requirement is fed on Day one, increasing to 100% by Day three. Adverse effects (e.g. development of diarrhoea), bodyweight and body condition score should be monitored and the amount of calories adjusted up or down as appropriate. The use of illness factors to modify the calculation is no longer recommended.

Monitoring the emergency patient

An example of a monitoring chart is shown in Figure 7.18. The example shown has had treatments up to 1800 hours. The other side of the sheet includes areas to write comprehensive notes and to monitor findings.

Although many advanced monitoring techniques are now available in veterinary practice, the most important monitoring tool is the serial physical examination. The following parameters should be recorded at regular intervals (up to every 15 minutes in unstable patients, through to every 6-8 hours in stable patients):

- Pulse rate
- Pulse quality
- Mucous membrane colour
- Capillary refill time
- Respiratory rate
- Respiratory effort
- Temperature
- Demeanour
- Bodyweight (every 12 hours).

7.18 Example of monitoring chart.

ICU Treatment Sheet

THE ROYAL VETERINARY COLLEGE
UNIVERSITY OF LONDON

Label

Case No.:
Name:
Species: Cat
Breed:
Sex:
Age:
Clinician:

Owner:
Address:
Tel:
Ref Practice:
Ref Tel:
Ref Fax:

PROBLEM LIST
Urethral obstruction
Bradycardia
Hyperkalcaemia

Date: 31 / 5 / 07   Weight: am   pm: 4·2 kg
Clinician: A VET   Signature:
Clinician tel: 0208 1234567   Bleep: 13
Student:

P Catheter site (L) ceph   Date placed 31 / 5 / 07
Checked ✓ NEW   Code status (R) . DNR

DAILY ORDERS
place iv catheter ☑
sedate (ket/diazepam) /unblock ☑
place indwelling u cath ☑

DIAGNOSTIC TESTS
PCV/TS/venous blood gas ☑
urinalysis ☑
Haem/biochem ☑

Weight 6am _____ kg

	6	7	8	9	10	11	12	13	14	15	16	17	18	19	20	21	22	23	0	1	2	3	4	5	6	7	8
MM / CRT / PULSES / HR											✓	✓		✓													
RR / EFFORT											✓	✓		✓													
Temp											✓	✓		✓													
PCV / TS											✓	✓															
Nova											✓	✓															
continuous ECG																											
Calcium gluconate 10% 1ml/kg slow iv											✓																
0.9% NaCl 20ml/kg bolus iv											✓																
0.9% NaCl @ 20ml/hr																											
check + record urine output q4													✓														
Walk / Carry / Hoist / Trolley																											
Food																											
Water																											
Notify >																											
Notify <																											

TIME	T	P	R	MM	CRT	PCV	TS	Na	K	BG	Lac	Creat	UOP (ml/kg/hr)
4pm	35·7	120	30	pale pink	25	30	68	153	8·8	7·6	4·0	637	
5pm	36·6	150	28	pale pink	1·5s	26	62	151	7·2				
7pm	37·1	160	24	pink	1·5s								
8pm												3·2	

RM080795

The significance of changes in these parameters is discussed in the relevant body system sections above. Other monitoring techniques that can be considered include:

- Urine output
- Urine specific gravity
- Blood pressure
- Pulse oximetry
- ECG
- Central venous pressure
- Serial electrolyte and blood gas parameters.

It is vital that any parameter monitored is recorded accurately. Successful management of emergency patients often involves several members of staff and it is essential that the patient's status is accurately communicated between different staff members.

Emergency patients often require a lot of effort but can be some of the most rewarding patients to nurse.

Further reading

Adams W and Niles J (1999) Management of a critical care unit. In: *BSAVA Manual of Advanced Veterinary Nursing*, ed. A Hotston Moore, pp. 85–112. BSAVA Publications, Cheltenham

Battaglia A (2000) *Small Animal Emergency and Critical Care: A Manual for the Veterinary Technician*. WB Saunders, Philadelphia

Boag A and Nichols K (2007) First aid and emergency nursing. In: BSAVA Textbook of *Veterinary Nursing, 4th edn*, ed. Lane DR *et al.*, pp. 351–387. BSAVA Publications, Gloucester

Campbell A and Chapman M (2000) *Handbook of Poisoning in Dogs and Cats*. Blackwell Publishing, Oxford

King L and Boag A (2007) *BSAVA Manual of Canine and Feline Emergency and Critical Care, 2nd edn*. BSAVA Publications, Gloucester

8

Practical fluid therapy

Paula Hotston Moore

This chapter is designed to give information on:

- Causes of fluid imbalance in the body
- Appropriate fluid choices for a compromised patient
- Calculation of fluid requirement
- Assembly of fluid therapy equipment
- Positioning and restraint of the animal in order to receive fluid therapy
- Administration of fluid therapy
- Monitoring the patient during and after fluid therapy
- Identification of problems resulting from fluid therapy
- Health and safety aspects of fluid therapy

Fluid requirements of the healthy patient

The healthy patient requires sufficient fluid on a daily basis in order to maintain life and function adequately. This amount is known as the maintenance requirement. There are known figures for this:

Maintenance requirement = 50–60 ml/kg/24 hours

Figure 8.1 gives an example of calculating the maintenance requirement for a dog.

How much fluid does a 25 kg Labrador require over a 24-hour period?

Maintenance requirement = 50–60 ml/kg/24 hours
Taking 50 ml/kg as the requirement:
50 ml x 25 kg = 1250 ml

Answer: 1250 ml is required for a 25 kg Labrador over a 24-hour period.

8.1 Calculation of maintenance requirement.

A healthy animal obtains its fluid requirement from metabolism, diet and drinking water. Metabolism of carbohydrate and fats provides the body with water. Depending on the type of diet, a greater or lesser amount of water will be present: dry diets contain less water than tinned diets. An animal fed a dry diet is likely to drink more water than one fed on a moist, tinned diet. Drinking water is available to the animal via its water bowl and is accessible to most animals by way of streams, rivers, garden ponds, rainwater puddles and also from other sources, depending on its lifestyle.

When an animal is not able to source water, its fluid requirements are not met. Possible reasons for inadequate fluid intake include:

- Animal unable to drink due to illness
- Anorexia
- Lethargy
- Unconsciousness
- Facial trauma
- Disease of pharynx or oesophagus
- Drinking water not provided.

For example, if an animal is anorexic it is not obtaining its usual amount of fluid from food.

Alternatively, the animal may be unable to drink and therefore will not gain its normal amount of water from drinking.

Fluid is lost from the healthy animal's body by natural (insensible) losses that occur on a daily basis: breathing, panting, sweating, urinating and defecating. The amount of fluid taken into the body must equal the amount of fluid lost from the body in order for the animal to maintain its correct fluid levels and be able to function normally. In the healthy animal these fluid levels are maintained on a daily basis. Normal fluid intake must match normal fluid losses. It is only when factors interfere with these normal functions that there becomes an imbalance of fluid within the body. Further details on the theoretical aspects can be found in the *BSAVA Textbook of Veterinary Nursing*.

Indications for fluid therapy

Fluid therapy is an essential part of supportive therapy. An animal will require fluid therapy if it is unable to take in sufficient fluid to maintain its normal levels, or if fluid is lost abnormally from the body.

Reasons for abnormal fluid losses include:

- Vomiting
- Diarrhoea
- Excessive wound discharge
- Other discharges (e.g. vaginal discharge during open pyometra)
- Diabetes
- Renal disease
- Effusions (e.g. ascites).

The animal is not able to function normally with insufficient levels of fluid and over a period of hours it will become metabolically unstable should fluid levels remain unbalanced. Administration of fluid therapy restores the normal fluid balance within the body, thus allowing the animal to function adequately.

Assessing hydration

If an imbalance in fluid levels is suspected there is a variety of ways in which to assess how much fluid has been lost. These figures will always remain as estimates, since accurate determination of exactly how much fluid has been lost is not possible. There are several common methods of assessing hydration levels:

- Clinical examination
- Measurement of packed cell volume (PCV)
- Monitoring bodyweight
- Measurement of known losses
- Monitoring urine output
- Measurement of urine specific gravity
- Measurement of blood urea nitrogen and creatinine levels.

One or more of these methods is employed in any given situation, depending on the facts that are available at the time.

Clinical examination

The patient is examined for signs of fluid loss. Parameters that indicate fluid loss are: dry mucous membranes, sunken eyes, loss of skin elasticity, general demeanour and delayed capillary refill time.

- Mucous membranes are moist in the healthy animal.
- Eyes should appear open, bright and alert.
- Skin elasticity is measured by 'tenting' the skin along the dorsal neck:
  - In the healthy animal the skin will return to its normal position almost immediately
  - In the dehydrated animal, the skin remains tented or takes longer to return to its normal position.
- The general demeanour of the patient gives a general indication of its wellbeing:
  - The healthy patient will be bright, alert, responsive and interested in its surroundings
  - A dehydrated patient is lethargic, less responsive and not interested in its surroundings.
- Capillary refill time (CRT) is assessed by pressing down on the mucous membranes of the lips or gums to blanch them (see Figure 7.14):
  - Normal capillary refill time is <2 seconds
  - In the dehydrated animal a capillary refill time of >2 seconds is often apparent.

There are established clinical signs associated with varying levels of dehydration that are universally recognized (Figure 8.2).

Dehydration level	Clinical signs
< 5%	Not detectable
5–6%	Subtle loss of skin elasticity
6–8%	Marked loss of skin elasticity Slightly prolonged capillary refill time Slightly sunken eyes Dry mucous membranes
10–12%	Tented skin stands in place Capillary refill time >2 seconds Sunken eyes Dry mucous membranes
12–15%	Early shock Moribund Death imminent

8.2   Clinical signs associated with dehydration.

Measurement of packed cell volume

Packed cell volume (PCV) measures the proportion of red blood cells in a given volume of blood (see also Chapter 10).

- The normal PCV range for a dog is 39–55%.
- The normal PCV range for a cat is 24–45%.
- The normal PCV range for a rabbit is 34–50%.

As the individual animal's own normal value is not often known, a 'typical' value of 45% for a dog, 35%

for a cat and 40% for a rabbit is taken. In a dehydrated patient, the PCV will increase. It is possible to calculate the estimated level of dehydration according to the percentage rise in PCV of the patient (Figure 8.3). For every 1% rise in PCV, the animal requires 10 ml of fluid/kg bodyweight.

If a 4.5 kg dehydrated cat has a PCV of 54%, how much fluid can it be estimated has been lost?

Normal cat PCV = 35%
Current PCV = 43%
Increase = 8%
For every 1% increase in PCV, animal requires 10 ml fluid/kg
8% increase in PCV = 8 x 10 ml x 4.5 kg = 360 ml

Answer: 360 ml of fluid

8.3 Use of packed cell volume (PCV) to estimate fluid loss.

Monitoring bodyweight

If the animal's bodyweight prior to illness or dehydration is available, this figure is used to estimate fluid requirement. A comparison is made of the bodyweight prior to illness with that of bodyweight after illness; the fluid loss is then calculated on the basis that 1 kg is equal to 1 litre of fluid (Figure 8.4).

Prior to illness, a Border Terrier weighed 12 kg. Following an episode of vomiting and diarrhoea, the same animal was found to weigh 11.2 kg. How much fluid can it be estimated to have lost?

Difference in bodyweight = 12 kg – 11.2 kg = 0.8 kg (800 g)
1 kg = 1 litre, therefore 800 g = 800 ml

Answer: 800 ml

8.4 Use of bodyweight in calculation of fluid loss.

Comparison of bodyweight is not often used since few owners know their healthy animal's accurate bodyweight.

Measurement of known losses

In the literature there are previously calculated figures for fluid losses that occur with vomiting and diarrhoea. It is estimated that for every episode of vomiting an animal loses 4 ml/kg and for every episode of diarrhoea an animal loses 4 ml/kg (Figure 8.5). These figures are rough estimates since the actual volumes of fluid lost in episodes of vomiting and diarrhoea can be very variable, depending on the disease processes involved.

In order to use this method of estimating fluid loss, a detailed history must be sought from the owner.

Monitoring urine output

In the healthy animal, normal urine output is 1–2 ml/kg/hour. Urine output will decrease during dehydration. Measurement of urine output is accurately monitored by collecting urine, using either an indwelling urinary catheter or regular emptying of the bladder by urinary catheterization. The urine is measured and, if found to be lower than 1–2 ml/kg/hour, fluid losses are estimated.

Measurement of urine specific gravity

Specific gravity indicates the concentration of a solution. Urine specific gravity is measured to assess fluid hydration levels and kidney function. A refractometer is used (see Chapter 10). A dehydrated animal with normal kidney function will have a raised urine specific gravity because of the body's ability to concentrate urine and conserve fluid. Normal values for urine specific gravity are:

- Dog 1.015–1.040
- Cat 1.015–1.050
- Rabbit 1.003–1.036.

Measurement of blood urea nitrogen (BUN) and creatinine levels

Animals that become dehydrated will have increases in urea and creatinine levels. This is due to the animal becoming shocked and reduced blood flow to the kidneys. Similar changes will be seen in animals with renal failure but these animals will not concentrate their urine. Normal values for BUN are:

- Dog 3.1–9.2 mmol/l
- Cat 5.5–11.1 mmol/l
- Rabbit 4.6–10.4 mmol/l.

Average values for creatinine are:

- Dog 30–90 µmol/l
- Cat 26–118 µmol/l
- Rabbit 88 µmol/l.

A 12 kg dog has vomited twice and had one episode of diarrhoea. Estimate the fluid loss.

Vomit = 2 x 4 ml/kg x 12 kg = 96 ml
Diarrhoea = 1 x 4 ml/kg x 12 kg = 48 ml
Total = 144 ml

Answer: estimated fluid loss = 144 ml

8.5 Estimate of fluid loss due to known losses.

Calculating fluid requirements

First, the amount of fluid that is lost is estimated using one of the methods outlined above. Having estimated the amount of fluid lost, it is then possible to calculate how much fluid should be administered to the patient. Practically this means that the information required is: how many drops of fluid are to be given in how many seconds via a burette or giving set, or how many ml/h via a drip pump? This information enables the veterinary nurse to adjust the fluid giving set to deliver the required amount of fluid.

The following mathematical steps are followed in this calculation.

1. Calculate the amount of fluid (ml) lost as previously discussed.
2. Calculate the maintenance requirement (ml) as previously discussed.
3. Calculate total amount of fluid (ml) to be administered (add fluid lost to maintenance requirement).
4. Decide over how many hours the fluid is to be given.
5. Calculate how much fluid (ml) will be administered per hour, i.e. total fluid (ml) to be administered divided by total number of hours.
6. Calculate ml/minute (ml/hour divided by 60 minutes).
7. Calculate drops per minute (ml/minute x giving set rate, which is found on giving set packaging; standard giving set rate is 20 drops per ml).
8. Calculate 1 drop every x seconds (60 divided by drops/minute).

Worked examples of these calculations are given in Figures 8.6 and 8.7.

Usually, pre-existing fluid losses are administered at an increased rate over a period of 6–8 hours and then maintenance fluids are given.

A 14 kg Collie is found to be 10% dehydrated. The fluid is to be given over 8 hours. The giving set delivers 20 drops/ml. Calculate the drip rate to '1 drop every x seconds'.

1. Fluid lost = 10% of 14 kg dog = 10/100 x 14 kg = 1.4 kg
   1.4 kg = 1400 g = 1400 ml
2. Maintenance requirement = 50 ml/kg/day
   50 ml/kg x 14 kg = 700 ml
3. Fluid lost plus fluid maintenance = 1400 ml + 700 ml = 2100 ml
4. To be given over 8 hours, as stated:
   2100 ml ÷ 8 hours = 262.5 ml/hour
   262.5 ml/hour ÷ 60 minutes = 4.37 ml/minute
5. 4.37 ml/minute x giving set rate of 20 = 87.4 drops/minute
6. 60 ÷ 87.4 drops/minute = 0.68 (round up to 1)

Answer: 1 drop every 1 second.

8.6   Calculation of fluid rate: Example 1.

A 5 kg cat requires fluid at twice maintenance. Fluid is to be given via a burette over 24 hours. Calculate the drip rate to '1 drop every x seconds'.

1. Fluid required = twice maintenance = 2 x 50 ml/kg x 5 kg = 500 ml
2. 500 ml over 24 hours = 500 ml ÷ 24 hours = 20.83 ml/hour
3. 20.83 ÷ 60 minutes = 0.34 ml/minute
4. 0.34 ml/minute x giving set rate of 60 (standard giving set rate for a burette) = 20.4 drops/minute
5. 60 ÷ 20.4 drops/minute = 2.94 (round up to 3)

Answer: 1 drop every 3 seconds.

8.7   Calculation of fluid rate: Example 2.

Oral administration of fluids

Animals that are mildly dehydrated and are not in shock may be given oral fluids to overcome dehydration. This oral route of fluid administration is not suitable for animals that are more severely dehydrated and already shocked, because absorption from the gastrointestinal tract is reduced (see Chapter 7).

For animals that are drinking voluntarily, oral rehydration solutions can be provided instead of drinking water. In other cases, oral rehydration solutions can be provided through assisted or tube feeding methods.

Commercial oral rehydration fluids are available; they are often in powder form and are mixed with water. These fluids contain both water and electrolytes. The animal can be encouraged to drink at regular intervals, or the fluid can be syringed into the animal's mouth. Not all fluids are able to be administered orally and in situations where gastrointestinal function is limited the fluid is not absorbed efficiently. Often a patient will not be able to drink sufficient amounts of fluid to maintain its fluid requirements, particularly in cases where dehydration is also present. It is then that an alternative route of fluid administration becomes necessary.

Fluids used for replacement

It is usually recommended to 'replace like with like'. This statement means that whatever fluid has been lost from the body should be replaced with fluid of the same type. For example, a cat that has had a road traffic accident and lost blood should receive blood during its fluid therapy. Similarly, an animal that has lost electrolytes and fluid through vomiting should receive those same electrolytes and fluid during administration of fluid therapy.

There are a number of fluids available commercially. This chapter will not provide an exhaustive list; instead it will explain the differences between the types of fluid and reasons for administering one type of fluid rather than another.

Fluid used in intravenous fluid therapy can be divided into three groups: blood, colloids and crystalloids.

Blood

Blood is used in cases such as severe anaemia, severe haemorrhage or where there is a clotting problem such as in von Willebrand's disease. Blood must be collected from a donor animal and then infused into a recipient.

Blood donors

The donor animal is likely to be an animal known to the veterinary practice and of a good temperament – possibly an animal belonging to a staff member or owned by a client living close to the surgery. The blood donor must be in good health, have previously been screened and known to be negative for infectious diseases, and have a normal packed cell volume. Donor dogs should weigh a minimum of 25 kg and cats a minimum of 4 kg and should not be obese.

Permission from the owner must always be sought. RCVS guidelines (March 2007) indicate that it is a recognized veterinary practice to take blood from a donor 'with the intention of administering the blood or its products where there is an immediate or anticipated clinical indication for the transfusion.' This is usually done within an individual veterinary practice or between local practices: if performed on a larger commercial scale, a licence would be required. Blood is collected from the donor's jugular vein into a blood collection bag (Figure 8.8) containing an anticoagulant, often citrate phosphate dextrose (CPD). The patient does not usually require sedation. One unit (400 ml) is collected from dogs and up to 50 ml from a cat.

Ideally blood donors and recipients should be cross-matched to avoid a blood transfusion reaction, but in many veterinary practices this is not possible due to the time needed for such tests to be undertaken. Cats certainly should be cross-matched or blood typed prior to donation as a transfusion reaction is more likely (Figure 8.9). Dogs, however, may tolerate one transfusion without side effects.

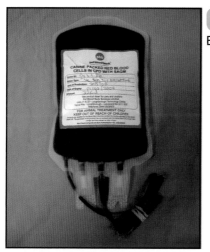

8.8 Blood bag.

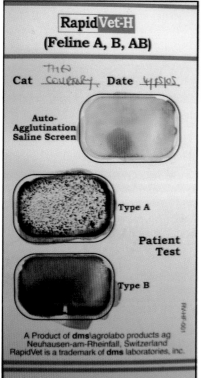

8.9 Cat blood type card.

Blood transfusion

Blood is administered to the patient via a blood administration set (Figure 8.10). This has a filter to remove any clots.

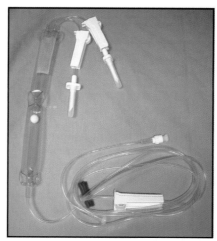

8.10 Blood administration set.

Initially blood is administered at a rate of 0.25 ml/kg/hour for the first 15 minutes; this is then increased to 20 ml/kg/hour over a period of 2–4 hours. The patient must be monitored closely for signs of a blood transfusion reaction such as urticaria, muscle tremors, tachycardia or convulsions. If a transfusion reaction is suspected the blood infusion is stopped immediately and the veterinary surgeon's advice sought. A transfusion reaction is most likely to occur within the first hour of the patient receiving blood.

Colloids

Colloids (Figure 8.11) are also known as plasma expanders. They remain in the vascular space for longer than crystalloids, as their osmotic potential is so great that colloids draw fluid out of the interstitial and intracellular spaces, into the plasma. Colloids expand and maintain the vascular volume.

Colloid type	Example product names	Duration of action	Rate of fluid administration
Gelatins	Haemacell	Up to 6 hours	Dog: up to 90 ml/kg/hour Cat: up to 60 ml/kg/hour
	Gelofusine	Up to 6 hours	Maximum dose: 20 ml/kg/24 hours
Starch (hetastarch, pentastarch)	elo-HAES, HAES-steril, Hemohes	24–36 hours	Maximum dose: 20 ml/kg/24 hours

8.11 Colloid solutions.

Colloids are used either when rapid restoration of the intravascular volume is required or as a second choice when blood is not available. They are likely to be used in situations of shock or when the circulating blood volume needs to be increased to replace recent losses. Examples of situations requiring colloid fluid replacement include:

- Road traffic accidents (shock and possible blood loss)
- Internal haemorrhage
- External haemorrhage
- Surgery where blood loss is anticipated
- Hypovolaemic shock.

Colloids are used in conjunction with standard fluid administration giving sets and equipment. At the time of writing, colloids are only available in units of 500 ml.

Oxyglobin

Oxyglobin (bovine haemoglobin glutamer-200) is a plasma volume expander that contains haemoglobin, which improves oxygen delivery by increasing the oxygen content of the blood. Oxyglobin has the advantages of not requiring cross-matching and does not require a donor animal. Its cost is often prohibitive: it is an expensive product and is therefore not accessible to all clients. Another disadvantage of Oxyglobin is that it affects some laboratory tests for several days following administration; in addition it alters mucous membrane colour, turning membranes brown.

Crystalloids

Crystalloids (Figure 8.12) are a group of water-based fluids, containing a selection of fundamental electrolytes. Whilst administered intravenously and thus entering the intravascular space, crystalloids spread quickly into the extracellular fluid within the body.

Information regarding each individual crystalloid and which electrolytes are included is found on the data sheet pertaining to each fluid. The veterinary nurse must be familiar with the key crystalloids widely available on the UK market, and in particular those used within their own place of work.

Electrolytes

In deciding which crystalloid fluid to use, the veterinary surgeon will establish which electrolytes have been lost from the patient and then select a crystalloid fluid that contains the electrolytes that need to be replaced. It is possible to establish which electrolytes have been lost either by measuring blood parameters or by estimating losses from the clinical history.

Electrolytes are the ions dissolved in body fluids. The most important are sodium (Na^+), potassium (K^+), chloride (Cl^-) and bicarbonate (HCO_3^-) (Figure 8.13).

In choosing a crystalloid fluid, the main considerations are:

- Whether sodium or chloride electrolytes have been lost
- Whether the patient is acidotic or alkalotic
- Whether potassium is being lost or there is an excess of potassium within the body
- Whether hypoglycaemia is present.

Crystalloid fluid	Constituents	Clinical indications
Hartmann's solution (lactated Ringer's solution)	Na^+, Cl^-, small amounts of potassium and calcium, lactate	Diarrhoea Correction of metabolic acidosis
0.9% Sodium chloride (normal saline)	Na^+, Cl^-	Vomiting Correction of metabolic alkalosis Urinary tract obstruction
5% Dextrose	Dextrose	Water loss
0.18% Sodium chloride and 4% dextrose (dextrose saline)	Small amounts of Na^+ and Cl^- and 4% dextrose	Water loss
Ringer's solution	Na^+, Cl^-, small amounts of potassium and calcium	Pyometra Severe vomiting
Darrow's solution	Na^+, Cl^-, potassium (smaller amounts) and lactate	Severe diarrhoea
Hypertonic saline	High levels of Na^+ and Cl^-	Severe haemorrhage Hypovolaemia

8.12 Crystalloids.

Electrolyte	Normal range in dog (mmol/l)	Normal range in cat (mmol/l)	Causes of deficiencies	Signs of deficiencies	Causes of increased levels	Signs of increased levels
Potassium	3.8–5.8	3.7–4.9	Anorexia, gastrointestinal disturbances, renal failure	Inappetence, weakness, cardiac abnormalities	Urinary tract obstruction, diabetic ketoacidosis, renal failure, Addison's disease	Bradycardia, cardiac arrest, collapse
Calcium (ionized)	1.0–1.5	1.0–1.5	Hypoparathyroidism, eclampsia	Twitching, seizures	Neoplasia (especially lymphysarcoma), Addison's disease	Polyuria/polydipsia, renal failure, vomiting, lethargy
Bicarbonate	17–24	17–24	Ketoacidotic diabetes, acute renal failure	Rapid deep respiration	Iatrogenic	

8.13 Electrolytes.

The fluid containing the electrolytes that have been lost from the body is preferred. A crystalloid fluid containing lactate is metabolized in the body into bicarbonate, which is useful in treating metabolic acidosis. Therefore, the ideal crystalloid fluid for a patient with metabolic or respiratory acidosis is one containing lactate, such as Hartmann's solution or Darrow's solution. Conversely, using a crystalloid that contains lactate is not preferred in a patient with alkalosis. Acid–base balance (Figure 8.14) is covered in more detail in texts such as the *BSAVA Textbook of Veterinary Nursing.*

Type of imbalance	Causes
Respiratory acidosis	Hypoventilation, e.g. in anaesthetic depression, ruptured diaphragm, pneumothorax, pleural effusion, bronchitis
Respiratory alkalosis	Hyperventilation, e.g. in pain, stress, hyperthermia, excessive IPPV
Metabolic acidosis	Examples: acute renal failure, ketoacidotic diabetes, vomiting and diarrhoea, shock
Metabolic alkalosis	Examples: vomiting, pyloric obstruction, over-infusion of solutions containing bicarbonate

8.14 Causes of acid–base imbalances.

It is then decided whether potassium is being lost or is accumulating within the body. If potassium levels in the body are low, administering a crystalloid that contains potassium will replenish the potassium levels. If there is an excess of potassium in the body, it will become harmful to administer a fluid that contains potassium. Crystalloids should be checked for their potassium levels in considering which fluid to administer.

In hypoglycaemic animals, dextrose saline is usually selected to maintain blood glucose levels.

Routes of administration

Dogs and cats

Intravenous route

The most commonly chosen route through which to administer fluid therapy to the sick cat or dog is the intravenous route. This allows fluid to be administered directly into the intravascular space, improves general circulation, replaces lost fluids and is able to be administered continuously. The vein frequently used is the cephalic, but the saphenous, jugular, femoral and ventral tail veins can also be used (Figure 8.15). The cephalic is often the favoured vein as it is easily accessible and well tolerated by the patient. The saphenous vein is used as a second choice when the cephalic is unable to be used: for example, in cases of injury to the foreleg or difficulties with access. The alternative veins shown in Figure 8.15 are also used; the choice of vein is largely left to personal preference and the accessibility of the vein, depending on each individual clinical situation. The jugular vein is chosen for rapid infusion and in critically ill animals.

The equipment (see later) is selected and prepared. The patient is then suitably restrained, the vein raised by an assistant and the fluid administered into the vein via an intravenous catheter (see Figure 8.22).

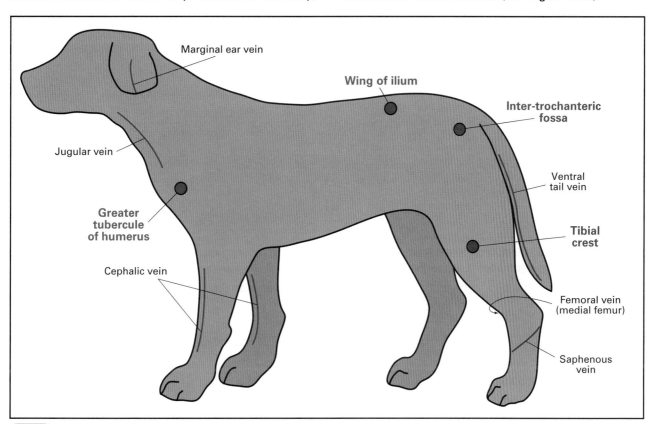

8.15 Location of veins used for intravenous fluid therapy and sites of intraosseous administration (●).

Intraosseous route

Fluid is occasionally administered by the intraosseous route. This route is particularly useful in neonates, where administration into a peripheral vein is more difficult, or in cases where peripheral veins become unavailable due to collapse of the circulatory system. The intraosseous route is still useful for fluid therapy in these situations since the veins within bone marrow remain unaffected in dehydration or circulatory collapse. The intraosseous route is contraindicated in cases of septic shock, fractured bones and pneumatic bones of birds.

Sites used for intraosseous administration of fluid are the tibial crest, the intertrochanteric fossa of the femur, wing of the ilium, tibial tuberosity and greater tubercle of the humerus (see Figure 8.15). In adult cats and dogs, specialized intraosseous needles are used (Figure 8.16). In neonates and small species, spinal needles or hypodermic needles are used.

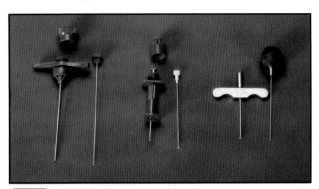

8.16   Intraosseous needles.

Osteomyelitis is a potential complication of fluid administered by this route; therefore as soon as an intravenous route becomes available, intraosseous fluids are discontinued and the intravenous route is used instead.

Subcutaneous, intraperitoneal and oral routes

Occasionally the subcutaneous route is used to administer fluids. This site is less useful in cats and dogs, as only small amounts of fluid can be administered and there is a prolonged amount of time between administration and absorption of the fluid. Fluid administered straight into the intravascular space is absorbed at a quicker rate and is then able to restore circulation.

Fluid is sometimes administered by the intraperitoneal route, but again this has a slower absorption time. Intraperitoneal fluid administration is reserved for patients where other routes are not available.

Oral fluids are occasionally administered as a method of rehydration. If an animal is able to drink voluntarily, the oral route should be maintained.

Other species

Rabbits

In rabbits, fluid is administered via the same routes as those used for cats and dogs. In addition, the marginal ear vein on the lateral aspect of the pinna is frequently used for intravenous access. The marginal ear vein is superficial and readily accessible in rabbits.

Other small mammals and reptiles

Common species routinely presented in veterinary practice include rats, hamsters, guinea pigs and reptiles, all of which have small superficial veins so that it is frequently impractical to use the intravenous route for administration of fluids. Instead, fluid is given via the intraosseous or intraperitoneal routes. The subcutaneous route is often readily accessible in smaller species but is less suitable in shocked patients, due to compromised circulation. (See *BSAVA Textbook of Veterinary Nursing* for more details.)

Administration equipment for fluid therapy

Methods of fluid administration by various routes are listed in Figure 8.17.

Route of fluid therapy	Method of administration
Intravenous	Intravenous catheter
Subcutaneous	Needle and syringe
Intraperitoneal	Needle and syringe
Intraosseous	Intraosseous catheter or spinal needle

8.17   Methods of fluid administration.

Catheters

Over-the-needle catheters

Over-the-needle intravenous catheters (Figure 8.18) are commonly used for intravenous administration of fluid into a peripheral vein. This type of catheter has a metal stylet over which the catheter slides. The metal stylet pierces the vein and is then removed; the catheter itself, through which the fluid is administered, remains in the vein.

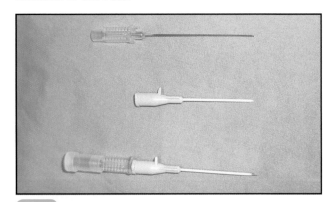

8.18   Over-the-needle catheters.

The largest possible diameter of catheter is used, to allow fluid to flow quickly through and because a larger lumen is less likely to get blocked. These types of catheter are colour coded according to their size (in gauge of diameter), but the codes vary between manufacturers. For peripheral veins, typical sizes would be 24 gauge for a rabbit, 21 gauge for a cat and 18 gauge for a 25 kg Labrador.

Through-the-needle catheters

Through-the-needle catheters are used for administration of fluid into the jugular and central veins. They have a metal stylet, through which the catheter is fed. This type of catheter is long and is able to be kept in place more easily in veins that are more mobile. Various through-the-needle catheters are available; their placement techniques vary slightly and the manufacturer's guidelines should be followed.

Luer mounts

Both over-the-needle and through-the-needle intravenous catheters have a luer mount at the free end to which a variety of other equipment (e.g. fluid administration set, three-way tap, syringe, bung) can be fitted. The equipment has either a male or female luer mount, which fits into another piece of equipment also having a luer mount. This sizing system allows items of equipment to be compatible and to connect with each other simply.

Butterfly and hypodermic needles

Butterfly needles (also known as scalp vein sets) are used less commonly to administer intravenous fluid. They are not ideal, since the metal needle is likely to irritate or puncture the vein when left *in situ*, allowing perivascular administration of fluid. Butterfly needles should not be used in administration of intravenous fluid therapy over a prolonged period, but are occasionally used to administer a large bolus of fluid.

Similarly, a standard hypodermic needle and syringe are not used for intravenous fluid administration.

Administration sets

There is a wide variety of fluid administration sets (also known as giving sets) available. They are all based on a basic design; some have differing ports or flow-control settings. The coiled type allows the patient to move more freely about its kennel and tends to become less twisted. The type of administration set used solely for administration of blood has a filter within the flow chamber to filter out any clots. The drip factor of a standard fluid administration set is 20 drops/ml.

Burettes

A burette (Figure 8.19) is used in situations where a smaller, accurate amount of fluid is administered, such as in patients with a lower bodyweight (neonates, cats, exotics). The standard drip factor for a burette is 60 drops/ml.

Extension sets

If a patient requires a greater length of tubing than the standard administration set allows, an extension set is used. The extension set is simply a length of tubing which, when connected between the catheter and administration set, gives extra length to the whole system. This is used when the fluid bag is situated some distance from the patient and more tubing is necessary. The extension set has no effect on the speed at which fluid is administered.

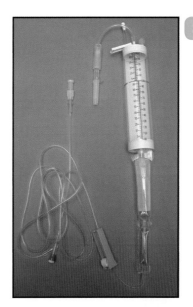

8.19 Burette.

Ancillary equipment

Three-way taps

A three-way tap is sometimes connected to the intravenous catheter and is then available for injection of drugs.

Bungs

A bung placed into the intravenous catheter can be used when the patient temporarily does not require fluid to be given. An example of this is if a patient is walked outside to urinate: it is easier to manage and possibly more comfortable for the patient to be disconnected from the administration set whilst moving around. Alternatively the patient may be removed from intravenous fluids for a short period of time, for example to allow it to have free access to drinking water. The administration set can easily be reconnected when necessary.

T-connectors

A T-connector is sometimes connected to the intravenous catheter (see Figure 8.22d) and allows injection of drugs into the catheter. The administration set can be disconnected from it since it also acts as a bung. In addition, it reduces the need to handle the intravenous catheter and therefore the risk of introducing infection to the catheter site.

Infusion pumps and syringe drivers

An infusion pump (Figure 8.20) is used to provide an accurate, continuous flow of fluid over a set period of time. The fluid administration set is fed through the infusion pump and the pump is programmed with the fluid rate to be given over a set period. An alarm will sound to alert staff if the tubing becomes blocked or fluid runs out. An infusion pump allows accurate flow of fluid and identifies any administration problems immediately. The infusion pump can be either hung from a drip stand or attached to the kennel door.

There is a selection of syringe drivers (Figure 8.21) and pressure bulb syringes commercially available, but they are not in common use. These administer fluid under pressure and are more suitable for small volumes of fluid than are drip pumps.

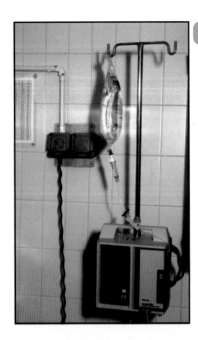

8.20   Infusion pump.

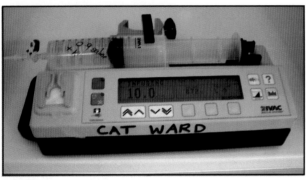

8.21   Syringe driver.

Preparation of equipment for intravenous fluid therapy

To prevent hypothermia, all fluid must be warmed to (but not exceeding) body temperature prior to administration to the patient. Fluid is warmed either by being heated in a warm-water bath, or placed in a warming cabinet or incubator, or by using thermal fluid heating jackets.

It is vital that the equipment used in administering fluid remains sterile. When preparing equipment, attention must be given to keeping equipment clinically clean. A common mistake is to allow the ends of the administration set to become contaminated against table ends or the floor. Care must be taken to keep all equipment away from possible contaminants.

All equipment should be gathered prior to the commencement of fluid administration and expiry dates should be checked for currency. Supplementary equipment is selected according to individual needs, such as:

- Scissors or electric clippers
- Scalpel blade for cutting down on to the vein (if preferred)
- Skin preparation solution
- Bandaging materials
- Solution of heparin anticoagulant.

Heparinized saline

Heparin is used for flushing the catheter to prevent blockage.

Heparinized saline is prepared by adding 5 ml of 1000 IU/ml heparin to 500 ml of sterile saline.

The required amount of heparinized saline is then drawn into a sterile syringe and needle and is used to flush the intravenous catheter immediately after it has been placed and after each new bag of fluid is connected.

Approximately 1–2 ml of heparinized saline is routinely used to flush the catheter.

Connecting the bag of fluid to the administration set

1. Gather together all equipment required.
2. Wash hands with a surgical scrub solution.
3. Check that administration set and bag of fluid are in date.
4. Examine fluid bag for cloudiness or floating particles. Should these be seen, select an alternative bag of fluid.
5. Warm bag of fluid to 37°C as previously discussed.
6. Remove bag of fluid from outer packaging.
7. Hang fluid bag on drip stand or from a suitably raised object.
8. Twist off the wings on the giving set port on the bag of fluid.
9. Remove fluid administration set from outer packaging. Handle carefully to ensure that the two ends of the tubing are not contaminated by coming into contact with a non-sterile surface (e.g. floor, tabletop, patient).
10. Turn off the fluid administration set by turning the flow regulator.
11. Using a gentle twisting action, insert the spiked end of the fluid administration set into the giving set port in the bag of fluid.
12. Slowly squeeze the fluid collection chamber two or three times to fill it approximately one-third to one-half full of fluid.
13. Allow fluid to flow slowly along the tubing by turning on the administration set. This flushes air from the length of the tubing. This is performed with a small bowl or kidney dish placed underneath the tubing to collect a small amount of leaked fluid. Avoid an excess of fluid escaping from the administration set: as the fluid slowly flows to the end of the tube, turn off the administration set to stop the flow of fluid.
14. To prevent an embolism from air being introduced into the patient's vein, ensure that there are no significant air bubbles remaining in the administration set.
15. The end of the administration set is hung over the drip stand or infusion pump, ready for use.

 WARNING
Remember that fluid bags and administration sets are for single use only.

Insertion of intravenous catheter into a vein

A strict aseptic technique is vital in placing the intravenous catheter. All equipment is selected first.

1. An assistant restrains the patient either standing, or in lateral or sternal recumbency.
2. Hair is clipped away from the site to expose the vein.
3. The vein is raised by the assistant and the vein visualized.
4. Hands are washed using a routine skin-cleansing solution.
5. The skin surrounding the vein is surgically cleaned using a standard surgical preparation technique, with a routine skin cleanser. The site is now prepared and ready for insertion of the catheter.
6. Hands are surgically cleaned using a standard scrub-up technique and sterile gloves worn by the person inserting the intravenous catheter.

Steps in placement of an over-the-needle intravenous catheter are as follows:

1. Raise surgically prepared vein in order that the vein can be visualized.
2. Slowly introduce the intravenous catheter into the vein (Figure 8.22a).
3. Stop inserting as soon as blood appears in the chamber of the catheter (this is known as blood flashback) (Figure 8.22b).
4. Hold the stylet still and feed the catheter along the length of the stylet, into the vein (Figure 8.22c).
5. Withdraw the stylet.
6. Connect a three-way tap to the catheter or bung/stopper.
7. Secure the catheter in place using pre-cut lengths of zinc oxide tape (Figure 8.22d).
8. Flush the catheter with heparinized saline.

The catheter is now ready to be connected to the chosen fluid administration equipment (e.g. T-connector/fluid administration set/extension set).

After the administration equipment has been attached and it is certain that fluid is flowing freely, the vein is monitored to check that fluid is not being administered perivascularly. Should perivascular administration occur, swelling above and around the vein becomes immediately obvious. In this case, administration of the fluid must stop and the catheter must be reinserted.

Once inserted and connected, the intravenous catheter is bandaged in place. The purpose of the bandage is to prevent contamination of the catheter site. A small amount of padding is used, covered by conforming non-adhesive bandage, which is held in place by zinc oxide tape or a tertiary layer of adhesive bandage.

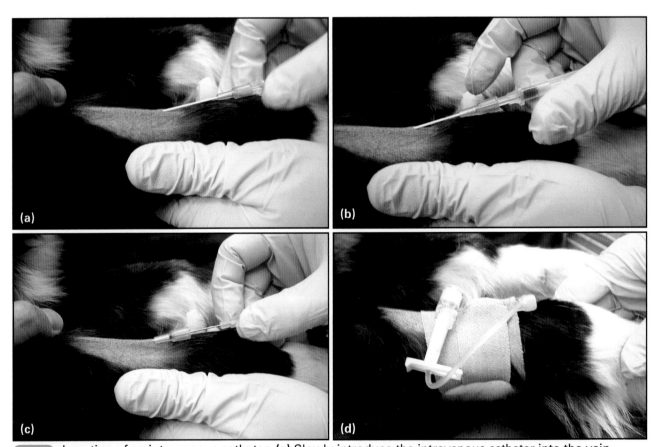

8.22 Insertion of an intravenous catheter. **(a)** Slowly introduce the intravenous catheter into the vein. **(b)** Stop inserting the catheter as soon as 'flashback' appears in the catheter chamber. **(c)** Feed the catheter along the length of the stylet into the vein. **(d)** Connect a T-port to the intravenous catheter and secure in place.

General care of intravenous catheter and fluid line

An intravenous catheter must only be left in place for 48 hours, after which the catheter must be removed and replaced in a different vein. Once in place, the catheter is checked at regular intervals – at least four times daily. This involves removing the bandage so that the catheter site can be viewed fully.

- Evidence of perivascular injection of fluid is shown by a swelling above and around the catheter insertion point, as described above.
- Any dislodging of the catheter from its original position or any kinking in the catheter length should be noted.
- Evidence of bruising around the vein indicates that the catheter needs to be removed.
- If the area around the catheter is painful to the patient, this signifies a problem and should be investigated further.
- The join between the catheter and the fluid administration set is checked for a secure connection.

If any of the above complications are noted, the fluid should be turned off and the catheter removed. A new catheter site is identified. The catheter is flushed with heparinized saline, (as described above) immediately after placement and also after drugs are injected through the catheter or a new bag of fluid is administered.

- The bandage covering the catheter is examined for soiling. If soiled, the bandage should be replaced.

- The fluid administration set is checked along its length to ensure that it is not twisted or kinked. This is usually easily remedied by untwisting the tubing or splinting the patient's limb to prevent bending at the joint, which is often a cause of kinking in the fluid administration line.
- Patient interference will be seen in the form of chewing the administration set or the bandage covering the catheter. The patient should be fitted with an Elizabethan collar to prevent further interference.
- The general demeanour and comfort of the patient should be recorded. A patient that is lethargic, unresponsive or generally quiet must be fully examined to investigate the causes.

Monitoring during fluid therapy

A patient undergoing fluid therapy must receive 24-hour nursing care. In addition to the standard hospitalization sheet (see Figure 5.11), a fluid record chart (Figure 8.23) must be completed.

- The plan of treatment administered to the patient should be recorded, with particular attention to the fluid therapy, and any amendments to the initial plan should also be recorded, as and when they occur.
- All fluid administered to the patient should be recorded, together with details of urine output, biochemical laboratory test results, general patient observations and any other drugs to be administered.

FLUID MONITORING CHART

Patient details   Animal Name: ....   Breed: ....   Age: ....

Sex: ....   Weight: ....   Case/Hospital no: ....   Vet: ....

Owner details: Owner Name: ....   Owner address: ....

....   Owner contact tel no: ....

FLUID THERAPY PLAN: Name of fluid: ....   Total amount of fluid to be given: ....

Fluid rate: ....   Drugs to be administered: ....

Date/time/ initials	Catheter & giving set checked	Intravenous line patent?	Bright/alert/ responsive?	Urine	Faeces	Problems	Approx amount of fluid remaining	Fluid rate (drop/second or ml/hour)

8.23 Example of a fluid monitoring chart, to be used in conjunction with a standard hospitalization sheet (see Figure 5.11).

All personnel nursing the patient must be vigilant in completing the fluid record chart to ensure that all details are fully recorded. This enables all veterinary staff to be fully aware of the progress of the patient and how much fluid has been given in total.

- The patient should be closely monitored for general signs of wellbeing (e.g. patient response to voice and touch), taking into consideration the individual's presenting problem.
- Rectal temperature, pulse and respiratory rate are recorded.
- Capillary refill time, skin turgor and colour of mucous membranes are noted.
- Chest sounds are auscultated and evidence of râles (abnormal sounds arising from the lower respiratory tract) must be brought to the attention of the veterinary surgeon immediately.
- Urine output must be accurately monitored in the patient receiving fluid therapy. In critically ill patients, an indwelling urinary catheter is placed and a closed drainage system is used to record urine output. Alternatively, the patient could be allowed to urinate freely and a rough estimate made of urine passed. This is not an accurate method of recording urine output and one to be avoided during administration of fluid therapy. Normal urine output of 1–2 ml/kg/hour is restored once the patient becomes rehydrated.
- Blood biochemistry and packed cell volume (PCV) are measured to monitor the patient's response to fluids. Since PCV is raised during dehydration, it should lower as the patient's hydration levels stabilize.

The intravenous catheter and fluid administration set should be closely monitored for problems, as discussed previously. The fluid therapy plan should be revised twice daily and any changes should be recorded on the patient's fluid monitoring sheet.

Complications during fluid therapy

In a patient with normal circulatory and renal function, over-transfusion of fluid is a possible but unlikely complication of fluid therapy. Excess fluid is lost from the body via the urinary system; thus an excess of fluid may accumulate if renal function is impaired. A patient showing signs of circulatory disease may have an existing build-up of fluid and therefore fluid overload during fluid therapy is possible.

Signs of over-transfusion of fluid include:

- Oedema of body tissues
- Râles
- Dyspnoea
- Lethargy
- Moist cough
- Tachypnoea
- Pulmonary oedoma.

Should over-transfusion be suspected, fluid administration must be ceased and the advice of a veterinary surgeon sought immediately. Attentive monitoring of the patient, together with urine output measurement, is likely to guard against over-transfusion of fluid.

Further reading

Bowden C and Masters J (2003) *Textbook of Veterinary Medical Nursing*. Butterworth-Heinemann, Oxford

Hotston Moore P (2004) *Fluid Therapy for Veterinary Nurses and Technicians*. Butterworth-Heinemann, Oxford

Welsh E and Girling SJ (2007) Fluid therapy and shock. In: *BSAVA Textbook of Veterinary Nursing, 4th edn*, ed. DR Lane *et al.*, pp. 388–411. BSAVA Publications, Gloucester

Orpet H and Welsh P (2002) *Handbook of Veterinary Nursing*. Blackwell Science, Oxford

9

Medical nursing

Rachel Lumbis

This chapter is designed to give information on:

■ Common infectious diseases
■ Diseases of body systems
■ The nursing role in medical diseases
■ Nursing geriatric, recumbent or soiled patients
■ Dealing with anorexic patients and providing assisted feeding
■ Administration of enemas
■ Urinary catheterization
■ Physiotherapy
■ Medical nursing of exotic pets

Introduction

The approach to any animal presented with a medical condition should always start with the collection of a detailed history, followed by a thorough physical examination. This provides the necessary information required to determine if the animal has a systemic disease or a disease affecting only one body system, and in some cases allows a diagnosis to be reached.

The veterinary nurse's role may include assisting the veterinary surgeon in collecting the information required from the clinical examination and participating in the diagnostic procedures being carried out. In addition, the veterinary nurse has a major role to play in providing patient care, administering treatment and monitoring for signs of improvement or deterioration. These are extremely important and valuable responsibilities; therefore it is vital that nurses are familiar with the information required to carry out their job efficiently and professionally.

In this chapter general principles will include exotic pets. Specific conditions will relate only to dogs and cats, though further information on the care and medical nursing of exotic pets is given at the end of the chapter. Treatments and diagnostic tests suggested throughout the chapter are described in further detail in Chapters 3, 10 and 11.

Medical diseases

A medical disease may be defined as a pathological condition of a part, organ, or system of an organism requiring, or amenable to, treatment by medicine as opposed to surgery. Conditions can result from various causes, such as infection, genetic defect or environmental stress, and are characterized by an identifiable group of signs or symptoms.

An aide-mémoire that helps in the broad categorization of medical diseases is the acronym DAMNIT-V:

■ **D**egenerative
■ **A**nomalous anatomy (congenital / hereditary / acquired)
■ **M**etabolic
■ **N**utritional & Neoplastic
■ **I**nfection & Inflammation & Immune-mediated
■ **T**rauma & Toxic
■ **V**ascular.

Consideration should be given to all body systems. All relevant information should be documented in order to obtain a full history and clinical picture.

Methods of disease control include the following:

- Select suitable animals for breeding
- Ensure adequate life-stage nutrition
- Prevent access or exposure to toxins
- Avoid trauma
- Ensure adequate ventilation (6–12 air changes per hour, depending on the number of animals within each air space)
- In the case of dogs and cats, relative humidity should be less than 55% and temperature between 15 and 24°C
- All areas accessible to animals must be easy to clean.

Chapter 5 gives information on basic animal management. Further advice for clients on disease control can be found in Chapter 2.

Clinical examination and history taking

The clinical examination of the patient provides essential information about its state of health. To detect abnormalities, a routine systematic method of examination is required and this involves practice and thoroughness. All findings, both normal and abnormal, should be recorded. Patients should undergo initial observation on arrival at the veterinary surgery, prior to disturbance.

Taking a patient's history

It is common for a history to be obtained prior to a physical examination. Usually, much of the relevant information is already known, but there are occasions when the veterinary nurse will be required to acquire further details. For instance, in the event of an emergency, specific details about the patient's recent history will be required (see Chapter 7).

As with the physical examination itself, it is of paramount importance that the veterinary nurse adopts a systematic approach and established routine to avoid missing any vital details. All information, both normal and abnormal, must be recorded.

A history should include:

- Routine history:
  - Age, breed, sex and sexual status (e.g. neutered or entire)
  - Vaccination status
  - Details of antiparasitic treatment
  - Dietary history – food being fed, amount, frequency, etc.
  - Environmental factors and lifestyle
- Medical history:
  - Description of past medical problems and any treatment received
  - Details of current drug therapy – type, dose, etc.
  - Description of current medical problem(s)
  - Determination of functional integrity of unmentioned body systems (e.g. frequency of urination).

Emphasis should be placed upon trying to establish:

- What the owner perceives to be the most concerning problem
- The duration, speed of onset and dynamics of the illness as perceived by the owner
- Character of emissions; changes in health status, behaviour, appetite, bodyweight, condition, etc.

Initial observation

Initial observation should include:

- General demeanour
- Urine and faecal output
- Presence of vomit
- Presence of blood.

Temperature, pulse and respiration

Figure 9.1 gives TPR data for small animals.

- T: temperature – record in degrees Celsius and degrees Fahrenheit
- P: pulse – note rate, rhythm and character
- R: respiration at rest – record rate, depth and manner.

Performing a clinical examination

A methodical approach to performing a clinical examination is set out in Figure 9.2.

Animal	Temperature (°C)	Pulse (beats/min)	Respiration (breaths/min)
Dog	38.3–38.7	60–100	10–30
Cat	38.0–38.5	160–200	20–30
Neonatal dogs and cats	35.5–36.1	200–220	15–35
Ferret	38.8	200–250	30–40
Rabbit	38.5–40.0	180–300	30–60
Chinchilla	38–39	100–150	45–80

9.1 TPR data for dogs, cats and small mammals. (continues) ▶

Animal	Temperature (°C)	Pulse (beats/min)	Respiration (breaths/min)
Guinea pig	39–40	190–300	90–150
Gerbil	38.0	300–400	90–140
Hamster	36.0–38.0	280–412	33–127
Rat	37.5–38.0	260–450	70–150
Mouse	37.5	500–600	100–250

9.1 (continued) TPR data for dogs, cats and small mammals.

Body area	Normal findings	Abnormal findings
General	Healthy body condition and weight. No signs of injury or masses	Signs of malnourishment. Muscle atrophy. Wounds. Matting of the fur. Alopecia or areas of hair loss. Penetrating foreign bodies. Enlarged lymph nodes. Emaciation or obesity
Head and neck	Free from discharges. No signs of fractures. Symmetry and complementary (balanced) conformation	Presence of aural, nasal or ocular discharge or haemorrhage. Swelling, pain or crepitus (could indicate fracture). Asymmetry or non-complementary conformation
Ears, eyes and nose	All free from discharge or haemorrhage. Central eyeball position. Palpebral reflex. Pupils responsive to light	Haemorrhage from the ears. Constricted or dilated pupils. Nystagmus. Difference in size of pupils. Nictitating membranes (third eyelids) drawn across the eye(s). Abnormal colour of conjunctival mucosa or bruising to sclera. Unilateral or bilateral epistaxis. Swelling of nasal bones
Mouth	Odour free. Mucous membranes pink. Capillary refill time (CRT) of 1–2 seconds. Moist mucous membranes	Malodour (could be indicative of dental disease or kidney failure). Pale = severe shock or haemorrhage. Brick red = toxic or septicaemic patient. Cyanotic = severe dyspnoea. Yellow = (jaundice) liver damage. Prolonged CRT could indicate low blood pressure or haemorrhage. Tacky or dry mucous membranes. Profuse salivation (could indicate poisoning). Check for oral ulceration or redness, which could occur following ingestion of poisons
Thorax	Auscultation of heart, normal heart rate and rhythm. Normal respiratory rate and effort. Heart rate should be in synchrony with femoral pulse rate	Tachycardia, bradycardia, heart murmur. Palpation of prescapular and axillary lymph nodes. Listen to any wounds to detect hissing sound on inspiration, indicating penetration of the pleural cavity. Dyspnoea, tachypnoea, bradypnoea, apnoea. Thoracic trauma, e.g. fractured ribs, ruptured diaphragm, intercostal muscle damage
Abdomen	Normal carriage, musculature and integument	Haemorrhage from the penis. Bruising or swellings of the abdominal wall. Signs of pain – hunched or praying position
Spine and limbs	No signs of abnormalities or injury. Conscious proprioception. Full range of movement. Normal gait – soundness and coordination. Normal carriage, symmetry and musculature	Signs of deformity, swelling or pain. Deformities in spinal column. Absence of conscious proprioception (could be indicative of spinal damage). Lameness, flaccid or spastic paralysis. Quadriplegia, hemiplegia, paraplegia. Hyperaesthesia
Pelvis	Stability	Signs of instability, pain, crepitus or deformity
Perianal region	Normal temperature. Anus and external genitalia clean and free from discharge. Voluntary tail movement. Tail held high	Hypothermia, hyperthermia. Lesions or discharge. Enlarged prostate in male dogs. Abnormalities such as cryptorchism or monorchism in males. Incorrect tail carriage/flaccid tail. Bloody or purulent discharge. Signs of pyometra in females. Signs of diarrhoea, haemorrhage or parasitic worms

9.2 Performing a clinical examination.

Infectious diseases

An infectious disease is one caused by microorganisms that can successfully invade and grow in the host's tissues. Organisms responsible for causing disease include bacteria, protozoa, fungi and viruses. For an infection to survive, it must be transmitted. The mode of transmission (see Chapter 2) is an important factor in understanding the disease. Common canine and feline infectious diseases are described and illustrated in Figures 9.3 to 9.8.

Canine infectious disease	Incubation period	Method of infection	Target tissues	Clinical signs	Complications	Nursing care	Treatment
Parvovirus (canine parvovirus) ⚠	3–5 days	Ingestion following direct or indirect contact. Large amounts of virus found in faeces	All rapidly dividing cells, including bone marrow, intestine and other lymphoid tissue. Myocardium in unprotected neonatal puppies	Sudden death from myocarditis rarely seen due to good levels of maternal antibody. Gastroenteritis now most common form: acute vomiting, diarrhoea, anorexia, abdominal pain, dehydration	Malabsorption. *Be aware of zoonotic risk – can cause upset stomach in humans.* Also a disease affecting ferrets	Isolation procedures. Barrier nursing. Provide and maintain therapy as prescribed. Monitor vital signs and record episodes of vomiting and diarrhoea. Discuss with owner the implications for multi-dog households. Clean and disinfect affected areas	Intravenous fluid therapy using Hartmann's solution. Antibiotics. Anti-emetics
Leptospirosis (*Leptospira canicula* and *L. icterohaemorrhagiae*) ⚠	Approx. 7 days	Penetration through skin, mucous membranes, cuts, transplacental and venereal. Direct and indirect spread possible. Urine a major source of infection	Kidneys (*L. canicula*) Liver (*L. icterohaemorrhagiae*)	Acute vomiting, anorexia, polydipsia. Initially oliguria, then polyuria. Pain over kidneys Sudden death in unweaned puppies. Acute vomiting, anorexia, abdominal pain, jaundice, petechial haemorrhage on mucosa, collapse	Excretion of organisms may persist for weeks following recovery	Precautions required for zoonotic disease. Isolation procedures. Barrier nursing. Provide and maintain therapy as prescribed. Monitor vital signs. Maintain fluid lines. Maintain a clean and stable environment. Clean and disinfect affected areas. Careful disposal of waste – excretion of organisms via urine	Intravenous fluid therapy using Hartmann's. Possibly whole blood. Antibiotics. Anti-emetics
Lyme disease (*Borrelia burgdorferi*) and ehrlichiosis (*Ehrlichia* spp.) ⚠	Variable: acute to extended	Vector – deer tick (*Ixodes dammini*)	Kidneys (fatal). CNS. Joints	Lameness ± swollen joints, fever, lymphadenopathy, anorexia, lethargy		Precautions required for zoonotic disease. Barrier nursing. Prevention of ticks. Client education regarding avoidance of endemic areas	Antibiotics to treat the bacterial infection. NSAIDs to control pain relief when polyarthritis is a clinical sign
Kennel cough complex (*Bordetella bronchiseptica*, parainfluenza virus, herpesvirus, reovirus and secondary bacterial agents)	5–7 days	Aerosol spread and inhalation. Dogs in direct contact or within same air space.	Upper respiratory epithelium	Dry 'hacking' cough, pyrexia, occasional retching, mucopurulent nasal discharge, possibly ocular discharge	Chronic infection, bronchopneumonia	Isolation procedures. Barrier nursing. Provide and maintain therapy as prescribed. Advise owners regarding in-contact dogs. Clean and disinfect affected areas	Antibiotics. Cough suppressants
Infectious canine hepatitis (canine adenovirus)	5–9 days	Ingestion, following direct or indirect contact. Organisms found in saliva, vomit, faeces and urine	Hepatocytes, vascular endothelium, other lymphoid tissue and bone marrow	Sudden deaths in unweaned puppies, acute vomiting, bloody diarrhoea, pyrexia, anorexia, abdominal pain, petechial haemorrhages on mucous membranes	Corneal oedema or 'blue eye', glomerular nephritis	Isolation procedures. Monitor vital signs and record episodes of vomiting and diarrhoea. Provide and maintain therapy as prescribed. Care of intravenous fluid lines. Clean and disinfect affected areas	Intravenous fluid therapy using Hartmann's. Whole blood where bleeding is extensive. Antibiotics. Anti-emetics. Intestinal protectants
Distemper (morbillivirus) ⚠	7–21 days	Inhalation or ingestion following direct or indirect contact. Virus found in ocular and nasal discharge, urine and faeces	Epithelial cells of respiratory and alimentary tract. Nervous system and other lymphoid tissue, including bone marrow	Anorexia, pyrexia, vomiting, diarrhoea, coughing, ocular and nasal discharges, tonsillitis, hyperkeratosis of pads and nose, nervous signs including chorea, muscle tremors and seizures	Nervous signs developing years after initial infection: seizures, chorea, old dog encephalitis. Dental disease (see Figure 9.6)	Barrier nursing. Isolation procedures. Monitor vital signs and record episodes of vomiting and diarrhoea. Maintain fluid lines. Provide and maintain therapy as prescribed. Bathe discharge from eyes and nose. Clean and disinfect affected areas	Intravenous fluid therapy using Hartmann's, antibiotics, anticonvulsants, anti-emetics, antidiarrhoeal agents

9.3 Canine infectious diseases. ⚠ indicates a zoonosis.

Disease/Infection	Incubation period	Method of infection	Target tissues	Clinical signs	Client advice	Nursing care	Treatment
Feline panleucopenia, also known as feline parvovirus (parvovirus)	2–7 days	Ingestion following direct or indirect contact. Virus found in body secretions, i.e. saliva, vomit, faeces and urine. Transplacental	All rapidly dividing cells, especially intestine, bone marrow and other lymphoid tissue	Acute vomiting, anorexia, abdominal pain, followed by fluid diarrhoea, dehydration and weight loss. Fetal infection leads to cerebellar hypoplasia and ataxia after birth	Advise owner regarding in-contact cats	Prevent spread of infection to other cats – isolation. Clean and disinfect affected areas. Provide and maintain therapy as prescribed	Intravenous fluid therapy using Hartmann's, antibiotics, antiemetics, intestinal protectants
Feline leukaemia virus (FeLV) (retrovirus)	Months to years	Virus excreted in saliva, urine, faeces and milk. Transmission by direct contact, including biting and mutual grooming	Immune system, bone marrow, intestines, salivary and lacrimal glands, urogenital tract	Associated with infection of the haemopoietic system	40% of affected cats will eliminate the virus and recover. 30% develop a low immunity and show symptoms of infection. 30% develop a latent infection	Advise owner regarding prevention – recommend vaccination. Prevent spread of disease – isolation, barrier nursing	None
Feline infectious anaemia (FIA) (Mycoplasma haemofelis)	Not known, may have carrier states	Cat bites, fleas, in utero, via milk	Red blood cells	Sudden onset of acute haemolytic anaemia, tachycardia, tachypnoea, pallor of mucous membranes, weakness, collapse	Flea control. Prevent cat fights. Neuter entire male cats	Provide and maintain therapy as prescribed. Observe vital signs during hospitalization period. Ensure stress-free environment. Assist owner with flea eradication	Systemic tetracyclines, blood transfusions if severe, clear flea infestations
Feline upper respiratory tract disease (FURTD), also known as cat flu (feline calicivirus, feline herpesvirus, Bordetella and other bacteria)	2–10 days	Aerosol spread by direct or indirect contact. Viruses found in large numbers in ocular/nasal secretions and exhaled breath	Upper respiratory tract epithelium (Figure 9.7)	Pyrexia, paroxysmal sneezing, serous then mucopurulent ocular and nasal discharge (Figure 9.8), blepharospasm. Anorexia (some cases)	Advise vaccination. Prevent contact with other cats	Prevent spread of infection – isolation. Clean and disinfect affected areas. Encourage patient to eat – warm food, feed highly palatable diet, hand feed, appetite stimulants. Provide and maintain therapy as prescribed. Maintain fluid lines. Bathe ocular and nasal discharges	Correct dehydration if present, antibiotics, enteral feeding if anorexic
Feline pneumonitis (Chlamydophila felis) ⚠	4–10 days	Direct contact via ocular discharge	Upper respiratory tract, ocular mucous membranes, nasal epithelium	Pyrexia, serous then mucopurulent ocular and nasal discharge, sneezing, blepharospasm, anorexia	Be aware of zoonotic risk – application of basic hygiene standards will prevent any slight possibility of cross-transmission to humans. Consequences for in-contact cats. Advise vaccination	Prevent spread of infection – isolation. Maintain strict levels of hygiene to avoid cross-contamination to other animals. Carriers of the disease remain an outlet for further infection. Provide and maintain therapy as prescribed	All in-contact cats should be treated with ocular tetracyclines and/or systemic tetracyclines
Feline immuno-deficiency virus (FIV) (retrovirus)	Variable, from weeks to months	Cat bites – high level of virus in saliva	Lymphoid tissue. Bone marrow	Associated with immunosuppression. Chronic gingivitis, chronic URTD, non-regenerative anaemias, development of FeLV, FIP, FIA, toxoplasmosis and other infections, chronic weight loss	Advise screening of other cats in the household. Isolation of infected cats. Advise owners regarding male cat aggression, roaming and fighting	Provide and maintain therapy as prescribed. Isolation of infected and non-infected cats	None. Treat secondary infections symptomatically
Feline infectious peritonitis (FIP) (coronavirus)	Variable	Oronasal route	Vascular endothelium, peritoneum, pleura, eye, meninges, kidneys	Wet/effusive form (approximately 60%): ascites, hydrothorax, pericardial effusion, anorexia, weight loss, diarrhoea

Dry/non-effusive form (approximately 40%): clinical features often vague, non-specific and variable. Weight loss and inappetence common presenting signs. Other clinical signs dependent on which organs have been affected and how much damage has been done. May affect eyes, abdomen, CNS, liver, kidneys | Found mainly in young cats – 80% of cats that develop FIP are under 2 years old. Often affects pedigree breeds. Multi-cat households, cats that have been in rescue establishments/boarding catteries or those attending shows are more likely to become infected. Effusive FIP (the acute form) usually occurs within 3–6 weeks of a stressful event in a cat's life | Provide advice on prevention. No certain way to prevent an infected cat from developing FIP, but the following points may help: minimize stress for the cat – do not re-home it and avoid putting it into a cattery. Where possible do not breed from an infected cat. Any mating that has produced kittens that have developed FIP should not be repeated. Kittens are usually protected from the virus until they are 5–6 weeks of age therefore they should be isolated after this time until they are sold | FIP is usually fatal and no treatment has proved to be reliable. A vaccine has been developed against feline coronavirus but it is not available in the UK. Therapy largely symptomatic and consists mainly of fluid replacement and nutritional support |

9.4 Feline infectious diseases. ⚠ indicates a zoonosis.

Disease	Incubation period	Method of infection	Target tissues	Clinical signs	Complications	Nursing care	Treatment
Rabies (rhabdovirus) ⚠ **Fatal zoonotic disease**	2 weeks to 4 months. Mean period of 3 weeks depending on site and severity of bite wound and dose of virus	Biting, but virus can cross mucous membranes. Saliva contains large amount of virus therefore great care is required when handling animal with suspected rabies	Neuromuscular junction, nervous system	Furious form: hyperexcitability, aggression, depraved appetite, aimless walking, development of paresis and dysphagia with facial asymmetry. Finally, seizures. Dumb form: little observed until progressive paralysis	Disease of worldwide importance. In most of Europe rabies is found principally in foxes. In other parts of the world, notably Indian subcontinent, the dog is a major reservoir. If a human is bitten by a suspect rabid animal, the wound should be washed immediately and aggressively with a 20% soap solution, quaternary ammonium compound or ethanol	Where rabies is suspected, ensure safety of personnel. Do not allow animal to be handled unless essential. Ensure animal is isolated and safely locked up. Rabies is a notifiable disease in the UK: *anyone* who knows or suspects that an animal has rabies must report it immediately to the police or their local veterinary divisional office. The animal should be kept in a cage and euthanasia should *not* be performed until further instructions are received from the relevant authorities	None – always fatal. Vaccination effective at preventing rabies and should be used in all dogs and cats where the disease is endemic. Inactivated vaccines available in UK as part of Pet Travel Scheme (see Chapter 2)
Salmonellosis (*Salmonella*) ⚠	2–7 days, though carrier status may occur	Contact with contaminated food or water and from exposure to infected faecal material	Gastrointestinal tract, CNS, placenta, respiratory tract	Acute gastroenteritis, diarrhoea ± vomiting, anorexia, depression, dehydration as consequence of water and electrolyte losses, pyrexia	Higher incidences reported in kennels and breeding establishments – may relate to higher stocking densities, poor hygiene or staff spreading infection via hands, boots, clothing or food bowls	Human infection from pet animals rare but *Salmonella* spp. zoonotic therefore usual precautions must be taken. Wash hands regularly. Wear protective clothing. Dispose of all infected material (should be incinerated). Disinfect premises and all affected areas	Dependent on severity of symptoms. Intravenous fluid therapy, antibiotics if signs of systemic disease
Toxoplasmosis (*Toxoplasma gondii*) ⚠	2–5 weeks	In cats, indirect, via ingestion of tissue cysts found in the intermediate host (rodent). Ingestion of oocysts from cat faeces causes infection in dogs, sheep and humans	Muscle tissue and brain possible, placental tissue in sheep and humans	All species: lethargy, depression, anorexia, pyrexia, weight loss, neurological signs, ocular disease, lymphadenopathy. Abortion in sheep and humans	Cats can also infect sheep (via sheep feed) causing abortion in ewes. Aborting ewes and their lambs are a high zoonotic risk. Shedding of toxoplasmosis by cats is made worse by immunosuppression (e.g. FeLV and FIV)	Important zoonosis; especially important in immunosuppressed individuals. Promote strict hygiene precautions. Educate clients: • Pregnant women should not handle cat litter • Ensure all meat is cooked thoroughly • Wear rubber gloves when gardening • Prevent cats from hunting • Cover children's sandpits	Antibiotics

9.5 Infectious diseases affecting both dogs and cats. ⚠ indicates a zoonosis.

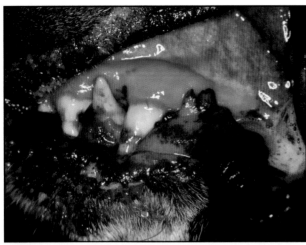

9.6 Yellowing of teeth as a result of enamel hypoplasia due to distemper during tooth development. (Reproduced from *BSAVA Manual of Canine and Feline Infectious Diseases*. © Dr Ian Ramsey)

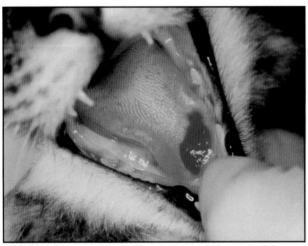

9.7 Tongue ulceration in a cat infected with feline calicivirus. (Reproduced from *BSAVA Manual of Canine and Feline Infectious Diseases*)

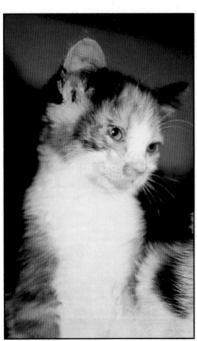

9.8 Ocular and nasal discharge in a kitten with cat flu. Feline herpesvirus was isolated from this kitten. (Reproduced from *BSAVA Manual of Canine and Feline Infectious Diseases*)

Methods of infectious disease control

Clients must be correctly advised regarding methods of infectious disease control. This is especially important to breeders, owners of boarding kennels and those who have multi-pet households. Measures should include the following:

- Have isolation/quarantine facilities to prevent direct contact; have separate equipment (including bowls and kitchen utensils) for this area
- Ensure that staff/owners are aware of procedures to follow when in contact with quarantined animals
- Maintain hygiene to prevent fomite contamination and insect vectors
- Avoid overcrowding and increase ventilation
- At first signs of disease, seek appropriate treatment
- Vaccinate all newcomers and maintain booster vaccinations
- Undertake parasite control.

In addition, the veterinary practice should educate clients by means of well-pet clinics, vaccine reminders, and advice on nutrition, worming and flea control (see Chapter 2).

Hygiene

The best way to minimize infection within the hospital environment is to practise good hygiene (see Chapter 4):

- Wash and disinfect all equipment thoroughly
- Clean all surfaces regularly
- Do not rely on disinfectant to kill all infective agents – remove all organic matter first
- Use correct dilution factors for disinfectants
- Use disposable bedding if possible
- Keep personal hygiene standards high – wash hands between patients or use alcohol-based hand hygiene products
- Prepare food away from where waste is stored
- Keep vermin under control.

Patients that are most likely to spread disease should be cleaned out and treated after all other patients in the isolation facility.

- Each patient in isolation should be allocated its own equipment (food bowl, water bowl, etc.). This should be washed and disinfected separately from others. Bedding should all be disposable and discarded into clinical waste.
- Barrier nursing must be instigated in all patients with infectious diseases. Clear notices should be displayed to prevent inadvertent cross-contamination.
- Veterinary nurses should be allocated solely to the isolation facility and not allowed to nurse patients in the general ward.

Further information on disease control and prevention can be found in Chapters 2 and 4.

Zoonoses

Zoonoses (see Figures 9.3, 9.4, 9.5, 9.9, 9.36 and 9.37) are diseases that are transmissible between vertebrate animals and humans; they may produce different symptoms in humans. The risk of catching a zoonotic disease varies according to the individual's occupation, frequency and type of contact with animals and geographical location. In a veterinary practice the risk is inevitably higher than in most environments, as staff regularly come into contact with animals and their waste products.

Important nursing considerations for animals with suspected or confirmed zoonoses are as follows:

- Hygiene prophylaxis – strict attention must be paid to hygiene. Always take preventive measures: wash hands thoroughly after handling animals with *any* disease. It might turn out to be zoonotic even if it initially looks unlikely
- Protection from zoonotic disease is a high priority. Personal protective equipment (PPE), such as disposable gloves, aprons and foot covers, should be worn. The amount of such clothing should be upgraded according to the degree of risk anticipated
- Veterinary nurses should be allocated solely to the isolation facility and not allowed to nurse patients in the general ward; exposure should be kept to a minimum, as far as possible
- Ensure that the very young and old are not exposed to animals with possible zoonotic infections
- Seek medical advice quickly if exposed to a zoonotic disease
- Carrier animals are a potential source of infection with zoonotic disease
- Ensure that adequate prophylactic protection is implemented when there is a known possible risk (e.g. rabies vaccines for nurses dealing with bats in the UK).

Educating clients about disease risks from pets

Clients should be given the following advice:

- Do not allow animals to lick human faces or mouths – this is especially important when children are playing with animals
- Never let animals eat or drink off utensils used for human food consumption
- Clean and prepare animals' feeding utensils in a separate area to human ones
- Pregnant women should be vigilant about personal hygiene after contact with animals
- Prevent cats from contaminating children's sandpits
- Keep gardens and kennel runs clear of faeces.

Diseases of the respiratory system

It is important for the veterinary nurse to be able to differentiate between upper (URTD) and lower respiratory tract disease (LRTD) (Figure 9.10).

Nasal discharge
Aetiology
Nasal discharges can be:

- Serous – early bacterial, viral and fungal infection or allergy
- Mucopurulent – established infections, foreign body, tumour (Figure 9.11), allergy
- Epistaxis (nose bleed) – trauma, tumour, clotting defect, severe bacterial or fungal infection
- Unilateral – localized disease
- Bilateral – systemic disease or advanced local disease.

Nursing care

- Obtain detailed history from owners.
- Advise owners as to possible causes of nasal discharge.
- Advise owners of diagnostic procedures that may be used.
- Assist veterinary surgeon in carrying out procedures and treatment.
- Keep nares clean and free from discharge.
- Encourage animal to eat (especially important in cats).
- Prevent and discourage animal from pawing at its face or rubbing its nose on the ground.
- Isolate and barrier nurse if an infectious disease is suspected.

Disease	Cause	Route of transmission
Viral diseases		
Rabies	Rabies virus	Saliva
Bacterial diseases		
Salmonellosis	*Salmonella* spp.	Faecal contamination
Campylobacterosis	*Campylobacter* spp.	Faecal contamination
Leptospirosis	*Leptospira* spp.	Urine
Fungal diseases		
Ringworm	*Microsporum* spp., *Trichophyton* spp.	Direct contact
Parasitic diseases		
Toxocariasis	*Toxocara* spp. roundworms	Faecal contamination
Hydatid disease	*Echinococcus granulosus* tapeworm	Faecal contamination
Cheyletiellosis	*Cheyletiella* spp. mites	Direct contact
Scabies	*Sarcoptes scabiei* mite	Direct contact

9.9 Examples of zoonotic diseases.

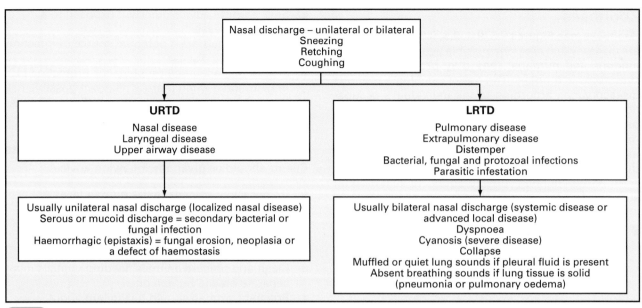

```
                    Nasal discharge – unilateral or bilateral
                                  Sneezing
                                  Retching
                                  Coughing
```

URTD	**LRTD**
Nasal disease Laryngeal disease Upper airway disease	Pulmonary disease Extrapulmonary disease Distemper Bacterial, fungal and protozoal infections Parasitic infestation
Usually unilateral nasal discharge (localized nasal disease) Serous or mucoid discharge = secondary bacterial or fungal infection Haemorrhagic (epistaxis) = fungal erosion, neoplasia or a defect of haemostasis	Usually bilateral nasal discharge (systemic disease or advanced local disease) Dyspnoea Cyanosis (severe disease) Collapse Muffled or quiet lung sounds if pleural fluid is present Absent breathing sounds if lung tissue is solid (pneumonia or pulmonary oedema)

9.10 Differentiating upper from lower respiratory tract disease.

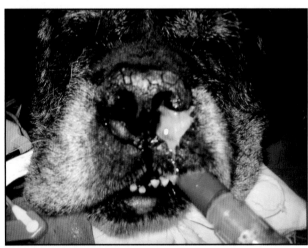

9.11 Mucopurulent nasal discharge from a dog with a nasal tumour. (Reproduced from *BSAVA Textbook of Veterinary Nursing, 4th edition*)

Coughing

Aetiology

Coughing may be associated with:

■ Chronic bronchitis
■ Cardiac failure
■ Neoplasia
■ Airway foreign bodies
■ Tonsillitis, pharyngitis, tracheitis
■ Tracheal collapse
■ Pulmonary oedema
■ Pulmonary haemorrhage
■ Lungworm infection (*Oslerus osleri*, *Aelurostrongylus abstrusus*)
■ Bronchopneumonia.

Treatment

This depends on the underlying cause, but may include:

■ Cardiac drug therapy
■ Diuretics
■ Antibiotics
■ Anthelmintics
■ Antitussives
■ Corticosteroids
■ Environmental improvements in air temperature, humidity and quality
■ Bronchodilators.

Drug therapy is described in further detail in Chapter 3.

Nursing care

■ Differentiate the problem from kennel cough (see Figure 9.3).
■ Obtain detailed history from owners in order to ascertain possible causes.
■ Examine the throat and mouth – check for ulcers or inflammation and ensure that they are clean and patent.
■ Remove the collar and use a harness or 'Halti' if upper respiratory disease is suspected.
■ Prepare drug therapy as prescribed.
■ Feed soft food (by hand if required).
■ Note capability of transmitting airborne disease.
■ Keep patient isolated from other patients, preferably in glass-fronted kennel.
■ Provide TLC.
■ Perform coupage (see Physiotherapy, later).
■ Change environmental temperature and humidity as necessary.

Acute respiratory failure

Acute respiratory failure is the inability of the respiratory system to perform gaseous exchange well enough for the blood and tissues to remain adequately oxygenated. This situation is classified as an emergency and requires first aid measures and appropriate medical treatment to prevent deterioration and a potentially fatal outcome.

Aetiology

Acute respiratory failure may be associated with:

- Airway obstruction: airway foreign body, laryngeal paralysis, tracheal collapse
- Neoplasia
- Pleural effusion
- Trauma
- Lung disease
- Respiratory muscle paralysis
- Failure of the respiratory control centre – brain injury, drug or anaesthetic overdose
- Pneumothorax, haemothorax, pyothorax, chylothorax
- Ruptured diaphragm
- Gastric torsion
- Infections: tetanus, botulism, bacterial and viral pneumonias
- Paraquat poisoning.

Clinical signs

These may include some or all of the following, depending on the underlying cause:

- Change in character of breathing – dyspnoea, tachypnoea, apnoea, orthopnoea
- Open-mouth breathing
- Cyanosis
- Tachycardia with a weak, thready pulse
- Collapse, unconsciousness and death.

Treatment

Procedures for treatment of airway obstruction are given in Chapter 7 and in the *BSAVA Manual of Advanced Veterinary Nursing*.

Nursing care

- Ensure that airway is patent.
- Increase environmental oxygen content.
- Provide manual ventilation if necessary.
- Ensure that pulmonary function is adequate to maintain animal, e.g. enforced cage rest to reduce respiratory demands.
- Provide treatment and administer drug therapy as prescribed by the veterinary surgeon.
- Provide circulatory support.

Chronic pulmonary failure

Chronic pulmonary failure is caused by a more gradual progressive impairment of lung function. If left untreated, it can lead to acute respiratory failure and the associated symptoms of respiratory distress.

Aetiology

Chronic pulmonary failure may be associated with:

- Chronic bronchitis/bronchiectasis
- Lungworms
- Foreign bodies
- Pulmonary oedema
- Pulmonary neoplasia
- Asthma (in cats)
- Pleural effusions
- Pneumonia.

Clinical signs

These include:

- Reduced exercise tolerance
- Chronic cough
- Breathlessness
- Increased respiratory noise.

Nursing care

- Provide treatment and administer drugs as prescribed by veterinary surgeon.
- Restrict exercise.
- Monitor and maintain a suitable temperature – avoid exposure to extremes of temperature.
- Maintain a clean environment.
- Humidification of inspired air helps to prevent drying of the mucous membranes and aids removal of mucus, therefore it is important to monitor and maintain a suitable humidity.
- Administer coupage to help to loosen mucus (see 'Physiotherapy' section, below).
- Place overweight animals on a diet as this will significantly improve lung and airway function.

Diseases of the circulatory system

Heart disease may be:

- Congenital
- Acquired.

Heart failure may be:

- Acute
- Chronic.

Congenital heart defects

Congenital heart defects are malformations that are present at birth. In dogs and cats, they occur as isolated defects (most common) or in various combinations. Purebred animals have a higher prevalence of congenital defects.

Nursing care

- Administer fluid therapy – especially if there has been a reduced fluid intake.
- May need treatment for aspiration pneumonia, to include coupage.
- May need tube feeding to increase nutrient uptake – gastrostomy tube is preferable.
- If tube feeding is not required, feed liquid food or soft food balls little and often and from a height. This will help prevent regurgitation and aspiration pneumonia, and may be especially important after surgery. Warming the food and hand-feeding may help overcome inappetence.
- Provide a stress-free environment.
- Administer drug therapy as prescribed.
- Ensure that the animal is taken for frequent short walks rather than one long walk.

Diagnostic tests

Heart defects can be detected using the following:

- Auscultation
- Ultrasound (most important)
- X-ray
- ECG
- Evaluation of clinical features
- Angiocardiography.

There are many possible congenital heart defects that may occur in puppies and kittens. The commonest types are:

- Patent ductus arteriosus
- Pulmonary stenosis
- Aortic stenosis
- Ventricular septal defects
- Mitral and tricuspid dysplasia
- Tetralogy of Fallot
- Persistent right aortic arch.

Patent ductus arteriosus (PDA)

- Most common congenital heart defect in dogs.
- Fetal blood vessel between aorta and pulmonary artery remains patent.
- Blood shunts from left to right (Figure 9.12).
- Machinery murmur on auscultation.
- Clinical signs dependent on extent of shunting but include weakness, dyspnoea, exercise intolerance, cough and cyanosis.
- Prognosis excellent with surgery but this may be cost-prohibitive.

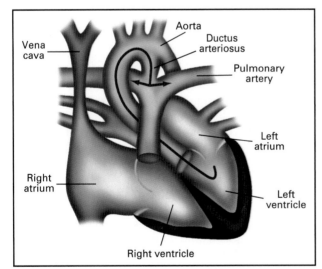

9.12 Patent ductus arteriosus (PDA). Blood flows from the left ventricle, into the aorta, and then into the pulmonary artery (instead of going to the body where it is needed).

Pulmonary stenosis

- Narrowing of the blood vessel leaving the right side of the heart through the pulmonary artery.
- Obstructs the blood from leaving the right ventricle.
- High pressure build-up on right side of heart.

- A heart murmur might be detected at routine auscultation in a young animal; otherwise, they may present later with signs of right-sided heart failure.
- Prognosis dependent on severity of the stenosis. Patients with a mild PS may have a normal life span, but animals with severe PS often die within 3 years of diagnosis.

Aortic stenosis

- Common in Boxer dogs.
- Narrowing of the blood vessel leaving the left side of the heart through aorta.
- High pressure build-up on left side of heart.
- No clinical signs until left-sided heart failure occurs, which could prove fatal.
- Prognosis in animals diagnosed with a severe stenosis is guarded. Those with a mild stenosis are more likely to be asymptomatic and live longer.

Ventricular septal defects

- A hole exists between right and left ventricles.
- Size of hole determines clinical signs exhibited.
- Generally blood shunts from left to right; congestive heart failure (CHF) likely to occur (Figure 9.13).
- Clinical outcome dependent on size of hole – surgery needed to close larger defects.
- Animals with a moderate-size defect can have a fairly normal life span whereas those with a large defect are likely to develop left-sided heart failure. Occasionally, spontaneous closure of the defect can occur within the first 2 years of life.

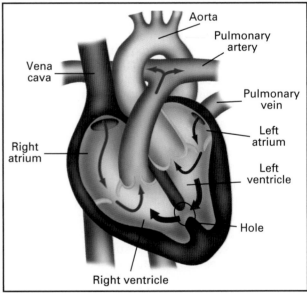

9.13 Ventricular septal defect. Blood flows from the left to the right heart through a hole in the septum, causing congestive heart failure.

Mitral and tricuspid dysplasia

- Deformity of the atrioventricular valves.
- Allows regurgitation of blood between ventricles and atria.

- Can lead to heart failure.
- Common cause of heart disease in young dogs, especially Golden Retrievers.
- Treatment consists of medical management for signs of CHF. Prognosis is usually guarded to poor, but some dogs survive for several years.

Tetralogy of Fallot

- Condition where several defects exist together: pulmonary stenosis, ventricular septal defect, dextraposed aorta and right ventricular wall hypertrophy (Figure 9.14).
- Clinically causes cyanosis, exercise intolerance, systolic murmur and heart failure.
- Definitive surgical repair requires open heart surgery.
- Prognosis depends on severity of the condition. Mildly affected animals or those that have undergone successful surgery may live for 4–7 years. Prognosis is otherwise poor and sudden death at an earlier age is common.

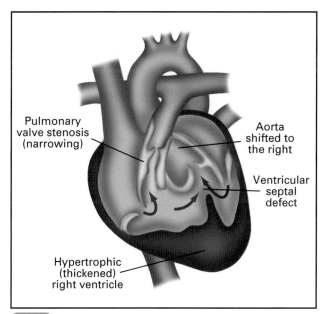

Pulmonary valve stenosis (narrowing)

Aorta shifted to the right

Ventricular septal defect

Hypertrophic (thickened) right ventricle

9.14   Tetralogy of Fallot.

Persistent right aortic arch (PRAA)

- Causes vascular ring anomaly, trapping oesophagus at level of heart base.
- Clinically causes oesophageal obstruction to passage of solid food.
- Post-weaned puppies exhibit 'regurgitation' following eating; may swallow without difficulty but may cough due to aspiration of food on regurgitation.
- Clinical signs include dysphagia, regurgitation and can lead to aspiration pneumonia.
- Prognosis is usually good following surgical intervention, but some dogs experience persistent regurgitation despite successful surgery.

Acquired heart defects

Acquired heart defects develop over time.

Endocardial disease

- Chronic degeneration of the heart valves.
- Leads to regurgitation of blood into left atrium, causing congestion and heart failure.
- Clinical signs include lethargy, pyrexia, shifting lameness, anorexia and detection of a new heart murmur.
- Prognosis is poor due to permanent damage of the heart valves.

Myocardial disease

Dilated cardiomyopathy (DCM)

- Seen in large breeds of dog and may develop in cats as a result of taurine deficiency.
- Often idiopathic and results in systolic failure, reduced efficiency of myocardium to contract.
- Goals of treatment to control signs of congestive heart failure, increase cardiac output and improve pulmonary function, achieved through thoracocentesis and drug therapy.
- Prognosis is generally guarded to poor.

Hypertrophic cardiomyopathy (HCM)

- Most common form of heart disease in cats.
- Caused by thickening of heart wall and results in diastolic failure, reduced ability of myocardium to relax and fill with blood.
- Stress and activity levels should be minimized.
- Main goals of treatment to facilitate ventricular filling, often achieved using drug therapy.
- Prognosis depends on several factors, including response to therapy and disease progression.

Pericardial disease

- Often seen in medium-sized and large breed dogs and results in fluid accumulation inside pericardium, preventing heart from expanding.
- Prognosis is good once the fluid has been drained (pericardiocentesis); however, if the effusion recurs the pericardium may have to be surgically removed.

Nursing care

- Keep the patient calm.
- Assist with diagnostic tests.
- Blood tests for haematology and biochemistry.
- Record an ECG of diagnostic quality.
- Administer drugs as directed by veterinary surgeon.

Acute heart failure

Cardiac arrest due to truly acute heart failure is rare in dogs and cats. Acute heart failure occurs if the heart is unable to pump enough blood to meet metabolic demands.

Aetiology

Acute heart failure may be associated with:

- Congenital defects
- Myocardial disease
- Arrhythmias
- Hypoxia for any reason.

Many of these can be related to chronic heart disease.

Clinical signs

These may include:

- Sudden onset, often during exercise
- Collapse
- Unconsciousness (flaccid collapse)
- Pallor or cyanosis of mucous membranes may be observed
- Very weak or undetectable pulse
- Spontaneous recovery, which may be complete or include a period of lethargy.

Diagnostic tests

All or some of the following may be used to reach a diagnosis:

- Auscultation
- Radiographs of thorax
- ECG measurements
- Blood gas analysis
- Blood pressure measurements
- Ultrasound.

Treatment

- Establish and maintain patent airway.
- Provide oxygen (see Chapter 7).
- Apply cardiac massage at 60 compressions per minute.
- Administer drugs as prescribed by veterinary surgeon.
- Apply defibrillation if appropriate.
- Administer fluid therapy (see Chapter 8).
- Monitor for signs of congestive failure.

Nursing care

- Protect from stressful environment and events.
- Administer oxygen.
- Provide cage rest.
- Keep warm.
- Assist veterinary surgeon to deliver care, treatment and administer drugs.
- Regularly monitor and record vital signs.

Chronic heart failure

Aetiology

The heart is a muscular pump. When this muscle fails, cardiac output falls and clinical signs develop. Pooling of blood develops in the venous system and vascular beds such as the lungs or body tissues, causing congestion. The location of congestion depends on whether pump failure is left- or right-sided.

Causes of congestive heart failure

Myocardial disease:
- **Dilated cardiomyopathy (systolic failure)**
- **Hypertrophic cardiomyopathy (diastolic failure).**

Arrhythmias

Taurine deficiency in cats

Pressure overload:
- **Resistance to outflow of blood increases the force of contraction needed and muscle hypertrophy increases pressure in the ventricle.**

Volume overload:
- **Excess volumes of blood entering the chamber cause myocardial stretching.**

Clinical signs

In addition to general clinical signs, left- and right-sided congestive heart failure have specific features (Figure 9.15).

General	
Tachycardia, weak pulse, pallor of mucous membranes, tachypnoea, coughing, exercise intolerance, weight loss	
Left-sided heart failure	**Right-sided heart failure**
Poor venous return from lungs	Poor venous return to heart
Pulmonary congestion and oedema	Congestion of liver, spleen and intestines
Tachypnoea and coughing	Hepatomegaly
	Ascites

9.15   Clinical signs of congestive heart failure.

Diagnostic tests

Chronic heart failure may be detected using:

- Auscultation
- Radiographs of thorax and abdomen
- ECG measurements
- Blood pressure measurements
- Blood gas measurements
- Ultrasound examination.

Treatment

- Treatment of underlying cause where known.
- Cage rest.
- Cardiac drugs (see Chapter 3).
- Dietary management (salt reduction).
- Control of obesity.

Nursing care

- Provide suitably stress-free environment.
- Provide and maintain therapy as prescribed by veterinary surgeon.
- Monitor vital signs.
- Attend to dietary requirements – control weight and avoid high salt intake.

- Restrict exercise.
- Patients for whom pulmonary oedema and congestion are a problem should be observed regularly – ensure that they are not recumbent for long periods of time.
- Ensure that owner brings pet in regularly (every 3–6 months) to monitor for signs of disease or deterioration.

Blood pressure

A measurement of blood pressure indicates the pressure exerted on the walls of the blood vessels by the blood and is dependent on the blood volume (Figure 9.16). There are minor differences in blood pressure in dogs and cats depending on the animal's age (Figure 9.17), sex, diet and level of physical fitness. In dogs, blood pressure also depends upon breed; this is not the case in cats. Blood pressure may be adversely affected by loss of circulating blood volume (see Chapter 7), or as a result of vascular, cardiac, renal or other systemic disease.

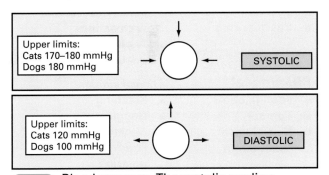

9.16 Blood pressure. The systolic reading indicates the blood pressure within the arteries after ejection from the ventricles (when the myocardium contracts). The diastolic reading indicates the blood pressure within the arteries when the myocardium relaxes. The systolic reading is higher than the diastolic reading.

Species	Age	Average normal systolic pressure (mm Hg)
Cat	1 year	123
	5 years	141
	11 years	158
Dog	<6 months	108
	1 year	127
	5 years	141
	12 years	145
Rabbit		90–130

9.17 Average normal systolic blood pressure in the dog, cat and rabbit.

Blood pressure is usually measured using a non-invasive technique (Figure 9.18). An invasive technique (using arterial catheterization) provides a more accurate measurement. When measuring the blood pressure of an individual, a series of readings should be obtained. This allows rejection of any anomalies

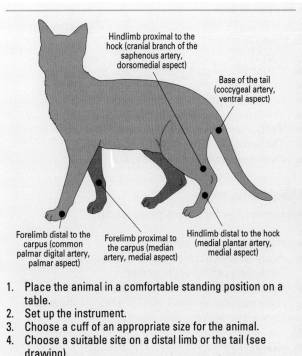

1. Place the animal in a comfortable standing position on a table.
2. Set up the instrument.
3. Choose a cuff of an appropriate size for the animal.
4. Choose a suitable site on a distal limb or the tail (see drawing).
5. Shave the transducer site and lubricate with gel.
6. Place transducer over the artery while listening for the pulse on the instrument's loudspeaker or earphones.
7. Inflate the cuff until the pulse stops. Then, while looking at the pressure dial, slowly deflate the cuff until the pulse restarts.
8. Take a number of readings over several minutes.
9. Record the measurement on the patient's record.

9.18 How to measure arterial blood pressure using a non-invasive technique.

and also allows the direction of any variations through a series of readings to be assessed.

Anaemia

Aetiology

Causes and types of anaemia are summarized in Figure 9.19.

Haemorrhagic anaemia
Acute blood loss: trauma, rupture of internal organs, clotting disorders
Chronic blood loss: haematuria, melaena, neoplasia, clotting disorders
Haemolytic anaemia
Immune-mediated
Mycoplasma haemofelis infection
Reactions to drugs (e.g. sulphonamides, anticonvulsants)
Non-regenerative anaemia
Bone marrow hypoplasia
FeLV or FIV infection
Toxaemic states (e.g. chloramphenicol, oestrogens)
Renal failure and erythropoietin deficiency
Neoplasia, including lymphosarcoma and leukaemias

9.19 Types of anaemia, with examples of causes.

Clinical signs

Clinical signs are dependent on cause and duration but may include:

- Pallor of mucous membranes
- Jaundice
- Obvious signs of haemorrhage
- Weakness, collapse
- Tachycardia and weak pulse
- Tachypnoea
- Exercise intolerance and lethargy.

Diagnostic tests

Anaemia may be investigated using:

- Physical examination
- Routine biochemistry and haematology, including reticulocyte count
- Check clotting factors: activated partial thromboplastin time (APTT) and prothrombin time (PT), and platelet count
- Coombs' test
- ANA (antinuclear antibody) test
- Bone marrow biopsy.

Treatment

- Control of active haemorrhage by pressure bandaging followed by surgical correction.
- Whole-blood transfusions in severe chronic cases when PCV is <0.15 l/l, and in all acute cases.
- Plasma expanders or oxyglobin used if whole blood unavailable (see Chapter 8).
- Correct underlying disease if present, e.g. renal disease.
- Erythropoietin in cases of renal disease and in some other cases of marrow hypoplasia.
- Stopping any drugs known to affect haematology.
- Immunosuppressive drugs for immune-mediated disease.
- Vitamin K1 for warfarin poisoning.
- Provision of adequate diet to ensure presence of all haematinics (substances, such as iron, folic acid and B vitamins, that are necessary for haemoglobin and red cell production).
- Administration of tetracycline for *Mycoplasma haemofelis*.

Nursing care

- Assist with administration of prescribed drug therapy.
- Monitor vital signs.
- Administer general care of trauma patients.
- Assist in carrying out diagnostic tests.
- Advise owners where poisoning is suspected, to prevent further intake.
- Keep patient calm and quiet.
- Avoid stress.
- Administer blood products and monitor closely for adverse reactions.
- Feed a diet high in iron and B vitamins.

Diseases of the alimentary tract

The alimentary tract comprises the mouth, oesophagus, stomach, intestines, rectum and anus.

Dysphagia

Dysphagia is when an animal is unable to swallow, although maintaining the desire to eat.

Oral	Clinical signs:
- Fractured jaw - Foreign body - Neurological dysfunction - Neoplasia - Dental disease	- Inability to pick up food - Food falls out of mouth - Food held in cheeks
Oesophageal	*Clinical signs:*
- Megaoesophagus - Stricture - Vascular ring	- Regurgitation, usually associated with eating - Aspiration pneumonia
Pharyngeal	*Clinical signs:*
- Foreign body - Tumour - Neurological dysfunction	- Retching - Gagging - Choking - Food appears at nostrils

Diagnostic tests

Dysphagia may be detected using:

- Observation of eating behaviour
- Examination of oral cavity and pharynx
- Radiographs of oral cavity, pharynx and oesophagus
- Barium swallow
- Endoscopy.

Treatment

- Identification and correction of underlying cause.
- Nutritional management (refer to Assisted feeding section later in this chapter).
- Antibiotics for aspiration pneumonia.

Nursing care

- Carry out drug therapy as prescribed by veterinary surgeon.
- Assist in establishing nutritional management and appropriate feeding procedures.
- Ensure no excitement or exercise before and after feeding.
- Observe for signs of complications (aspiration pneumonia).
- Assist with diagnostic procedures.

Anorexia

Anorexia is where an animal has lost the desire to eat.

Aetiology

Anorexia may be associated with:

- Nasal congestion (especially in cats)
- Systemic illness/disease
- Nausea.

Nursing care

- Offer food that is:
  - Highly palatable
  - Strong smelling
  - Warm
  - Soft.
- Do not force feed.
- Allow patient privacy to eat alone.
- Attempt hand feeding.

Vomiting

It is essential to make two important assessments in the patient presented with 'vomiting':

1. Is the patient vomiting or regurgitating?
2. If vomiting, is this primary gastric disease or secondary to systemic disease (Figure 9.20)?

Is the patient vomiting or regurgitating?

Vomiting
- **Often occurs many hours after eating**
- **Active abdominal effort**
- **May be preceded by lip smacking, salivation and signs of distress**
- **May contain digested food and bile**
- **Stomach contents are usually acid but if small intestine contents are expelled the pH may be increased**

Regurgitation
- **Often occurs suddenly and without warning**
- **Can occur soon after feeding but contents may remain in oesophagus for many hours**
- **No effort required – animal lowers head and volumes of material expelled**
- **Food contents undigested**
- **Oesophageal contents should have a neutral pH**

Diagnostic tests

Vomiting may be investigated using:

- History and physical examination of patient
- Abdominal radiography including barium studies (see Chapter 11)
- Routing haematology and biochemistry
- Endoscopy.

Primary

Acute and chronic gastritis
Gastric ulceration
Gastric neoplasia
Pyloric stenosis
Gastric foreign body

Secondary

Azotaemia associated with renal disease
Ketoacidosis and diabetes mellitus
Pyometra
Addison's disease
Hepatitis
Pancreatitis
Colitis

9.20 Examples of causes of primary and secondary vomiting.

Treatment

- Primary vomiting:
  - Identify and correct underlying cause (e.g. surgery to remove foreign body, correct pyloric stenosis or remove tumour).
- Secondary vomiting:
  - See sections for appropriate systemic diseases elsewhere in this chapter.
- Gastritis:
  - Nil by mouth
  - Intravenous fluid therapy using Hartmann's solution
  - Antiemetics
  - Gastric protectants such as sucralfate
  - Antacids such as cimetidine
  - Once vomiting stops, use low-fat veterinary diets and return slowly to normal diet.

Nursing care

- Provide and maintain therapy prescribed by veterinary surgeon.
- Provide a clean and comfortable environment, including absorbent/waterproof bedding and warmth.
- If no definitive diagnosis has been made, provide isolation facilities or choose a kennel that is easy to clean and disinfect.
- Keep kennel and patient clean of vomitus.
- Monitor vital signs.
- Assess hydration status and monitor and record patient's fluid intake and output.
- Monitor intravenous fluid therapy if applicable.
- Observe and record frequency of vomition.
- Observe for signs of progression/deterioration, especially dehydration.
- Inform owner of patient's progress.

Diarrhoea

Diarrhoea is the frequent evacuation of faeces that are unformed and more watery than normal. Two questions need to be answered:

- Is the diarrhoea associated with primary intestinal disease or is it secondary to systemic disease (Figure 9.21)?
- If the diarrhoea is primary, is it originating from the small or large intestine (Figure 9.22)?

Primary
Viral and bacterial infections
Hookworm and whipworm infections
Giardiasis
Inflammatory bowel disease (IBD)
Tumours: lymphoma, adenocarcinoma
Colitis

Secondary
Addison's disease
Azotaemia and renal failure
Liver disease
Pancreatic disease
Hyperthyroidism

9.21 Examples of causes of primary and secondary diarrhoea.

Sign	Small bowel	Large bowel
Weight loss	Present but increased appetite	Absent
Faecal volume	Increased (due to failure of absorption)	Reduced
Faecal frequency	Normal or increased	Increased May exhibit urgency to pass faeces
Faecal fat (steatorrhoea)	May be present	Absent
Faecal starch	May be present	Absent
Faecal blood	May have melaena	May have fresh blood
Faecal mucus	Absent	May be present

9.22 Small *versus* large intestine diarrhoea.

Diagnostic tests

Diagnosis of small and large intestinal diarrhoea (enteritis) may include some or all of the following procedures:

- Faecal analysis for:
  - Undigested food components, especially fat and starch
  - Parasitic and protozoan examination
  - Bacteriology for pathogens, especially *Salmonella* and *Campylobacter*
  - Serum folate, cobalamin estimations and TLI (trypsin-like immunoreactivity) test
- Endoscopic examinations and biopsy.

Treatment

General treatments for enteritis without concurrent vomiting include:

- Nil by mouth for 24–48 hours
- Maintenance of oral fluids to prevent dehydration
- Maintenance of electrolyte balance
- Antidiarrhoeal drugs
- Easily digestible diet (low fat and high biological value protein) for 5–7 days then a slow return to normal diet.

Antibiotics should only be used where definitive bacterial infection is confirmed.

Nursing care

- If no definite diagnosis has been made, provide isolation facilities, or choose a kennel that is easy to clean and disinfect.
- Instigate isolation/barrier nursing procedures.
- Provide a clean and comfortable environment, including absorbent bedding and warmth. For cats, ensure that a clean litter tray is available at all times.
- Ensure that dietary management is carried out correctly.
- Monitor and record the usual patient parameters.
- Observe for signs of progression/deterioration, especially dehydration and vomiting.
- Assess hydration status and monitor and record the patient's fluid intake and output. Monitor intravenous fluid therapy if applicable.
- Record all episodes of defecation – note consistency and volume.
- A soiled patient should be bathed immediately and then dried with disposable absorbent towel. Gloves and an apron should be worn and then disposed of in clinical waste.

Inflammatory bowel disease (IBD) and colitis

IBD is a relatively new term used to describe chronic enteritis that results in malabsorption of nutrients from the small intestinal lumen into the enterocytes. Patients with IBD must not be confused with patients with maldigestion (see Exocrine pancreatic insufficiency). Clinical signs of IBD usually reflect the predominant site of the disease (which can occur along the whole length of the gastrointestinal tract) and the extent of mucosal damage: vomiting; anorexia; weight loss; and diarrhoea.

Colitis is a common cause of chronic diarrhoea in dogs but not in cats. The aetiology of colitis is not frequently determined but may include:

- Bacterial infections, especially *Salmonella* and *Campylobacter*
- Parasitic infections with whipworms
- Food hypersensitivity reactions
- Secondary to colonic neoplasia.

Treatment

Treatment for IBD and colitis differs from the general regimes:

- Feeding of exclusively hypoallergenic diets (single protein), which are gluten-free
- Anti-inflammatory drugs
- Occasionally, antibiotics for bacterial overgrowth.

Nursing care is similar to that for diarrhoea.

Constipation

Constipation is a condition where faecal matter becomes impacted in the large intestine. The aetiology of constipation is long and varied and not necessarily directly associated with the alimentary tract (Figure 9.23).

Dietary
Too high or low a level of fibre in the diet
Feeding of bones
Orthopaedic
Pelvic fractures
Lumbar spinal lesions
Hindlimb instability
Colonic
Rectal strictures
Rectal foreign bodies (fur or hair balls)
Rectal tumours
Perineal rupture with rectal dilation
Megacolon
Anal sac disease or abscessation
Other
Neurological dysfunction
Prostatic hyperplasia

9.23 Causes of constipation

Clinical signs

Constipation may be associated with the following clinical signs:

- Failure to pass faeces
- Passage of small amounts of very hard faeces
- Vomiting
- Tenesmus or dyschezia (difficulty passing faeces, usually involving excessive straining)
- Haematochezia (presence of visible fresh blood in the faeces)
- Melaena (presence of visible partially digested blood in the faeces).

Diagnostic tests

The diagnosis of constipation may be made using all or some of the following tests:

- Careful physical examination of the patient
- Rectal examination
- Neurological examination
- Radiographs of the abdomen, vertebrae and pelvis, including contrast studies (see Chapter 11)
- Endoscopic examination.

Treatment

- Finding and correcting underlying cause.
- Alteration of diet and ensuring that bones are not fed.
- Stool-softening agents.
- Surgical correction of obstructions.

  Nursing care is similar to that for diarrhoea.

Gastrointestinal foreign body obstructions

Cats and, especially, dogs are prone to consuming foreign bodies, which lodge in the alimentary tract (Figures 9.24 and 9.25).

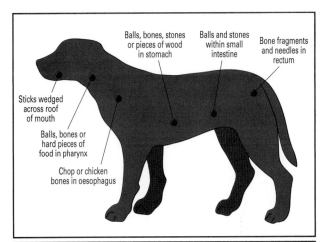

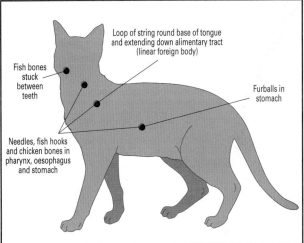

9.24 Common types of foreign body found in the alimentary tract.

Clinical signs

These depend on the location of the foreign body and may be summarized as follows:

- *Oral* – salivation, pawing at mouth, dysphagia
- *Pharynx* – dysphagia, salivation, gagging, retching and dyspnoea
- *Oesophagus* – regurgitation
- *Stomach* – can be asymptomatic (unless in pylorus, when acute vomiting occurs); secondary enteritis and colitis can develop
- *Proximal small intestine* – acute vomiting with or without secondary enteritis
- *Distal small intestine* – chronic or intermittent vomiting with or without secondary enteritis
- *Rectum* – tenesmus, dyschezia, haematochezia and constipation.

Diagnostic tests

Diagnosis depends on the nature of the foreign body and its location. The following procedures may be used to detect foreign bodies:

■ Oral examination
■ Rectal examination
■ Radiographs and contrast studies (Figure 9.25)
■ Endoscopy
■ Exploratory laparotomy.

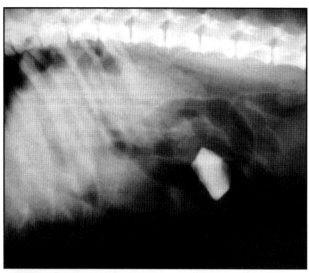

9.25 Radiograph showing radiodense foreign body in the intestine of a dog.

Treatment

Treatment depends on the location of the foreign body, but usually involves some form of surgical intervention or endoscopic retrieval. Nursing care should be as appropriate for clinical signs (see above).

Hepatic disease

Hepatitis (inflammation of the liver) is a general term used to describe most forms of hepatic disease. The causes of hepatitis are numerous, but usually involve a bacterial or viral infection. As with all potentially infectious diseases, barrier nursing should be instigated until a definitive diagnosis is made.

Classification

Primary hepatic disease may be:

■ Caused by infections (e.g. infectious canine hepatitis (ICH), leptospirosis)
■ Toxic, due to the ingestion of chemicals
■ Drug-induced (e.g. anticonvulsants, azathioprine)
■ Hereditary – copper accumulation
■ Associated with a portosystemic shunt.

Hepatic disease may also be *secondary* to metastatic malignant disease, Cushing's disease (hyperadrenocorticism) or diabetes mellitus.

Clinical signs

Clinical signs (Figure 9.26) are frequently non-specific and could equally be associated with disease of another body system; other clinical signs, including jaundice, are more specific.

Non-specific
Vomiting and diarrhoea
Weight loss
Polydipsia and polyuria
Anorexia
Specific
Anterior abdominal pain
Jaundice
Ascites
Bleeding tendency
Hepatomegaly
Encephalopathy

9.26   Clinical signs of hepatic disease.

Jaundice

An increase in plasma bilirubin level (hyperbilirubinaemia) eventually results in yellow discoloration of the skin and mucous membranes. This is known as jaundice. There are many causes and generally they are divided into three different categories.

Pre-hepatic:
Associated with haemolysis of red blood cells.

Hepatic:
Due to various hepatic diseases.

Post-hepatic:
Associated with bile duct obstruction.

Diagnostic tests

Diagnostic procedures are described in more detail in the *BSAVA Manual of Advanced Veterinary Nursing.* They include:

■ Clinical signs
■ Blood biochemistry (elevation in liver enzymes)
■ Abnormal liver function tests
■ Ultrasonography
■ Liver biopsy.

Treatment

■ Dietary management.
■ Antibiotics.
■ Anti-inflammatory drugs.
■ Intravenous fluid therapy.
■ Water-soluble bile acids (ursodeoxyonalic acid).

Nursing care

■ Where infection is suspected, provide isolation/barrier nursing.
■ Provide nutritional support. Most hepatic patients need an energy-dense diet containing moderate amounts of protein with a high biological value and increased levels of water-soluble vitamins. These patients are often anorexic and so may require hand-feeding or tube-feeding.

- Provide and maintain therapy prescribed by veterinary surgeon and assist with diagnostic or surgical procedures as required.
- Patients are likely to require intravenous fluid therapy – this must be monitored and recorded accurately.
- Monitor all vital signs and report progress to veterinary surgeon – the mucous membranes may be jaundiced and ascites may develop.
- Advise owner of animal's progress.

Pancreatic disease

The pancreas is composed of two types of tissue:

- Exocrine tissue (>90%) – produces digestive enzymes
- Endocrine tissue (<10%) – produces the hormones insulin and glucagon.

Diseases of the exocrine pancreas can be divided into:

- Pancreatitis (acute and chronic forms)
- Exocrine pancreatic insufficiency (EPI)
- Exocrine tumours.

Pancreatitis

Acute pancreatitis is more common in dogs; chronic pancreatitis is more common in cats.

Aetiology

The aetiology of pancreatitis is extensive and includes:

- Obesity
- High-fat diets
- Drug therapy
- Trauma
- Surgical manipulation
- Ascending infection (especially in cats)
- Secondary to hepatic disease (especially in cats)
- Bile duct obstruction (especially in cats).

Clinical signs

- Sudden onset of anorexia and pyrexia.
- Acute vomiting.
- Depression.
- Anorexia.
- Pyrexia.
- Anterior/cranial abdominal pain.
- Dehydration, shock and collapse.
- Later, diarrhoea may be observed.

Diagnostic tests

Diagnosis of pancreatitis is difficult and a variety of tests may be required in order to reach a definitive diagnosis. Diagnostic procedures are given in more detail in the *BSAVA Manual of Advanced Veterinary Nursing* and include:

- Clinical findings
- Radiography to reveal dilated duodenum and local peritonitis in anterior abdomen

- Serum amylase, lipase and trypsin-like immunoreactivity (TLI) test
- Leucocytosis and shift to the left
- Ultrasonography of the pancreas.

Treatment

- Nil by mouth for 3–5 days (includes oral fluids) – even the sight or smell of food can stimulate release of pancreatic enzymes, which exacerbates the pancreatitis.
- Aggressive intravenous fluid therapy using Hartmann's solution.
- Antibiotics.
- Analgesics.
- Low-fat diet with replacement enzymes.
- Restoration of bodyweight to normal.
- Maintaining in the long term on low-fat diets.

Nursing care

- Manage feeding and fluid therapy, as above.
- To prevent stimulation of pancreatic enzymes, patient should be isolated or removed from kennels when others are being fed.
- Monitor vital signs and report any progression.
- Keep kennel clean of any vomitus and provide a comfortable environment.
- Provide and observe response to initiation of feeding.
- Pancreatitis is an extremely painful condition and peritonitis may develop as a complication.
- Ensure that medical treatment prescribed by the veterinary surgeon is carried out and recorded. Drugs that may be used include analgesics and antibiotics.
- Assist with diagnostic procedures as required – blood and faecal samples may be required.

Exocrine pancreatic insufficiency (EPI)

One consequence of chronic pancreatitis is EPI. This condition is rare in cats but relatively common in dogs. The damage to the pancreas results in a loss of functional cells and a total lack of digestive enzyme production. Subsequent maldigestion occurs as the animal is unable to digest food.

Aetiology

EPI may occur:

- As a result of a hereditary deficiency in exocrine tissue, especially in German Shepherd Dogs
- As a congenital condition in young dogs
- Following repeated episodes of pancreatitis with destruction of exocrine tissue.

Clinical signs

Signs of EPI include:

- Ravenous appetite
- Coprophagia
- Marked weight loss despite polyphagia
- Chronic large volume diarrhoea
- Steatorrhoea
- Poor condition.

Diagnostic tests

EPI may be detected using:

- Faecal analysis to detect undigested fat and starch (see Chapter 10)
- Serum trypsin-like immunoreactivity (TLI) test.

Treatment

- Low-fat diets.
- Replacement enzyme supplement given with food.
- Antibiotic for secondary bacterial overgrowth.

Nursing care

- Provide dietary management and supplementation of food with pancreatic enzymes.
- Feed a low-fat highly digestible diet.
- Feed small frequent meals.
- Monitor faecal consistency, amount and colour.
- Prevent faecal soiling.
- Monitor weight.
- Assist with diagnostic tests.
- Advise owner on use of prescribed treatment.

Advice to owners

- Owners of obese animals should be counselled about their pet's diet.
- Indicate how condition will improve:
  - Faecal character will improve within 48 hours
  - Weight gain will occur slowly over several weeks
  - Ravenous appetite will be last to improve.
- Offer encouragement to owner at repeat visits, as compliance is essential to success.
- There is no cure for EPI and so the disease needs to be managed using medication and diet. It is especially important that clients receive accurate information on how to manage the disease correctly, in order to allow their pet to live a normal life.

Renal disease

Renal disease results in the failure of the kidneys to perform their normal function. Renal disease may occur suddenly (acute renal failure) or develop gradually over a period of time (chronic).

Renal disease

Acute renal failure (ARF)
Causes include:
- **Mercury poisoning**
- **Ethylene glycol poisoning (antifreeze)**
- **Gentamicin administration**
- **Sulphonamide administration**
- **Leptospirosis**
- **Hypovolaemia following haemorrhage**
- **Addison's disease**
- **Congestive heart failure**

Nephrotic syndrome
- **End-stage kidney disease**

Chronic renal failure (CRF)
Causes include:
- **Progression from ARF**
- **Nephrotoxins**
- **Congenital disease**
- **Systemic lupus erythematosus (SLE)**
- **Progression from glomerulonephritis**

Glomerulonephritis
Causes include:
- **Antibody/antigen complexes in infection**
- **Immune-mediated disease, such as SLE**
- **Endocrine disease, such as Cushing's disease and diabetes mellitus**

Clinical signs, diagnosis, treatment and nursing care of renal failure are given in Figure 9.27.

Acute renal failure (ARF)	Chronic renal failure (CRF)
Clinical signs	
Relate to uraemia: sudden onset anorexia, depression, anuria or oliguria followed by polydipsia and polyuria, vomiting, dehydration, halitosis	*A loss of 75% of kidney function is required for signs to develop.* Anorexia, weight loss, lethargy, vomiting and diarrhoea, polydipsia and polyuria, non-regenerative anaemia, halitosis and oral ulceration
Diagnostic features	
Sudden increases in blood urea and creatinine, hyperkalaemia, metabolic acidosis, hyperphosphataemia. Urinalysis may reveal isothenuria, proteinuria, haematuria, casts and/or oxalate crystals; low urine specific gravity	Increases in blood urea, creatinine and phosphorus, altered Ca:P ratio to >1:4. Urinalysis may reveal isosthenuria, casts, haematuria, proteinuria. Anaemia. Usually low urine specific gravity
Treatment	
Identify and remove underlying cause (antifreeze or drugs), intravenous fluid therapy using 0.9% saline or 5% dextrose saline, diuretics once dehydration is corrected, correct electrolyte disturbances, antiemetics, H2 blockers, promote urine production, monitor urine production carefully – look for production >2ml/kg bodyweight per hour, antibiotics	Intravenous fluid therapy, antiemetics, antibiotics, dietary management using low phosphorus and protein diets, phosphate binders in food, anabolic steroids or erythropoietin to stimulate bone marrow, ACE inhibitors (benazepril licensed for this use), vasodilators (e.g. enalapril)

9.27 Clinical signs, diagnosis, treatment and nursing care of renal failure. (continues) ▶

Acute renal failure (ARF)	Chronic renal failure (CRF)
Nursing care	
Barrier nurse if an infectious cause is suspected. Advise owner if infections or poisons are implicated. Monitor vital signs and record all episodes of vomiting. Administer fluid therapy. Monitor hydration status. Monitor and record urine production (normal = 1–2 ml/kg/hour). Administer drugs as prescribed and assist with diagnostic procedures. Assist in establishing nutritional management of patient and feed a low-protein, low-phosphorus diet. Encourage animal to eat if inappetent. Keep animal clean and provide a comfortable environment and TLC	

9.27 (continued) Clinical signs, diagnosis, treatment and nursing care of renal failure.

Nephrotic syndrome

This is classified as end-stage kidney disease and requires supportive care. Clinical signs and diagnostic tests are very similar to those observed and performed in cases of chronic renal failure but also include the following.

Clinical signs

- May have signs of systemic disease.
- Ascites, subcutaneous oedema and hydrothorax.
- Severe weight loss.

Diagnostic tests

Nephrotic syndrome may be detected through:

- Hypoproteinaemia associated with albumin loss
- Severe proteinuria.

Treatment

- Plasma expanders (colloids).
- Diuretics for oedema, with care.

Lower urinary tract disease

Cystitis

Aetiology

Causes of cystitis include:

- Trauma
- Calculi (Figures 9.28 and 9.29)
- Ascending infections, especially in females
- Secondary to diabetes mellitus
- Secondary to neoplasia
- Secondary to immunosuppression (animals with Cushing's disease (hyperadrenocorticism), FIV, FeLV or those receiving steroid treatment).

Clinical signs

Cystitis may have the following signs:

- Increased urinary frequency
- Urinary tenesmus
- Dysuria
- Incontinence
- Polydipsia.

Diagnostic tests

Cystitis may be detected using:

- Urinalysis, very important (see Chapter 10) – catheterized or cystocentesis
- Urine culture and sensitivity testing, ideally following cystocentesis
- Tests for underlying causes
  - Blood tests
  - Radiography (Figure 9.29)
  - Ultrasonography.

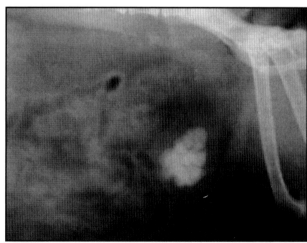

9.29 Radiograph revealing multiple radiodense calculi in the urinary bladder of a dog. These were subsequently found to be struvite calculi.

Type	Urine pH	Breeds commonly affected	Radiodensity	Location
Struvite	Alkaline	Many breeds; often secondary to other causes of cystitis	Radiodense	Bladder/urethra
Oxalate	Acid/alkaline	Miniature Schnauzer, Yorkshire Terrier Persian, Burmese, Himalayan cats	Variable	Urethra
Urates	Acid/alkaline	Dalmatian, Bulldog, Yorkshire Terrier	Radiolucent	Bladder
Cystine	Acid	Dachshund, English Bulldog	Radiolucent	Bladder

9.28 Urinary calculi. See also Figure 10.26.

Treatment

- Antibiotics (selected following sensitivity results).
- Dietary management if calculi are present, to aid dissolution and prevent recurrence.
- Surgery to remove calculi or tumours.
- If appropriate, increase urine production by adding salt to diet and encourage water intake.

Nursing care

- Administer and maintain therapy as prescribed.
- Collect samples for urinalysis.
- Prevent urine scalding (regular washing and application of barrier cream).
- Ensure that dietary management is carried out.
- Encourage exercise to allow regular urination.

Urinary incontinence

Urinary incontinence is an inability to control urination. The condition may be mild (with dribbling of urine) or complete (no control at all).

Aetiology

Causes of urinary incontinence include:

- Sphincter mechanism incompetence (SMI) – mainly in older bitches
- Tumours (e.g. transitional cell carcinoma)
- Prostatic disease
- Neurological defects
- Hypoplastic bladder
- Cystitis
- Behavioural problems.

Clinical signs

Signs of urinary incontinence include:

- Passage of urine when recumbent or mobile
- Wetness around the perineum
- Signs of cystitis
- Urine scalding of the perineum and hindlimbs.

Treatment

- Identify and treat underlying cause (surgical or medical treatments).
- Treat secondary cystitis.

Nursing care

- Administer and maintain therapy as prescribed.
- Use barrier creams to prevent urine scalding.
- Use incontinence pads for bedding.
- Offer frequent opportunities for passage of urine.
- Clip and clean perineal region.
- Offer advice to owner.

Feline lower urinary tract disease (FLUTD)

Previously known as feline urological syndrome (FUS), this disease includes a number of conditions that affect the lower urinary tract in cats.

Aetiology

The exact cause of FLUTD is unclear but the following may play a part:

- Nutritional factors
- Infectious disease
- Trauma
- Neurogenic causes
- Neoplastic disease
- Congenital abnormalities
- Iatrogenic causes (e.g. stressful situations).

Clinical signs

Signs of FLUTD include:

- Signs of cystitis and sometimes urinary tract obstruction
- Dysuria
- Anuria and secondary azotaemia
- Haematuria
- Azotaemia
- Tenesmus
- Distended bladder.

Treatment

- Identification and treatment of underlying cause where possible.
- Antibiotics.
- Urinary acidifiers.
- Dietary management – low magnesium, phosphorus in particular.
- Behavioural treatments (e.g. feline pheromone diffusers).

Nursing care

- Administer and maintain therapy as prescribed.
- Monitor urine production.
- Monitor for signs of dysuria and uraemia.
- Collect samples for assessing progress of case.

Diseases of the nervous system

Disorders of the nervous system can cause a wide variety of signs, depending on the site of the problem. An accurate history and thorough neurological examination are necessary. From the initial assessment it may be possible to define the problem as:

- Diffuse
- Focal or multifocal
- Symmetrical or asymmetrical
- Painful or nonpainful
- Progressive, regressive or static
- Mild, moderate or severe.

Seizures

Several terms are used to describe seizures, including 'fits' and 'convulsions'. Epilepsy is a term used to describe a central nervous disorder in which an irritable focus leads to disordered brain activity and tonic/clonic spasms. Seizures may be primary, or secondary to systemic disease (Figure 9.30). Continuous seizures are called *status epilepticus*.

Primary
Infections, both viral or bacterial
Trauma with increased intracranial pressure
Congenital conditions such as hydrocephalus
Epilepsy
Brain tumours

Secondary
Hypoglycaemia
Portosystemic shunts
Hypocalcaemia
Hypokalaemia
Uraemia
Poisons such as metaldehyde

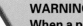 **9.30** Examples of causes of primary and secondary seizures.

Clinical signs

- *Preictal* – just before the fit, the animal will usually be asleep or resting and will awaken suddenly, appearing restless and anxious.
- *Ictal* – the actual fit: collapse, tonic and clonic activity, salivation, jaw champing, vocalization, voiding of urine and faeces are all possible.
- *Postictal* – following the fit the animal may appear exhausted, dazed and anxious again. This will last for variable periods of time.

> ⚠ **WARNING**
> **When a pet dog or cat is having a seizure, the owner is likely to be highly distressed. The veterinary nurse should take command, calm the owner and give advice on what action is required. This information is often conveyed over the phone and therefore needs to be clear and precise.**
>
> - **Do not handle or attempt to restrain the animal.**
> - **Stay with the animal but only observe.**
> - **Attempt to time how long the fit lasts for.**
> - **Provide a quiet and dimly lit room.**
> - **Remove children and others from the vicinity of the room.**
> - **Remove any objects that may injure the animal during the fit.**
> - **Do not drive the animal to the surgery during its fit.**
> - **Only when the fit has finished should the animal be driven to the surgery for examination.**

Treatment

- Identify and correct the underlying cause.
- Where epilepsy is diagnosed, start anticonvulsant treatment.

Opinion varies as to when anticonvulsants should be started. Usually if the animal has epilepsy and has a fit more frequently than every 3 months, then anticonvulsants should be prescribed.

Nursing care

- Advise the owner on how to deal with an animal having a seizure (see above).
- Administer drugs as prescribed by the veterinary surgeon.
- Advise owner on:
  - Safe handling and storage of anticonvulsants
  - Recording episodes of fits
  - Looking out for recurrence of fits, which may manifest as minor episodes, initially called 'petit mal', rather than typical fits.
- Assist with the collection of blood samples to help monitor treatment.

Loss of consciousness

This is sometimes known as syncope or fainting. Unlike a seizure, syncope is a flaccid collapsing episode, with none of the activity observed with seizures. It should not be confused with seizures – there is no tonic or clonic muscle activity, and the animal is unable to be aroused or respond to normal stimuli.

Aetiology

Loss of consciousness may be caused by:

- Cerebral anoxia
- CNS trauma
- Cardiopulmonary disease
- Barbiturate poisoning
- Heatstroke
- Airway obstruction
- Hypocalcaemia
- Narcolepsy
- Addison's disease (hypoadrenocorticism)
- Vagal collapse (especially in Boxer dogs).

Clinical signs

The signs of syncope are:

- Sudden onset, with no preictal phase
- Flaccid collapse for variable periods of time
- Occasionally associated with exercise
- Cyanosis or pallor of mucous membranes
- Other signs of systemic disease
- Spontaneous recovery.

Diagnostic tests

Syncope may be detected by:

- Assessing cardiopulmonary function: ECG, radiography, ultrasonography, blood gases
- Biochemical profile for metabolic disease
- Neurological examination, if due to primary CNS disease.

Nursing care of the unconscious patient

- Check for patent airway and mucous membrane colour.
- Supply oxygen and artificial respiration.
- Send for veterinary surgeon.
- Monitor vital signs.
- Assist veterinary surgeon in collecting blood samples.
- Assist veterinary surgeon with additional therapy as required.

Paresis and paralysis

When the spinal cord is injured it may result in *paresis* (a deficit in voluntary movement in one or more limbs) or *paralysis* (a complete loss of voluntary movement).

Definitions

Monoplegia – one limb affected
Hemiplegia – limbs on one side affected
Tetraplegia or quadriplegia – all limbs affected

Spinal cord injury is most likely following:

- Trauma such as road traffic accidents
- Intervertebral disc protrusion
- Neoplastic lesions.

Clinical signs

- Paresis or weakness of one or more limbs.
- Paralysis of one or more limbs.
- Urinary and/or faecal incontinence.
- Lack of skin sensation (panniculus reflex).
- Loss of tail function.

Diagnostic tests

Paresis/paralysis may be detected by:

- Physical examination of the patient
- Radiographic examination of the vertebral column with contrast studies (see Chapter 11)
- CSF tap (cerebrospinal fluid sampling)
- Neurological examination, including:
  - Withdrawal reflex: noxious stimulus to foot results in withdrawal and awareness
  - Anal reflex: observe if anal sphincter contracts when inserting thermometer
  - Panniculus reflex: pin prick on skin along flank results in skin twitching
  - Patellar reflex: hold hindlimb partially extended and tap patellar ligament – limb should extend, but not excessively
  - Tail function: pin prick for sensation – no tail wagging with motor loss
  - Conscious proprioception: knuckle each paw – animal should immediately correct so pads touch floor
  - Assess muscle tone in limbs
  - Assess ability to urinate and defecate.

Nursing care

- Help the veterinary surgeon to carry out neurological examination.

- Monitor vital signs.
- Assist with radiographic procedures.
- Prevent pressure sores by frequent turning and suitable bedding (see 'Nursing the recumbent patient' below).
- Avoid excess movement that may damage spine.
- Assist in emptying bladder and rectum.
- Prevent urine and faecal soiling.
- Apply physiotherapy as directed (see 'Physiotherapy' section below).
- Ensure that adequate nutrition is provided.

Endocrine diseases

Diabetes mellitus

Diabetes mellitus (DM), also known as sugar diabetes, is caused by a relative or absolute deficiency of insulin and is a disease of considerable complexity. It can be categorized into two idiopathic types, type 1 and type 2, sometimes referred to as insulin-dependent diabetes mellitus (IDDM) and non-insulin-dependent diabetes mellitus (NIDDM), respectively. There is a third type, which is secondary diabetes.

Idiopathic diabetes mellitus

Type 1
Insulin-dependent (IDDM):
- **More common in dogs (and young people)**
- **Occurs when the immune system destroys the insulin-producing beta cells in the islets of Langerhans within the pancreas**
- **Can also be caused by hypoplasia of the islet cells in the pancreas**
- **Loss of islet cells can also be caused by pancreatitis, autoimmune disease, toxicity or neoplasia**
- **Results in a total absence of insulin production and therefore renders the patient dependent on insulin injections.**

Type 2
Non-insulin-dependent (NIDDM):
- **More common in cats (and older people)**
- **Can occur in obese animals or those under the effects of some hormones**
- **Caused by decreased sensitivity of tissues to the actions of insulin**
- **The pancreas may produce no, too little, normal or excessive amounts of insulin, but the insulin fails to achieve its normal action**
- **Can often be treated without using insulin although most cats and dogs do require insulin for successful treatment.**

Secondary diabetes mellitus

- **Occurs as a result of an underlying disease or disorder, or drug therapy.**
- **Treatment may or may not be necessary for diabetes as well as the associated condition.**

Clinical signs

Uncomplicated diabetes:

- Polyphagia
- Bright alert animal
- Weight loss
- May be obese
- Recurrent urinary tract infections.

Ketoacidosis:

- Anorexia and depression
- Vomiting and diarrhoea
- Dehydration
- Ketotic breath
- Cataract formation (dogs).

Both:

- Poluria
- Polydipsia.

Feline diabetes mellitus

- **Cats with insulin resistance are typically of normal weight or obese with a normal appetite and clinically well.**
- **They may become transiently diabetic at times of stress or concurrent illness, recovering for a time only to relapse later.**
- **Cats are frequently hyperglycaemic as a result of stress in a hospital environment and handling to obtain a blood sample. Sampling at home or use of fructosamine assays are suitable alternatives.**

Diagnostic tests

Diabetes mellitus may be detected by:

- Clinical findings
- Cataracts in dogs
- Glucosuria
- Ketonuria
- Hyperglycaemia
- Elevated fructosamines.

Fructosamine assays

Fructosamine assays should be used to assess glycaemic control because:

- **Fructosamine is a more specific indicator of pancreatic endocrine activity than glucose**
- **It is not affected by acute increases in blood glucose, such as stress.**

The normal range for serum fructosamine is 225–450 µmol/litre.

- **High fructosamine levels indicate poor glycaemic control over the previous 3 weeks.**
- **Low fructosamine levels suggest excessive glycaemic control over the past 3 weeks.**

Initial stabilization and monitoring

- A newly diagnosed diabetic patient is usually hospitalized for assessment of a glucose curve (Figure 9.31). This involves taking a blood sample at least every 4 hours to observe the effect, and duration of action, of the insulin.
- Urine is sampled 2–3 times daily to monitor ketonuria and observe trends in glucosuria.
- Insulin (intermediate or long-acting) is administered once or twice daily.
- The patient should be fed at the same time as insulin administration and then again 6–8 hours later if one dose of insulin is given.
- The patient should be fed at the same time as insulin administration if two doses of insulin are given.

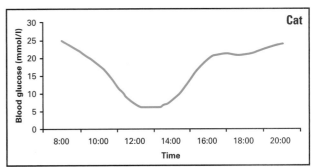
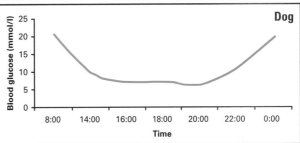

9.31 Ideal blood glucose curves for a stable diabetic cat and dog (insulin administered at 8 am). A stable diabetic cat is able to maintain a blood glucose range of 5–15 mmol/l for most of each 24-hour period. A stable diabetic dog is able to maintain a blood glucose range of 5–12 mmol/l for most of a 24-hour period. (Data courtesy of Intervet, UK)

Treatment

Routine management

- Once an effective insulin protocol has been established, there should be no need to change the patient's routine.
- Any changes to a routine should be continued for a minimum of 3 days to allow the patient to adjust before assessing the response.
- Alterations in insulin dose should be based on glucose curves or fructosamine levels. Urine samples are only useful as indicators of urinary tract infections (and possibly ketone levels) in long-term management.
- Feed one-half of daily food ration.
- Administer insulin.

- Feed remainder of diet 8 hours later.
- Repeat each day.
- Once stable, diabetic bitches should be spayed as insulin requirements can change at different stages in the hormone cycle.

Ketoacidosis

This may be the first time that a diabetic animal presents. If untreated the diabetic animal may develop diabetic ketoacidosis (DKA). This is a result of excessive breakdown of fats within the body. Ketones (energy source derived from fat breakdown) are produced in the liver. These cause metabolic acidosis and exacerbate the existing condition. *DKA is a life-threatening condition and must be treated promptly.*

- Nil by mouth.
- Intravenous fluids, such as Hartmann's solution then 0.9% saline.
- If necessary, supplementation with potassium, bicarbonate or phosphorous.
- Soluble insulin.
- Monitor blood glucose, sodium and potassium.

Insulin

The function of insulin is to assist in the transport of glucose from the blood into the tissue cells. In DM the blood glucose levels are markedly elevated, while the tissues are starved of glucose. Some cases of DM are transient, while other patients may require insulin

for the remainder of their lives. The types of insulin licensed for dogs and cats and the appropriate doses are shown in Figure 9.32.

Insulin storage and administration

- All types of insulin should be stored in a refrigerator at 4°C.
- Gently agitate the insulin bottle before withdrawing the insulin – *do not shake the bottle.*
- Never swab the top of the bottle or injection site with isopropyl alcohol as it may inactivate the insulin.

Insulin overdose, or hypoglycaemia
Causes:

- Usually error in calculation of dose or administration
- Animal refusing to eat after being given correct insulin dose
- Insulin peaking before main meal in afternoon
- Animal abnormally active, leading to abnormally high energy (glucose) use.

Clinical signs

Low blood glucose can be fatal, so it is extremely important to recognize the associated signs, which are often subtle in the early stages and include:

ISOPHANE AND LENTE INSULINS
- Administered by subcutaneous injection
- Their peak effect occurs about 8 hours post-injection and lasts for about 24 hours
- Ideal for most dogs and can be used in the long-term management of diabetes

NEUTRAL INSULINS
- Also called soluble insulins
- Can be administered i.v., i.m. or s.c.
- They have a quick onset of action but a short duration of activity (only 2 hours)
- Used primarily for the treatment of life-threatening ketoacidotic emergencies

There are two types of veterinary insulin licensed for dogs and cats:

100 IU/ml bovine insulin
- Use 1 ml insulin syringe marked in black
- Available in three forms: neutral, lente and protamine zinc

40 IU/ml porcine insulin
- Use 1 ml insulin syringe marked in red
- Available as a mixed insulin

PROTAMINE ZINC INSULINS
- Peak effect occurs 8–12 hours after administration by s.c. injection and lasts for up to 36 hours
- Usually used in the long-term management of diabetes and ideal for dogs, particularly those that metabolize insulin quickly
- As most cats metabolize insulin at a faster rate than dogs, protamine zinc insulins are the preferred treatment for cats

MIXED INSULINS
- A mixture of amorphous zinc and protamine zinc insulins
- Used to alter the duration of circulating insulin levels
- Amorphous zinc insulin peaks at three hours after injection and lasts for 8 hours
- Protamine zinc insulin peaks more slowly

9.32   Insulin types and dosages.

- Muscle tremors
- Restlessness
- Unusual movements or behaviour (some animals become very quiet and stop eating)
- Ataxia and incoordination
- Weakness
- Collapse
- Unconsciousness
- Death.

Treatment

- Dependent on clinical condition of the animal
  - If conscious, give a high sugar solution or food
  - If unconscious, seek immediate veterinary assistance for intravenous glucose infusion
- May need to change time of main meal if insulin is peaking early
- Glucose curve (± fructosamine assay) to assess stability.

Factors to consider when hospitalizing a diabetic patient

- Maintenance of a diabetic patient requires a strict routine.
- Keep stress levels to a minimum otherwise a false hyperglycaemia may be recorded (especially in cats).
- Diabetic animals undergoing anaesthesia are starved as usual but given half their usual dose of insulin on the morning of the procedure. They should be fed as soon as possible after recovery from anaesthesia and the remaining insulin dose given.
- If blood glucose levels are low, a glucose saline infusion may be administered during anaesthesia and blood glucose levels retested following surgery.
- Encourage the patient to eat. Refer to owner for advice on normal diet and routine.

Dietary management

A high-fibre or protein diet should be used.

- Such a diet helps to treat obesity (if this is an issue).
- It helps to slow down glucose absorption from intestine and so reduce postprandial glucose surges.
- Diet should contain adequate protein of high biological value (BV), fat and carbohydrate for calories.
- Carbohydrate must be complex and not simple sugars; therefore semi-moist foods should *not* be used.
- Titbits should not be fed.
- The same amount should be fed at the same time each day and a strict regimen is essential in order to keep the condition stable. This is more important than what is being fed.
- Obese diabetic patients should be dieted by feeding two-thirds of the dietary requirements for their ideal weight.
- Fresh water must always be available.

Exercise

- Moderate exercise (similar from day to day) should be provided.
- If the patient is obese, exercise should be increased gradually as the animal's weight falls to normal.
- There should be no major changes in exercise from day to day.
- Strenuous and sporadic exercise can cause severe hypoglycaemia and should be avoided.

Complications of diabetes

- Persistently high levels of glucose in the blood may cause damage to nerves, resulting in weakness and muscle wasting (usually of the hindlegs). This is most common in cats.
- High blood glucose levels (hyperglycaemia) causes changes in the lens of the eye. Water diffuses into the lens, causing swelling and disruption of the lens structure and resulting in opacity (cataracts). This is more common in diabetic dogs than cats. Control of high blood glucose levels can help to prevent or delay the onset of diabetic cataracts.

Diabetes insipidus

Diabetes insipidus (DI), also known as 'water diabetes', results from a failure either of the pituitary gland to produce antidiuretic hormone (ADH) ('central diabetes insipidus') or of the kidneys to respond to ADH ('nephrogenic').

Clinical signs

Animals appear generally healthy in other respects but show the following signs:

- Polyuria – affected animals pass very large volumes of urine, often with incontinence
- Urine produced is very dilute
- Specific gravity (SG) <1.008
- Secondary polydipsia due to fluid loss.

Diagnostic tests

Other causes of polyuria/polydipsia (PU/PD) should be ruled out. All parameters on routine blood screens should be normal, although there may be evidence of dehydration (mildly elevated PCV and plasma protein). Urine SG is low (<1.010 but often <1.003). The water deprivation test (WDT) and ADH test are outlined in Figure 9.33.

Treatment

Central diabetes insipidus

- Daily supplementation of exogenous ADH (desmopressin, vasopressin or DDAVP).
- Usually administered as intranasal drops or drops into the conjunctival sac from where it is easily absorbed.

Water deprivation test (WDT)

This test assesses the ability of the patient to concentrate its urine. It should be performed with great care and never in patients with renal dysfunction.

It is vital that the following contraindications are observed:

- The patient has high blood urea (indication of possible kidney dysfunction)
- The patient has a high blood calcium concentration
- There are signs of any other disease that may explain the clinical signs
- The patient cannot be monitored adequately for the entire period of the test.

In order for the WDT to have any value a strict protocol must be adhered to:

1. Weigh the patient and calculate 5% of its bodyweight.
2. Empty the urinary bladder, measure and record the specific gravity (SG).
3. Place animal in a kennel and withhold all food and water.
4. Every hour, empty bladder, measure SG and weigh patient.
5. Stop when urine SG reaches 1.025–1.030 or when the patient has lost 5% of its bodyweight, or sooner if patient becomes distressed.
6. If SG >1.025, after this test, animal is normal. If SG <1.020, after this test, suspect DI.
7. Once test is finished, allow free access to water.

ADH response test

- Once animal is rehydrated, repeat test as above but give ADH injection.
- If urine SG increases, then animal has central DI.
- If SG does not increase, then animal has nephrogenic DI.

9.33 Water deprivation and ADH response tests.

Nephrogenic diabetes insipidus

- Difficult to treat.
- Animal will not respond to ADH.
- Thiazide diuretics may decrease urine volume by increasing the reabsorption of salt.

Nursing care

- Assist veterinary surgeon with diagnostic tests.
- Assist in collection of samples as required.
- Administer therapy and medication as prescribed.
- Ensure that water is freely available at all times (except during water deprivation or ADH response tests).
- Measure water intake on a daily basis.
- Take patient outside regularly to allow opportunity to urinate and defecate.
- Advise owner on condition and treatment regime.

Hyperadrenocorticism (Cushing's disease)

Hyperadrenocorticism (HAC), often referred to as Cushing's disease, is a common endocrine disorder of dogs. It results from excessive production of adrenal steroid hormones, particularly cortisol, and is normally caused by either a pituitary or an adrenal tumour.

Canine hyperadrenocorticism (Cushing's disease)

- **Normally affects middle-aged to elderly dogs, uncommon in animals less than 6 years.**
- **Both males and females can be affected, however it is more common in females.**
- **It is particularly common in poodles, terriers and Dachshunds.**

Pituitary-dependent:
From excessive secretion of adrenocorticotropin (ACTH) from the pituitary gland. Accounts for 85–90% of cases

Iatrogenic:
Prolonged treatment/excessive administration of glucocorticoids, e.g. prednisolone tablets

Adrenal-dependent:
Unilateral tumour of the adrenal gland, which excretes excess cortisol. This type accounts for about 10% of cases

Clinical signs

Clinical signs can be dramatic and may include:

- Polydipsia
- Polyuria
- Polyphagia
- Alopecia, mainly affecting flanks, thighs and abdomen (due to effect of cortisol on hair cycle)
- Calcinosis cutis (deposition of calcium in the skin)
- Abdominal distension
- Pot-bellied appearance
- Exercise intolerance
- Panting
- Persistent infections, due to suppression of immune system
- Muscle weakness and atrophy
- Urinary tract infection
- Secondary diabetes mellitus.

Diagnostic tests

Cushing's disease may be detected by:

- Elevations in alkaline phosphatase, cholesterol, alanine aminotransferase and glucose
- Neutrophilia, lymphopenia and eosinopenia
- Ultrasonography of adrenal glands
- Endocrine screening tests.

Endocrine screening tests for hyperadrenocorticism

ACTH stimulation test:
Identifies >50% of dogs with adrenal-dependent disease and approximately 85% of those with pituitary-dependent disease. Also used for monitoring treatment.

Low-dose dexamethasone screening test (LDST):
Identifies almost all cases of adrenal-dependent disease and 90–95% of pituitary-dependent disease.

High-dose dexamethasone screening test (HDST): Can be used to differentiate between adrenal- and pituitary-based disease when a diagnosis of hyperadrenocorticism has already been made.

Endogenous ACTH assay: High concentrations of ACTH are found in dogs with pituitary-dependant disease and correlate with the size of a pituitary mass.

Treatment

- Pituitary-dependent HAC normally treated medically with drug therapy, using trilostane. Medication levels should be monitored through repeat ACTH stimulation tests at regular intervals (see Chapter 3).
- Adrenal-dependent HAC ideally requires surgical removal of the affected adrenal gland, though medical management may be the only option for treatment.

Nursing care

- Monitor clinical signs.
- Monitor vital signs.
- Assist veterinary surgeon with diagnostic tests.
- Ensure that water is freely available.
- Take patient outside regularly.
- Administer medication following veterinary surgeon's instructions.

Hypoadrenocorticism (Addison's disease)

This is more common in dogs than in cats and is caused by a reduction or failure of glucocorticoid and mineralocorticoid secretion by the adrenal cortex, resulting in fluid and electrolyte imbalances. It can also occur in association with the overtreatment of hyperadrenocoticism (Cushing's disease).

Clinical signs

Clinical signs are often chronic and vague. Animals may continue for several years with non-specific signs of illness before a crisis develops.

Chronic:

- Anorexia
- Lethargy
- Weakness
- Vomiting
- Diarrhoea
- Polydipsia
- Polyuria
- Hypotension.

Acute (Addisonian crisis):

- **Life threatening!**
- Hypovolaemic shock
- Collapse
- Severe bradycardia
- Weak pulse
- Vomiting and diarrhoea.

Diagnostic tests

Diagnosis is not always easy, due to the exhibition of vague clinical signs. It is also common for animals to present in Addisonian crisis. The following tests may be used:

- Blood tests for haematology and biochemistry
  - Elevated BUN and creatinine (which can be easily confused with chronic renal failure (CRF)), sodium and potassium
  - Lymphocytosis, eosinophilia, neutropenia, anaemia
- Sodium:potassium ratio (<25:1)
- ACTH stimulation test for definitive diagnosis.

Treatment

- Acute conditions (Addisonian crisis):
  - Urgent medical treatment
  - Intravenous corticosteroids
  - Aggressive fluid therapy with a non-potassium containing fluid (0.45% NaCl)
  - Monitoring of electrolyte levels.
- Chronic conditions:
  - Medical management – administration of glucocorticoids and mineralocorticoids
  - Monitoring renal and electrolyte levels on a regular basis.

Nursing care

- Monitor vital signs.
- Assist with diagnostic tests.
- Administer medication as prescribed.
- Ensure water is freely available.
- Take outside regularly.
- Monitor clinical signs.

Hypothyroidism

This condition is most frequently seen in dogs and only rarely in cats. It is typically a disease of middle-aged medium-sized bitches. Breeds that are predisposed include Dobermann, Golden Retriever and Irish Setter. Patients have an underactive thyroid gland, leading to reduced production of thyroxine that, in turn, results in a reduction in metabolic rate.

Clinical signs

The classic signs of the condition (Figure 9.34) are:

- Anorexia
- Weight gain
- Marked lethargy
- Muscle weakness
- Bilateral alopecia
- Seborrhoea
- Hyperpigmentation
- 'Tragic' expression
- Bradycardia.

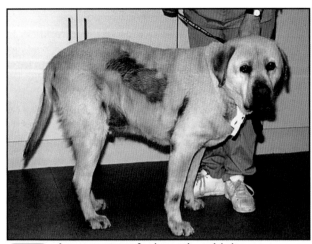

9.34 Appearance of a hypothyroid dog. (Reproduced from *BSAVA Manual of Canine and Feline Endocrinology, 3rd edition*)

Diagnostic tests

Diagnostic procedures are explained in more detail in the *BSAVA Manual of Advanced Veterinary Nursing*. They include:

- Measurement of thyroxine (T4) levels (free and total) in serum (usually very low)
- Measurement of thyrotropin (thyroid stimulating hormone, TSH) levels (high) and ratio
- TSH stimulation test to assess thyroid function (poor response).

Treatment

Treatment is simple and usually very effective:

- Thyroid replacement therapy using oral supplementation with a synthetic hormone
- Monitoring total T4 levels and cardiac function.

Nursing care

- Assist veterinary surgeon with diagnostic tests.
- Monitor vital signs.
- Administer medications as prescribed and directed.
- Feed an appropriate diet (animals are often overweight).
- Monitor clinical signs.

Hyperthyroidism

This condition is observed most frequently in cats (but rarely in those under 6 years of age) and is rarely seen in dogs. Patients have an overactive thyroid gland, commonly caused by a benign tumour. This leads to an excessive production of thyroxine, which results in a marked increase in metabolic rate.

Clinical signs

Classic signs of the condition include:

- Polyphagia
- Polydipsia and polyuria
- Weight loss

- Aggression, hyperexcitability, restlessness
- Occasionally chronic vomiting and diarrhoea
- Hypertrophic cardiomyopathy
- Tachycardia
- Palpable enlargement of the thyroid glands (goitre).

Diagnostic tests

Diagnosis is based on clinical features and the measurement of high T4 levels.

Treatment

- Methimazole, given daily, inhibits thyroid hormone production and affects tri-iodothyronine (T3) levels. Repeat blood tests are required to monitor the condition and ensure that the treatment regime is working effectively.
- Cardiac drugs are often required to treat hypertrophic cardiomyopathy (especially prior to surgery).
- Thyroidectomy – surgical removal of neoplastic thyroid gland(s).
- Radioactive iodine treatment:
  - This is a procedure that requires the use of special facilities, therefore patients are usually referred
  - Patients are kept in complete isolation with minimal human contact during treatment
  - Due to the nature of treatment, owner visits are not permitted
  - Once treatment is complete, cats are hospitalized for a further week until radiation/radioactivity levels have decreased
  - Following discharge, cats must remain isolated in one room at home for 1–2 weeks.

Nursing care

- Assist with diagnostic tests and monitoring tests.
- Monitor patient's vital signs and water intake.
- Administer and maintain therapy as prescribed.
- Assist with surgical procedures where appropriate.

Diseases of the musculoskeletal system

Nine per cent of the calcium and phosphorus in the body is found in bone. In addition, calcium is required for blood clotting and for nerve and muscle function. Phosphorus is used in enzyme systems throughout the body. The relationship between plasma calcium and phosphorus is important and is expressed as a ratio. Normally this is in the region of 1.5:1 (Ca:P).

Vitamin D, which is activated by the kidney, is required to:

- Assist in the absorption of calcium and phosphorus from the small intestine
- Reduce loss of calcium and phosphorus from the kidney
- Increase mineralization of bone.

Bone disease may be metabolic or non-metabolic.

Metabolic bone disease

Secondary nutritional hyperparathyroidism

Aetiology

- Caused by deficiency of calcium or excess of phosphorus in the diet.
- Most commonly associated with feeding 'all meat' diets.
- Often associated with young growing puppies of the giant breeds.

Parathormone (parathyroid hormone, PTH) controls the levels of calcium and phosphorus in the blood (Figure 9.35). If an animal is fed a diet low in calcium, it will develop hypocalcaemia. The parathyroid gland will then secrete PTH, which causes the breakdown of bones and release of calcium from the skeleton. Renal excretion of phosphorus is increased to restore the Ca:P ratio.

Clinical signs

Signs include:

- Depression
- Lameness
- Pain on locomotion
- Compression fractures and pathological fractures occurring following minor trauma
- Demineralization may lead to 'rubber jaw' and loosening of teeth.

Treatment

- Most effective treatment is dietary correction.
- Use a suitable commercial puppy food.
- *Do not* supplement a bad diet with calcium.

Metaphyseal osteopathy

This is also known as Möller Barlow's disease, juvenile scurvy or hypertrophic osteodystrophy. The true cause is not known but is thought to be associated with a deficiency in Vitamin C.

The disease affects the metaphysis, where a necrotic band develops next to the growth plate, followed by deposition of a band of osseous tissue in the metaphyseal and periosteal reaction. It occurs in young growing dogs, often of large breeds; clinical signs will disappear as the dog matures.

Clinical signs

Signs include:

- Often severe lameness and pain on movement
- Some dogs totally unable to walk
- Swollen and very painful growth-plate regions of all four limbs
- Pyrexia (often >40.5°C).

Treatment

- Powerful analgesics are required.
- Correct the diet to a commercial puppy growth diet.

Nursing care

- Ensure adequate fluid intake.
- Give nursing care to turn animal regularly.
- Ensure that urination and defecation are possible.

Rickets

Rickets is the term used in young animals for the condition termed osteomalacia in adults. The cause

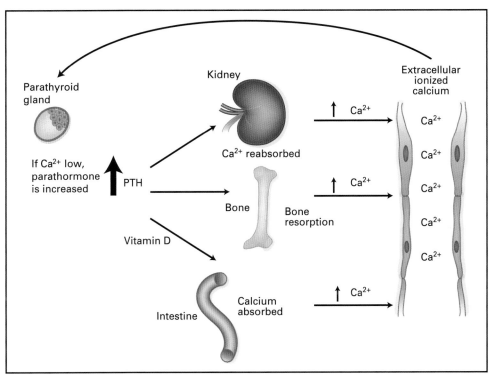

9.35 Influence of parathormone on blood calcium and phosphorus levels. (Reproduced from *BSAVA Textbook of Veterinary Nursing, 4th edition*)

is not fully understood but is thought to be due to dietary deficiency of vitamin D, calcium and phosphorus. This results in failure of mineralization around growth plates. It is most frequently observed in young growing dogs.

Clinical signs
Signs include:

- Marked enlargement of growth plates
- Bowing of limbs
- Enlargement of costochondral junction
- Lameness (less severe than metaphyseal osteopathy)
- Spontaneous fractures may occur.

Treatment

- Correct the diet to an appropriate puppy growth diet.
- Analgesics initially to control pain.

Nursing care

- Provide soft comfortable bedding.

Non-metabolic bone disease
Pulmonary osteopathy
Also known as Marie's disease or hypertrophic osteopathy, this is a condition of the bones of the lower limbs, especially forelimbs, associated with a thoracic mass. Bilateral painful soft tissue swelling of the lower forelimbs and lameness are often observed *before* thoracic signs develop. Marked periosteal proliferation occurs in the carpal and metacarpal bones and digits. There is no joint involvement. The reason for these changes is unknown.

Treatment

- Removal of the thoracic mass, although usually by the time limb changes occur the mass is inoperable.
- Euthanasia.

Osteomyelitis
This inflammation of the bone usually involves both cortex and medulla. The condition is classified as follows:

- Infectious causes:
  - Bacterial infections
  - Fungal infections
- Non-infectious causes:
  - Trauma to the bone
  - Fractures
  - Foreign bodies and implants.

Clinical signs
Signs include:

- Lameness
- Pyrexia

- Lethargy
- Inappetence
- Heat, pain and possible discoloration over site of affected bone
- Loss of limb function.

Diagnostic tests

- Radiographs reveal lytic areas in bone together with other areas of proliferation – must be differentiated from a bone tumour.
- Failure of fractures to heal is suggestive.
- Obvious bone fragments may be seen.

Treatment

- Identify and correct underlying cause.
- Remove bone fragments and foreign bodies surgically.
- A lengthy course of antibiotics where infection is present. The drug of choice is selected according to bacterial sensitivity.

Bone tumours
Several bone tumours may be observed in dogs and cats and are either primary (originating in the bone) or secondary (invasion of bone by tumour tissue from another source). The two most important are osteoma and osteosarcoma.

Osteoma

- **Benign slow-growing tumour.**
- **May cause mechanical interference with function if near a joint.**

Osteosarcoma

- **Highly malignant tumour with very aggressive growth characteristics, proving locally destructive and invasive.**
- **Initially spreads to local lymph node, then lung.**
- **More common in giant breeds (St Bernard, Great Dane, Dobermann) and dogs over 7 years of age.**
- **Approximately 75% of osteosarcomas occur in appendicular skeleton; remainder in axial.**
- **Most prevalent 'around' stifle and in hindlimb, 'away from' elbow in forelimb.**
- **Treatment of choice for dogs: wide surgical excision (amputation) in combination with adjuvant chemotherapy or radiotherapy.**
- **Prognosis remains guarded despite successful surgery, due to high incidence of metastasis.**

Arthritis
By definition, arthritis means inflammation of the joint. *Polyarthritis* indicates inflammation of several joints.

Classification of arthritis

DEGENERATIVE
Primary: ■ Aetiology unknown
Secondary: ■ Hip dysplasia
             ■ Cruciate ligament rupture

INFLAMMATORY
Infective: ■ Bacterial, viral, fungal and
                   mycoplasmal
Non-infective: ■ Crystal formation (gout)

IMMUNE-MEDIATED
Erosive: ■ Rheumatoid
                ■ Polyarthritis
Non-erosive: ■ Systemic lupus erythematosus
                  (SLE)
                ■ Polyarteritis nodosa
                ■ Drug-induced

Clinical signs

There is a variable degrees of lameness. Signs depend on the type of arthritis:

■ Degenerative: slow onset, improves with exercise, crepitus on movement
■ Infective: pyrexia and joint pain
■ Immune-mediated: multiple joint involvement, other signs of systemic disease or recent history of drug administration or vaccination.

Diagnostic tests

Diagnostic procedures are explained in more detail in the *BSAVA Manual of Advanced Veterinary Nursing* but include:

■ Radiographic changes to joint and periosteal regions around joint
■ Checks for systemic disease:
  – Routine blood tests
  – Coombs' test
  – Tests for antinuclear antibody and rheumatoid factor
  – Cytology of joint fluid.

Treatment

■ Identification and treatment of underlying cause.
■ Antibiotics in infective disease.
■ Immunosuppressive drugs in immune-mediated disease.
■ Non-steroidal anti-inflammatory drugs in degenerative disease.
■ Surgery to correct joint instability.
■ Weight and exercise management.
■ Physiotherapy and hydrotherapy.
■ Nutritional supplementation (e.g. glucosamine, chondroitin sulphate).

Nursing care

■ Assist with radiography.
■ Assist with laboratory tests, including the collection of blood samples and joint fluid.

■ Administer and maintain therapy prescribed by the veterinary surgeon.
■ Assist animal with locomotion in order to allow defecation and urination.
■ If patient is recumbent, turn frequently to prevent decubitus ulcers.
■ Perform physiotherapy where appropriate.
■ Maintain a clean environment.
■ Provide soft comfortable bedding.
■ Advise owner accordingly:
  – Diet if obese
  – Encourage frequent walks of short duration.

Muscle disease

Myositis refers to inflammation of the muscle. This may involve one muscle group or can be associated with multiple muscle groups (*polymyositis*). There are many causes of myositis, including infections and immune-mediated disease.

Myopathy, or muscle weakness and loss of function, may also occur with metabolic diseases, such as Cushing's disease and hypothyroidism (see above).

Diagnostic tests

Tests used in muscle disease include:

■ Routine blood tests for systemic disease
■ Muscle biopsy
■ Electromyography (EMG) to assist in detecting disease of muscle fibres and associated nerves.

Treatment

Treatment depends on the underlying cause but may include antibiotics, immunosuppressive drugs and treatment for metabolic disease.

Nursing care

■ Physiotherapy.
■ Observe patient for signs of pain and discomfort.
■ Administer drug therapy as prescribed.
■ Care for recumbent patients (see later).

Cutaneous disease

Parasitic skin disease

Parasitic skin diseases are summarized in Figure 9.36; information for clients is discussed further in Chapter 2 and diagnostic tests in Chapter 10.

Nursing care

■ Many parasitic skin diseases are zoonotic; therefore appropriate measures should be taken to avoid contamination.
■ Wear personal protective equipment when handling infected animals, to avoid spreading disease.
■ Many treatments used to treat parasitic skin disease are harmful to humans if inhaled or if they come into contact with skin.
■ There is potential for spread; therefore suitable disinfectant protocols must be implemented.

Ectoparasite	Appearance	Clinical signs	Distribution	Life cycle/transmission	Owner advice	Host-specific	Diagnostic test
Sarcoptes scabiei (canine scabies) ⚠	Adults – round-bodied mite	Intense pruritus. Alopecia, scales and crusts	Ventrum, ears and elbows, in epidermal burrows	Permanently resides on animal. Transmitted from animal to animal by close contact	Often transmitted via foxes. Exceedingly contagious	No (rarely)	Multiple skin scrapings required from elbow, ear or sites with papules
Trichodectes canis (dog biting louse) ⚠	Adults – biting lice with broad head. Chewing mouthparts on ventral aspect	Mild: carrier showing no sign. Severe: papules, crusts, seborrhoea sicca	Under matted hair and around body orifices	Permanently resides on animal. Transmitted from animal to animal by close contact	Insecticides will kill adult and nymphal stages, but eggs difficult to kill	Yes	Demonstration of eggs attached to hairs or visualization of adult louse through naked eye or skin scrape/brush
Ctenocephalides felis (cat flea); *Ctenocephalides canis* (dog flea). The cat flea is the most common species of flea affecting dogs and cats in the UK ⚠	Eggs – small brown laterally compressed. Flea dirt – brown granules turn red when wet	Pruritus. Acute – wheals and erythema. Chronic – seborrhoea, lichenification, alopecia	Dogs – dorsum (especially lumbosacral area). Cats – miliary (generalized) dermatitis or focal eosinophilic granuloma (pink plaque)	Majority of life cycle is off host. Eggs, larvae and adults present in environment	Regular flea treatment should be recommended, especially during spring/summer. Flea is intermediate host in tapeworm life cycle, therefore important to treat animals against both	No	Demonstration of adult flea or their faeces by combing animal's coat with fine-tooth comb over piece of damp white paper
Ixodes canisuga (dog tick); *Ixodes ricinus* (sheep tick); *Ixodes hexagonus* (hedgehog tick). The sheep and hedgehog ticks are the most common species seen on small animals in the UK ⚠	Flattened, ovoid, yellow-white to red-brown	Carrier shows no sign, or mild local irritation (especially if incompletely removed)	Usually over ears, face and ventral body	Feeds on animal. Animals infected from environment	Ticks should always be removed with care	No	Visualization of parasite by naked eye
Demodex canis (dogs); *Demodex cati* (cats) (demodectic mange) ⚠	Small, cigar-shaped burrowing mite	Causes mild erythema, alopecia and may be pruritic if secondary pyoderma present. May cause mange in hamsters and gerbils	Localized (especially face and forelimbs) or generalized	Small numbers found in normal animals and only become significant when animal's immune response is inadequate	*Demodex* mites are normal inhabitants of canine skin. Puppies can be infected from their mothers within first few days post whelping	Yes	Found deep within hair follicles so skin should be squeezed before performing deep skin scraping
Otodectes cynotis (ear mites) ⚠ (occasionally)	Adults – white dots visible to naked eye	Cause of otitis externa and may mimic flea allergy dermatitis if generalized. Head shaking	Common cause of ear problems but can also cause a generalized problem	Permanently resides on animal. Transmitted from animal to animal via close contact	Easily transmitted between animals in multi-pet households	No	Mites visible to naked eye. Superficial scrapings, smears of ear wax or sticky tape preparations helpful
Linognathus setosus (dog sucking louse) ⚠	Eggs – small, white and attached to hair ('nits'). Adults – sucking lice with typical fixed piercing mouthparts	Mild: carrier showing no sign. Severe: papules, crusts, seborrhoea sicca	Under matted hair and around body orifices	Permanently resides on animal. Transmitted from animal to animal by close contact	Drugs used for lice infestations must be applied directly to animal	Yes	Demonstration of eggs attached to hairs or visualization of adult louse through naked eye or skin scrape/brush
Cheyletiella parasitivorax ⚠	Mite commonly found on cats, dogs and rabbits. Adults – large white 'walking dandruff'. Eggs – loosely attached to hair	Extremely variable. Mild: carrier showing no sign. Severe: mild, non-suppurative dermatitis and scurf	Diffuse but usually more dorsal	Permanently resides on animal. Transmitted from animal to animal via close contact	All animals in household should be treated whether showing clinical signs or not	No	Superficial skin scrapes or sticky tape preparations or coat brushings useful
Neotrombicula autumnalis (harvest mite) ⚠	Small orange spider-like mites	Irritation, hypersensitivity and pedal dermatitis	Commonly found on feet and lower limbs	Free-living mites with only larval form being parasitic	Normally becomes problem in late summer and autumn	No	Larval stages bright orange and readily visible to naked eye
Notoedres cati (feline scabies) ⚠	Burrowing mite, resembles *Sarcoptes*	Pruritus, lichenification, crusting alopecia	Head, ears and neck; can be generalized	Permanently resides on animal	Easily transmitted from animal to animal via close contact	No	Single skin scrape of eyes, ear or face
Felicola subrostratus (feline biting louse) ⚠	Cat biting louse	Mild: carrier showing no sign. Severe: papules, crusts, seborrhoea sicca	Under matted hair and around body orifices	Permanently resides on animal. Transmitted from animal to animal by close contact	To reduce small risk of environmental spread, bedding should be washed or even burnt	Yes	Demonstration of eggs attached to hairs or visualization of adult louse

9.36 Parasitic skin diseases. ⚠ indicates a zoonosis.

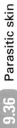

Ringworm

Also known as dermatophytosis, this is a fungal infection of the skin, hair and nailbed areas of dogs and cats. It is more common to see clinical disease in cats rather than in dogs. Infection is obtained by direct contact and indirect contact (fomites). Ringworm is an important zoonosis (Figure 9.37).

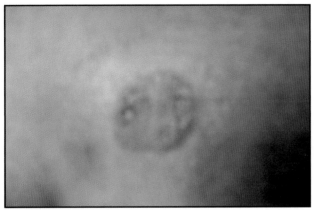

9.37 Dermatophytosis (ringworm) lesion on human skin.

There are two main types of organism involved:

■ *Microsporum canis* accounts for around 95% of feline disease and 50–80% of canine disease
■ *Trichophyton* spp. account for around 4% of feline disease and 12–60% of canine disease.

Clinical signs

■ **Cats:**
  – May initially appear as circular areas of alopecia, grey and crusting
  – May also appear as miliary dermatitis
  – May remain asymptomatic.
■ **Dogs:**
  – Initial circular rings of alopecia, grey and crusting
  – Most often seen around head and forelimbs
  – May become generalized.

Diagnostic tests

Diagnostic procedures are explained in more detail in Chapter 10. They include:

■ Plucking hairs for culture
■ Ultraviolet light fluorescence (Wood's lamp)
■ Skin scrapings to observe spores.

Treatment

■ Oral antifungals (e.g. itraconazole).
■ Clip hair from lesions in longhaired breeds.
■ Topical antifungals.

Nursing care

■ Wear gloves when handling patient for treatment.

■ Assist veterinary surgeon in carrying out diagnostic tests.
■ Administer and maintain therapy prescribed by veterinary surgeon.
■ Help to prevent self-trauma by animal.
■ Burn bedding where possible.
■ Disinfect with sodium hypochlorite, formalin or enilconazole solutions.
■ Advise owners:
  – This is a zoonotic disease, therefore medical attention should be sought if skin lesions develop in humans (Figure 9.37)
  – Limit handling of pet
  – Wear gloves and wash hands if direct contact occurs
  – Ensure that environment is cleaned and disinfected.

Hormonal alopecia

The conditions in this group are usually associated with one of the following:

■ Hypothyroidism
■ Hyperadrenocorticism (Cushing's disease)
■ Sertoli cell tumour (hyperoestrogenism)
■ Canine ovarian imbalances (hypo- and hyperoestrogenism)
■ Feline hormonal alopecia.

Clinical signs

■ The majority of cases have bilateral alopecia, usually starting on the flanks.
■ There is rarely pruritus. The skin is unreactive unless there is secondary infection.
■ There are frequently other signs of systemic disease.

Diagnostic tests

Diagnosis depends on finding and correcting the underlying cause:

■ Blood tests
■ Hormonal assays.

Pyoderma

Pyoderma is more common in the dog than in the cat. There is frequently an underlying cause for its development, such as demodicosis or immunosuppression. Pyoderma may be classified according to its depth in the skin (Figure 9.38).

Feline pyoderma is associated with cat bites: oral bacteria are 'injected' under the skin, leading to cellulitis. It usually involves a limb, with swelling, pain and pyrexia.

Treatment

■ Identifying and correcting underlying cause.
■ Culture and sensitivity of purulent material (usually *Staphylococcus aureus*).
■ Long-term antibiotics.

Surface dermatitis
Acute moist dermatitis and skin fold dermatitis
Frequently involves the side of the face, or hindquarters
Associated with ear infections and anal sac disorders
Significant self-trauma involved in aetiology
Skin fold dermatitis due to anatomical problem with folding of skin preventing proper ventilation
Seen mostly in Sharpei, Pug and Pekingese

Superficial dermatitis
Impetigo, puppy dermatitis or juvenile dermatitis
Often seen on ventral abdomen of puppies
Multiple yellow pustules
Also occurs as folliculitis where the hair follicle is involved
Ring formations develop, giving moth-eaten appearance
Formations spread out radially

Deep pyoderma
Pododermatitis (i.e. affecting feet)
Paws become swollen and painful and exude pus
Fistulas and sinus tracts may be seen
Furunculosis associated with ringworm and *Demodex* infection
Very serious deep-seated infection that may be generalized

9.38 Some types of pyoderma.

Allergic skin disease

Various forms of allergic skin disease are seen in dogs and cats.

Urticaria

Urticaria (hives) is a condition characterized by focal superficial oedematous swellings over the skin surface, with erection of hairs at each site.

- Lesions single or multiple and variably pruritic.
- Induced by drugs, vaccines, insect bites/stings, blood transfusions, foods, plants and other factors.
- Dogs more commonly affected than cats.
- Diagnosis based on presentation and known cause.
- Treat by removing cause and giving anti-inflammatory drugs.

Atopic dermatitis

Atopy is the term used to describe a disease condition arising from the allergic reaction to environmental particles.

- Large number of known antigens, including house mites, fungi, pollens and dander.
- Usually affects dogs from 1–3 years of age.
- Intense pruritis, especially around eyes, feet, axilla and ventral abdomen.
- May have otitis externa and ocular discharge.
- Miliary lesions may develop, especially along the back.
- Diagnosis through intradermal skin testing.
- Treatment is lifelong antihistamines, anti-inflammatory drugs, shampoos, and desensitization or exclusion of allergens.

Contact dermatitis

- May be induced by soaps, detergents, chemicals of any kind.
- Develops about 5 weeks after initial exposure.
- Pruritus and erythema involving feet, ventral abdomen and face.
- Diagnosis by patch testing with suspect agents.
- Treatment involves avoiding contact with known agents.

Food hypersensitivity

- May occur due to consumption of proteins in food such as beef, pork, milk and eggs.
- Pruritic skin disease and/or chronic vomiting and diarrhoea may occur.
- Diagnosis on clinical presentation, use of elimination diets.
- Treatment requires avoidance of initiating agents.

Nursing patients with special requirements

Nursing the geriatric patient

Elderly patients may be diagnosed with various and often multiple conditions that may require medical or surgical management. Geriatric nursing also involves caring for the ageing animal in both health and disease, which may sometimes prove challenging.

Elderly animals must be treated with extra care, for whatever reason they are admitted. After all, these are generally the patients that are least able to compensate for any shortfall in nursing care. They also often take longer to recover from medical interference.

In general, giant breeds of dog tend to age more rapidly than smaller breeds and cats tend to age less rapidly than dogs. Animals that may be described as 'geriatric' or 'senior' include:

- Large-breed dogs aged 6 years and older
- Smaller-breed dogs aged 8–9 years and older
- Cats aged 9 years and older.

As animals enter old age they have a decreased ability to adjust to change. There is a reduction in body cells (as those that wear out are not readily replaced) and the surviving cells do not work as efficiently as before. The two main factors responsible for these changes are:

- Ageing – physical and behavioural changes
- Accumulated injury.

These factors, along with common disease problems associated with ageing (see Figure 9.39) must be taken into consideration when nursing a geriatric patient.

Ageing

Physical factors that are reduced in geriatric animals include:

- Stamina and agility
- Metabolic rate (an average 20% decrease, which often leads to obesity, exacerbating many other geriatric disease processes)
- Muscle mass (less efficient cells, and decreased replacement leading to atrophy)
- Bone mass
- Immune responses (therefore increased susceptibility to disease, including neoplasia)
- Sense of smell, taste, sight and hearing
- Hair (becomes sparse, dull and listless, and white hairs appear on muzzle)
- Elasticity of the skin, some thickening of the skin, callus formation
- Ability to produce melanin (nose may become pinker).

Behavioural changes seen in geriatric animals include:

- Forgetting basic obedience and house training
- Irritability when disturbed
- Slower reactions to stimuli
- Development of sleep disorders

- Less adaptable to change
- Disorientation
- Inappetence.

Accumulated injury

Injuries sustained during a lifetime plus an age-related loss of functional reserve mean that maximum organ function is reduced with age. This becomes apparent when the animal is stressed due to:

- Severe exercise
- Changes in routine (e.g. hospitalization, boarding kennels)
- Changes in environmental temperature
- Acute illness
- Anaesthesia
- Inadequate nutrition
- Dehydration.

Diseases

A number of diseases associated with decreased cell and organ function are commonly seen in geriatric animals (Figure 9.39).

Digestive system	
Oral cavity	Increased dental calculus. Periodontal disease leading to atrophy and retraction of the gums, with increased tooth loss. Infected teeth can lead to absorption of bacteria/uraemia/decreased saliva production. Tumours
Oesophagus	Loss of muscle tone
Stomach	Reduced hydrochloric acid secretion, resulting in vomiting and flatulence and intermittent diarrhoea
Liver	Decreased hepatocyte numbers leading to reduced liver function, biliary and intestinal secretions. Impaired intestinal motility
Intestine	Decreased rate of intestinal epithelial renewal leading to decreased lipid absorption. Decreased villous height and width thus decreased areas for nutrient absorption
Anal glands	Impaction due to increased thickness of fluid, irregular defecation, decreased bulk of faeces
Cardiorespiratory system	
Heart	Cardiac output decreased by 30% in last third of animal's lifespan. Fibrous thickening of the valves (endocardiosis). Red cell counts and haemoglobin levels decrease. Reduced peripheral circulation
Lungs	Atrophy of secretory structures may cause obstructive lung disease. Chronic bronchitis. Increased susceptibility to infection. Reduced ability to expel air. Alveolar capillary membrane has reduced diffusing capacity. Atrophy and weakening of respiratory muscles. Loss of elastic tissue. Increased pulmonary fibrosis, eventually leading to increased intrapleural pressure, decreased cardiac output and ultimate right-sided cardiac failure
Urinary system	
Kidneys	Reduced function. Scarring of medulla and cortex. Decreased glomerular filtration rate as a result of interstitial pressure, reduced renal perfusion and altered permeability of glomerular membrane.
Bladder	Incontinence due to reduced bladder sphincter tone particularly in spayed bitches. Chronic cystitis from incomplete bladder emptying
Endocrine system	
	Decreased secretion of hormones by thyroid glands, testes and ovaries. Geriatric hormonal activity may affect skin and coat condition, and encourage weight gain. Lethargy
Reproductive system	
	Mammary gland tumours. Pyometra in entire bitches and queens. Testicular atrophy. Testicular tumours. Pendulous prepuce due to oestrogen secretion from Sertoli cells or androgen deficit. Prostatic hyperplasia. Prostatic disease – enlarged due to hypertrophy, infection, cysts and neoplasia. Perineal rupture
Musculoskeletal system	
	Loss of muscle mass. Deterioration of neuromuscular function. Loss of bone mass. Thinner cortices of long bones. Split and fragmented cartilage. Thickened synovial fluid and joint capsules. Osteophyte formation. Arthritis – wear and tear of joints

9.39 Common problems associated with ageing in the main body systems. (continues)

Nervous system and special sense organs	
General	Chronic hypoxia of the brain. Sleep disorders. Neuromuscular disorders. Depression. Reduced reaction to stimuli. Reduced response to pain
Eye	Impaired sight. Retinal atrophy. Iris atrophy. Cataracts. Increased density of the lens (nuclear sclerosis). Increased tear viscosity. Increased susceptibility to infection.
Ear	Chronic otitis. Wax accumulation. Impaired hearing
Nose	Decreased sense of smell
Hair and skin	
	Prolonged healing time of skin. Reduced general condition. Thinned coat. Greasy skin. Calluses and pressure sores. Increased frequency of sebaceous gland adenomas, cysts, lipomas, skin tumours. Hyperkeratinized footpads. Nails, including dew claws, often become overgrown and sometimes malformed, due to reduced exercise and cell dysfunction. Warts

9.39 (continued) Common problems associated with ageing in the main body systems.

Nutrition

Dietary needs

The gastrointestinal tract of a geriatric animal may have reductions in muscle tone, ability to absorb nutrients and provision of gastric juices. The diet must be adjusted accordingly and should be fed in divided meals, two to four times daily. The animal may also need encouragement to eat.

Dietary factors to consider include:

- Increased palatability
- Increased digestibility
- Fibre (aids digestive tract function and used to control obesity, but may reduce the palatability of the diet)
- Carbohydrate levels to maintain normal body weight
- Sufficient vitamins, minerals and essential fatty acids (EFA)
- Reduced energy content
- Feeding a high-quality protein to help to reduce muscle mass loss, but not high levels of protein in cases where there is existing renal disease
- Reduced calcium and phosphorus to avoid excessive intake
- Freely available fresh water.

Further adjustments should be made for a patient with concurrent disease:

- Obesity – reduce fat
- Cardiac disease – reduce sodium
- Renal disease – reduce phosphorus
- Liver disease – increase vitamins B, C, D and K.

Monitoring water intake

Water intake may be slightly increased in older animals, because of reduced organ efficiency, but water should always be freely available. If the water intake is significantly elevated or decreased, the veterinary surgeon should be notified. Owners can be taught how to monitor fluid intake at home and should be instructed to contact the surgery if there are any marked changes. *Polydipsia* is usually defined as a water intake >100 ml/kg bodyweight/24 hours.

Calculating an animal's water intake

1. Calculate the average daily water requirement for the patient (40–60 ml/kg/day).
2. Measure out the water required, rounded up to the nearest half litre, and give to the animal.
3. Replenish with fresh measured water if required.
4. Measure any water left after 24 hours and calculate the animal's actual water intake.

It should be noted that the amount of moisture contained within the food provided (e.g. canned versus dry) will influence the animal's daily water intake.

Exercise

A change in exercise regime may be required in the geriatric pet, due to reduced stamina or concurrent disease. Short and frequent exercise is beneficial as it helps to maintain joint movement and muscle tone and to reduce adhesions and stiffness, and will also help to control obesity.

When walking:

- Allow frequent opportunity for urination and defecation
- Observe frequency of urination and defecation
- Note any respiratory change or coughing
- Look for lameness or stiffness of gait
- Avoid sudden changes in routine.

In lethargic or hospitalized patients, passive physiotherapy of the limb joints (see later) may help to maintain joint mobility and muscle tone.

Mental stimulation

The elderly patient may tend to sleep more, be less mentally alert, and more likely to be 'disobedient'. Often they will need more attention than younger adult animals, which can be time-consuming for both owners and nurses. However, mental stimulation can be very effective in those that are seemingly withdrawn.

Methods of mentally stimulating patients include:

- Exercise and access to fresh air
- Daily grooming
- Physiotherapy
- New and interesting toys
- Provision of a varied environment
- Television, radio or music (especially if animal is left alone)
- Supervised socialization with other animals and people
- Hand-feeding.

Grooming

Older pets tend to be less fastidious about grooming and require assistance from the owner and nurse to maintain cleanliness and a well groomed look. This process provides regular mental stimulation for the patient and improves the bond between the handler and the animal. The following points should be borne in mind.

- Handle gently but confidently, taking care as older animals are more likely to become irritable and snap at handlers.
- Over-enthusiastic grooming may be uncomfortable for pets with arthritis or reduced muscle mass.
- Grooming prevents matting, stimulates skin and sebaceous glands and maintains the coat in good order.
- Increased sebum production causes the coat to lose its gloss, making it appear greasy and resulting in the accumulation of dirt more quickly. This can cause an unpleasant odour.

Grooming also provides the opportunity to check for:

- Discharges (regular cleaning of eyes, ears, prepuce and vulva)
- Nail health (nails, including dewclaws, often become overgrown and sometimes malformed)
- Skin lesions or growths
- Parasites.

Bedding

The special needs of a geriatric patient in relation to bedding should be considered. These include:

- Increased need for sleep
- Increased need for warmth
- Peripheral circulation not as efficient in the geriatric and calluses or bedsores may occur
- Incontinence.

Appropriate adaptations include:

- Raising the bed and placing in a draught-free area
- Providing warmth and insulating bedding
- Providing cushioned or thick bedding (e.g. PCV-covered foam, synthetic fleece, blankets) to give support
- For patients with normal bladder control: providing beanbags
- For incontinent patients: providing bed with urine-proof base and washable bedding.

Thermoregulation

Elderly patients have a reduced ability for thermoregulation. Poor circulation often warrants the provision of additional heating. It is important to maintain a comfortable atmosphere away from draughts and to prevent extremes in environmental temperature. See 'Nursing the recumbent patient', below.

Hospitalization of the geriatric patient

Hospitalization periods should be kept to a minimum, as geriatric patients are less adaptable to change and become stressed when taken out of their normal environment. They may also be susceptible to nosocomial infection (an infection acquired within a hospital environment).

- Remember that many geriatrics are blind, deaf, arthritic (in any combination); therefore reference should be made to owners regarding individual degrees of sight, hearing, ambulation, etc.
- Provide a hospital environment that is conducive to their needs and try to reduce stress.
- Follow patient's normal routine as far as possible with regard to feeding, walking, etc.
- Ensure that canine patients are given frequent but short trips outside to help to reduce incontinence problems and reduce stiffness.
- Observe closely for signs of chronic disease.
- Monitor vital signs on a regular basis.
- Physiotherapy can be used as a supportive therapy.

> **WARNING**
> - **Blind patients should be spoken to before being approached, so that they are aware of the handler's presence.**
> - **Deaf patients should be approached through their line of sight.**

Special considerations relating to anaesthesia and surgery are covered in Chapters 12 and 13.

Advice to owners

It is important to remember that clients are usually very bonded to their older pet; after all, they are likely to have owned them for many years and will probably consider them part of their family.

Advice concerning a geriatric pet may be complicated. After discussing care and treatment with the owner, advice should be backed up with leaflets and written instructions.

Factors to discuss with the owner include:

- Exercise
- Urination and defecation
- Eyesight and hearing
- Feeding and water intake
- Behaviour
- Mental stimulation
- Bedding
- Grooming
- Veterinary care.

Veterinary care

- Owners should be encouraged to get their elderly pets checked every 6 months as part of a geriatric healthcare programme. These checks may detect problems early, before advanced disease or disabilities become apparent and more complex to control.
- The importance of regular worming and the need for continued protection against infectious diseases through vaccination should be emphasized.
- Owners should always be encouraged to discuss changes in their geriatric pet's behaviour. All too often such changes are attributed solely to old age, which may result in failure to detect their true cause.
- If oral hygiene is neglected, the animal may experience pain and discomfort leading to dull and depressed behaviour, sometimes misinterpreted by the owner as being a sign of old age and therefore often ignored. Regular dental care can make all the difference to an elderly pet's quality of life (Figure 9.40).

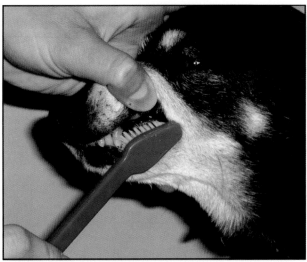

9.40 Good oral hygiene is especially important in geriatric patients.

Nursing the recumbent patient

A recumbent patient is one that is unwilling or unable to rise. Problems occur because of this inability and the fact that the patient is in the same position for prolonged periods of time.

Causes of recumbency include:

- Spinal trauma (e.g. disc protrusion)
- Fractures (e.g. pelvis, limbs)
- Electrolyte imbalances, head injuries, shock
- Debilitating medical disease (e.g. Cushing's syndrome, cardiac disease)
- Neurological disorders (e.g. coma)
- Anaesthesia or sedation
- Paraplegia.

Problems associated with recumbent patients, as discussed below, are more easily prevented than cured.

Nursing care

- Choose a kennel of adequate size so that the patient can lie comfortably. Waterproof bedding is ideal, with absorbent bedding material placed on top.
- Recumbent patients may be hospitalized in the same kennel for some time so ensure that they can see some activity to keep them stimulated.
- Monitor and record the usual parameters (TPR and especially urine and faecal output). Any abnormalities should be recorded and reported.
- Provide a concentrated highly digestible diet, placed within easy reach of the patient. Patients who are recumbent due to a medical condition are likely to be depressed and may require hand feeding. Water must be available at all times; intake should be monitored.
- Prevent decubitus ulcers, hypostatic pneumonia and soiling. Ensure that the patient is clean and dry every time it is turned (see below).
- Even if the patient is incontinent, dogs should be taken outside on a regular basis to provide a change of environment.
- If the patient has an indwelling catheter, this should be cared for accordingly.
- Carry out physiotherapy techniques.

Hypostatic pneumonia

When a patient is recumbent for long periods, blood pools in the lower lung. The alveoli tend to collapse, causing oxygen deficiency and static blood supply. This in turn is an ideal medium for growth of microorganisms causing pneumonia.

Prevention

- Turn the laterally recumbent patient every 2–4 hours.
- Alternate lateral recumbency with supported sternal recumbency for periods of 30 minutes. Patients can be supported using sandbags, rolled-up blankets or towels, or beanbags.
- Encourage active assisted or supported exercise.
- Give respiratory physiotherapy – positioning, postural drainage, coupage and vibrations (see section on physiotherapy, below).
- Record all treatments, including time in each position.

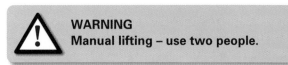

⚠ **WARNING**
Manual lifting – use two people.

Clinical signs

- Increased rate and depth of respiration.
- Increased effort of respiration.
- Abdominal breathing.
- Increased lung sounds, gurgling – moist breathing.
- Depression.
- Signs of restlessness or discomfort.
- Pale or cyanotic mucous membranes.
- Slow capillary refill time.

Treatment

If hypostatic pneumonia develops, the veterinary surgeon must be informed immediately so that treatment may be given promptly.

Decubitus ulcers

Decubitus ulcers, also known as pressure sores or bedsores, occur on areas with little subcutaneous fat and over bony prominences (Figure 9.41). Pressure on these areas in the recumbent patient is almost continuous, resulting in a decreased local blood supply and anoxia of tissues. This results in red sores on bony prominences, inflammation and possible ulceration or bleeding. The patient may demonstrate signs of pain or restlessness.

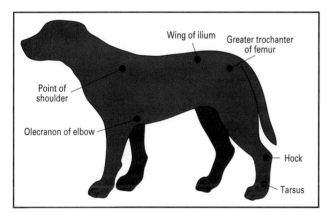

9.41 Sites liable to decubitus ulcer formation.

Prevention

- Turn or reposition patient every 2–4 hours.
- Provide supportive and comfortable bedding, such as PVC-covered foam mattresses, synthetic fleece or bubblewrap (multiple layers of bedding are sufficient if PVC foam beds are not available).
- Practise physiotherapy (orthopaedic and neurological, massage).
- Pad and bandage potential problem areas.
- Pay close attention to hygiene.
- Check problem areas twice daily.

Treatment

- Inform the veterinary surgeon.

Nursing care

- Clip the area.
- Clean with a mild antiseptic and then dry thoroughly.
- Apply a soothing barrier or therapeutic cream.
- Provide extra padding or bedding.

Problems associated with urination and defecation

Constipation, diarrhoea, urinary retention, urinary incontinence and patient soiling are some of the problems encountered with the recumbent patient.

Constipation

Due to decreased circulation, decreased activity, decreased intake of food and water and administration of opioid analgesics, constipation may occur.
    Factors to consider:

- A patient should pass faeces at least once every 48 hours. If this does not occur, the veterinary surgeon should be informed
- Diet may need to be adjusted to try to reduce the occurrence. High-fibre diets are of benefit in the prevention but not in the treatment of constipation
- Treatment may be prescribed by the veterinary surgeon (e.g. oral liquid paraffin or an enema).

Diarrhoea

Faecal incontinence may occur in a patient with neurological disease, nerve damage due to trauma, or debility. Factors to consider:

- Treatment of the cause
- Adjusting the diet – feed a diet that contains high-quality protein and is low in fat
- Nursing of the soiled patient (see later).

Urinary incontinence

Urinary incontinence may occur in a patient with neurological disease, nerve damage due to trauma, or debility. Factors to consider:

- Nursing of the soiled patient (see later)
- Catheterization (see later).

Because a debilitated patient is unable to rise, urine is retained for long periods. When it is eventually released, the patient may appear 'incontinent'. A bladder sphincter weakness can develop. Regular supported exercise and encouragement to urinate may be all that is required to keep the patient clean and comfortable.

Urine scalding

Urine scalding and soiling can often be prevented (see later). If urine scalding occurs, dermatitis (inflammation of the skin) will be evident.

Urine retention

Urinary retention may be due to nerve damage, trauma or obstruction of the lower urinary tract.
    Factors to consider:

- Catheterization (see later)
- Cystocentesis.

Temperature control

Debilitated patients may not be able to maintain a normal body temperature.

- Recumbent patients are not exercising and therefore do not generate sufficient body heat. Core body temperature and peripheral circulation are reduced, leading to poor perfusion of tissues and cold extremities.

- Anorexic patients are at risk due to the lowering of the metabolic rate.
- Soiled patients may also be at risk if they are not kept clean, warm and dry.

Hypothermia is shown by: abnormally low body temperature, pale mucous membranes, reduced pulse rate, cold extremities, and depression. Treatment of hypothermia may include the provision of extra warmth and measures to reduce heat loss from the patient (detailed above). The veterinary surgeon may request warmed intravenous fluids.

Measures that can be employed to reduce heat loss include the following.

- Keep the patient out of draughts.
- Provide warm and insulating bedding (e.g. synthetic fleece, bubblewrap, space blankets).
- Keep the kennel area at the correct temperature (e.g. 18–21°C for hospitalized patients).
- Provide a safe heat source (e.g. infrared heat lamp).
- Physiotherapy – both massage and passive and active exercise (see section on physiotherapy) can help to maintain body temperature.
- Monitor the patient's body temperature regularly.
- Warm intravenous fluids to body temperature prior to administration.

Musculoskeletal problems

Muscle tone and joint movement are maintained during normal exercise. Due to lack of exercise, recumbent patients lose muscle tone and muscle mass. In addition, joint movement may be compromised and limb oedema may occur. The result may be reduced long-term function and mobility. Physiotherapy used from the onset of recumbency enhances the patient's chance of successful rehabilitation.

Physiotherapy techniques (see later) used to support recumbent patients include:

- Massage – effleurage, petrissage and friction
- Passive exercise and active movement.

Inappetence or inability to eat or drink
Feeding

- Feed a high-quality palatable diet, with high digestibility and low bulk.
- Ensure that the patient can actually reach the food: offer food by hand if necessary, or try positioning the patient in supported sternal recumbency to allow better access to the feeding bowl.
- Appetite stimulation may be tried.
- Enteral tube feeding may be required.

Fluids

- Water should be freely available and offered every 2 hours if the patient is able or unwilling to drink.
- Water may be carefully and slowly syringed into the patient's mouth, taking care to avoid aspiration (Figure 9.42).

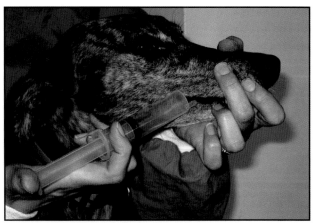

9.42 Syringing water carefully into the patient's mouth.

- Monitor water intake (normal range 40–60 ml/kg bodyweight/24 hours).
- Monitor hydration status – skin tenting, colour and feel of mucous membranes, capillary refill time (see Chapter 8).

Skin and coat problems

The recumbent patient may be unwilling or unable to groom itself. Matting can occur and lesions may be undetected. Regular grooming is required, together with a check of nail length and a look for skin lesions or parasites.

Depression

Mental stimulation is vital for the recumbent patient. In a busy surgery it is often difficult to give extra care, but taking time and giving encouragement during nursing procedures can help to prevent depression.

The veterinary surgeon may consider sending a depressed patient home to be nursed. It is vital to give the owner an accurate and detailed explanation of nursing care and therapies, with written back-up.

Nursing the soiled patient

Patients can become soiled with: food; urine; faeces; vomit; blood; saliva; discharges from the vagina or prepuce; or wound exudates. The hospitalized patient should be observed regularly and given immediate care when soiling occurs. This will reduce complications and make the animal feel more comfortable. The following general measures may be taken to reduce the likelihood of soiling:

- Provide a large enough kennel so that the animal can move away from the soiled area
- Provide absorbent bedding
- Observe patient regularly
- Remove any soiled bedding immediately
- Clean the soiled kennel appropriately and, when dry, supply fresh bedding
- Sponge down or bathe the patient, dry carefully and return to the clean kennel.

Food and discharges

Any soiling with food should be cleaned and dried immediately. Discharges should be bathed on a regular basis and protective cream applied as required.

Urinary soiling and scalding

Urine soiling may occur during recovery from anaesthesia, with recumbent or incontinent patients, or when patients are given insufficient opportunity to urinate. Repeated soiling can lead to urine scalding. The general rules above apply, in addition to the following points.

- Opportunity to urinate:
  - Dogs: supported towel-walking to the run may be necessary for some patients
  - Cats: assist them to the litter tray at regular intervals with support; and, unless contraindicated (e.g. urethral blockage), gentle steady pressure can be exerted on the bladder to encourage urination.
- Record urination on record sheet and note the colour, clarity, odour, straining and frequency.
- Catheterization may be indicated.
- Look for signs of urine scalding, bathe any affected areas with mild antiseptic solution and dry thoroughly.
- Barrier cream can be applied to help to reduce or treat urine scalds.

Faeces

- If faecal soiling occurs, adequate and immediate cleansing of the patient is required.
- Hair may need to be clipped, and barrier cream applied to the perineal region.
- Monitor hydration status and weight changes.
- In severe cases intravenous fluids may be prescribed.

The following should be observed and recorded about the faeces when nursing a patient with diarrhoea:

- Content: mucus, blood, endoparasites
- Colour
- Consistency
- Straining.

Vomit

Nursing of the vomiting patient requires good nursing skills in both observation and care of the patient. The following observations should be made:

- Content: food, bile, blood
- Frequency of vomiting
- Association with feeding
- Hydration status.

In caring for the vomiting patient:

- General rules for reduction of soiling apply
- The mouth and gums can be bathed with tepid water
- Medication and intravenous fluids may be prescribed by the veterinary surgeon
- When feeding is recommended, it should be introduced slowly, offering small frequent meals of bland food.

Blood, saliva and exudate

General rules of the soiled patient apply, keeping the patient clean, dry and comfortable.

Soiling from exuding wounds can be reduced by using appropriate absorbent dressings with regular dressing changes. Monitor the wound for signs of infection.

Bathing the soiled patient

The first consideration is whether the patient is well enough for a bath. Weak, geriatric or hypothermic patients may be better with a sponge-down to reduce stress and loss of body heat.

Bathing procedures for dogs

- Prepare a warm dry kennel for after bathing.
- Look for skin lesions; record and report as necessary.
- Brush out coat.
- Clip any matted hair (with permission from owner or veterinary surgeon).
- Select a mild shampoo.
- Ensure that the water is at body temperature before the patient is placed in the bath or under the shower hose.
- Never leave a patient unattended in the bath.
- Rinse out shampoo thoroughly.
- Squeeze excess water from the coat.
- Dry carefully with towels.
- Ensure adequate restraint before using a hairdryer, which should be turned first to low power to ensure tolerance by the patient.
- Heat lamps may be used to aid drying.
- When the patient is completely dry, barrier cream can be applied to problem areas if required.

WARNING
Cats with soiling problems should only be sponged down, as they become very stressed if bathed.

Nursing the anorexic patient and assisted feeding

When an animal that is not eating is admitted to the veterinary practice it may require assisted feeding, ranging from appetite stimulation to parenteral feeding, depending on the clinical condition. It is important to differentiate initially whether the patient is anorexic or dysphagic.

- Anorexia:
  - There is a lack or loss of appetite due to pyrexia, pain, weakness or stress
  - Animals may refuse to eat because they are hospitalized; in some cases it may be appropriate to send them home for treatment of the disease process
  - With an anorexic patient, appetite stimulation can be tried initially before progressing to the more complicated techniques.
- Dysphagia:
  - The patient may have the desire to eat but is physically unable to do so. This is often due to a mechanical or neurological order.

> **WARNINGS**
> - It is inappropriate to use appetite stimulation methods for a dysphagic animal. Enteral feeding should be used until the disorder is repaired or treated.
> - Prior to assisted feeding, it is essential that the patient is adequately hydrated and that any electrolyte disturbances are corrected.
> - With *all* methods of assisted feeding, it is vital that bodyweight is monitored carefully.

Appropriate choice of feeding procedures is illustrated in Figure 9.43.

- **Enteral feeding** entails using the gastrointestinal tract to provide nutritional support to patients who are unable or unwilling to eat. It is the best choice if the gastrointestinal tract is functioning normally, as it keeps the gut working – if the gut works, use it. Techniques for enteral feeding are explained in detail in the later section on 'Medical nursing techniques'.
- **Parenteral feeding** is the administration of the essential nutritional needs of the patient via the intravenous route. It is used where the gastrointestinal tract is non-functional.

Appetite stimulation

In some cases an inappetent or anorexic patient may be persuaded to eat. Some of the methods shown in Figure 9.44 may be tried. An animal in pain may be unwilling to eat and pain relief may be indicated. Short-term medical appetite stimulants may also be prescribed by the veterinary surgeon.

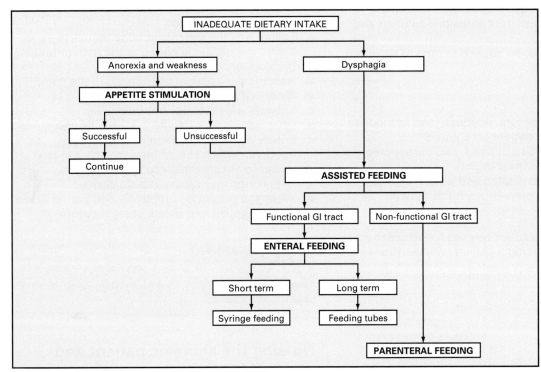

9.43 Appropriate choice of feeding procedures.

9.44 Methods of appetite stimulation.

Medical nursing techniques

Enteral feeding techniques

Syringe feeding

Syringe feeding (force feeding) can be tried with conscious patients who have the ability to swallow normally and who have a functioning gastrointestinal tract. Syringe feeding can be used on a short-term basis for cooperative patients, to stimulate the appetite and encourage the patient to start eating on its own. Soft tinned foods can be given into the mouth as a bolus (Figure 9.45), or liquidized food mixed with water can be given carefully with a syringe (Figure 9.46).

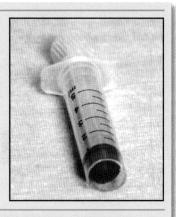

1. Place core boluses on the tongue via an adapted 5 or 10 ml syringe (right)
   or
   Food can be placed in the pharyngeal area to stimulate the swallowing reflex.
2. Allow the patient to swallow before further feeding.

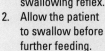 How to give a bolus feed.

1. Liquidize food and mix with water.
2. The filled syringe is always directed towards the roof of the patient's mouth and the food introduced slowly. This stimulates the swallowing reflex and reduces the chance of aspiration.
3. Place the syringe behind the canine tooth and administer slowly, with the patient's head in a normal/horizontal position
   or
   Hold the side pocket of the gum open and syringe liquidized food into it, push the gum against the teeth and allow the animal to swallow.

9.46 How to give a liquid syringe feed.

Tube feeding

Administration of nutrition into the gastrointestinal tract can be achieved using a number of methods of tube feeding (Figure 9.47):

- Naso-oesophageal – placed in the caudal oesophagus via the ventral meatus
- Pharyngostomy – placed in the caudal oesophagus via the pharynx
- Gastrostomy – placed straight into the stomach via laparotomy or percutaneous endoscope
- Jejunostomy – placed into the jejunum via laparotomy or endoscope.

Feeding tubes are measured in French gauge (FG or F), in which 1 FG unit is equal to 0.33 mm.

Care of feeding tubes

- Prior to feeding, flush tube with sterile saline to check for blockages.
- Keep any skin incisions clean and dry.
- Keep the tube capped to prevent entry of air and introduction of infection.
- Following feeding, flush the tube with sterile saline to prevent food drying in the tube, causing a blockage.
- Prevent patient interference.
- Flush the mouth regularly with water and dry afterwards.
- Monitor patient closely for signs of complications.

Complications of tube feeding

- **Occlusion of the tube**
- **Vomiting, diarrhoea**
- **Oedema, haemorrhage**
- **Aspiration of food**
- **Hypoglycaemia**
- **Peritonitis.**

If a feeding tube becomes occluded, flushing with a few millilitres of a carbonated drink may relieve the blockage.

Naso-osophageal tube

Equipment:

- Naso-oesophageal tube – made of polyurethane (PU), polyvinylchloride (PVC) or silicone. The widest possible tube should be selected.
  - 3.5–6 FG for cats
  - 5–10 FG for dogs
- Sedative if required (under veterinary direction)
- Local anaesthetic drops or spray
- Pen
- Water-soluble lubricant
- 5 ml syringe and 21 gauge needle
- Sterile water
- Elastoplast or zinc oxide tape
- Cyanoacrylate glue or suture material
- Scissors
- Elizabethan collar
- 20 ml syringe to administer feed.

Placement

This is outlined in Figure 9.48.

Care and maintenance of the tube

- Clean the patient's face, eyes and mouth.
- Ensure that the tube does not cause the animal any distress – apply lidocaine drops if necessary.
- The position of the tube must be checked regularly. It should be located in the oesophagus, just cranial to the cardiac sphincter, to prevent reflux and weakening of the sphincter muscle.

Indications	Contraindications	Complications	Advantages	Disadvantages
Naso-oesophageal tube				
Anorexia. Oral food intake reduced for more than 3 days. Loss of >5% bodyweight. Where a general anaesthetic is contraindicated. When long-term enteral feeding is required (7–10 days)	Non-functional gastrointestinal tract, oesophageal disease, persistent vomiting, unconsciousness	Occlusion of the tube. Regurgitation of the tube (particularly in cats). Patient interference. Ingestion of part of the tube. Diarrhoea (due to bacterial overgrowth or increased water intake, or feeding too quickly)	Easy to place. Can be used for up to a week. Animal still able to eat and drink with tube in place. Inexpensive	Small-gauge tube so only certain liquid feeds can be used
Orogastric (stomach tube)				
Usually a repeated method, not indwelling. When rapid feeding is required. For neonates during first few days of life. Anorexia in exotic species. Particularly useful in chelonians suffering from post-hibernation anorexia	Oral trauma, pharyngeal trauma	Aspiration pneumonia if tube is misplaced. Mouth must be kept open throughout feeding to prevent patient from chewing the tube	Useful in neonates and exotics. Relatively easy procedure. Can be placed whilst animal is conscious. Requires little or no maintenance	Not well tolerated by adults. Short-term use only – can be used for 2–3 days. Requires cooperative patient as the tube is passed
Pharyngostomy tube				
Facial, mandibular or maxillary disease, trauma or surgery. Long-term support required	Pharyngeal trauma, non-functional gastrointestinal tract, persistent vomiting, unconsciousness	Interference with epiglottal function. Oedema. Infection at site of skin puncture. Haemorrhage. Occlusion of the tube. Aspiration of food. Patient interference	Useful for short- to mid-term use. Easy to administer any liquidized food into the oesophagus	Requires general anaesthesia so unsuitable for weak/unstable animals. Can be easily dislodged. Stoma site can become infected. Limited to liquid diets. Most useful for short-term feeding (<14 days). May induce gagging. Can be associated with partial airway obstruction
Gastrostomy tube; percutaneous endoscopically placed gastrostomy (PEG) tube				
Upper gastrointestinal tract must be by-passed. Anorexic patients. Placed either surgically, by endoscopy, or percutaneously	Malabsorption in digestive tract, non-functional gastrointestinal tract, persistent vomiting	Hyperglycaemia. Occlusion of the tube. Infection at site of skin puncture. Patient interference. Peritonitis	Large-diameter tube. Easy to feed. Any liquidized food may be fed. Can be left *in situ* for months at a time; special low-profile tubes available for prolonged feeding. Patient tolerance excellent	Requires general anaesthesia. Specialized equipment required (endoscope). Should remain in place for minimum of 5–7 days to ensure adequate adhesions form between stomach and abdominal wall
Jejunostomy tube				
Upper gastrointestinal tract must be by-passed. Long-term support required	Non-functional lower GI tract, malabsorption	Infection. Digestive tract complications	Can be used long term. Useful if upper GI tract needs to be by-passed	Requires general anaesthesia. Predigested and very simple nutritional units must be delivered to avoid severe digestive tract complications. Prolonged hospitalization usually required. Expensive. High maintenance

9.47   Types of feeding tube.

1. Apply local anaesthetic drops to one of the external nares (medial aspect) and leave for a few minutes.
2. Pre-measure the tubing against the outside of the patient to the 9th–10th rib and mark it with the pen.
3. The patient is restrained in sternal recumbency.
4. The patient's head is restrained in a normal position as the tube approaches the pharynx. This helps to prevent tracheal intubation.
5. The end of the tube is lubricated and introduced into the anaesthetized naris, directed caudoventrally and medially.
6. As soon as the tip reaches the septum (after about 2 cm) the nares are pushed dorsally. This opens the ventral meatus of the nasal cavity and ensures passage of the tube into the pharynx.
7. The tube is then angled downwards and slightly inwards and advanced slowly into the caudal oesophagus up to the pre-measured line.

> ⚠️ **WARNING**
> **Check that the tube is correctly placed by introducing 3–5 ml of sterile water via the tube. If coughing occurs the tube is probably down the trachea rather than the oesophagus. Pull back tube and reposition. Incorrect placement is more likely if the patient is sedated, due to suppression of the cough reflex. Radiographs of the lateral chest and auscultation for borborygmi may be indicated to ensure correct placement. If the tube is passed into the stomach there is a risk of reflux oesophagitis and vomiting.**

8. When the tube is correctly placed, apply two sticking plaster butterflies to the external tubing.
9. Stick the tapes with superglue to the hair (or suture to the skin) along the bridge of the nose and over the frontal region of the head. With cats, the tube and tapes must not interfere with their whiskers, as this will reduce their tolerance of the tube.
10. Occlude the end of the tube with a bung or cap.
11. Apply a properly fitted Elizabethan collar.

9.48 Placement of a naso-oesophageal tube.

Removal of the tube

Once the animal has started to eat sufficient amounts of food voluntarily, the tube can be removed:

- Release the sutures or glue attachments
- Keep the tube sealed to prevent aspiration of any contents, with the cap in place or a finger over the end of the tube, and then gently pull it out.

Pharyngostomy tube

A pharyngostomy tube is surgically placed whilst the patient is under general anaesthesia. It is inserted through the lateral wall of the pharynx and into the oesophagus. Pharyngostomy tubes have a larger bore than naso-oesophageal tubes, which means that more concentrated food can be passed into the stomach. Pharyngostomy tubes are less popular in practice, due to the need for a general anaesthetic and interference with oropharyngeal function, particularly in cats.

Equipment:

- Pharyngostomy tube
  - 10–12 FG for cats and small dogs
  - 5–10 FG for larger dogs
- Scalpel handle and blade
- Blunt dissecting scissors
- Mouth gag
- Sutures
- Zinc oxide $1/4$ inch tape.

Placement of a pharyngostomy tube

1. The patient is given general anaesthesia.
2. Clip the left side of the neck, caudal to the mandible, and prepare it for surgery.
3. Measure the tube and mark it to the 9th–10th rib, so that it will sit in the caudal oesophagus.
4. The veterinary surgeon passes the tube through an incision made in the skin just behind the mandible, through the oropharynx.
5. With a mouth gag in place, the tube is manipulated to redirect it into the oesophagus.
6. It is then sutured into place using butterfly tapes.
7. The tube must be capped.

Care and maintenance of the tube

- Keep the incision site and surrounding area clean and dry.
- The position of the tube must be checked regularly. It should be located in the oesophagus, just cranial to the cardiac sphincter, to prevent reflux and weakening of the sphincter muscle.

Removal of the tube

- Release the sutures.
- Keep the tube sealed to prevent aspiration of any contents, and gently pull it out.
- The wound is left to heal by granulation.

Gastrostomy tube

Gastrostomy tubes are one of the preferred methods of assisted nutrition in animals that are unable or unwilling to eat. They are placed surgically, at laparotomy, or percutaneously and endoscopically (percutaneous endoscopic gastrostomy – PEG) (Figure 9.49). A general anaesthetic is required for either method of placement. These tubes are well tolerated by the patient. They must be left *in situ* for at least 5–7 days and can remain in place for months.

Equipment:

- Mouth gag
- Endoscope
- Endoscopic forceps or snare
- Depezzar mushroom-tipped catheters, 16–24 FG
- Dilator (e.g. pipette tip)
- Surgical kit
- Suture material
- 14 gauge intravenous catheter
- Bandage
- Elizabethan collar.

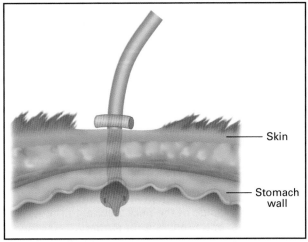

 Diagrammatic representation of a gastrostomy tube inside the animal.

Placement of a gastrostomy tube

1. Patient is given a general anaesthesia and prepared for surgery.
2. The endocope is passed into the stomach with the tip placed against the wall.
3. The veterinary surgeon makes a stab incision through the skin and passes an intravenous catheter into the stomach.
4. A suture is passed through the catheter and pulled back up the oesophagus and into the mouth.
5. A Depezzar catheter is passed down the oesophagus and into the stomach with the attached suture.
6. It is pulled through the stab incision, sutured to the skin and a bandage into place. A properly fitted Elizabethan collar is applied.

> **⚠ WARNING**
> - **Do not feed the patient on the day of PEG tube placement. A seal must be allowed to form in order to prevent the leakage of food.**
> - **The following day, check that the tube is in the correct position prior to feeding, by passing Gastrografin through the tube and taking a radiograph.**

Care and maintenance of the tube

- The stoma may discharge a little for the first few days and should be cleaned once or twice daily and a sterile dressing applied.
- Keep the incision and the skin around the catheter clean and dry.
- Regularly check the clip keeping the tube in place. If it loosens, the stomach contents could leak into the abdominal cavity leading to peritonitis.

Removal of the tube

- Gastrostomy tubes should be left in place for a minimum of 5–7 days to allow adhesions to form between the stomach and abdominal wall.

- Sometimes the tube may be pulled out through the incision intact.
- In some cases removal involves a general anaesthetic, cutting off the catheter at skin level, and endoscopy to remove the section left in the stomach.
- The wound is left to heal by granulation.
- Withhold food for 24 hours after removal.

Jejunostomy tube

A jejunostomy tube is a feeding tube that is surgically placed in the mid to distal duodenum or proximal jejunum, bypassing the stomach. Continuous feeding of easily digestible diets through the jejunostomy tube requires prolonged hospitalization. This procedure is rarely used, due to the cost of placement, associated high maintenance and possible complications.

Care and maintenance of the tube

- Keep the incision site and surrounding area clean and dry.
- Predigested and very simple nutritional units must be delivered, to avoid severe digestive tract complications.

Calculation of nutritional requirements for enteral tube feeding

Calculation of the volume of food to be administered over 24 hours for enteral feeding is based on the patient's calorific requirement divided by the calorific content of the food. This is taken as the number of kcal/ml or kcal/g in a selected commercial diet.

Resting Energy Requirement (RER) is the energy required over a 24-hour period by a sick patient in a comfortable stress-free environment such as a veterinary hospital ward. It replaces the term BER (Basal Energy Requirement) which is more suitably applied to the energy requirements of anaethetized patients. RER is calculated using the following equations:

- Bodyweight <5 kg (cats) or >40 kg (giant dogs): RER (kcal) = 60 x bodyweight (kg)
- Bodyweight 5–40 kg (most dogs): RER (kcal) = 30 x bodyweight (kg) + 70

'Illness factors' are factors by which RER may be increased in certain disease conditions. However, the use of illness factors may result in detrimental overfeeding of patients, leading to increased complications. The use of illness factors is therefore discouraged.

> **Example**
>
> *For a 10 kg hospitalized Border Terrier who has a severe infection:*
>
> **Bodyweight = 10 kg**
> **Resting energy**
> **requirement (RER)**   = (30 x bodyweight) + 70
> = (30 x 10) + 70
> = 300 + 70
> = 370 kcal
> ▶

Calories required	= 370 kcal/24 hours
Calorific content of selected food	= 2 kcal/ml
Food requirement	= calories required ÷ calorific content
	= 370 ÷ 2
	= 185 ml food/day

Once patients are more active and usually eating by themselves, their feeding requirements can be increased. Maintenance energy requirement (MER) is the amount of energy required by a moderately active animal in its daily search for and utilization of food.

- Dogs: MER = 2 x RER
- Cats: MER = 1.4 x RER.

Under certain conditions MER is increased, for example:

- Gestation: 1.1–1.3 x MER
- Working: 1.25–2.5 x MER
- Lactation: 2–4 x MER
- Cold or heat: 1.2–2 x MER
- Growth: 1.5–3 x MER
- Obese or geriatric: 0.6–0.8 x MER.

More information on feeding healthy pets can be found in Chapter 2.

Tube feeding regimes
Diet

- The prepared food must be fine enough to pass through the tube without occluding it. The food must include:
  - Water
  - Protein of high biological value (BV)
  - Energy as carbohydrate and fat (to satisfy BER calculations)
  - Vitamins and minerals.
- Depending on the patient's condition, veterinary enteral diets should be used, or veterinary diets suitable for the specific debility, liquidized and mixed with water.
- All daily nutritional requirements over 24 hours should be divided into four to six meals per day.
- Food should be introduced gradually and the amounts adjusted as follows:
  - Day 1 = about one-third of the nutritional need, diluted with water 1:3
  - Day 2 = about two-thirds of the nutritional need, diluted with water 3:1
  - Day 3 = full amount of nutritional need (the total food calculated for a 24-hour period).

Maximum quantities per bolus feed

When *commencing* bolus enteral feeding, a maximum of 20 ml feed/kg bodyweight should be given. This can be gradually increased over 2–3 days:
Dogs: 45 ml/kg
Cats: 1–1.4 kg bodyweight – 35 ml/kg;
1.5–4 kg – 30 ml/kg; 4.1–6 kg – 22 ml/kg

Feeding technique
The technique for feeding a patient with an enteral feeding tube in place is given in Figure 9.50.

1. Use large 20 ml or 50 ml sterile syringes for feeding.
2. Warm food to body temperature.
3. Position the patient either standing or sitting, or in sternal or right lateral recumbency.
4. The tube should be flushed with 5–10 ml of water before and after feeding each time, to avoid blockages.
5. Over the first few days start with frequent small amounts of food. Gradually increase amount and decrease frequency.
6. Feed in boluses slowly over about 15 minutes to allow for comfort and gastric dilation and to reduce the chance of vomiting or aspiration pneumonia.
7. Continuous feeding is thought to be more beneficial (particularly in the acute patient) and this can be done using continuous infusion systems that control the rate of feeding.

For any enteral feeding, the following information should be recorded:

- Baseline parameters before and during feeding
- The time of the feed and the volume of food given
- Any regurgitation or vomiting
- Any other observations, deviations or abnormalities.

9.50 How to feed a patient with an enteral feeding tube in place.

Parenteral feeding
Total parenteral nutrition (TPN) is the delivery of nutrition via the intravenous route and is applicable to those animals that are temporarily unable to assimilate adequate nutrients from the gastrointestinal tract. It is relatively uncommon in veterinary medicine outside of referral practices, because:

- It uses the jugular vein
- It is expensive
- It needs constant monitoring
- Severe metabolic effects can occur.

This subject is covered in more detail in the *BSAVA Manual of Advanced Veterinary Nursing*.

Enemas
An enema is a fluid preparation that is passed through the anus into the rectum and colon to stimulate evacuation of faecal matter, or to introduce fluid preparations for diagnostic or therapeutic purposes.

Indications

- Constipation or impaction due to:
  - Nature of faecal matter (e.g. furballs, bones)
  - Obstruction of faecal passage (e.g. enlarged prostate, neoplasia, anal diverticulum)
  - Inability to pass faeces (e.g. recumbency, pelvic nerve damage, gastrointestinal problems – megacolon).

- Diagnostic or surgical procedures to:
  - Empty colon prior to endoscopy or radiography
  - Introduce contrast media for radiographic examination of the colon (e.g. barium enema)
  - Empty colon prior to surgery of the pelvis, colon or anal regions.
- Therapeutic purposes to:
  - Administer drugs.

Basic equipment and solutions

Basic equipment includes:

- Gloves
- Protective clothing
- Lubricant
- Enema administration equipment or micro-enema (see below)
- Enema preparation (Figure 9.51), warmed
- Litter tray for cats, or outside run for dogs.

Equipment

There is a choice of equipment for administration of an enema (Figure 9.52). The most commonly used items in practice are the proprietary micro-enema and the enema pump (Higginson's syringe, Figure 9.53).

Solution	Quantity	General points
Warm water	*Cats*: 5–10 ml/kg *Dogs, small–medium*: 20–30 ml/kg *Dogs, large*: 30–40 ml/kg Repeat every 20–30 minutes if necessary	Cheap, easy to use and non-irritant
Soap and water Obstetrical lubricant and water Glycerine and water Olive oil and water	5–10 ml/kg	Strong soap solutions and hot water enemas irritate the mucosa and should not be used
Liquid paraffin	5–10 ml/kg every 1–2 hours	Cheap and effective but very messy
Proprietary agent (e.g. Microlax; see Figure 9.53)	As directed by manufacturers	Easy to administer
Phosphate enema (see Figure 9.53)	As directed by manufacturers	May cause hypocalcaemia therefore not recommended for use in cats and small dogs
Contrast medium (e.g. barium sulphate)	5–15 ml/kg	Used for radiographic contrast studies. Barium should not be used if suspected bowel rupture or perforation – use water-soluble iodine-containing contrast medium (e.g. Gastrografin) instead
Saline	1–2 ml/kg Do not repeat for up to 12 hours	Use with care in cats and small dogs

9.51 Solutions used for enemas.

Equipment	Description and method
Micro-enemas (e.g. Microlax; see Figure 9.53)	Comes in tube with long nozzle for direct insertion into rectum
Enema pump (Higginson's syringe; see Figure 9.53)	Open-ended tube of the enema pump is inserted into chosen enema preparation. Bulb is squeezed gently to draw fluid through pump. Repeat until enema preparation starts to come through rectal insertion nozzle. Once nozzle is lubricated it is ready for use
Hose and funnel	Hose is filled with enema preparation. Funnel is attached to outer end of hose. Enema solution is poured in, allowing gravity to fill rectum
Hose and 50 ml syringe	Syringe and hose are filled with enema preparation. Hose end is lubricated and inserted into rectum. Syringe is gently depressed, pushing enema into rectum
Foley catheter	Used for barium enemas, with attached enema bag. After insertion of catheter into rectum the bag is squeezed, forcing barium into rectum, or suspended above animal, allowing barium to flow by gravity. Barium is then allowed to run back into bag
Cuffed rectal catheter	Device for humans but can be used to give barium enema with barium bag attached

9.52 Enema administration equipment.

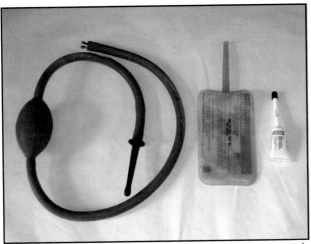

9.53 Higginson's syringe, phosphate enema and Microlax.

Technique

The method for administering an enema is described in Figure 9.54.

Ensure that the procedure is as stress-free and comfortable as possible. Always provide the patient with reassurance and encouragement.

1. Gather all equipment together before starting the procedure.
2. Warm enema preparation to body temperature.
3. Fill enema administration equipment with enema preparation.
4. Lubricate nozzle prior to insertion into the rectum.
5. Ensure adequate restraint. Hindquarters may need to be slightly raised.
6. Lift tail.
7. Insert tip of nozzle gently.
8. Administer enema slowly and gently – *stop if there is resistance, never force an enema preparation.*
9. Allow patient free exercise and observe for evacuation of bowels.
10. After the procedure, clean and dry perineal region (oil-based enemas are particularly messy) and record the result of the enema on the hospital sheet or patient record.

9.54 Administration of an enema.

Urinary catheterization

A urinary catheter is a narrow tube inserted via the urethra into the bladder to obtain a sample, maintain drainage or measure urinary output. Urinary catheterization may be indicated for a number of reasons:

- Diagnostic:
  - Biochemical analysis, when a sample cannot be obtained by free flow
  - Bacteriology, where a sterile urine sample is required
  - Introduction of radiographic contrast media
- Medical:
  - Maintenance of bladder drainage in neurological disorders
  - Measurement of urinary output
  - Relief of urinary incontinence, to prevent soiling
  - Introduction of drugs
- Obstruction:
  - Patient comfort – to drain the bladder or when there is partial obstruction
  - To check for urethral patency
  - Urethral obstruction – hydro-propulsion may be used
- Surgical:
  - Preoperative bladder drainage
  - Postoperative bladder drainage to prevent pressure on the bladder wound

Contraindications:

- Vaginitis
- Open pyometra
- Complete obstruction of urethra or bladder neck.

Equipment

The equipment required (Figure 9.55) varies depending on the species, size and sex of the patient. Typical uses and special features of catheters for dogs and cats are listed and illustrated in Figures 9.56 to 9.59.

General, non-sterile
Appropriate restraint (sedation if required)
Clippers
Antiseptic solution – to clean vulva or prepuce
Water-based lubricating jelly, or local anaesthetic gel
Kidney dish
General, sterile
Gloves
Catheter
Universal container
10 ml or 20 ml syringe
Three-way tap
Positive contrast agent, as required
Foley catheter (additional requirements)
Stylet and spigot (see Figure 9.67)
Lubricant, must be water-based
Sterile water, syringe and needle (for balloon inflation)
Elizabethan collar
Speculum for bitch catheterization, as required (see Figure 9.60)
Jackson cat catheter (additional requirements)
Suture material
Elizabethan collar

9.55 Equipment required for urinary catheterization.

	Plain plastic (dog)	Foley	Metal (bitch)	Tieman (bitch)
Sizes	6, 8, and 10 FG	8–30 FG	6, 8, 10, and 12 FG	8, 10, and 12 FG
Length	50–70 cm	30–40 cm	20–25 cm	43 cm
Material	Flexible nylon	Soft latex rubber with polystyrene core	Silver-plated brass	Polyvinyl chloride (PVC)
Features	Straight, some rigidity, two lateral eyelet drainage holes	Balloon inflated with sterile water lies behind eyelets at tip of catheter	Straight metal, curved tip	Curved tip
Luer connector	*Yes*	*No* Spigot adapter required to create luer mount, for attaching syringe or sterile drip administration set. Medical urine collection bags have adapter attached	Some do	*Yes*
Use	*Dog* and *bitch*	*Bitch*	*Bitch*	*Bitch*
Re-use	Disposable	Disposable – the balloon may be weakened after use and catheters must only be used once	Sterilize using an autoclave	Disposable
Advantages	Transparent, ease of use	Indwelling	Can be autoclaved and reused	Transparent
Disadvantages	May be too long for use in bitches	*Very* flexible. Stylet required. Place stylet in eyelet hole at the tip of the catheter and lie it *alongside* the catheter to facilitate placement. Petroleum-based lubricant will damage this catheter	General anaesthesia required for safe introduction. Risk of urethral trauma	Over-flexible, can be difficult to introduce
Indwelling	*Adaptations for the male dog*: attach zinc oxide butterflies to external catheter for suturing to prepuce	*Yes*. Held in position by balloon inflated with correct amount of sterile water (written on side arm of catheter). When the catheter is correctly placed the balloon lies at *neck of the bladder* and is then inflated. The water is introduced via a side arm, with one-way valve, which runs up side of the catheter from the balloon to catheter end. Resistance to inflation indicates that catheter is not properly placed	*No*	*No*
Notes	If indwelling: flush catheter every 4 h with sterile water to ensure patency	*Deflate* balloon *before* removing catheter *Flush* catheter every 4 h with sterile water to ensure patency. Urine will not flow down the catheter until *stylet is removed* after placement	Rarely used	

9.56 Dog and bitch catheters and their use in veterinary practice. See also Figures 9.57 and 9.58.

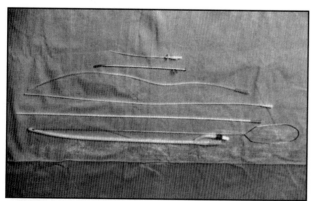

9.57 Types of urinary catheter. From top to bottom: Jackson cat catheter; metal bitch catheter; Tieman bitch catheter; Portex dog catheter 6 FG; Portex bitch catheter 8 FG; Foley catheter with stylet in place.

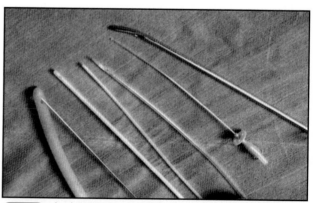

9.58 A closer view of the tips of the urinary catheters. From left to right: Foley catheter with stylet in place; two plain plastic dog catheters; Tieman bitch catheter (with curved tip); Jackson cat catheter; metal bitch catheter.

	Plain plastic	**Jackson (cat)**	**Silicone cat**	**Slippery Sam**
Sizes (FG)	3 and 4	3 and 4	3.5	3–3.5
Length (cm)	30	11	12	14 and 11
Material	Flexible nylon	Flexible nylon	Medical-grade silicone	PTFE (Teflon)
Features	Straight, some rigidity, two lateral eyelet drainage holes	Metal stylet in lumen of catheter to aid placement (removed once catheter is correctly placed)	Very similar in design to standard Jackson cat catheter	Very similar in appearance to conventional cat catheter
Luer connector	Yes	Yes	Yes	Yes
Use	Tom and queen	Tom and queen	Tom	Tom
Indwelling	No	Yes in tomcats (circular nylon flange at proximal end enables catheter to be sutured to prepuce)	Yes	Yes
Advantages	Transparent Easy to use	Indwelling	All lubricants compatible Suitable for long-term use Smooth catheter sheath ensuring ease of placement	Indwelling Wire guide supplied to aid introduction Proximal fitting enables syringe attachment
Disadvantages	More flexible			
Reuse	Disposable	Disposable	Disposable	Disposable

9.59 Cat catheters and their use in veterinary practice. See also Figures 9.57 and 9.58.

Size of catheter

The catheter must be:

- Of sufficient length to reach the bladder (to ensure good drainage)
- Wide enough so that urine will not flow down the outside of the catheter.

> **The external diameter of a catheter is measured using French gauge (F, or FG).**
> *1 unit FG = 0.33 mm*
> **For example, a 6 FG catheter has an external diameter of 2 mm.**

Storage and reuse of catheters

Catheters should be stored flat in sterile packaging, in a cool dry place. No heavy weights should be placed on top. Plastic catheters are disposable but some may need to be re-sterilized. Damaged catheters must be disposed of immediately.

If the catheter is to be reused:

1. Check for damage (e.g. kinks).
2. Flush forcefully with cold water.
3. Wash in warm detergent solution.
4. Rinse.
5. Dry, pack, label and autoclave (or sterilize using ethylene oxide).

Specula

A speculum (Figure 9.60) may be used during catheterization of the bitch, to aid in viewing the urethral orifice. Specula that can be used include:

- Auriscope with light source within the auriscope handle
- Catheterization speculum (an adapted auriscope with one edge removed)
- Sim's vaginal speculum
- Human rectal speculum
- Human nasal speculum (two flat blades that separate when the handles are pushed together)
- Home-made speculum from a syringe case.

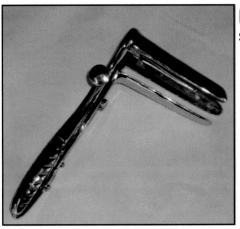

9.60 Speculum.

A light source is useful (a pen torch may be used if no light source can be attached).

Specula must always be cleaned and sterilized after use. All except the adapted syringe case can be autoclaved.

1. Rinse first with cold water, flushing out any debris.
2. Wash with mild detergent.
3. Rinse, dry, pack, label and autoclave.

Catheterization technique

General principles for urinary catheterization are listed in Figure 9.61. Methods for cats (tom and queen) and for male dogs are given in Figures 9.62 and 9.63. Sedation under veterinary direction may be required for some patients, particularly cats.

- Adequate restraint is essential, to minimize contamination and reduce urethral trauma.
- A good aseptic technique with sterile equipment is essential when catheterizing a patient, to protect staff from zoonoses and the patient from infection.
- Ensure sterility – if pre-packed, check that equipment is sterile, that the packaging has not been damaged or opened and that it is not past its use-by date.
- Check catheters for any damage and check that they are fully patent.
- Ensure that the correct catheter type and size are used.

---

1. Gather all equipment together before starting the procedure.
2. Clip hair and clean skin around vagina or prepuce with antiseptic solution.
3. Before removing catheter from packaging, measure against the patient the length needed to reach the bladder.
4. Wash/scrub hands and put on gloves.
5. Assistant opens outer packaging of catheter.
6. Operator removes catheter in inner sterile packaging.
7. Operator must snip the end off the inner packaging and push out the tip of the sterile catheter.
8. Assistant lubricates the end.
9. Operator pushes back the inner packaging as the catheter is advanced into the urethra, maintaining sterility.
10. *Never force a catheter.* If there is any resistance, *stop*.
11. When urine starts to flow down the catheter, stop.
12. Depending on the reason for catheterization, attach either syringe or three-way tap, suture in place, inflate balloon, or collect urine sample.

9.61   General principles for urinary catheterization.

Tomcat

1. General anaesthesia or heavy sedation.
2. Position in right lateral recumbency, tail deflected.
3. Extrude penis by applying gentle finger pressure on either side of prepuce.
4. Advance catheter tip with slight rotation, along urethra, parallel to vertebral column.
5. Advance catheter into bladder.
6. Suture in position if appropriate.

Queen

1. General anaesthesia or heavy sedation.
2. Position in lateral recumbency.
3. Lubricate catheter.
4. Pass blind along vaginal floor and guide ventrally into urethral orifice.
5. Advance catheter into bladder.

9.62   How to catheterize tomcats and queens.

---

1. Restrain patient in lateral recumbency or standing.
2. Wash hands and put on gloves.
3. Extrude penis by retracting prepuce.
4. Prepare catheter; cut top off plastic wrapper.
5. Lubricate end of catheter.
6. Insert catheter gently but firmly into extruded penis by feeding from remaining plastic wrapper.
7. Advance into bladder – stop if there is any resistance.
8. Stop when urine is seen.

Resistance may be found at any of the common sites of urethral obstruction: neck of bladder, prostate, ischial arch, and caudal to os penis.

9.63   How to catheterize a male dog.

Catheterization of the bitch

Catheterizing a bitch can be done either by using the fingers to locate the urethral orifice (Figure 9.64) or by locating and viewing it using a speculum and light source (Figure 9.65). The digital method can be straightforward in larger bitches, but a vaginal 'scope may be necessary for those that are too small. Whatever method is used, care should be taken to reduce trauma by gently lubricating equipment and handling the patient gently.

---

1. Position patient either standing or in lateral recumbency, with tail held securely deflected.
2. Scrub hands and put on sterile gloves.
3. Lubricate gloved left index finger and insert between lips of vulva into the vestibule in a dorsal then cranial direction.
4. Locate urethral orifice as raised pimple on ventral floor.
5. Move finger just cranial to urethral orifice.
6. Use right hand to guide catheter under left finger along its length and into urethral orifice.
7. Advance catheter into bladder.
8. If inserting a Foley catheter, inflate the balloon (maximum quantity of water that should be used is printed in ml on arm of catheter).
9. Resistance will be felt if catheter is not in bladder.
10. Remove stylet and urine will be seen.

9.64   How to catheterize a bitch, using the digital method (described for a right-handed person).

---

1. Lubricate the speculum.
2. Insert the speculum in a dorsal then cranial direction.
3. Visualize the urethral orifice on the ventral floor of the vestibule.
4. Advance the catheter through the speculum into the urethral orifice.
5. If the patient is in dorsal recumbency, draw the hindlimbs caudally.
6. Advance the catheter into the bladder.
7. If inserting a Foley catheter, inflate the balloon (maximum quantity of water that should be used is printed in ml on arm of catheter).
8. Resistance will be felt if catheter is not in bladder.
9. Remove stylet and urine will be seen.

9.65   How to catheterize a bitch using a speculum. This technique can be carried out with the patient in a standing position with the tail securely deflected, or in dorsal recumbency with the hindlimbs initially drawn cranially.

Complications of urinary catheterization

Complications that may occur following urinary catheterization include:

- Cystitis
- Infection
- Bladder/urethral trauma
- Patient resistance
- Blockage of indwelling catheters.

If blood is seen at catheterization, when multiple catheterization is used, or when an indwelling catheter is placed, prophylactic antibiotics may be prescribed by the veterinary surgeon. After catheterization, urine production should be observed for colour, odour, clarity and haematuria, and any straining or frequent urination with little urine produced. Observations should be recorded and reported to the veterinary surgeon.

Catheter management and measuring urine output

Urine output can be monitored by placement of an indwelling catheter and collecting and measuring urine produced by the patient.

- A urine collection bag can be attached to the catheter (Figure 9.66).
- The catheter can be sealed with a bung or spigot (Figure 9.67) and the bladder emptied at regular intervals.
- A collection bag should be of adequate size for the potential urine output of the patient, and the contents of the bag should be measured and emptied at regular intervals.

Urine collection bags	Catheter attachment
Medical urine collection bag (intended for human use)	Foley catheter – these collection bags have an incorporated spigot, which fits directly on to the Foley catheter
Sterile administration set and empty drip bag	Can be attached to any catheter with a luer connector. A Foley catheter must have a spigot adapter (either plastic or metal) for connection

9.66 Urine collection bags.

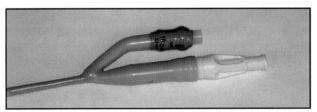

9.67 Spigot attached to a Foley catheter.

Normal urine output is calculated at 1–2 ml/kg bodyweight/hour.
A urine output of <1 ml/kg/hour should be reported immediately to the veterinary surgeon.

- Patients who have sealed indwelling catheters must have the bladder emptied at regular intervals.
- Record details of urine collected and time of emptying bag or bladder.
- Indwelling catheters can remain *in situ* for up to 10 days unless problems arise.

Physiotherapy

Physiotherapy is the use of physical or mechanical agents to treat pain and movement dysfunction as they relate to the muscles, joints and nerves of the body. Physiotherapy can be used as preventive therapy, to reduce losses, and as a treatment to promote recovery and build up physical strength and mobility. It must be carried out under the direction of a veterinary surgeon. Qualified medical and veterinary physiotherapists are available to provide extra guidance to veterinary nurses. Physiotherapy may be carried out at floor or table level. Table level is often more comfortable for the operator but extra restraint of the patient is needed. The different forms of physiotherapy are outlined in Figure 9.68.

Passive exercise	
Massage	Range of motion exercise Stroking Effleurage Petrissage Friction Percussion/coupage
Active exercise	
Active assisted exercise	Use slings/towel
Active exercise	Light support initially but eventually progressing without support
Active restricted exercise	Hydrotherapy
Electrotherapy	
Electrotherapy	Ultrasound Laser Muscle stimulation Transcutaneous electrical nerve stimulation (TENS)
Other	
Contrast bathing	Application of heat and cold together
Application of heat	Superficial hyperthermia
Application of cold	Local hypothermia

9.68 Forms of physiotherapy.

WARNING
- **The patient must be in a comfortable position and handled in a quiet and reassuring manner.**
- **All physiotherapy sessions should be started slowly and built up as the patient improves.**

Respiratory physiotherapy

Respiratory therapy is particularly useful in the treatment of the recumbent patient and of patients with pulmonary disease. Lung disease or decreased exercise can result in a reduction of lung volume and reduced ability to clear pulmonary secretions. The aims, physiological effects and benefits of respiratory physiotherapy are listed in Figure 9.69.

Aims	Physiological effects	Results
↓ Respiratory effort ↑ Lung volume, therefore ↑ oxygen uptake and gaseous exchange ↑ Secretion clearance To make the animal more comfortable	↑ Lung volume ↑ Oxygen uptake and gaseous exchange ↑ Secretion clearance	↑ Oxygen supply to the alveoli ↓ Pooling of secretions Animal comfort

 Aims, physiological effects and benefits of respiratory physiotherapy.

> **WARNINGS**
> - **Patients must be well hydrated before treatment.**
> - **Respiration and mucous membrane colour must be monitored throughout.**

Positional physiotherapy

The position of the patient can help to increase lung volume, improve ability to clear secretions, and prevent or treat hypostatic pneumonia. Different positions allow different lung volumes to be attained:

- Standing – maximum expansion of the ribs, diaphragm and lungs
- Sternal recumbency or sitting – reasonable expansion of the lungs
- Lateral recumbency – least expansion of the lungs.

If only one lung is affected by the disease the affected lung should be uppermost, allowing the lower lung greater expansion. If both lungs are affected the animal should be repositioned on a regular basis.

How to use positional physiotherapy

1. Encourage the patient to stand at regular intervals.
2. Support the patient in sternal recumbency with sandbags, cushions or rolled-up towels.
3. Maintain each position for 10–15 minutes, three or four times daily.
4. Between treatment sessions, turn laterally recumbent patient on a regular basis every 2–4 hours throughout the day and night.

Postural drainage

Postural drainage uses gravity to assist with clearance of secretions. The area of the lungs to be treated is positioned uppermost, and the patient's head should be slightly lower than its body. Secretions drain into the main bronchial airways and are then coughed up by the patient.

Each position should be maintained for 10–15 minutes three or four times per day, but treatment must be discussed in detail with the veterinary surgeon.

Contraindications:

- Recent trauma or surgery to the head, neck, thorax or spine
- Pregnancy
- Obesity
- Breathlessness
- Neoplasia
- Sepsis.

Manual techniques

These should be performed in postural drainage positions. Treatment sessions should last 5–10 minutes and be carried out four or five times a day.

Percussion or coupage

Slow rhythmic clapping with cupped hands and loose wrists on the chest wall (Figure 9.70). This creates an energy wave that is transmitted to the airways, which loosens secretions and allows them to be coughed up.

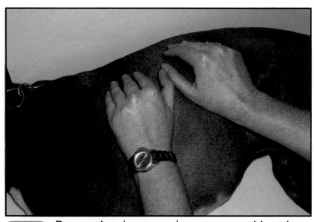

9.70 Percussion (coupage) uses cupped hands and loose wrists.

Vibrations

Fine oscillations of the hands on the chest wall directed inwards. These must be performed on expiration.

Gentle shaking

Coarse oscillations performed as above.

Contraindications:

- Thoracic surgery
- Trauma
- Osteoporosis.

Orthopaedic and neurological physiotherapy

Patients with orthopaedic and neurological disease or injuries may have physiotherapy consisting of physical agents (e.g. cold, heat) and/or mechanical agents (e.g. massage, exercise). The aim is to increase the blood supply to, and lymphatic drainage from, the affected area and to increase muscle strength and coordination.

Local hypothermia

Local hypothermia is the application of cold compresses to the affected area. It is used in acute phase injury, to help to minimize bruising and oedema, and to reduce pain in the first 48 hours following trauma.

Local hypothermia: 5–10 minutes every 4–6 hours

Physiological effects	Results
↓ Tissue temperature, vasoconstriction, ↓ nerve conduction, relaxation of skeletal muscle	Analgesia, ↓ oedema, ↓ bruising

Contraindications:

- Diabetes mellitus
- Peripheral vascular disease
- Ischaemic injury.

Superficial hyperthermia

This is the application of warm compresses to the affected body area. It is used to reduce evident swelling and bruising, and for alleviation of pain, 48–72 hours following trauma.

Superficial hyperthermia: 10–20 minutes, 4–6 times a day

Physiological effects	Results
↑ Tissue temperature, vasodilation, ↑ local circulation, ↑ metabolic rate	Relief of muscle tension, analgesia, ↓ oedema

Contraindication:

- Bleeding disorders.

Massage

Massage is used on the limbs to increase arterial, venous and lymphatic flow, facilitating nutrient delivery and waste removal from the tissues. Effleurage is used first, to relax the patient, followed by petrissage and friction techniques. When performing massage techniques, the hands should mould to the body contours.

Massage: 10–20 minutes, 2–3 times per day

Physiological effects	Results
Assisted venous return to the heart, ↑ lymphatic flow, ↑ muscular motion, ↑ tissue perfusion, maintained and improved peripheral circulation	↓ Oedema, ↓ muscle tension and spasm, temporary analgesia, ↑ muscle tone, ↑ movement through stretching of adhesions, ↓ heart rate

Contraindications:

- Infection
- Pyrexia
- Malignancy
- Fracture or sprain
- Some types of joint disease
- Haemarthrosis
- Acute inflammation.

Effleurage

The palms of the hands are passed continuously and rhythmically over the patient's skin, with long stroking movements in one direction only (Figure 9.71). One hand supports the limb and the other massages; the hands are alternated with each stroke.

Effleurage will stimulate the skin, disperse oedema and promote venous return.

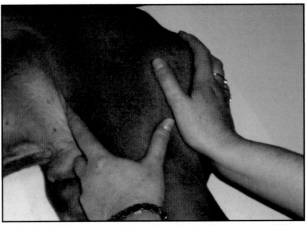

9.71 Effleurage of the hindlimb. The palm of the massaging hand is held flat, with a firm gliding movement pushing up from the distal to the proximal limb.

Petrissage

This is for muscular areas. Using both hands, the skin is lifted up and pressed down, the muscle is grasped and squeezed, rolled and released, moving the hands steadily over the area (Figure 9.72).

Petrissage will increase blood supply to the muscles, reduce muscle spasms and prevent or break down adhesions.

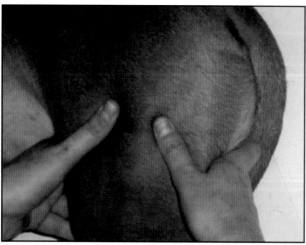

9.72 Petrissage of the hindlimb in a recumbent patient.

Friction

A series of small circular movements are made with the pads of the thumbs, one or more fingers or the heel of the hand, depending on the part of the body under therapy.

Passive exercise/movement

Passive exercise is where there is no active muscle action from the patient. The operator manually moves limbs and individual joints through as full a range as possible. Passive exercise must be performed with care, as manipulation may initially be painful. The therapy is used for its physiological effects in recumbent patients, and where movement at a joint has been compromised through injury or treatment – for example, where a limb has been immobilized after fracture and becomes weak and stiff through lack of use.

Passive exercise: 10–20 minutes, 2–3 times a day following massage

Physiological effects	Results
Stretched adhesions, maintained or improved blood and lymphatic flow, stimulated sensory nerves	Prevention or ↑ range of movement, prevention or improvement of contractures, improved microcirculation to muscles and joints, improvement of stiffness

The techniques are described and illustrated in Figure 9.73 and 9.74.

Contraindications:

- Fractures involving the joint
- Some types of joint disease
- Haemarthrosis (<5 days post-incident).

1. The patient should be comfortable, supported in lateral recumbency with the affected limb uppermost. Sandbags can be used to give additional support.
2. Use one hand to stabilize the limb above or below the joint during manipulation.
3. Use the other hand for manipulation of the joint.
4. Manipulate the distal joints of the limb first, i.e. put each toe through its full range of movement.
5. Then, working up the limb, put each joint through its full range of movement as far as the hip or shoulder.
6. Move the whole limb passively in a normal ambulatory fashion.
7. When the movement at a joint is restricted, gentle overpressure can be used at the end of the range of movement.
8. As treatment progresses, range of movement at the restricted joint improves slowly.

9.73 How to use passive exercise on the limbs. The aim is to move each joint individually through its full range. In recumbent patients the uppermost limbs are manipulated first. The patient can then be turned and the process repeated on other limbs.

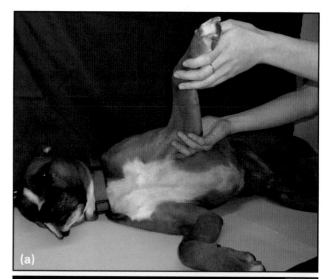

(a)

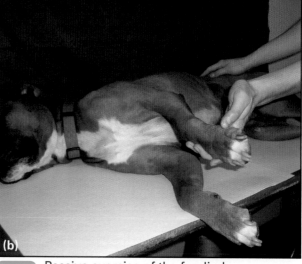

(b)

9.74 Passive exercise of the forelimb. **(a)** Abduction. **(b)** Adduction. (continues) ▶

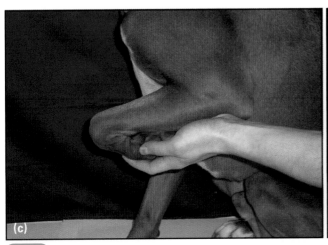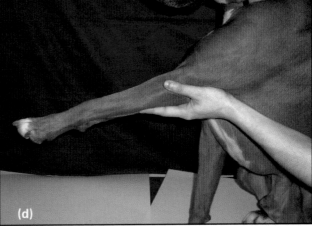

9.74 (continued) Passive exercise of the forelimb. **(c)** Flexion. **(d)** Extension.

Active movement

> **Active movement:** treatment sessions last from a few seconds, proceeding up to 10 minutes as the patient gains strength
>
> | Physiological effects | Results |
> | --- | --- |
> | ↑ Blood supply and lymphatic drainage, ↑ muscular tone | Gradual build-up of muscular tone and strength, improved balance and coordination, patient comfort and stimulation |

The different stages and exercise techniques used are shown in Figure 9.75. Each stage is started slowly, and must be achieved by the patient before going on to the next stage. The patient builds up strength and coordination. Although enhanced by using these methods, recovery can still be a slow process. It should not be rushed: the patient should be allowed to regain confidence with its increasing ability. It should be noted that as 'exercise' therapy is undertaken, the patient will have increased energy requirements and the diet may need to be adjusted accordingly.

Contraindications:

- Recent trauma
- Infection
- Pyrexia
- Malignancy
- Fracture sites
- Haemarthrosis
- Acute inflammation.

Hydrotherapy

The patient is exercised in water, which supports the animal while allowing it to move freely without bearing weight. As hydrotherapy treatment progresses and the patient has achieved active exercise in the water,

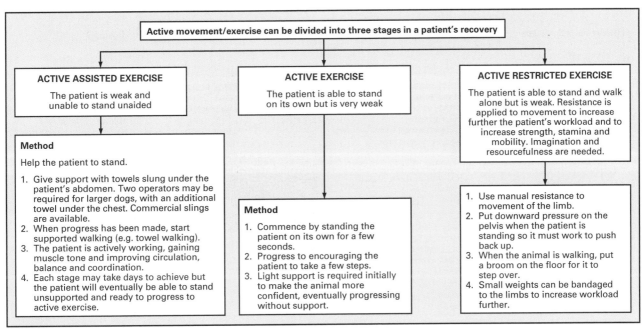

9.75 Stages of active exercise and movement.

it can be moved into resisted exercise: a whirlpool bath or water treadmill is used to offer resistance to movement, thus making the patient work harder. This is best performed in specially built professional units by suitably qualified and experienced staff.

Equipment for hydrotherapy includes:

- Sink, tub table or purpose-built pool filled with water (temperature 37–40°C)
- Waterproof clothing
- Towels and hairdryer
- Warm, draught-free kennel.

Guidelines for hydrotherapy

1. **Prepare a warm dry kennel for after therapy.**
2. **Gather equipment.**
3. **Check that water temperature is between 37 and 40°C.**
4. **Place the patient in the water, giving initial support.**
5. **Do not leave the patient.**
6. **Remove the patient at the end of the session, or immediately if fatigued.**
7. **To reduce the risk of hypothermia, dry the patient thoroughly before placing in prepared kennel.**

Contraindications:

- Cardiopulmonary disease
- Epilepsy
- Some skin conditions.

WARNING
Constant monitoring and support must be given while a patient is undergoing hydrotherapy.

Medical nursing of exotic pets

Exotic pets are now commonplace in veterinary practice, as owners increasingly seek veterinary attention for them. Knowledge of the common ailments of each species is essential for providing appropriate nursing care and for recognizing the individual needs of hospitalized patients. One of the most important considerations is that rabbits and rodents are prey animals and so must be housed away from potential predators such as dogs, cats and ferrets.

As with cats and dogs, exotics can be nursed back to health by providing nourishment, comfort and TLC. Although the principles of medical nursing are universal to all animals, certain procedures require adaptation due to species variation. Most exotic species have an innate fear of humans and any form of human contact is likely to induce a degree of distress. This must be taken into consideration when providing nursing care.

In order to nurse successfully the various species of mammal, reptile and bird that may be presented to veterinary practices, a sound knowledge of the anatomy and physiology of these species is required (see *BSAVA Textbook of Veterinary Nursing*, *BSAVA Manual of Exotic Pets* and the exotic species-specific Manuals).

Patient examination

Examination of the exotic patient should be performed using a systematic approach, as for a cat or dog. However, it will not always be appropriate or possible to take accurate TPR readings. These animals should be observed unobtrusively, avoiding unnecessary physical contact.

Common diseases

Common diseases of rabbits, other small mammals, birds and reptiles are shown in Figures 9.76 to 9.79.

Aetiology and pathogenesis	Clinical signs	Prevention (see also Chapter 3)	Nursing care	Treatment
Myxomatosis				
Caused by myxoma/poxvirus). Transmitted by insect vectors (mosquitoes, fleas, lice). Incubation period 5–14 days, but variable	Lethargy; pyrexia; depression; red and swollen eyes; oedematous lips, genitalia and anus. Progresses rapidly to death. In less virulent form, skin tumours develop in large numbers	Live vaccine given s.c and intradermally at ear base. Control insect vectors. Prevent contact with wild rabbits	Intensive nursing care. Maintain high environmental temperature (21–22°C). Regular cleaning of eyes and nares. Nutritional support. Provide and maintain therapy as prescribed. Care of intravenous fluid line	Supportive only; rarely successful. Fluid therapy, antibiotics to prevent secondary infection, and good nursing care may be successful in mild cases. Euthanasia is often the only humane course of action.
Viral haemorrhagic disease (VHD)				
Caused by a calicivirus. Incubation period 1–3 days. Highly contagious; spread directly and indirectly by insects and birds. Infection occurs by nasal, conjunctival and oral routes. Causes villous atrophy, especially ileum	Rapid course of disease. Pyrexia; depression; lethargy; anorexia. Some may show signs of tachypnoea, cyanosis, diarrhoea, convulsions, epistaxis. Death may occur. Many cases develop so rapidly that rabbit is found dead without having shown any apparent signs	Killed adjuvanted vaccine given at 10–12 weeks old; annual boosters recommended. Young rabbits should be bought from vaccinated stock only	Intensive nursing care. Relieve symptoms	None

9.76 Common diseases of rabbits. (continues)   ▶

Aetiology and pathogenesis	Clinical signs	Prevention (see also Chapter 3)	Nursing care	Treatment
Pasteurellosis				
Caused by bacterium *Pasteurella multocida*. Transmission by aerosol, direct contact or fomites. Main route of entry nasal exposure or via wounds. Many rabbits are carriers. Target tissues nasal cavity and tympanic bullae. Development of clinical disease triggered by stressors (malnutrition, overcrowding, transportation, corticosteroids). Rabbits with myxomatosis often develop secondary pasteurellosis	Nasal discharge; sneezing; conjunctivitis; dacrocystitis; bronchopneumonia; head tilt; abscesses; mastitis; genital infections; depression; anorexia; pyrexia; death	Currently no vaccine available. Isolate rabbits testing positive for infection. Antibiotics during periparturient period to prevent transmission from infected does to kits. Early weaning of kits at 4–5 weeks. Husbandry: good ventilation; good sanitation; and minimizing stress	Oxygen therapy. Monitor fluid therapy. Provide stress-free environment. Provide and maintain therapy as prescribed. Assisted feeding if anorexic	Systemic antibiotic therapy. Surgical removal of abscesses. Lancing, draining and flushing of abscesses
Encephalitozoonosis				
Caused by the microsporidian parasite *Encephalitozoon cuniculi*. Infected rabbits shed spores in urine, which are ingested or inhaled. Life cycle of parasite 3–5 weeks. Targets CNS, eye, liver, kidney	May be asymptomatic; carrier status occurs. Signs most often neurological: ataxia; torticollis; posterior paresis/paralysis; urinary incontinence; tremor; convulsion; death. Lens damage to eye. Chronic signs include weight loss and polyuria/polydipsia.	Fenbendazole several times a year according to anticipated risk. Good hygiene; raised food dishes; water bottles rather than bowls. Provision of clean grazing where multiple rabbits are kept outdoors (or wild rabbits have access). *E. cuniculi*-free breeding colonies are available	Quiet gentle care to minimize exacerbation of clinical signs. Assisted feeding. Administration of medication. Advice to owners on prevention and treatment.	Long course of fenbendazole. Systemic antibiosis. Dexamethasone in acute stages. Surgical lens removal has good prognosis. Neurological signs unlikely to resolve completely. Euthanasia if signs fail to resolve to a level where quality of life is good.
Fly strike (myiasis)				
Caused by flies that lay eggs on rabbit's skin. In warm conditions eggs hatch into larvae – in hours or days – that burrow into skin on the perineal region or into open wounds. Common in outdoor rabbits with perineal soiling due to urine scalding, diarrhoea or living in poor sanitary conditions	Depression; lethargy. Maggots visible	Good sanitation and husbandry. Regular cleaning of cage/hutch, especially in summer. Weight control – overweight rabbits are unable to groom and caecotrophs may accumulate around anus. Avoid overcrowded conditions. Use insecticides and insect growth inhibitors	Provide and maintain therapy as prescribed. Assist with antiparasitic treatment. Educate owners on prevention. Remove risk of urine and faecal soiling. Provide quiet and stress-free environment	Remove fly larvae. Thoroughly clean wounds. Fluid therapy. Antibiotic therapy. Analgesia. Treat for shock.
Dental disease				
Malocclusion of incisor and/or molar teeth may be congenital or result of insufficient dental wear or low dietary calcium. Spikes may form on the teeth, damaging oral soft tissues. Dental abscesses may form. Lacrimal duct function may be compromised	Weight loss; salivation; poor grooming; secondary gastrointestinal signs (diarrhoea, accumulation of caecotrophs); ocular discharge; facial abscessation; food impaction in mouth; pain on palpation of jaw or oral examination	Feeding fresh and dried natural herbage (hay, grass, vegetables) rather than concentrate or processed rations. (If using commercial mix, should be high in fibre and pelleted to prevent selective feeding.) Early detection of disease and suitable intervention	Assisted feeding before and after dental surgery, including use of nasogastic tubes. Regular cleaning of eyes, mouth and perineal areas. Give medication as directed. Advice to owners on correct feeding	Burring or removal of affected teeth. Antibiosis and analgesics as required. Euthanasia if disease is severe

9.76 (continued) Common diseases of rabbits.

Disease	Species affected	Aetiology	Clinical signs	Nursing care	Treatment
Barbering (fur chewing)	Mice, rats, gerbils, guinea pigs, chinchillas	Chewing of the fur, by other animals or as self-mutilation, is relatively common	Hair loss, most commonly at tail base and top of head. Loss of whiskers in rats	Adding complexity to environment, e.g. more shelters, can help	Reduction of stocking density; removal of dominant animal. Guinea pigs: need to ensure adequate supply of good hay
Proliferative ileitis (wet tail)	Hamsters, ferrets. Common in weanlings aged 3–8 weeks	Caused by the bacterium *Lawsonia intracellularis*, stress, weaning, dietary change	Diarrhoea; lethargy; anorexia; dehydration	Administration of drug therapy as prescribed. Maintain good sanitation and husbandry	Supportive care; antibiotic therapy; fluid therapy to correct dehydration. Prognosis is guarded

9.77 Common diseases of other small mammal pets. (continues) ▶

Disease	Species affected	Aetiology	Clinical signs	Nursing care	Treatment
Slobbers (dental disease/malocclusion)	Rabbits, chinchillas, guinea pigs	Common. May be due to incorrect feeding, genetics or trauma	Excessive salivation ('slobbers'); dysphagia; depression; drooling; pain (reluctance to move or aggression)	Advise owners on prevention and feeding a suitable diet. Provide assisted feeding. Administer therapy as prescribed. Feed grass and good quality hay	Regular burring every 6–8 weeks; treatment of inflamed gingivae, dental abscesses and periodontal disease. Analgesia and antibiosis
Traumatic injuries	All small mammals	Overcrowding and subsequent fighting; poor handling. Some species prone to falling off surfaces	Incoordination; collapse; hyperpnoea	Educate clients on correct handling techniques. Hand feeding. Provide supportive care	Warmth; fluid therapy; nutritional support; wound care
Cheek pouch impaction	Hamsters	Often caused by artificial foods or by cotton wool-type bedding materials	Large persistent swellings (bilateral or unilateral) on face	Provide supportive care. Monitor hamster closely during food intake	Manual removal of impaction or saline irrigation; treatment of superficial infection; investigation for dental malocclusion
Pododermatitis	Rodents, rabbits	Common in overweight animals housed on wire	Pressure sores on palmar and plantar surfaces of feet	Control weight in overweight animals. Improve cage substrate to increase padding	Treatment of pressure sores; may require surgical debridement; analgesia
Tyzzer's disease (*Clostridium piliforme*)	Gerbils, hamsters, rabbits, rats and mice	Poor hygiene; stress; overcrowding; recent transportation; concurrent disease	Watery diarrhoea; depression; weight loss; death. High morbidity and mortality in young rabbits	Assist with diagnostic procedures. Provide supportive care. Advise owners on prevention and good husbandry	Antibiosis, though poor response not uncommon. Treatment only palliative once clinical signs observed
Nutritional disease	Guinea pigs prone to hypovitaminosis C (scurvy) as unable to synthesize	More likely to be subclinical than an obvious nutritional deficiency	Malocclusion; lethargy; swollen joints; weight loss; death.	Client education on prevention – ensure that animals are fed a commercially prepared diet that is nutritionally balanced	Oral vitamin C; treatment of underlying infectious or parasitic disease
	Hypovitaminosis D3	Rodents: indoor-kept pet fed all-seed diet. Ferrets: all-meat diet and no calcium supplement	Rickets; well muscled heavy mammal with poorly mineralized bones; joint inflammation		Correction of dietary deficiency (calcium, vitamin D3) and any UV light deficiency

9.77 (continued) Common diseases of other small mammal pets.

Disease	Aetiology	Clinical signs	Nursing care	Treatment
Feather conditions	Infections; parasites; psychological disorder due to poor husbandry	Plucking of feathers from own body leaving only those on head untouched; dominant birds may sometimes pluck feathers from subordinate bird; feather loss or damage; irregular or abnormal moult	Prevent self-trauma. Provide bird with more attention. Regularly spray bird with water to prevent from getting too dusty and then over-grooming. Administer medication as prescribed	Dependent on cause: improved nutrition; enriched environment; treatment of underlying disease
Psittacine beak and feather disease (PBFD) Usually affects psittacine birds but can affect others. Usually young birds <3 years; common in young African Grey parrots	Viral disease. Transmitted by particles of feather dander	Abnormal feather growth; misshapen and crumbly beak; feather plucking; poor feather quality; secondary infections such as aspergillosis	Isolate birds that test positive. Barrier nursing. Assisted feeding. Warm food to room temperature prior to administration	No cure and no preventive treatment; many cases prove fatal. Probiotics and nutritional support. Isolation and retest in 6 weeks
Intestinal parasites Especially affects young birds aged 3–4 months; older birds may be carriers	Coccidial and other parasites	Diarrhoea; rapid loss of condition; anorexia; weight loss; dysentery; general debilitation; polydipsia	Monitor and maintain hydration status. Administer antiparasitic treatment as prescribed. Maintain strict hygiene standards	Fluid therapy; vitamin B supplementation; checking for stress or concurrent disease; antiprotozoal drugs
Ornithosis/psittacosis ⚠	*Chlamydophila psittaci*	Listless and dull; respiratory signs; depression; sinusitis; conjunctivitis; green diarrhoea; death	*Zoonotic risk – appropriate precautions must be taken and owners must be warned about associated implications* Reduce unnecessary exposure. Protective equipment including mask must be worn during contact. Strict hygiene standards must be adopted. Isolate affected birds	Treatment should be carried out under quarantine conditions. Parenteral treatment – antibiotics and vitamin A injections
Egg binding Commonest reproductive complaint of caged birds	Poor diet; overproduction of eggs and subsequent low blood calcium levels	Lethargy; dullness; deformed eggs; uterine rupture; depression; straining; bloodstained faeces	Provide suitable nesting material. Educate owners on prevention. Provide clean, quiet, warm, draught-free environment. Monitor hydration status	Manual expression or surgical removal of eggs; ovariohysterectomy; oxytocin; fluid therapy; treatment of hypocalcaemia; nutritional support

9.78 Common diseases of birds. ⚠ indicates a zoonosis. (continues) ▶

Disease	Aetiology	Clinical signs	Nursing care	Treatment
Regurgitation	Common in birds approaching weaning: indicates that more solid foods need to be added to diet. Younger birds regurgitate due to crop stasis, crop infection, GI obstruction, overfeeding and antimicrobial use. Breeding behaviour; pathological; toxicities; digestive difficulties; metabolic disease processes	Expulsion of small amounts of crop contents	Obtain detailed history from owners to determine type of regurgitation. Acute cases should be treated as emergency. Monitor hydration status. Provide supportive care	Dependent on cause; may be indistinguishable from vomiting. Fluid therapy; antibiotic/antifungal drops in infectious cases; toxin neutralizing compounds in poisoning cases; removal of foreign body

9.78 (continued) Common diseases of birds.

Disease	Species affected	Aetiology	Clinical signs	Nursing care	Treatment
Stomatitis (mouth rot)	Many reptiles but particularly seen in snakes and chelonians	Bacterial infections; local trauma; chronic stressors such as suboptimal ambient temperature; associated with anorexia, especially following hibernation; overzealous force feeding of anorectic reptiles; secondary to systemic process such as sepsis or viral disease	'Cheesy' white deposit in mouth; oedematous swelling of ventral neck; dysphagia; hypersalivation; occasionally dyspnoea; possible nasal discharge	Barrier nurse. Assisted feeding. Warm food to room temperature prior to administration	Mouth cleaned and debrided daily; topical antibiotic therapy if possible; systemic antibiotics; parenteral fluids
Salmonellosis ⚠	Amphibians, lizards, snakes	Salmonella: foodborne infection; can be shed intermittently by healthy reptiles. Soil and stagnant water are most common sources	Dependent on species infected. Septicaemia and sudden death; Mycobacterium lesions affecting integument, GI and respiratory tracts; abortion in pregnant animals; progressive weight loss; poor general condition	*Major zoonotic concern therefore appropriate precautions must be taken.* Use appropriate hygiene to prevent infection. Educate clients on personal hygiene	Antibiosis; fluid therapy; probiotics. Due to high zoonotic risk, euthanasia often recommended
Dysecdysis	Snakes and invertebrates	Difficulty in shedding skin may be multifactorial: sub-optimal environment; low relative humidity; lack of available water; malnourishment; ectoparasitism; systemic disease. Excessive sloughing may be due to endocrine disorders or hypervitaminosis A	Retained pieces of dried epidermis adhere to body	Address environmental issues and ensure correct conditions provided. Educate owners on prevention	Increase humidity by spraying or bathing to loosen dry skin
Nutritional disease		Hypovitaminosis A	Mucous membranes thicken and oral and respiratory secretions dry up, leading to poor functioning of ciliary mechanisms	Assist with correction of dietary deficiencies. Educate owners on prevention of nutritional diseases	Vitamin A supplementation
		Metabolic bone disease	Prominent bowing of limbs; weak bones; rickets; joint inflammation; lethargy		Correction of dietary deficiency (calcium, vitamin D3) and any UV light deficiency
		Thiamine deficiency (usually fish-eating snakes and terrapins)	Neurological disorders such as lack of coordination, convulsions; eventually death		Correction of dietary deficiency with vitamin B1 (thiamine)
Regurgitation	Common in snakes; rarely seen in chelonians and lizards	Improper ambient temperature; consumption of too large a meal; force feeding; rough handling, particularly after feeding; ingestion of foreign bodies; infectious causes (parasites, viruses); ulcers; neoplasia	Effortless expulsion of partially digested food. Usually occurs 1–3 days after consumption of a meal	Monitor temperature. Administer treatment as prescribed. Monitor hydration status. Control food intake	Dependent on cause. Correction of environmental temperature; treatment of infectious causes
Gout	Snakes, chelonians	Renal failure can lead to hyperuricaemia (elevated uric acid levels in bloodstream) resulting in formation of crystals in the body. Many factors can contribute to renal damage and gout: dehydration; excessive dietary protein; increased levels of dietary vitamin D3 and calcium	Joint inflammation if urates deposited in joints (articular gout). Organ failure if urates deposited on serosae of internal organs (visceral gout)	Monitor fluid therapy. Assisted feeding. Educate owners on correct dietary requirements	Fluid therapy; nutritional support. Euthanasia should be considered

9.79 Common diseases of reptiles. ⚠ indicates a zoonosis.

Nutritional support

General feeding of exotic pets is discussed in Chapter 2. This section will concentrate on assisted and supplementary feeding.

Rabbits

Assisted feeding is often necessary and should be instituted as soon as possible if a rabbit is anorexic. Anorexia for 2–3 days or more has serious consequences, including gastrointestinal hypomotility and stasis, mucosal atrophy and hepatic lipidosis.

Syringe or tube feeding, and the use of prokinetic drugs (see Chapter 3), are all important parts of the medical management of this species.

Nasogastric intubation is well tolerated in rabbits. A size 5–8 FG naso-oesophageal tube should be used. Correct placement of the tube should always be confirmed by taking a radiograph, as rabbits are unlikely to cough if the tube or saline is placed into the trachea. It is important to ensure that the patient cannot interfere with the tube, but it is vital that caecotrophy can still be performed. Recovery diet (Supreme Petfoods) with or without added puréed vegetables makes an ideal food suitable for syringe feeding rabbits, but it is too thick to use with a nasogastric tube, which is only suitable for solutions. General methods for tube feeding and the care of feeding tubes are described earlier in the chapter.

Frequency of feeding and the amount given varies with the type of diet selected. Rabbits should be fed approximately 2–3 times a day at a rate of 10–20 ml/kg bodyweight. A more accurate method is to calculate the rabbit's daily calorific requirement using the following equation:

**Resting energy requirement (RER) (kcal/day) =
70 x bodyweight (kg)**

Coprophagia is a normal and important process for rabbits and other herbivores. The first time food passes through the digestive system it is only partially digested and emerges as a caecotroph. This is immediately eaten and then fully digested. Rabbits that are unable to practise caecotrophy may suffer from weight loss and digestive disorders.

Birds

The provision of food and fluids via a crop tube is an easy method and one that a veterinary nurse can perform (see *BSAVA Manual of Practical Animal Care*). Rigid metal tubes are preferred when used gently. These tubes can be passed into the crop or oesophagus of the bird and palpated to ensure correct placement. Small birds such as budgerigars may only tolerate 1–2 ml but larger birds can accept up to 20 ml at a time.

Daily nutritional requirements for birds can be estimated using the following formula:

**Resting energy requirement (RER) =
K x bodyweight (kg)**

where K is a constant, set at 78 for non-passerine birds and 129 for passerine birds.

Once RER has been calculated, the metabolic energy requirement (MER) can be calculated as follows:

MER = 1.25 x RER

Daily weighing and assessment of body condition will ensure that enough calories are being given.

Reptiles

In reptiles, resting energy requirements (RERs) vary widely depending on activity level and environmental temperature, and so calculations are made at that animal's optimal environmental temperature. Energy requirements also vary according to the animal's stage of life.

**RER = 10 x bodyweight for all reptiles in general
MER = 1.5 x RER**

Assisted feeding methods are often used in reptiles to provide nutritional support and sometimes for fluid administration. Pharyngostomy and oesophageal tubes are often selected, due to the limited stress factor that is associated with them. It is important to remember that severely dehydrated patients may have existing gut pathology; therefore this route may need to be supplemented by others.

Further reading

Agar S (2001) *Small Animal Nutrition*. Butterworth-Heinemann, Oxford

Aspinall V (2003) *Clinical Procedures in Veterinary Nursing*. Butterworth-Heinemann, Oxford

Bowden C and Masters J (2003) *Textbook of Veterinary Medical Nursing*. Butterworth-Heinemann, Oxford

Flecknell P and Meredith A (eds) (2006) *BSAVA Manual of Rabbit Medicine and Surgery, 2nd edn*. BSAVA Publications, Gloucester

Gorman C (1995) *The Ageing Dog*. Henry Ling Ltd, Dorchester

Howarth S, Gear R and Bryan E (2007) Medical disorders of dogs and cats and their nursing. In: *BSAVA Textbook of Veterinary Nursing, 4th edn*, ed. DR Lane *et al.*, pp. 457–506. BSAVA Publications, Gloucester

Meredith A and Redrobe S (eds) (2002) *BSAVA Manual of Exotic Pets, 4th edn*. BSAVA Publications, Gloucester

Orpet H and Welsh P (2002) *Handbook of Veterinary Nursing*. Blackwell Science, Oxford

Ramsey IK and Tennant BJ (2001) *BSAVA Manual of Canine and Feline Infectious Diseases*. BSAVA Publications, Gloucester

Sirois M (2004) *Principles and Practice of Veterinary Technology, 2nd edn*. Mosby, St Louis

Tartaglia L (2002) *Veterinary Physiology and Applied Anatomy*. College of Animal Welfare, Oxford

Acknowledgements

The author and editors wish to thank Wendy Busby for her contribution to the *BSAVA Manual of Veterinary Nursing*.

10

Practical laboratory techniques

Clare Knottenbelt

> **This chapter is designed to give information on:**
>
> - Health and safety in the practice laboratory
> - Maintenance and use of laboratory equipment
> - Collection, preparation and preservation of samples
> - Techniques for the laboratory tests commonly performed in veterinary practice

Introduction

Laboratory tests are usually performed as part of an investigation of a clinical problem or as a routine health screen. Many laboratory tests can be performed 'in house' with relatively simple equipment, whilst others need to be sent to external laboratories for analysis. This chapter will describe how to perform the common in-house tests and procedures for external submission.

Health and safety

Before using the laboratory all staff should be advised of potential hazards and understand how to use the laboratory equipment. The following basic laboratory rules should be adhered to.

- Establish fire prevention and fire drill routines.
- Provide a first aid kit and train a staff member to act as a first aider.
- Always wear adequate protective clothing, including a white coat.
- Wash hands frequently and before leaving the laboratory.
- Do not eat or drink in the laboratory and do not pipette by mouth.
- Label all hazardous materials, clean up spillage immediately, dispose of waste correctly and keep the laboratory tidy.

Health and Safety risk assessment is covered in Chapter 1.

Waste disposal and infection control

Spillages should be cleaned up immediately; the laboratory should be kept tidy; and clinical waste should be disposed of appropriately. Glassware should be soaked in suitable disinfectants. Sharp objects, including disposable plastic instruments, should be placed in a 'sharps' bin. Samples and culture plates should be autoclaved and placed into yellow clinical waste bags. Waste in clinical waste bags, glass bins and 'sharps' bins is sent away to be incinerated at the appropriate temperature. See Figure 4.11 for details on waste categories and disposal.

General infection control is covered in Chapter 4.

Collection and submission of samples

Veterinary investigations frequently involve the collection and preservation of various samples. It is within the scope of the veterinary nurse to conduct or assist in sampling techniques, and to ensure that samples are collected and preserved in a reliable and safe manner.

When collecting samples from any patient the following points should be remembered:

- Health and safety rules must be adhered to, ensuring cleanliness and personal hygiene for protection of both the patient and the handler
- Use sterile equipment, including needles, containers and catheters

- Gather all equipment *before* starting the procedure
- Ensure adequate restraint of the patient
- Label samples immediately after collection, with the owner's name, animal identification, date and the nature of the sample
- Examine fresh samples whenever possible
- Store samples correctly if they cannot be examined immediately
- Complete a laboratory analysis form for each patient with details of patient, type of sample, *a full clinical history* and laboratory request
- Record all results accurately and retain records for future reference
- Many tests are easy to do in practice, allowing rapid results to be obtained whilst the owner waits
- Regular quality control tests should be carried out on in-house laboratory equipment and results should be recorded
- Samples for an outside laboratory must include a laboratory analysis form (as above) and be prepared, packaged and posted correctly.

Preservation equipment and materials

The preferred method of sample preservation should always be confirmed with the external laboratory prior to sample collection. Methods of preservation commonly used are listed in Figure 10.1.

Universal containers and vacutainers

Figure 10.2 lists the anticoagulants required for various blood tests. Each tube is manufactured with the appropriate amount of anticoagulant for a given amount of blood. Tubes should therefore be filled to the level identified by a line or arrow on the side of the tube. Over-filling can result in clot formation, whilst under-filling may affect some blood parameters. Once filled, the tube should be gently rolled to ensure that blood is thoroughly mixed with the anticoagulant. Shaking the tube may result in haemolysis (rupture of red cell membranes). Serum gel tubes contain a gel that both promotes rapid clot formation and forms a layer between the serum and clot, therefore speeding up serum preparation. The expiry date on any tube should be checked before use.

Vacutainers were originally designed for human use, with the blood taken directly from the patient into the vacutainer. In small animals this process increases haemolysis and the excessive vacuum may collapse the vein against the needle. When using vacutainers, blood should be collected into a syringe and the blood placed in the vacutainers after removing the cap. Injection of blood through the cap will result in haemolysis.

Sample material	Sample types	Preservation required
Blood	Whole blood or plasma	Anticoagulant essential (Figure 10.2)
	Serum	None, separate once clot has formed (Figure 10.7)
	Blood smear	Air-dried smear essential
Urine	Urinalysis sample	Thymol, toluene or HCl unless examined within 30 minutes (Figure 10.23)
	Sediment	Formalin or thymol
	Culture	Boric acid
Faeces	Routine faecal analysis	Refrigerate if cannot be performed immediately
	Culture	Refrigerate if cannot be performed immediately
Body tissue	Histopathology	10% formalin essential
	Fine needle aspirate	Air-dried smear essential

10.1 Preservation of common samples.

Anticoagulant	Sample	Tests	Universal[a]	Vacutainer[a]
EDTA (ethylene diamine tetra-acetic acid) (combines with calcium to prevent clotting, causing least distortion of cells)	Whole blood	Haematology	Pink/red	Lavender
None	Serum	Biochemistry Bile acids	White/clear	Red
Serum gel	Serum	Biochemistry Bile acids	Brown	
Lithium heparin	Plasma	Biochemistry Electrolytes	Orange	Green or green/orange
Fluoride oxalate/fluoride (inhibits glucose-using enzymes)	Whole blood	Blood glucose	Yellow	Grey
Sodium/potassium citrate	Whole blood	Coagulation tests Platelet counts	Lilac	

10.2 A guide to anticoagulants in vacutainers and universal containers for blood samples. [a] Colour codes should always be checked, as some manufacturers may differ.

Large sterile containers

Urine and faeces should be submitted in sterile containers. Faecal containers often have a sterile spatula attached to the lid to make faecal collection easier. Some urine containers are designed like a syringe, to minimize the risk of aerosol formation and contamination during pouring.

Slide storage

Unfixed slides that cannot be examined immediately should be stored to prevent desiccation. This can be done by sealing the sample in a plastic bag.

Refrigeration

Storage at 4°C preserves whole blood and fresh tissue samples in the short term and is preferable to storage at room temperature. Storage for longer than 24–48 hours should be avoided whenever possible.

Freezing

Freezing preserves serum and plasma samples indefinitely. Freezing is the method of preservation for some histological examinations and for some non-routine blood tests such as measurement of ACTH levels. Checks should always be made with the laboratory before freezing a sample. Storage at –10°C will preserve samples for up to one week; lower temperatures (–15°C to –20°C) will preserve samples indefinitely. Frozen samples should be thawed slowly at room temperature.

Formol saline and formalin

These chemicals preserve cell structure after collection and are therefore used for tissue samples for histopathology. It is important to avoid skin contamination and inhalation when handling these chemicals.

Swabs and transport media

Swabs are used for the collection of small amounts of biological material, usually for identification of microorganisms. Specific transport media are required to preserve certain virology and bacteriology samples. The correct transport medium must be used, so checks should always be made with the external laboratory first.

Labelling and paperwork

Each sample should be labelled with the owner's name, the animal's name or reference number, the type of sample collected and the date of collection (e.g. 'Fluffy Brown – Urine 24/2/07').

An appropriate submission form should accompany every sample submitted to an external laboratory. If a submission form is not available, similar information should be provided in an accompanying letter. This information ensures that the laboratory performs the appropriate test and is able to interpret the results. Forms should be placed in a plastic envelope to prevent contamination should the container break in transit.

Information required by external laboratories

- **Name and address of submitting veterinary surgeon**
- **Owner's name**
- **Animal's name or reference number**
- **Species, breed, age and sex (M, MN, F, FN)**
- **Date of sampling and time of collection**
- **Clinical history, including presenting signs, and current treatments**
- **Types of samples collected (including type of preservatives used)**
- **Site(s) of sample collection**
- **Test or examination required**

Postage and packaging

Samples that are not preserved, packed or posted appropriately may be damaged in transit. Damaged samples can produce inaccurate results and it is therefore extremely important to ensure that samples arrive in the best possible condition.

- Check the information supplied by the laboratory to ensure that the correct types of sample are being sent.
- Do not post samples on a Friday, as they will sit in a warm post box all weekend.

The following are rules for postage of pathological samples, and *must* be adhered to.

- The sender must ensure that the sample will not expose anyone to danger (COSHH 1988).
- A *maximum* sample of *50 ml* is allowed through the post, unless by specific arrangement with Royal Mail.
- Samples must be labelled correctly with time, date, owner and animal identification, and nature of the sample (e.g. 'heparinized plasma').
- *Primary container* must be leak proof and must be wrapped in enough absorbent material to absorb the complete sample if leakage or breakage occurs.
- The wrapped sample is then placed in a *leak-proof plastic bag*.
- This is placed in a *secondary container* (e.g. polypropylene clip-down container or cylindrical metal container).
- Seal the correctly completed *laboratory form* in a plastic bag for extra protection and place with sample.
- Place in a *tertiary container* (strong cardboard or grooved polystyrene box), approved by Royal Mail, and seal securely.
- *Outer packaging must be labelled conspicuously*: 'FRAGILE WITH CARE / PATHOLOGICAL SPECIMEN / ADDRESS OF LABORATORY / Address of sender.
- Send by *first-class letter post* (*not* parcel post).

WARNING
If the Royal Mail's conditions are not complied with the sender is liable to prosecution.

Laboratory equipment

Using a microscope

Figures 10.3 and 10.4 describe how to set up and use a microscope.

---

1. Place the lowest power objective into position and turn the light intensity switch (rheostat) to a low setting before switching on the light.
2. Place the slide or counting chamber into the mechanical stage and adjust the position so that the lens lies over the area you want to examine.
3. Adjust the distance between the two eyepieces so that you can see a single image and increase the light intensity as necessary.
4. Use the coarse and fine focus to bring the object into focus.
5. Adjust the condenser and diaphragm to ensure optimal illumination.
6. Examine the object using the travelling knobs.
7. Once an area of interest has been identified, rotate the objective lenses to the next power and adjust the fine focus. It may be necessary to adjust the condenser, diaphragm and light intensity.
8. Oil immersion provides maximum magnification. If this is required, focus the object on a lower power then rotate the objective lens out of position. Place a drop of immersion oil over the area of interest and rotate the oil immersion lens into position.
   a. Always ensure that the lens is lying within the oil, otherwise the image will be distorted.
   b. Avoid contaminating the dry lenses with oil.
9. Areas of interest can be recorded using the two Vernier scales at any magnification.

10.3 Setting up and using a microscope.

Each scale consists of a main scale divided into millimetres and a Vernier plate with 10 divisions.

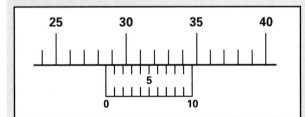

1. Observe where the division labelled 'zero' on the plate meets the main scale. If it falls between two divisions, record the lower number (28).
2. Note which of the plate divisions is aligned with a mark on the main scale (4).
3. The reading is recorded as the first number with the second number after the point 28.4).
4. Repeat the reading for the scale at right angles.
5. The readings are reported in same way as grid references on a map.

Always place the slide with the label to the right so that points can be relocated.

10.4 Reading the Vernier scale.

Care of laboratory equipment

The wiring (including the plug and fuse) of all electrical machinery should be checked regularly. Servicing, cleaning and lubrication should be performed following the manufacturer's guidelines. Quality control procedures should be performed on a regular basis to ensure that results continue to be accurate. Recording details of usage and servicing will ensure that all equipment is safe and reliable. Microscopes and automated analysers should receive special attention. Microhaematocrit centrifuges should be cleaned regularly, because when capillary tubes break they contaminate the rubber cushion with blood and glass. Cleaning and disinfection procedures must be established for incubators to ensure that bacterial contamination does not occur.

Maintenance and care of a microscope

- **Identify a position in the laboratory appropriate for the microscope, i.e. away from direct sunlight, sinks and vibrating machinery. Avoid moving the microscope from the chosen site if possible.**
- **Keep the microscope covered when not in use.**
- **Turn the light intensity switch (rheostat) down to minimum if the light is left on for a prolonged period and before switching it off.**
- **Clean the lenses with lens paper after using oil immersion.**
- **Lower the stage and turn the lowest power objective into position after use.**

Maintenance and care of automated analysers

- **Identify a position in the laboratory appropriate for the analyser, i.e. away from direct sunlight and sinks. Ensure that there is adequate space for consumables and that they are stored appropriately (some may require refrigeration or freezing).**
- **Room temperature should be monitored to avoid wide temperature fluctuations.**
- **Perform daily cleaning and quality control procedures as recommended by the manufacturer.**
- **Keep a record of all tests performed.**
- **Keep the machine free of blood contamination. Remove all contaminated consumables after each use and dispose of appropriately.**
- **Ideally keep machine covered when not in use.**

Blood samples

Blood samples for biochemical or haematological analysis are often required for diagnostic or monitoring purposes. Sampling, storage and postage procedures must be appropriate, otherwise inaccurate and unreliable results may be obtained. General rules for taking blood samples are given in Figure 10.5.

Equipment:

- Sterile needle and syringe
- Cotton wool/swab
- Surgical spirit
- Curved blunt-ended scissors, or clippers
- Sample tube(s) (see Figure 10.2).

Choice and preparation of needle and syringe

Needle sizes for blood sampling

Species	Needle size
Cat	23 gauge x 5/8"
Dog	20 or 21 gauge x 5/8 or 1"
Rabbit	23 gauge x 5/8"
Exotic species	23 or 25 gauge x 5/8"

As large a needle as practical for the patient should be used as this allows more efficient evacuation of blood and reduces the risk of haemolysis.

The syringe size should reflect the amount of blood required for analysis. The needle and syringe should be both sterile and dry, as dirty equipment will cause contamination of the sample and wet equipment will cause haemolysis.

1. The syringe and needle must be put together aseptically.
2. Turn the bevel of the needle uppermost in line with the graduations on the syringe so that it is possible to see the amount of blood obtained.
3. Break the seal on the syringe, by withdrawing and then depressing the plunger, before taking the sample so that it is easier to draw the blood once in the vein.
4. The syringe and needle (with needle guard in place) are now prepared and are placed with the other blood sampling equipment.

Choice of vein

The jugular is the best vein for obtaining a blood sample from dogs and cats. The cephalic and saphenous veins can also be used. In general, collection from a larger vein results in a better quality sample (Figure 10.6). In exotic species, the tail vein or the jugular is commonly used. In rabbits, the jugular or ear vein provides good venous access. For more information on blood collection from exotic pets see *BSAVA Manual of Exotic Pets*.

Technique	Reasons
1. Gather and correctly prepare equipment	Process should be smooth and efficient
2. Use appropriate restraint	Safety and good access to vein
3. Clip skin over vein and apply 70% alcohol (surgical spirit)	Prevents introduction of infection and improves visualization of the vein
4. Raise vein by occluding the movement of blood towards the heart	Allows the vein to fill up and swell, making sampling easier
5. Sample from the part of the exposed vein that is furthest from heart	Minimizes damage to the vein, making it suitable for later use if required
6. As blood starts to come back, apply gentle pressure on plunger	Too much pressure allows the blood to flow too fast and cells may haemolyse or the vein may collapse against the bevel of the needle
7. Once the sample is obtained, the vein is released and pressure is put on the insertion site for at least 15 seconds	Reduces haemorrhage or haematoma formation
8. Remove the needle from the syringe and the tops from the required blood tubes and decant the blood gently	Pushing blood back through the needle and over-zealous evacuation of the syringe cause haemolysis
9. Fill serum samples last	Serum is obtained from a clotted sample
10. Fill anticoagulant tubes accurately and replace cap firmly	Over-filling may induce clotting. Under-filling may give unreliable results, or alter cell size and morphology
11. Gently mix/roll	Over-enthusiastic mixing causes haemolysis
12. Label containers immediately	Avoids mixing up of samples from different patients
13. Dispose of all pathological and hazardous waste appropriately	In accordance with Health and Safety regulations
14. Complete laboratory forms as necessary	Ensures laboratory has appropriate information

10.5 Some general rules for taking blood samples.

Vein	Location	Advantages	Disadvantages
Jugular	Pair of large veins that return blood from the head and neck region to the heart. Run down either side of neck from approximately point of mandible to point of shoulder (see Chapter 8)	Larger needle can be used, reducing risk of haemolysis. Large volume of blood can be obtained relatively quickly. Can still obtain sample from animals with poor circulation or shock as veins carry high volumes of blood. Cephalic vein can be left free for anaesthesia or fluid therapy	Inexperienced staff may find it harder to identify vein. Can be difficult in obese patients
Cephalic	Runs down anterior aspect of each forelimb and is accessible distal to elbow (see Chapter 8)	Familiar vein for venipuncture and easily identified. Suitable for small samples from large dogs	Slower flow of blood means haemolysis and collapse of vein during sampling more common. Poor sampling techniques may prevent use of vein for intravenous treatments or catheter placement

10.6 Choice of vein for obtaining a blood sample from dogs and cats.

Sample preparation

Once the sample has been collected, it may need to be processed further before analysis can take place. If it cannot be examined immediately it will need to be stored. The type of sample collected depends on the type of analysis required.

Sample type

- **Whole blood – must be collected into specific anticoagulant before analysis.**
- **Plasma – produced by removing the cellular components from whole blood in anticoagulant.**
- **Serum – produced by allowing blood to clot (no anticoagulant) and removing the cellular components.**

Whole blood samples

Whole blood is used for haematological analysis (red blood cells, white blood cells, platelets, etc.). It should not be frozen, but can be stored in a refrigerator at +4°C for up to 48 hours. Previously chilled samples must be returned to room temperature before analysis.

Serum or plasma separation

Separation prevents contamination by red cell contents due to cell membrane rupture (haemolysis). Exposure to heat, cold or violent shaking enhances haemolysis. If a sample is to be posted to a laboratory, separation of serum or plasma is recommended (Figure 10.7).

Plasma samples

Blood is placed into heparin anticoagulant and the heparinized plasma is separated from the red cells. The sample should be labelled with the usual details and the words 'heparinized plasma'.

Serum samples

Blood is placed into a plain tube (no anticoagulant) and left to clot at room temperature (out of the sun). Once the clot has retracted (approximately 1–2 hours)

- Collect at least 2 ml of whole blood:
  - For plasma place in heparin tube. Plasma samples can be centrifuged immediately
  - For serum place in plain tube (containing no anticoagulant). Serum samples should be left for at least 1 hour at room temperature to ensure clot formation and separation (15 minutes is usually adequate).
- Carefully detach clot from the side of the tube with a swab stick.
- *Warning: clot disruption, sample warming or violent shaking will increase the risk of haemolysis.*
- Centrifuge at 3000 rpm for 5 minutes.
- Remove the supernatant (serum or plasma) and place into a tube containing no anticoagulant.
- If the sample is to be frozen, ensure that there is sufficient space in the tube for expansion during freezing.

10.7 Preparation of plasma and serum samples.

the serum is separated from the clot. The sample should be labelled with the usual details and the word 'serum'.

Storage of plasma and serum

Serum and plasma can be stored in the refrigerator at +4°C for up to a maximum of 48 hours, or frozen for longer periods. Different analytes are stable in samples for variable periods. Checks should be made with the laboratory to determine how long a sample can be stored. Samples that have been frozen or chilled should be returned slowly to room temperature before examination.

Problems with blood samples

The following factors affect blood sample analysis and may cause erroneous results.

- **Icteric samples** (sample yellow due to large amounts of bilirubin in the blood)
  - This is unavoidable in certain clinical situations such as liver disease but nevertheless will affect results of other parameters.

- **Lipaemic samples** (sample cloudy due to large amounts of lipid in the blood)
  - Collect a fasting sample (at least 12 hours).
- **Haemolysed samples** (serum pink or red due to damage to red cell membranes and release of haemoglobin). To reduce haemolysis:
  - Use dry sterile equipment
  - Take a jugular sample with a large needle
  - Avoid excessive vacuum on the syringe
  - Remove the needle before decanting the blood
  - Do not crush the last cells in the syringes
  - Mix sample tube carefully
  - Separate serum or plasma, as necessary, before posting.

Haematology

There a number of parameters given in haematology results. Some of these are measured directly, either manually or by the haematology analyser. Others are calculated from these measured parameters. Figure 10.8 outlines the different parameters and how they are assessed. Avian red blood cells are nucleated (see Figure 10.20b) and therefore cannot be assessed using automated haematology analysers.

Packed cell volume (PCV)

The PCV is the percentage of whole blood volume that is taken up by the red cells. The PCV will fall in patients with anaemia and may be elevated if the patient is dehydrated or has abnormally high red cell production. The PCV is measured by centrifuging a capillary tube of whole blood using a microhaematocrit centrifuge (Figure 10.9) and then calculating what percentage of the blood volume is red cells (Figure 10.10).

PCV is usually measured using blood collected into EDTA anticoagulant, but heparinized capillary tubes are available to allow blood to be collected directly from small veins (in exotic species) or a small nick made in the patient's skin. Figure 10.11 describes the method of determining PCV.

Red cell parameter	Definition	Unit	Method of measurement
Packed cell volume (PCV)	Proportion of blood volume that comprises red cells	% or l/l	Microhaematocrit centrifuge In-house haematology analyser
Red blood cell count (RBC)	Number of red cells per litre of blood	x 10^{12}/l	Haemocytometer In-house analyser
Haemoglobin (Hb)	Weight of haemoglobin per decilitre of blood	g/dl	In-house analyser
Mean cell volume (MCV)	Average volume of a single red cell	fl	$MCV = \dfrac{PCV\ (\%) \times 10}{RBC}$
Mean cell haemoglobin concentration (MCHC)	Average concentration of haemoglobin in 100 ml of red cells	g/dl	$MCHC = \dfrac{Hb\ (g/dl)}{PCV\ (l/l)}$

10.8   Measurement of red cell parameters in a practice laboratory.

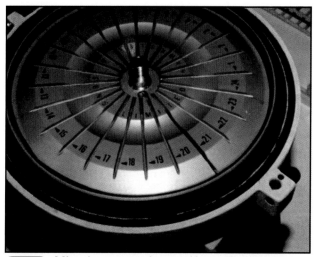

10.9   Microhaematocrit centrifuge. Tubes are placed on opposite sides of the centrifuge to ensure that the drum is balanced during spinning.

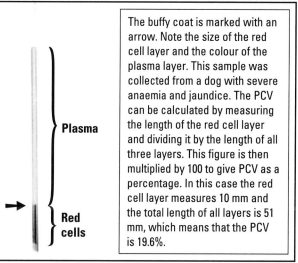

The buffy coat is marked with an arrow. Note the size of the red cell layer and the colour of the plasma layer. This sample was collected from a dog with severe anaemia and jaundice. The PCV can be calculated by measuring the length of the red cell layer and dividing it by the length of all three layers. This figure is then multiplied by 100 to give PCV as a percentage. In this case the red cell layer measures 10 mm and the total length of all layers is 51 mm, which means that the PCV is 19.6%.

Plasma

Red cells

10.10   Appearance of a capillary tube after centrifugation.

1.   Ensure that the contents of the blood tube are thoroughly mixed by inverting the blood tube.
2.   Three-quarters fill two capillary tubes by holding both the blood tube and the capillary tubes at an angle to enhance flow.
3.   Place a finger on the end of the capillary tube to prevent blood flowing out and plug the opposite end of the tube with soft clay.
4.   Place both capillary tubes on opposite sides of the centrifuge with the plug against the rubber rim of the centrifuge (see Figure 10.9). (Note the numerical position of each patient's samples.)
5.   Replace the metal cover and lock the centrifuge lid. Centrifuge at 10,000 rpm for 5 minutes and allow machine to come to a halt.
6.   Remove capillary tubes and measure PCV manually or using a Hawksley microhaematocrit reader. The sample will be divided into three layers: red cells, white blood cell layer (buffy coat) and plasma (see Figure 10.10).
7.   Calculate PCV in litres per litre (l/l) by measuring the size of the red cell layer and dividing it by the total length of all three layers. To convert this figure to %, multiply it by 100.
8.   Note size of buffy coat and plasma colour (red = haemolysis, yellow = jaundice) (see Figure 10.10).

10.11   Measurement of PCV using a microhaematocrit centrifuge.

Blood smear

Smears should be made as soon as possible after blood collection. Preparation of a blood smear is described in Figures 10.12 and 10.13.

Preparation of a good-quality smear is often difficult and requires practice.

Equipment required: 2 clean glass slides (A = smear slide, B = spreader slide), 1 capillary tube, blood sample in anticoagulant (usually EDTA)

1.   Ensure that contents of blood tube are thoroughly mixed by inverting blood tube.
2.   Using a capillary tube, place a single small drop of blood at one end of glass slide A.
3.   Holding glass slide A firmly on the work surface, place one end of slide B on the opposite end of slide A at an angle of 30–45°.
4.   Draw slide B back to the drop of blood and allow blood to spread out.
5.   Push slide B away from blood drop in a single rapid motion.
6.   Rapidly air-dry slide A.
7.   Check the quality of the smear and if adequate store or stain immediately.

How to recognize a good blood smear

■   Does it air-dry rapidly? (Thick smears will take longer to dry.)
■   Does it have a feathered (irregular) edge in the shape of a semi-circle?

Both these factors indicate that the blood has been spread out sufficiently to produce a monolayer (i.e. one cell thick), which makes examination of cell structure easier.

Remember: Good smears are a result of lots of practice so always prepare a number of smears and only submit the best.

10.12   Preparation of a blood smear (see also Figure 10.13).

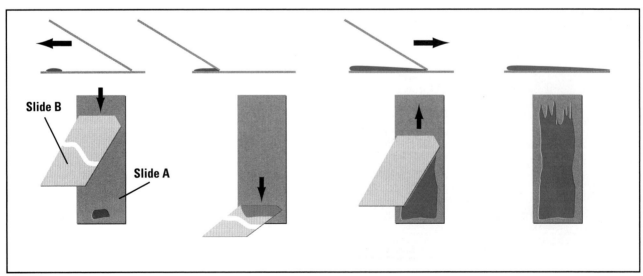

10.13   Preparing a blood smear by the draw back and push away method.

Common faults in blood smears and how to avoid them (see also Figure 10.14)

Fault	How to avoid
Too thick	Use smaller drop of blood
Too thin	Use larger drop of blood and/or faster spreading motion
Alternating thick and thin bands	Ensure spreading motion is smooth and avoid hesitation
Streaks along length of smear	Ensure edge of spreader is not irregular or coated with dried blood Ensure no dust on slide or in blood
'Holes' in smear	Ensure slide is free of grease
Narrow thick smear	Ensure blood is allowed to spread right across spreader slide before making smear

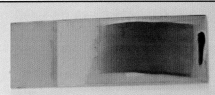

A good smear with a visible feathered edge.

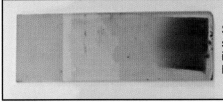

Smear is too short because insufficient blood was used.

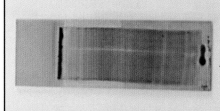

Smear is too long (too much blood) and has thick and thin bands (not spread smoothly).

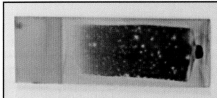

There are holes visible in the smear. This occurs when the slide is greasy, usually following handling.

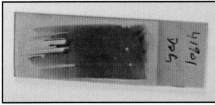

The feathered edge is very streaked, which may be due to uneven contact or dirt on the spreader slide.

10.14 Examples of good and bad blood smears. (Adapted from *BSAVA Manual of Canine and Feline Clinical Pathology, 2nd edition*)

The smear should be dried rapidly, or fixed by immersion in absolute methanol for 5 minutes, to prevent changes in cell morphology. Once dried the smear can be stored for 2 weeks; fixed smears can be stored indefinitely. Slides should be transported in slide holders to prevent breakage.

Examination of a stained blood smear provides information about red and white cell morphology (structure), differential white cell counts and platelet counts and may allow identification of blood parasites such as *Mycoplasma haemofelis* (the organism responsible for feline infectious anaemia).

Blood smears are commonly stained (Figure 10.15) using Leishman's (see Figure 10.19) or Diff-Quik (see Figure 10.20a). The use of different stains such as Giemsa may identify particular types of cells such as reticulocytes (immature red cells) or parasites such as *M. haemofelis*. Once stained, the slide is examined microscopically under both low power and oil immersion (Figure 10.16). Permanent preservation of stained smears allows them to be kept for prolonged periods.

Leishman's stain

1. Place the air-dried slide on a slide rack and cover with Leishman's stain. Leave for 1–2 minutes to fix.
2. Pour on distilled water (using twice the volume of the stain present on the slide) and gently rock the slide to mix the water with the stain.
3. Leave for 15 minutes before washing and flooding the slide with distilled water.
4. Leave the distilled water on the slide for 1 minute (the smear should start to appear pink).
5. Pour off the water.
6. Allow to dry in an upright position.

Giemsa stain

1. Dip the air-dried slide in methanol for a few seconds to fix the cells.
2. Flood slide with Giemsa and leave for 30 minutes.
3. Wash slide in distilled water.
4. Allow to dry in an upright position.

Diff-Quik stain

This stain can also be used for cytology samples, including fine needle aspirates.

1. Dip the air-dried slide into the fixative solution (fast green in methanol) five times.
2. Dip the slide five times into stain solution one (eosin, which is red) and then into stain solution two (thiazine dye, which is purple).
3. Rinse the slide with distilled water.
4. Leave to dry.

When performing a platelet count it may be necessary to dip the slide seven times in the second stain solution to achieve adequate staining.

10.15 Common stains for blood smears.

1. Examine the smear under low power:
    - Assess quality of the smear and find an area where the red cells rarely touch each other (monolayer)
    - Get a general impression of the numbers of white cells present
    - Check for clumping of white cells and platelets at the feather edge.
2. Place a drop of immersion oil on the area currently under examination.
3. Examine smear under oil immersion:
    - Count the numbers of neutrophils, lymphocytes, eosinophils, basophils and monocytes in 200 white cells. The percentage of each cell type is calculated by dividing the number counted by 2
    - Assess red cell morphology (strength of colour, size and shape of cells, size and shape of central pallor)
    - Perform platelet count (count number of platelets in 10 microscopic fields and multiply by 1.5).

10.16 Examination of a blood smear.

Permanent preservation of a blood smear

- **Either place DPX glue on the tail section of the smear and place a coverslip on top**
- **Or use acrylic spray to preserve the whole smear.**

Note: **If glue is used to hold the coverslip, the glue must be allowed to dry before the slide is examined.**

It should be noted that, with the introduction of in-house haematology analysers, examination of blood smears has become extremely important as many of these analysers cannot accurately differentiate the various white blood cell types if there is any change in cell size or morphology. In feline blood, machines sometimes mistake large platelets for red blood cells, providing a result that suggests that there is a reduction in platelet numbers (thrombocytopenia). Examination of a blood smear will confirm the actual platelet count.

White blood cells

White blood cell counts can be performed in the laboratory using dilution in a Unopette to destroy the red cells (Figure 10.17). A haemocytometer is used to count the white cells (Figure 10.18). The percentages of the different types of white cells and other nucleated cells (such as normoblasts) are established by counting the numbers of each cell type in 200 nucleated cells found on a blood smear stained with Leishman's. Differential counts can then be calculated. For example: neutrophil count = (number of neutrophils counted ÷ 200) x total white blood cell count.

Equipment required: Unopette disposable pipette (correct size for WBC); Unopette reservoir of diluent; haemocytometer; blood sample in anticoagulant (EDTA)

Note: The diluting fluid for WBC is 2 ml acetic acid mixed with 1 ml of 1% gentian violet and 97 ml of saline (this fluid results in destruction of the red blood cells).

1. Draw up 25 millilitres of blood (i.e. fill the WBC Unopette pipette), holding the pipette at an angle of 45 degrees.
2. Place pipette in Unopette reservoir of diluent (produces a dilution of 1 in 20).
3. Invert the reservoir to rinse pipette and thoroughly mix contents. Leave for at least 10 minutes to ensure that all the red cells are haemolysed.
4. Reverse pipette and discard the first few drops.
5. Fill the haemocytometer. Using low power (x10), count all white cells seen in squares W, X, Y and Z on the haemocytometer (Figure 10.24). Ignore any white cells touching the bottom and right-hand sides of the square but include those touching the top and left-hand sides.
6. Multiply the total count for all 4 squares by 50 to get the number of white cells/mm³ (equivalent to the number x 10⁶/l).

10.17 White blood cell count using a Unopette.

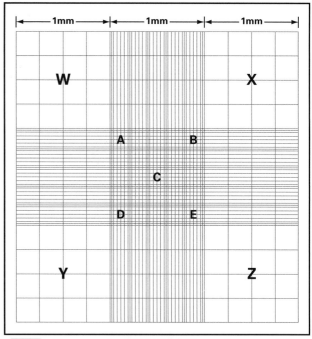

10.18 Haemocytometer grid. To perform a white cell count, the numbers of white cells in the squares marked W, X, Y and Z are totalled and multiplied by 50. When a red cell count is being performed the squares marked A, B, C, D and E are totalled and divided by 100. *Note*: When performing a red cell count, dilute blood to 1 in 200 with 3% sodium citrate and 40% formol saline.

Figures 10.19 and 10.20 demonstrate the appearance of cells found in routine blood smears. White cell morphology varies between species and with the type of stain used.

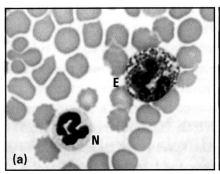
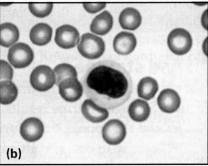
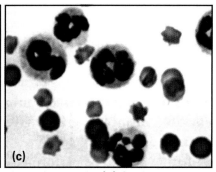

10.19 Appearance of the common white blood cells following staining with Leishman's. **(a)** Canine eosinophil and neutrophil. Note the granular appearance in the cytoplasm of the eosinophil. Both cells have a segmented nucleus. **(b)** Canine lymphocyte. Note the large rounded nucleus with little cytoplasm. **(c)** Feline neutrophils. Note the segmented nuclei. Some of these neutrophils are giant neutrophils, which are produced in association with severe inflammation.

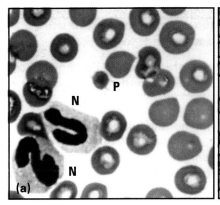
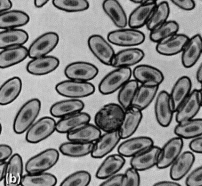

10.20 **(a)** Feline blood smear stained with Diff-Quik. Note the appearance of the neutrophils (N) and platelets (P). Platelets can sometimes be hard to see; if this is a problem, the slide should be dipped into the final stain (purple) seven times instead of five as this increases platelet staining. **(b)** Blood smear from a bird. The red cells are nucleated, which makes it difficult for automated analysers to differentiate them from white blood cells. (b, Courtesy of John Chitty)

Biochemistry

Biochemical analysis is usually performed on serum or heparinized plasma, which has been separated. Since stress or recent feeding can significantly affect the results of biochemical tests, samples should be collected after a 12-hour fast and patient handling should attempt to minimize stress. The presence of lipaemia (cloudy serum due to the presence of fat) and haemolysis (red serum due to red cell destruction)

results in a number of parameters being falsely elevated or decreased. Wherever possible, serum or plasma for biochemical analysis should be separated and examined to ensure that lipaemia and haemolysis are not present. Cats are particularly prone to stress associated with blood collection, resulting in high blood glucose and an increase in white blood cells (neutrophils and lymphocytes). Figure 10.21 lists the conditions associated with common changes in biochemical parameters.

Parameter	High levels	Low levels
Total protein	Dehydration; infection/inflammation; feline infectious peritonitis (FIP); some types of neoplasia	Protein loss (kidney, intestines, skin loss); liver failure; infectious exudate (e.g. pyometra, peritonitis)
Albumin	Dehydration	Protein loss (kidney, intestines, skin loss); liver failure; infectious exudate (e.g. pyometra, peritonitis)
Globulin	Dehydration; infection/inflammation; feline infectious peritonitis (FIP); liver inflammation; some types of neoplasia	Overwhelming infection
Alkaline phosphatase [a]	Young growing animal; steroid administration (dogs); hyperadrenocorticism; liver disease; bone tumours	Not significant
Alanine aminotransferase	Liver disease	Not significant
Bilirubin	Haemolytic anaemia; liver disease; bile duct obstruction	Not significant

10.21 Interpretation of biochemical abnormalities. [a] Treatment with corticosteroids can result in elevations of alkaline phosphatase in the dog. This phenomenon is not seen in the cat. (continues) ▶

Parameter	High levels	Low levels
Creatinine	Kidney disease; dehydration	Muscle wasting
Urea	Kidney disease; dehydration	Low protein diet; liver failure
Glucose [b]	Diabetes mellitus; stress (cats)	Insulin overdose; insulinoma; liver tumour/failure; sample storage
Calcium	Lymphosarcoma; hypoadrenocorticism; kidney failure; hyperparathyroidism; some tumours	Eclampsia; hypoparathyroidism
Inorganic phosphate	Kidney failure; hypoparathyroidism	Hyperparathyroidism
Potassium	Acute renal failure; urethral obstruction; hypoadrenocorticism	Chronic anorexia; kidney disease
Total thyroxine	Hyperthyroidism	Hypothyroidism; any chronic disease

10.21 (continued) Interpretation of biochemical abnormalities. [b] The stress associated with blood sampling can result in an increase in blood glucose levels in the cat.

Urine

Urine collection is a commonly used diagnostic tool in veterinary practice. Veterinary nurses need to be able to advise an owner how to obtain a free flow sample, and assist the veterinary surgeon with cystocentesis. The advantages and disadvantages of different urine collection techniques are shown in Figure 10.22. The tests that can be successfully carried out on the sample will be influenced by the type of urine sample container and preservative selected (Figure 10.23); the correct choice is therefore imperative.

Method of collection	Advantages	Disadvantages
Free-flow (midstream)	Easy and can be performed by owners Useful for routine monitoring (e.g. diabetic patients)	Contamination by surface bacteria, cells and discharges very likely Unsuitable for bacteriology Relies on patient urinating sufficient volumes Does not guarantee complete bladder emptying
Catheterization	Minimizes contamination from external genitalia and urethra Useful for collection of small volumes of urine from the bladder Guarantees complete bladder emptying	Cannot be used in patients with infections of the genitalia or lower urinary tact May cause damage to the urethra in patients with obstructions Sample will not be completely sterile
Cystocentesis	Sterile method of urine collection (best for bacteriology) Allows urine to be collected from patients with urethral obstruction	Requires adequate restraint Requires palpable or adequately filled bladder (unless ultrasound guidance is available) Cannot empty bladder completely May result in blood contamination Must be performed by veterinary surgeon Bladder palpation must be avoided after the technique

10.22 Advantages and disadvantages of different methods for urine collection.

Preservative	Comments	Type of analysis
Thymol	Will preserve urine for 24 hours	Biochemistry (except glucose) and sediment – but kills bacteria
Toluene or HCL	A thin layer over the surface – TOXIC	Biochemistry
Boric acid	Provided in commercial sample bottles Use 200 mg to 10 ml of urine	Bacteriology
Formalin	1–2 ml formalin to 15 ml of urine – TOXIC	Sediment (kills bacteria and alters protein results)

10.23 Preservatives that can be used in urine samples. (*Urine samples should be examined fresh.*)

Collection of urine samples

Free-flow samples

This technique is useful for many parameters, but it is unsuitable when a sample is required for bacteriology. A midstream sample gives the best representation of bladder contents and reduces contamination. The initial flow is likely to contain surface bacteria and preputial, prostate or vaginal fluids.

Equipment:

- Gloves
- Dogs: a shallow clean dish (kidney dish) or commercial urine collecting receptacle
- Cats: a litter tray, either empty or with 'washable litter' (see below)
- Sterile universal container.

It is important to ensure that containers and litter trays used for urine sample collection have been thoroughly rinsed and have not been cleaned with bleach, as this will alter the pH.

Technique

- Dog: keep on a lead and attempt to catch a midstream sample of urine in the dish.
- Cats: use an empty litter tray, or a tray filled with pre-washed and disinfected fish tank pebbles, or commercial pebbles.
- Decant urine into universal container and test urine as soon as possible.

If a urine sample cannot be obtained in this manner, gently squeezing the bladder (manual expression) may encourage patients to urinate. Patients must have at least 10–15 ml of urine in the bladder if this technique is to be successful. *Nurses should always check with a veterinary surgeon before using this method, as it is contraindicated in cases of urinary obstruction or local trauma.*

1. Palpate caudal abdomen to locate and determine size of bladder.
2. Apply gentle constant pressure (may be required for a few minutes before the patient will urinate).
3. Collect urine.

Catheterization

A urinary catheter is passed up the urethra and into the bladder to obtain a urine sample. Catheterization minimizes contamination from the external genitalia and urethra and therefore is preferred over free-flow samples if bacteriological examination is required. This method can also be used when there are small amounts of urine within the bladder, or when complete emptying of the bladder is required.

Catheterization is contraindicated if vaginitis or open pyometra are evident as infection may be introduced into the bladder.

Equipment:

- Gloves
- Sterile catheter
- Cotton wool and antiseptic

- Kidney dish
- Speculum (bitches – optional)
- Sterile urine sample bottles.

Technique

1. Once the patient has been catheterized, the initial flow of urine is directed into a kidney dish.
2. A midstream sample is taken directly into a sterile universal sample bottle and the lid is secured.
3. The sample is labelled appropriately.

Cystocentesis

Cystocentesis is the removal of urine directly from the bladder using a needle and is performed *by a veterinary surgeon.* Cystocentesis prevents the sample becoming contaminated by the urethra or genitalia and is therefore used to obtain a sample for bacteriology. It can also be used to drain the bladder in an obstructive emergency. Blood contamination of the sample can be a problem if the needle enters a blood vessel.

Equipment:

- Gloves
- Clippers
- Aseptic technique
- Sterile syringe
- Three-way tap
- Sterile needle (usually 21 gauge x 1–1½-inch, depending on size and obesity of the patient)
- Sterile urine sample containers.

Patient preparation

- Cats:
  - Position and restrain the animal, usually standing or in lateral recumbency (standing is usually better tolerated)
  - Clipping is not routinely performed for this procedure in cats.
- Dogs:
  - Position and restrain the animal, usually in dorsal recumbency
  - Clip an area 5–8 cm square around the midline of the caudal abdomen
  - Prepare skin aseptically.

Technique

The veterinary nurse's role is to assist prior to and following the actual procedure.

1. The bladder is palpated, and held steady through the abdominal wall.
2. In dogs, the needle is inserted to one side of the midline and directed slightly caudally into the bladder. In cats, the bladder is stabilized and the needle is inserted into the body of the bladder with the needle directed slightly caudally.
3. The plunger is withdrawn to obtain a sample.
4. The needle is removed from the skin, and pressure is applied at the site of penetration to prevent leakage of urine.

5. The contents of the syringe are evacuated into sterile universal containers and labelled immediately.

Note that bladder palpation should be avoided after cystocentesis.

Preservation and storage

Urine samples should be examined *immediately*, or within 30 minutes of collection. Storage of urine results in increased pH and bacterial number and spontaneous crystal formation. Bacteria in the urine utilize any glucose present and may therefore mask glucosuria. Crystals multiply and cells lyse in samples stored in a refrigerator (4°C). Samples can be preserved with the use of certain chemicals (see Figure 10.23).

Urine examination

A number of tests are routinely performed on urine. The method of each test is summarized in Figure 10.24. A refractometer should be used to measure urine specific gravity as dipstick estimations of specific gravity are inaccurate. Microscopic examination should be performed on freshly prepared sediment. If cytological examination is required, air-dried smears are stained; for crystals a wet preparation is examined. Common findings and their clinical significance are described in Figure 10.25.

Examination	Method
Visual inspection	Assess colour and turbidity (cloudiness)
Specific gravity (SG)	1. To calibrate refractometer, place distilled water beneath plastic cover of refractometer. 2. Adjust until SG = 1.000 and then dry refractometer. 3. Place urine under plastic cover of refractometer. 4. Read SG (the point where blue area turns to white; in the example (right) the SG is 1.024). 5. Rinse and dry refractometer. *Note*: Dipstick assessment of SG is inaccurate
Dipstick analysis (pH, glucose, ketones, protein, bilirubin)	1. Invert urine sample to ensure thorough mixing. 2. Cover all squares on dipstick with urine and note time. 3. Read dipstick results at times indicated on barrel. *Note*: Dipstick SG is inaccurate and dipsticks will not detect all types of ketones
Microscopic examination of sediment	Examine as soon as possible after collection 1. Centrifuge 10 ml at 2000 rpm for 5 minutes. 2. Remove supernatant and re-suspend sediment by tapping tube. *Wet preparation:* ■ Place a drop of suspension on a slide and stain with new methylene blue if necessary ■ Place a cover slip over the urine *Dry preparation:* ■ Make a smear using a drop of re-suspended sediment ■ Rapidly air-dry and stain with Leishman's stain

10.24 Summary of the tests used in routine urinalysis.

Abnormalities	Appearance	Significance
Cells		
Pyuria	Large numbers of WBC, usually neutrophils	Suggests urinary tract inflammation. Look for bacteria
Haematuria	Large numbers of RBC. May be crenated (star-shaped) or lysed, depending on urine concentration	Bleeding into the urogenital tract
Epithelial cells	Flat, irregular squamous cells with a small nucleus	Normal cells shed from the urethra, vagina or vulva
Transitional cells	Round small epithelial cells	May suggest urinary tract infection or neoplasia if found in large clumps

10.25 Appearance and clinical significance of common findings on microscopic examination of urine sediment. Further details can be found in the BSAVA *Manual of Canine and Feline Nephrology and Urology*. (continues) ▶

Abnormalities	Appearance	Significance
Casts (*worm-shaped structures*)		
Hyaline	Colourless, cylindrical	Mild tubular inflammation; pyrexia. Least significant type of cast
Cellular	Contain RBC, WBC, epithelial cells or a mixture	Renal tubular disease
Granular	Contain remnants of epithelial cells and WBC resulting in a granular appearance	Significant inflammation
Waxy	Opaque and wider than hyaline casts	Various renal diseases
Crystalluria (*Figure 10.26*)		
Struvite (triple phosphate)	Colourless 'coffin-lid' Alkaline urine	Common in normal cats and dogs. Associated with infection or calculi in some cases
Calcium oxalate	Colourless 'envelopes' or small stars Acid urine	May be normal. Associated with calculi or ethylene glycol toxicity
Calcium carbonate	Yellow to colourless spherules or dumbbells	Rare in dogs and cats. Common in herbivores
Ammonium urate	Yellow-brown 'thorn apples'	Normal in Dalmatians. Associated with calculi and liver failure
Uric acid	Prisms or rosettes	Common in Dalmatians, may be normal in other pets. Associated with calculi

10.25 (continued) Appearance and clinical significance of common findings on microscopic examination of urine sediment. Further details can be found in the *BSAVA Manual of Canine and Feline Nephrology and Urology.*

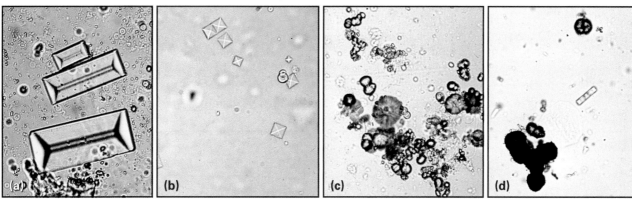

10.26 Microscopic appearance of some of the common urinary crystals. **(a)** Struvite (triple phosphate) crystals. **(b)** Calcium oxalate crystals. **(c)** Calcium carbonate crystals. **(d)** Ammonium urate crystals.

Faeces

Faecal samples may be required to aid diagnosis in gastrointestinal disease and it is important that samples are collected and examined fresh to obtain accurate results. Faeces are routinely examined for undigested food material and endoparasites. Faecal culture is performed to identify selected faecal pathogens such as *Salmonella* and *Campylobacter*.

It should be noted that many faecal pathogens and some faecal parasites are zoonotic. Extra care should be taken when handling the faeces of animals with suspected zoonotic diseases.

Collection

The sample can be obtained per rectum but, more commonly, freshly passed faeces are collected (Figure 10.27).

Equipment required: Suitable sterile container; gloves; perhaps a disposable spatula

1. Collect a *fresh* sample.
2. Fill container as full as possible – this *reduces desiccation of faeces or parasites, and reduces bacterial growth.*
3. Label the container (if an owner is collecting the sample, pre-labelling the container is useful).
4. Sample should be examined immediately, or refrigerated if this it not possible.
5. All the equipment used should be returned for disposal as clinical waste if infectious disease is suspected.

10.27 Collection and storage of freshly passed faeces.

Collection of samples per rectum

Per rectum collection of faecal samples ensures that fresh uncontaminated faeces are obtained for immediate examination. This procedure is, however, uncomfortable for the patient.

1. Clean and lubricate the perineal area (to prevent introduction of skin cells/bacteria).
2. Lubricate a gloved finger and insert it gently into the rectum – do not use force.
3. Obtain sample and fill and label container.

Storage

If faeces cannot be examined immediately, they should be stored in an airtight container or in the refrigerator. Faecal swabs for bacteriology can be stored in the refrigerator prior to despatch to an external laboratory.

Examination

Figure 10.28 describes the method and indications for in-house tests performed on faeces. Figure 10.29 shows the appearance of common faecal parasites.

Examination	Indications	Method
Gross examination	Preliminary assessment	Assess: ■ Consistency and colour ■ Presence of mucus or fat ■ Presence of specific material (worms, foreign material, undigested food)
Direct smear	Parasitic burden Undigested starch or muscle fibres	1. Place one drop of saline and one drop of faeces on slide. 2. Mix thoroughly, remove any large pieces of faecal material. 3. Smear and heat-fix, or cover with a cover slip. 4. Stain by placing a drop of stain at corner of cover slip and allow to spread. 5. Use 2% Lugol's iodine for starch (blue–black). 6. Use eosin, new methylene blue, Wright's for undigested muscle fibres. 7. Look for worm eggs under low power and protozoa under medium power (Figure 10.29).
Faecal flotation	Worm eggs Protozoa	1. Mix faeces with saturated sugar or zinc sulphate ($ZnSO_4$) solution [a]. (*Note*: Zinc sulphate flotation must be used for *Giardia* as other suspensions will cause destruction of this organism). 2. Ova and cysts will rise to surface, but centrifugation will improve sensitivity. 3. Examine supernatant within 15 minutes if looking for *Giardia*.
Faecal fat	Undigested fat	1. Mix one drop of fresh faeces with one drop of Sudan III on a glass slide. 2. Examine microscopically. 3. Undigested fat will be seen as orange droplets.

10.28 Common faecal examinations. [a] $ZnSO_4$ solution is made by mixing 331g of $ZnSO_4$ in 1 litre of water.

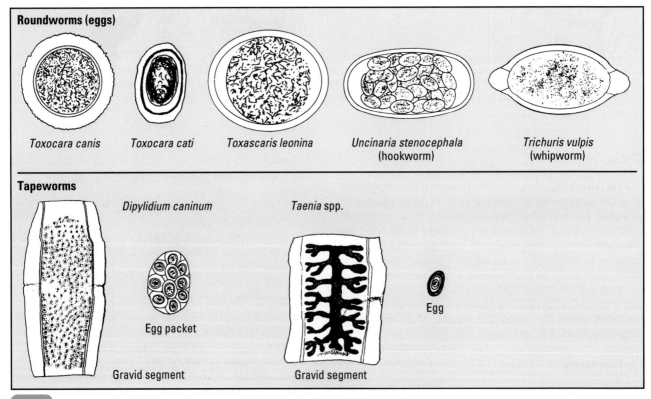

Roundworms (eggs)

Toxocara canis Toxocara cati Toxascaris leonina Uncinaria stenocephala (hookworm) Trichuris vulpis (whipworm)

Tapeworms

Dipylidium caninum Taenia spp.

Egg packet

Egg

Gravid segment Gravid segment

10.29 Identification of the common intestinal parasites of dogs and cats.

Body fluids

Body fluids are often needed for diagnostic purposes and the veterinary nurse's role is to help to prepare the patient and assist the veterinary surgeon. Samples may be submitted for cytology (EDTA), protein analysis (heparin or plain) or bacteriology (sterile plain tubes or swabs). *Collection of all body fluids must be performed by a veterinary surgeon* and they should be collected aseptically to avoid introducing infection.

Abdominal/peritoneal paracentesis

Equipment:

- Sterile 21–23 gauge needle x 1–2 inches
- Sterile 10–20 ml syringe
- Three-way tap
- Sample tubes (plain and EDTA)
- Kidney dish to drain fluid for therapeutic reasons
- Clippers.

Patient preparation

1. Clip ventral abdomen from the umbilicus caudally about 7.5 cm and about 5 cm either side of the midline.
2. Scrub using aseptic surgical technique.
3. Position patient in dorsal or lateral recumbency, or standing.
4. The needle is inserted to one side of midline slightly behind the umbilicus and suction is applied to obtain a sample.

Thoracocentesis

Equipment:

- Sterile 18 gauge x $^3/_4$–1-inch needle (or over-the-needle catheter). In cats, 21 gauge butterfly catheters are often used
- Sterile syringe and three-way tap
- Tube to attach to drainage luer of three-way tap and feed into a bowl of water (recommended to reduce chance of air entering the chest)
- Clippers
- Scalpel blade and suture (for over-the-needle catheter only)
- Kidney dish for removal of fluid for therapeutic reasons
- Sample tubes (plain and EDTA).

Patient preparation
Sedation may be required.

1. Place patient in lateral or ventral recumbency or standing.
2. Clip costal area on the right side two-thirds of the way down the chest for fluid, over the 7th to 10th ribs.
3. In dogs, local anaesthetic is injected subcutaneously and into the intercostal space.
4. Scrub using aseptic surgical technique.

The site for thoracocentesis is the 7th intercostal space (entering the skin over the 8th intercostal space).

Cerebrospinal fluid (CSF)

Cerebrospinal fluid samples are sometimes taken to aid diagnosis of neurological problems.

 WARNING
This technique is contraindicated in head trauma and increased intracranial pressure.

The area most commonly sampled is between the occipital crest and cervical vertebra 1; less commonly, the area between the 6th and 7th lumbar spaces (dog), and the lumbosacral space (cat) are used.

Equipment:

- 20 gauge 1–3-inch hypodermic or spinal needle, depending on patient size
- Clippers
- Sample tubes (EDTA and plain).

Patient preparation
General anaesthesia is required.

1. Place the patient in lateral recumbency.
2. Clip from occipital protuberance of skull to behind lateral wings of C1.
3. Prepare the site aseptically.
4. The patient is placed with neck flexed without twisting, and held straight in all planes and very still.

Arthrocentesis

This technique is used to collect joint fluid, which is normally clear or slightly yellow.

Equipment:

- Sterile 23–25 gauge x 1-inch needle
- 2 ml syringe
- Clippers
- Sample tubes and clean slides.

Patient preparation
General anaesthesia is required.

1. Position the patient in lateral recumbency with joint in flexion.
2. Clip adequately around joint.
3. Prepare clipped area aseptically.

Sample submission

- Decant sample from syringe into selected sample tubes.
- Label appropriately, including source of sample.
- For in-house analysis: smear sample on to slide and stain with Leishman's for cytology.
- For external laboratory: centrifuge sample, pipette off the supernatant and decant the deposit (concentrated cells and bacteria) into suitable tube.

Fine needle aspiration

Fine needle aspirates are often collected from lymph nodes and skin lumps. They can also be collected by veterinary surgeons from internal organs or masses, usually under ultrasound guidance (see also Chapter 13).

Equipment:

- Sterile 25 gauge x 1-inch needle (longer needles may be required for internal organs or masses)
- 5 ml or 10 ml syringe
- Clippers and spirit
- Clean slides.

Technique

This is described in Figure 10.30.

Skin and hair sampling

Skin sampling is used both for definitive diagnosis and for assessment of treatment protocols in dermatoses. Dermatological diagnosis is frequently achieved by performing a number of diagnostic tests to eliminate various causes. The common dermatological tests are described in Figures 10.31 to 10.33. Skin parasites that can be diagnosed using some of these methods are described in Figures 10.34 to 10.36 and illustrated in Figure 10.37. Since some external parasites and fungal infections are zoonotic (i.e. can be transmitted from animals to humans), knowledge of the life cycle, host specificity and zoonotic risk allows appropriate advice to be given to persons likely to come into contact with the affected animal. Skin swabs may be collected (Figure 10.39) and stained with Gram stain (Figure 10.40).

---

1. Lay out at least five slides on a clean surface and draw back an empty 10 ml syringe.
2. Clip the area to be aspirated and clean with spirit.
3. Immobilize the mass if possible (aspirates of body organs should be performed with ultrasound guidance).

Needle-only technique:
1. Insert the needle into the mass and move it rapidly in and out (to ensure cells are broken away from the tissue).
2. Remove the needle and attach to a syringe containing 10 ml of air.

Fine needle aspirate with suction:
1. With the needle attached to the syringe, insert the needle into the mass.
2. Draw back on the syringe to the 5 ml mark (this should be quite difficult because of negative pressure created).
3. Whilst maintaining suction, move the needle around within the mass.
4. Release suction before removing the needle from the mass.
5. Remove needle from end of syringe, draw 10 ml air into the syringe and reattach to the needle.

Making the smear:
1. With the bevel of the needle facing down squirt out the contents of the needle on to one end of a clean slide.
2. Make a smear or a squash preparation.

10.30 How to obtain a fine needle aspirate.

Test	Indications	Equipment	Technique
Hand-held lens examination	Fleas, flea dirt, lice, and *Cheyletiella*	Low-power hand-held magnifying lens	Examine skin and hair with lens
Wood's lamp	Some strains of *Microsporum canis* fluoresce when exposed to ultra violet (u/v) light	Wood's lamp (ideally double tube); gloves; protective clothing; dark room	Allow lamp to warm up (5–10 minutes). In a dark room, expose hairs for 3–5 minutes (some are slow to respond). 50% of *Microsporum canis* will fluoresce apple green in colour. If positive, perform hair plucking and culture on dermatophyte test medium, Sabouraud's medium, or send to outside laboratory. *Note:* Some bacteria, skin debris or certain drugs may fluoresce and give false positive results.
Coat brushing	Fleas, lice, *Cheyletiella*, dermatophytes (ringworm)	Fine-toothed comb; paper for collection of material; microscope slides; liquid paraffin; pipette; cover slips; microscope	Stand the patient over paper. Groom animal's coat with comb. Examine debris with hand-held magnifying lens. Place some debris on a slide with a drop of liquid paraffin and apply a cover slip. Examine under low power microscope. Use damp cotton wool to examine suspected flea dirt (turns reddish brown at edge of dirt). Samples for an outside laboratory should go into paper packs, e.g. Dermpacks
Mackenzie brush	Dermatophytes or spores of dermatophytes	Mackenzie brush; growth medium	*Sterile* toothbrush is brushed through coat to collect hairs. Press toothbrush on to dermatophyte test medium or Sabouraud's medium for culture

10.31 Common skin and hair sampling procedures. (continues) ▶

Test	Indications	Equipment	Technique
Skin scraping	For detection of all mites, particularly those living deep in the skin	Scissors or clippers; liquid paraffin; pipette; scalpel blade (size 10 or 15); microscope slides; cover slips; microscope	See Figure 10.32. Potassium hydroxide is sometimes used as it decolorizes skin and hair; however, it is caustic and kills the mites, making them hard to see
Hair plucking	Samples for fungal culture or trichograms, dermatophytes (ringworm), occasionally *Demodex*	Broad-rimmed epilation forceps; slides; liquid paraffin; gloves	Look for hairs immersed in scale and crust. Pluck single, entire hairs from the edges of lesions, using epilation *For in-house examination:* Place hair on slide. Add liquid paraffin or stain (lactophenol cotton blue or Quink black/blue ink). Examine under microscope. Affected material including hair shaft will stain blue *For an outside laboratory:* Place hair sample in clearly labelled paper envelope
Sticky tape preparation	Lice and *Cheyletiella*	Scissors or clippers; clear sticky tape (19 mm wide); liquid paraffin; microscope slides; microscope	See Figure 10.33
	Malassezia and bacteria	As above plus: Scotch tape 19 mm – other tapes unsuitable for staining Diff-Quik or Rapi-Diff stains; tissues; microscope; immersion oil	See Figure 10.33
Impression smears	Cytological assessment or *Demodex*	Microscope slide; microscope	Slide is pressed directly against lesion and smeared. Air-dry slide. Stain for cytology. Examine under microscope
Fine needle aspiration	*Demodex*, bacteria, cytology	Sterile 5 ml syringe; sterile 25 gauge needle; microscope slides; cover slip; microscope	Aspirate pustule or nodule contents using a sterile syringe and needle. Express contents on to slide. Smear or place cover slip on top. Examine under microscope
Skin biopsies	Histopathology, dermatophytes, *Malassezia*, bacteria and occasionally mites	Biopsy punch or scalpel blade and handle; sterile swabs; 10% formalin in wide-mouthed container; shiny card; sterile needle; suture material and instruments	See Figure 10.38

10.31 (continued) Common skin and hair sampling procedures.

Sedation under veterinary direction if required (e.g. for scrapes from face, feet or painful lesions).

1. Select areas of lesional skin (erythema, papules, scaling, alopecia).
2. Clip hair *carefully* with scissors or clippers, taking care *not* to touch the skin surface.
3. Pipette a drop of liquid paraffin on to skin or scalpel blade.
4. Gently pinch up skin at selected site to help extrude mites/bacteria.
5. Hold skin flat and taut and scrape with the scalpel blade at angle of 90 degrees to the skin until capillary ooze is seen. ***Always scrape several sites.***
6. Transfer scraping on to microscope slide(s). If the material on the slide is too thick it will be difficult to see anything. Divide material between slides.
7. Add a small amount of liquid paraffin and apply cover slip.
8. Clean scrape sites with dilute antiseptic.
9. Examine slide(s) first under low power (x4) magnification to increase scanning speed. Use with condenser low, and light beam diaphragm half-closed to closed to optimize contrast.
10. Increase magnification to x10 and systematically examine slide.

Note: Some types of mite are found in small numbers in normal animals. Some mites require collection of deep skin scrapes, whilst others can be detected on superficial skin scrapes (see Figure 10.34).
The appearance of the common mites is described in Figure 10.35 and illustrated in Figure 10.37.

10.32 Preparation and examination of a skin scraping.

For lice and *Cheyletiella*:	For *Malassezia* and bacteria:
1. Select areas of dry scaly skin and scurfy hair. 2. Clip hair carefully avoiding skin surface. 3. Apply sticky surface of adhesive tape to skin and base of hairs. 4. Add a small drop of liquid paraffin to a microscope slide. 5. Place tape (sticky side down) on to microscope slide. 6. Examine immediately using low power objective.	1. Select area of greasy, erythematous skin (axillae, inguinal and interdigital regions). 2. Clip hair *carefully*. 3. Apply sticky surface of adhesive tape several times to skin. 4. Stain sticky tape with Diff-Quik (Figure 10.15). 5. Attach tape, sticky side down, to microscope slide. 6. Cover with paper tissues and exert gentle pressure to remove excess fluid. 7. Examine immediately using x40 or x100 under oil immersion.

10.33   Sticky tape preparations.

Mite	Host	Diagnostic test	Significance
Demodex canis	Dog	Found deep within the follicles, so skin should be squeezed before performing deep skin scraping	Small numbers found in normal dogs. Many mites and immature forms confirm infection
Demodex cati	Cat	Found deep within the follicles, so skin should be squeezed before performing deep skin scraping	Rare
Sarcoptes scabiei	Dog	Lives in epidermal burrows, so multiple deep scrapings required. Take multiple skin scrapings from elbow, ear or sites with papules	Presence of even one mite is diagnostic
Notoedres cati	Cat	Single skin scrape of eyes, ear or face	Causes feline scabies (mange)
Cheyletiella	Cat Dog	Can be seen with naked eye as walking dandruff. Superficial skin scrapes or sticky tape preparations or coat brushings useful	Always significant and can be zoonotic
Otodectes	Cat Dog	Mites visible to naked eye. Superficial scrapings, smears of ear wax or sticky tape preparations helpful	Common cause of ear problems, but can also cause generalized problem

10.34   Diagnosis and significance of mites of the dog and cat.

Parasite	Parasite appearance	Clinical signs	Usual distribution
Ctenocephalides fleas	**Eggs:** small brown laterally compressed **Flea dirt:** brown granules turn red when wet	Pruritus **Acute:** wheals and erythema **Chronic:** seborrhoea, lichenification, alopecia	**Dogs:** dorsum (especially lumbosacral area) and ventrum **Cats:** milliary (generalized) dermatitis or focal eosinophilic granuloma (pink plaque)
Diptera (flies)	**Larvae:** many forms	**Mild:** local wheal **Severe:** 'fly-strike'	Anus, genitalia, wounds, etc.
Linognathus louse	**Eggs:** small, white, attached to hair ('nits') **Adults:** sucking lice with typical fixed piercing mouth-parts	**Mild:** asymptomatic carrier **Severe:** papules, crusts, seborrhoea sicca	Under matted hair and around body orifices
Trichodectes louse	**Adults:** biting lice with broad head; chewing mouth-parts on ventral aspect	**Mild:** asymptomatic carrier **Severe:** papules, crusts, seborrhoea sicca	Under matted hair and around body orifices
Cheyletiella fur mite	**Eggs:** loosely attached to hair **Adults:** large white 'walking dandruff'	**Mild:** asymptomatic carrier **Severe:** mild, non-suppurative dermatitis	Diffuse but usually more dorsal
Sarcoptes scabies mite	**Adults:** round-bodied mite	Intense pruritus Alopecia, scales and crusts	Ventrum, ears and elbows
Notoedres cati feline scabies mite	Resembles *Sarcoptes*	Pruritus Lichenification, crusting, alopecia	Head, ears and neck, occasionally generalized
Otodectes ear mite	**Adults:** white dots visible to naked eye	**Ears:** otitis externa **Generalized:** may mimic flea allergic dermatitis	Ears, occasionally generalized

10.35   Microscopic appearance, distribution and clinical signs of common external parasites of dogs and cats. (continues) ▶

Parasite	Parasite appearance	Clinical signs	Usual distribution
Demodex demodectic mange mite	**Adults:** small cigar-shaped mites Four stages of life cycle may be present	Mild erythema, alopecia May be pruritic if secondary pyoderma present	Localized (especially face and forelimbs) or generalized
Ixodes tick	**Adults:** flattened, ovoid, yellow-white to red-brown	Asymptomatic carrier or mild local irritation (especially if incompletely removed)	Ears, face and ventral body

10.35 (continued) Microscopic appearance, distribution and clinical signs of common external parasites of dogs and cats.

Parasite	Common name	Incidence	Appearance and significance
Found on ferrets			
Ctenocephalides felis	Cat flea	Common	
Otodectes cynotis	Ear mite	Common	
Found on rabbits			
Cheyletiella parasitovorax	Fur mite 'walking dandruff'	Very common (also found on chinchilla)	Scaling ++, 'dandruff' ++
Spillopsyllus cuniculi	Rabbit flea	Common	Small dark fleas; carry myxomatosis virus. May occur transiently on cats
Psoroptes cuniculi	Rabbit ear mite	Common	Cause scaling ++, debris in external canal and pain ++
Dipteran flies	Blue-bottles	Common	Maggots cause fly strike
Listrophorus gibbus	Fur mite	Not common	Not very pathogenic
Haemodipsus ventricosus	Lice	Not common	Pruritus ++
Found on guinea pigs			
Trixacarus caviae	Guinea pig mite	Common	Pruritus ++, scaling +, hair loss. Clinical signs often secondary to hypovitaminosis C
Gliricola porcelli, Gyropus ovalis	Lice	Not very common	Puritus and hair loss once infestation significant
Found on hamsters			
Demodex criceti		Common	Hair loss and scaling usually secondary to immunosuppression
Found on rats and mice			
Notoedres muris	Mange mite	Very common	Scabs over ears and shoulders
Radfordia affinis, Myobia musculi	Fur mites	Quite common	Fur loss, pruritus
Found on birds			
Cnemidocoptes pili	Scaly face mite of budgerigars	Common	Scaling of all featherless areas (also causes 'scaly leg' in poultry)
Dermanyssus gallinae	Red mite	Common in poultry, less so in other birds	Lives off the birds; feeds on them at night. Causes pruritus and loss of condition/anaemia
Ornithonyssus sylvarium	Northern mite of canaries	Common in colony situations	May cause death of whole nests of young birds (can also affect poultry)
Various species	Feather lice	Common	Mainly seen in wild birds
Found on reptiles			
Ophionyssus natricis	Snake mite	Common in colonies	Causes pruritus. Hard to see as they are under scales
Various species	Ticks; leeches (aquatic hosts)	Rare	Seen only on recently imported animals

10.36 Common ectoparasites of small mammals, birds and reptiles.

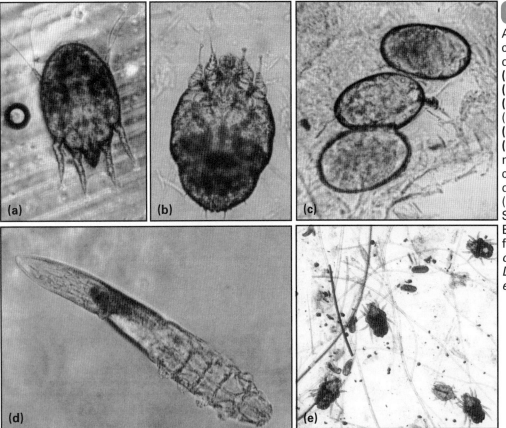

10.37 Appearance of the common mites of the dog and cat. **(a)** *Otodectes*. **(b)** *Sarcoptes* adult. **(c)** *Sarcoptes* eggs (high magnification). **(d)** *Demodex*. **(e)** *Cheyletiella yasguri* mites and eggs collected from the dorsum of a Boxer. (a–d, © A. Foster/ S. Shaw, University of Bristol; e, reproduced from *BSAVA Manual of Small Animal Dermatology, 2nd edn.*)

1. Clip hair carefully, avoiding skin.
2. Collect sample, using biopsy punch or an elliptical incision.
3. Blot off excess fluid with a sterile swab (so that it does not slip off the card).
4. Using a sterile needle, place dermal layer in contact with shiny card.
5. Place in 10% formalin immediately (cells deteriorate very quickly if left exposed to air).
6. Close skin with a single suture.

10.38 How to obtain a skin biopsy sample.

Equipment required: sterile 25 gauge needle (for pustules); sterile bacteriological swab; slides (for in-house examination)

1. Select lesions or areas where bacterial infection is suspected. Intact pustules are better than open lesions as there is less contamination.
2. Select correct type of swab with transport medium (for bacteriology).
3. If the pustule is intact, rupture it with a sterile needle.
4. Break the seal and remove swab without touching the edges, handling the lid only.
5. Rub the tip over or into the affected area.
6. Replace in the tube immediately.
7. Label the tube.
8. Make smear sample for examination, or package and dispatch to outside laboratory.

10.39 Collection of skin swab samples.

1. Prepare a heat-fixed smear.
2. Flood the slide with crystal violet and leave for 1 minute.
3. Wash off stain with Lugol's iodine, holding the slide at an angle.
4. Flood slide with Lugol's iodine and leave for 1 minute.
5. Pour off iodine and rinse with distilled water.
6. Hold the slide at a slight angle and pour on 95% alcohol until the stain no longer discolours the alcohol.
7. Immediately rinse the slide under running tap water to prevent excessive decolorization.
8. Flood with carbol fuchsin (which acts as a counter-stain) for 1 minute.
9. Rinse the slide and gently blot dry.

10.40 Method of performing a Gram stain.

Bacteriology

Bacteriology smears

Smears can be prepared from fluid samples, from swabs or from bacterial colonies grown on culture plates. The shape and staining characteristics will identify the type of bacterium. Appropriate antibiotics can often be selected on the basis of bacterial shape and appearance on Gram staining. Specific stains are used to identify families of bacteria. For example, Ziehl–Neelson stain is used to identify acid-fast bacteria such as the mycobacteria responsible for tuberculosis.

Bacterial culture

Many bacteria can be grown on blood–agar plates at 37°C. The plate is inoculated using a heat-sterilized metal loop to spread the sample across the plate. It is important to ensure that the loop has cooled before allowing it to contact the sample, since heat may destroy the bacteria within the sample. Streaking is used to ensure that the concentration of bacterial colonies is low enough in some areas of the plate to allow single colony identification (Figure 10.41). Some bacteria produce distinct colonies, which can be identified by their appearance on an agar plate.

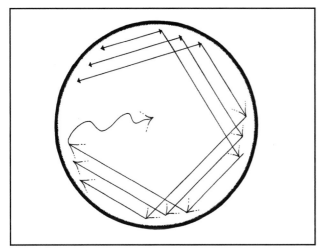

10.41 Inoculating an agar plate using the streaking method. The loop should be flamed and cooled between each 'streaking'.

Virology samples

Virus detection is now commonly performed in veterinary practice. Desktop kits are available for detecting feline leukaemia virus, feline immunodeficiency virus and canine parvovirus. External laboratories can perform tests for many other viral diseases. The tests available for commonly encountered viruses are listed in Figure 10.42.

Histopathological and biopsy samples

Samples of body tissue can be submitted for histopathological examination, but must be preserved immediately to be suitable for examination. For routine histopathological examination, either neutral buffered formalin (10% solution of 40% formaldehyde and buffers in distilled water) or 10% formol saline (40% formaldehyde in saline) can be used, but neutral buffered formalin is generally preferred as it reduces artefacts. Tissue samples should be small (<1 cm square) as poor cell preservation, resulting in cell death and destruction (necrosis), will occur if larger samples are preserved by this method. Each tissue sample should be placed in at least ten times the volume of formalin. For example: a piece of liver 1 cm square should be placed in a minimum of 10 ml of formalin. 'Fixing' a sample often causes it to swell slightly and harden; therefore the neck of the container must be wide enough to ensure that the sample can be removed with ease.

Equipment:

- Surgical kit
- Preservative – a minimum of *10 times the volume* of the sample
- Bowl containing preservative – for fixing the sample before transfer to sealed container (a minimum of 24 hours to fix) if required
- *Wide-necked* container.

It must be remembered that samples to be submitted by standard post cannot exceed 50 ml in volume.

Cadavers for postmortem examination

Cadavers should be chilled and transported to the laboratory as soon as possible. Autolysis (postmortem decomposition) will occur if the temperature and humidity are not reduced and the cadaver is not examined quickly.

Virus	In-house tests available	Samples required for external testing
Feline leukaemia virus (FeLV)	Desktop kits available for testing blood or saliva. Plasma or serum tests are more accurate than those using whole blood	Whole blood in heparin
Feline immunodeficiency virus (FIV)	Desktop kits available for testing blood. Plasma or serum tests are more accurate than those using whole blood	Whole blood in heparin
Feline infectious peritonitis (FIP)	None	Serum and/or abdominal fluid for coronavirus antibody titres
Feline calicivirus (FCV)	None	Oropharyngeal swab (in viral transport medium)
Feline herpesvirus (FHV)	None	Oropharyngeal swab (in viral transport medium)
Feline panleucopenia	Canine parvovirus faecal antigen test may detect virus in some cases	Serum (two samples 4 weeks apart) and/or faeces
Canine parvovirus	Canine parvovirus faecal antigen test	Serum and faeces
Canine distemper virus (CDV)	None	Serum (two samples 4 weeks apart)

10.42 Tests available for the common viral diseases of the dog and cat.

Toxicology

Each toxin suspected may require the collection of specific samples. It is therefore vital that the external laboratory performing the tests is contacted to ensure that the correct samples are submitted. In general the following guidelines apply.

- Specimens must be collected fresh and free from environmental contamination.
- Sample containers must be sterile and chemical free.
- Label with the usual details and the practice name and address.
- Freeze all samples (except those for histopathology) and post on ice to the laboratory.
- Accurate historical and clinical records must be sent with the samples.

Further reading

Bush BM (1975) *Veterinary Laboratory Manual*. William Heinemann Medical Books, London

Bush BM (1991) *Interpretation of Laboratory Results for Small Animal Clinicians*. Blackwell Science, Oxford

Day MJ, Mackin A and Littlewood J (2000) *BSAVA Manual of Canine and Feline Haematology and Transfusion Medicine*. BSAVA Publications, Gloucester

Harvey JH (2001) *Atlas of Veterinary Hematology: Blood and Bone Marrow of Domestic Animals*. WB Saunders, Philadelphia

Kerr M (2002) *Veterinary Laboratory Medicine, 2nd edn*. Blackwell, Oxford

Meyer D and Harvey J (1998) *Veterinary Laboratory Medicine. Interpretation and Diagnosis, 2nd edn*. WB Saunders, Philadelphia

Villiers E and Blackwood L (2005) *BSAVA Manual of Clinical Pathology, 2nd edn*. BSAVA, Gloucester

Ward A and McTaggart D (2007) Laboratory diagnostic aids. In: *BSAVA Textbook of Veterinary Nursing, 4th edn*, ed. DR Lane *et al*., pp. 317–350. BSAVA Publications, Gloucester

Acknowledgements

The author and editors wish to thank Wendy Busby for her contribution to the *BSAVA Manual of Veterinary Nursing*.

11

Diagnostic imaging techniques

Anne Ward and John Prior

> **This chapter is designed to give information on:**
>
> ■ Veterinary radiography health and safety
> ■ The principles of radiography
> ■ Routine radiographic procedures
> ■ Patient positioning
> ■ Contrast techniques
> ■ Film processing
> ■ Care of radiographic equipment
> ■ Assessing radiographic quality
> ■ Other diagnostic imaging techniques

Veterinary radiography health and safety

There is widespread use of X-rays for diagnostic purposes and a growing use of X-rays, beta rays and gamma rays for therapeutic purposes in veterinary practice. These essential tools can present a considerable potential for people in practices to be exposed to radiation.

Exposure to ionizing radiation can result in deleterious effects that may manifest not only in the exposed individual but could affect their descendents, hence the need for strict protective measures and guidelines. Such effects are either 'somatic' or 'genetic'.

Somatic effects are characterized by changes that occur within the organs of the exposed individual. These changes may occur within a few hours or up to many years later and it is cautiously assumed that any exposure to radiation may entail some risk; such risk is proportional to the dose received, even down to the lowest dose. Somatic exposure in veterinary medicine is quite uncommon; however, the possibility of genetic effects is much more of a concern, due to the lower doses used in veterinary radiology.

Protective measures need to ensure that any exposure is kept as low as reasonably achievable as even the smallest of radiation doses may have the ability to cause chromosomal damage within germ cells (genetic effects).

There are three main aspects of radiography that must be considered:

■ Personnel working with the X-ray equipment
■ Personnel within the vicinity of veterinary X-ray facilities and the general public
■ The animal being radiographed.

In each of these it is essential for guidance and implementation of measures to control the potential for exposure. The Acts and Regulations of particular importance to veterinary radiography are:

■ Ionizing Radiation Regulations 1999
■ Code of Practice
■ Guidance notes for the protection of persons against ionizing radiations arising from veterinary use (ISBN 085951 300 9 HMSO)
■ Local Radiation Rules and Regulations
■ Health and Safety at Work etc. Act 1974
■ Collection and Disposal of Waste Regulations 1988
■ Control of Substances Hazardous to Health (COSHH) 2002
■ Hazardous Waste Regulations 2005.

The Controlled Area

The radiography room is a Controlled Area when any X-ray equipment is switched on at the electrical supplies and X-ray production has been enabled. The Controlled Area consists of restrictions and barriers set at a distance of 2 metres or less when dealing with small animal radiography and 6 metres or less for large animal radiography. Radiography is not performed outside this area.

When entering the Controlled Area the guidelines set out in Figure 11.1 must be followed. In particular:

- Only staff wearing dosemeters and external persons whose presence the Radiation Protection Supervisor (see below) considers essential may enter the Controlled Area whilst radiography is being carried out. Students who have read the local rules are regarded as members of staff
- Persons under 18 years of age are not allowed into the radiography room when the X-ray equipment is switched on at the mains electrical supply and X-ray production is enabled
- Staff who are or become pregnant must inform their mentor and the Radiation Protection Supervisor immediately so that their duties may be reviewed if necessary
- No one may enter the X-ray room when an exposure is being made.

---

1. Only properly trained and qualified staff should operate the X-ray machine.
2. All non-essential persons should be removed from the room.
3. No pregnant women should be allowed within the radiographic area.
4. No persons under the age of 18 are allowed to be involved.
5. Avoid holding animals at all costs; implement the use of chemical or physical restraints.
6. No part of a person is allowed within the primary beam, even with protective clothing on.
7. Collimate as much as possible to reduce scatter radiation.
8. Wear protective clothing or, preferably, use a protective screen.
9. Check equipment regularly for cracks, holes and tears and replace if necessary.
10. Store protective equipment appropriately (e.g. no folding).
11. Monitoring for radiation exposure is essential for any person involved with radiography.
12. All persons are to adhere to the safety policies set up within the practice.

11.1 Guidelines for conduct involving veterinary radiography.

RPAs and RSAs

A **Radiation Protection Adviser** (RPA) is appointed external to the practice and either holds a diploma in radiology or has knowledge of radiation physics with an interest in veterinary radiography, as set out by the Approved Code of Practice. It is the RPA's responsibility to draw up a set of 'local rules'. These local rules have to provide information and guidelines on:

- Details of equipment
- Restrictions of Controlled Area
- Restraint of patients.

All staff should have a copy of a '**written system of work**', which provides a step-by-step list of procedures for performing radiography in the practice. This is monitored by a **Radiation Protection Supervisor** (RPS), who is usually the practice's principal, senior partner or head nurse and who ensures that radiography is being performed correctly and that all personnel are adhering to all relevant practice policies.

The role of the RPS involves:

- Initial training specific to the role of an RPS
- Ensuring compliance with the arrangements made by the RPA under the current Ionizing Radiation Regulations
- Supervision of the arrangements set out in the local rules
- Possession of sufficient authority to allow them to supervise all the radiation protection aspects of the work in areas subject to local rules (though it is not necessary for the RPS to be present at each individual exposure)
- Attending standardization training to maintain the currency of their role
- Knowing what to do in an emergency
- Knowing where to seek more information or advice.

Safe radiography

- Use of ionizing radiation should be justified.
- Exposures are kept as low as reasonably possible.
- Doses received by individuals do not exceed annual dose limits.
- Only suitably trained persons are to operate X-ray machines, under the direction of a veterinary surgeon.
- Persons operating the X-ray machine are responsible for ensuring the radiation safety of persons present.
- Non-essential personnel are excluded from the radiography room during radiography.
- The operator is fully aware of the radiation protection requirement and the radiographic techniques to be employed.
- After use, X-ray machines are switched off at the mains and secured against unauthorized use.

Dosemeters

The RPS is responsible for ensuring that employees receive adequate training and instruction about the care and use of dosemeters (also known as dosimeters) so that they are correctly worn and used. Suitable storage must be provided for dosemeters at all times as normal background radiation sources that people are exposed to in their everyday lives may produce a false reading with this equipment (see 'Care of radiographic equipment', below).

- Dosemeters must be worn at waist level on the trunk and under lead gowns when working in the radiography room.

- Dosemeters must not be exposed to excessive heat, sunlight, chemicals or pressure and must not be left in the X-ray room.
- All monitored personnel must take great care of their dosemeters and ensure that they are returned at the appropriate time for renewal.
- Loss or damage of dosemeters must be reported to the RPS immediately.

There are various types of dosemeter. The most common ones seen in veterinary practice are the film badge and the thermoluminescent dosemeter (TLD).

Film badge dosemeters

These offer a permanent record of exposure by means of a small piece of film that is sensitive to radiation, just like normal radiographic film (Figure 11.2). Once developed, exposed areas increase in optical density (i.e. blacken) in response to any incident radiation. The developed film is physical evidence of radiation exposure and can be stored for future review should there be any query over exposure.

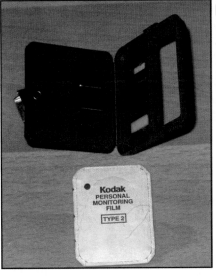

11.2 Film badge with the film removed and protected within its own envelope.

Thermoluminescent dosemeters

These are small devices used to measure radiation exposure. Visible light that is emitted from a crystal within the detector is measured when heated – hence the term thermoluminescent. The amount of light emitted is dependent on the ionizing radiation exposure. There are two main types of TLDs, both of which consist of a small crystal (either calcium fluoride or lithium fluoride) and a heating filament within a small glass bulb. The calcium fluoride TLD is used to record gamma exposure whereas the lithium fluoride TLD is used to record gamma and alpha exposure.

Other types of dosemeter

Pocket dosemeters are available that provide the wearer with an immediate reading of their exposure to X-rays and gamma rays. As the name implies, they are commonly worn in the pocket.

Other styles can include collar dosemeters and fingertip dosemeters, which allow the monitoring of the areas of the body that are more susceptible to the effects of radiation.

Protective clothing

It is important that any protective clothing is designed to provide protection against secondary radiation.

Flexible and lightweight lead sheeting can be used to protect personnel from exposure to X-ray radiation. This durable fabric is waterproof and free of any pinholes, thereby providing a uniform distribution of pure lead particles. The material needs to be handled carefully and appropriately to avoid any compromise of this protection (see 'Care of radiographic equipment', below). With a choice of lead equivalences of 0.25 mm, 0.35 mm and 0.5 mm, the variety of products available includes:

- Coat aprons (single- or double-sided, or miniature version for coverage of the reproductive organs)
- Skirt/tunic (Figure 11.3)
- Thyroid shield
- Protective eyewear
- Protective gloves
- Protective gauntlets
- Gonad shield
- Ovarian shield.

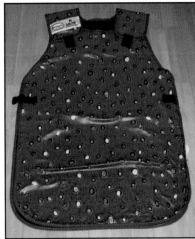

11.3 Lead tunics can come in a range of colours. Keeping this equipment flat at all times is imperative in order to avoid damage or cracks within the lead.

The X-ray room

A defined X-ray room or area for veterinary radiography should include:

- A space of adequate dimensions
- Radiation shielding provisions for persons within and outside the room or area
- Means of restricting access to the room or area
- X-ray warning signs (Figure 11.4) at all entrances
- Facilities for positioning and immobilizing the patient
- X-ray machine of adequate capacity and appropriate type to undertake the required radiographic procedure
- Low lighting (allows visibility of the light beam that indicates the path of the X-rays diverging from the tube head)
- Quiet environment (ensures a calm patient and that clear instructions can be heard by any persons in the immediate vicinity)

- Appropriate temperature, ventilation and humidity to help to avoid hypothermia (as patients may be sedated or anaesthetized) and provide a comfortable environment
- Notices stating that this is a 'Controlled Area', restricting movement, and highlighting that the area is designated for radiography
- Easy access to developing facilities.

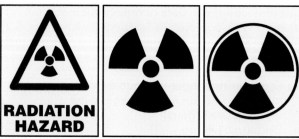

11.4 Various universally recognized X-ray radiation warning signs.

The X-ray machine

Portable machines allow transportation to an external source; mobile units allow the machine to be wheeled for storage purposes or for use in other areas of the practice. The larger, more powerful machines are usually fixed into position, ensuring the accuracy of the machine's location and consistency of the images being produced. A power supply and a suitable position within the Controlled Area is required whether the machine is portable, mobile or fixed.

X-ray machines are made up of three basic parts:

- The X-ray tube that produces the X-rays (usually protected in a lead case)
- Some form of collimation to focus and limit the size of the beam produced (usually a light-beam diaphragm)
- A control panel to vary the duration, intensity and penetrating power of the X-rays produced.

X-ray tube structure and production of X-rays

The physics of the production of X-rays cannot be fully covered in this manual and readers are referred to other texts. Only the basic principles of the production of X-rays in respect to their practical applications in veterinary radiography will be discussed here. Terms used in radiography are defined in Figure 11.5.

The entire range of wavelengths or frequencies of electromagnetic radiation, extending from gamma rays to the longest radio waves and including visible light, is known as the **electromagnetic spectrum** (EMS).

The energy in a **photon** of a given type of radiation is *directly* proportional to the **frequency** of the radiation and *inversely* proportional to its **wavelength** (Figure 11.6). This means that the longer the wavelength, the lower is the frequency and the lower the energy; and vice versa (short wavelength means high frequency and therefore high energy). The frequency is measured by the number of **cycles per second**. The higher the energy, the higher the **penetrating power** through matter and space. All members of the EMS have the same types of properties but at different intensities.

In 1895, Wilhelm Conrad Roentgen discovered that **X-rays** are produced as a result of the rapid deceleration of **electrons** that have been accelerated across an evacuated tube and made to collide with a target, producing heat when this occurs.

- The *source* of the electrons in an X-ray tube is a negatively charged (**cathode**) tungsten filament that is heated electrically. The heat produced in the filament, and therefore the number of electrons produced, varies according to the **current** or **milliamperage (mA)** applied to it.

Term	Definition
Film speed	The film speed refers to its sensitivity to light and X-rays. Speed is related to the size of the emulsion grains. Larger grains are more sensitive, producing faster emulsions than small grains
Grain size	The larger the film emulsion grain, the greater is the amount of light produced, but this produces reduced sharpness of images. Smaller grains, even though they produce less light, result in much better image definition
Photographic density	The amount of film blackening due to exposure to radiation. This is judged by how much light is transmitted through it
Contrast	The range of visible tones of grey on a radiograph. Tones range from white to black. Contrast is said to be *high* if the range of tones is small and *low* if the range is wide
Latitude	The ability of the film emulsion to respond to a range of exposures. An emulsion that produces a range of densities for a large range of exposures is said to have a *high* latitude. A *low* latitude is a small range of densities over a given range of exposure
Latent image	An invisible image on the X-ray film after it is exposed to ionizing radiation or light before processing
Milliamperage-seconds (mAs)	The number of X-rays produced over a given period. Calculated by multiplying the milliamperage (mA) by time (s)
Kilovoltage (kV)	Responsible for the accelerating force from the cathode to the anode, resulting in the penetrating power of the X-rays

11.5 Terminology relating to radiography.

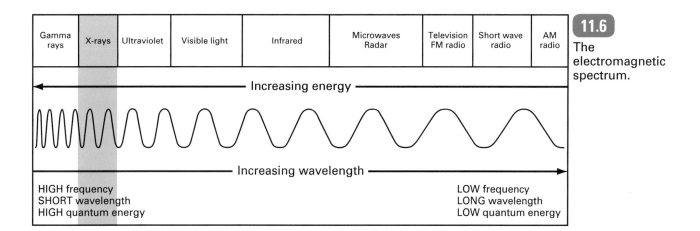

11.6 The electromagnetic spectrum.

- The *target* is a positively charged (**anode**) tungsten cone, often set in copper on a rotating molybdenum stalk (these metals help to dissipate heat).

The electrons are forced to accelerate from the cathode to the anode by the application of a **voltage**, measured in **kilovolts (kV)**, across the tube. The filament and target are enclosed in an evacuated glass envelope made of Pyrex to withstand the heat. The glass is surrounded by oil as a means of dissipating the heat produced and the whole structure is encased in lead to prevent the escape of the X-rays (Figure 11.7).

Collimation

A lead-lined aluminium box is located beneath the tube of most modern X-ray machines; it houses a series of adjustable lead plates that have bevelled edging to provide total closure. The lead plates together with a series of lights and mirrors form the light-beam diaphragm (LBD). This controls the angle of the primary beam and the area to be exposed; this is called collimation of the X-ray beam. Collimation focuses the beam on the area to be imaged, which acts both to improve the image produced and to reduce any danger to local personnel through exposure either directly to the beam or from 'scatter' from it. Practical collimation and the care of light-beam diaphragms are discussed later in this chapter. The light is usually set on a timer to avoid overheating of the bulb.

The control panel

Each X-ray machine has a panel of controls that allow at least some variation of the X-rays produced. These controls may include:

- **On/off switch**
- **Line voltage compensator** (keeps voltage constant at set levels)
- **Kilovoltage (kV)** – alters the potential difference across the tube, thus affecting the *speed* of the electrons across the tube: higher kV = faster electrons, which will create X-rays of greater energy and *greater penetrating ability*
- **Milliamperage (mA)** – indicates the current flowing to the filament; controls the *number* of electrons crossing the tube, affecting the *number of X-rays produced*
- **Time (s)** – determines the time when electrons can cross the vacuum and interact with the target; also controls the *number of X-rays produced*

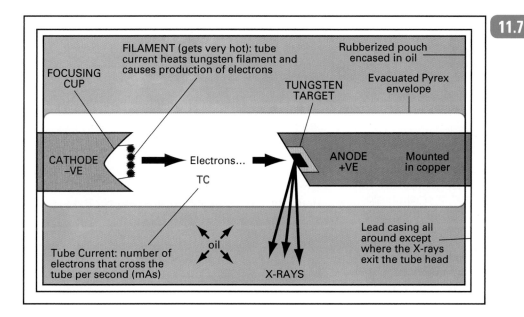

11.7 Components of a tube head.

The measurements *mA* and *s* (i.e. seconds) have the same effect and are often considered together as **milliamperage-seconds (mAs)**:

$$mA \times s = mAs$$

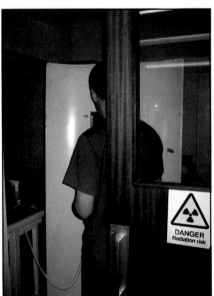

For example, an exposure of 100 mA for 0.05 seconds (5 mAs) produces the same number of photons as an exposure of 250 mA for 0.02 seconds (5 mAs).

- **Exposure button** – on a lead no shorter than 2 m long (Figure 11.8). Stationary anodes have a one-stage button that creates an exposure immediately, whereas rotating anodes have two stages: first the anode is rotated and then it is bombarded with electrons, creating an exposure (the spin and fire). Usually a warning light will illuminate when an exposure is made on X-ray machines.

11.8

The exposure button lead, in this case coming from the control panel on the left, allows the veterinary nurse to be positioned a safe distance away from the primary beam. A lead screen is giving additional protection. (Courtesy of E Mullineaux)

Timers

Timers include clockwork, synchronous and electronic types.

Clockwork timer

This is dialled or wound up to the time required. Although simple and cheap, this type of timer is not accurate; it can sometimes be found in smaller, older X-ray machines.

Synchronous timer

This has an electric motor and is more accurate than a clockwork timer: it allows a minimum exposure time of 0.1 seconds. This type is generally found in older X-ray machines.

Electronic timer

This type is found in modern machines. It allows very short exposure times, as low as 0.02 seconds.

Effects of changes in exposure factors

Two features of the X-ray beam can be controlled:

- The total *quantity* of X-rays produced
- The energy or penetrating power of these X-rays, which is referred to as the *quality* of the beam.

Quantity

Quantity of X-rays can be altered in two ways: by varying the current or the exposure time.

Varying the current

Varying the current (mA) alters the temperature of the cathode filament and thus the number of electrons in the cloud. The more electrons in the cloud, the more that are accelerated across the X-ray tube and the more X-rays that are consequently produced. The effect is to produce a blacker image without increasing patient penetration.

Changing the exposure time

Increasing the exposure time increases the number of electrons reaching the target, thereby increasing the number of X-rays produced. Doubling the exposure time doubles the number of X-rays produced.

- Quantity of X-rays produced = current (mA) x time(s) = mAs.
- *Increasing the current (mA) allows the exposure time to be reduced.*

Quality

Quality is varied by altering the **kV** setting. The higher the kV, the greater is the speed of the electrons moving across the X-ray tube and the greater are the energy and penetrating power of the resultant X-ray beam. Increased penetrating power is required for thicker, denser body areas. The effect on the film is to produce blacker images of lower contrast. A kV should be selected that just penetrates the densest part, giving the best possible contrast between structures.

- *Increasing the kV increases the quality and penetrating power of the X-rays produced.*

The 10kV rule

To achieve a required exposure, it is necessary to alter mAs and/or kV. For safety reasons in the practice, it is often preferable to increase the kV setting rather than extend exposure time.
Increasing the kV by 10 creates roughly the same effect as doubling the mAs .
Reducing the kV by 10 creates roughly the same effect as halving the mAs

Therefore, in practice, an increase of 10kV on an 'ideal' setting will allow the mAs to be halved. Conversely, reducing the kV by 10 on an 'ideal' setting would require the mAs to be doubled.

Interaction of X-rays with matter

Diagnostic X-rays produced by the X-ray machine and focused on the patient by a light-beam diaphragm can have several effects:

- They can be *absorbed* (**photoelectric effect**) into the patient's tissues (Figure 11.9a)
- They can be *scattered* (**Compton effect**) from the surface of the patient (Figure 11.9b)
- They can '*pass straight through*' the patient to interact with the X-ray cassette and produce an image (Figure 11.9c). Image production is affected by the film focal distance (see later).

In reality, when a radiograph of a patient is taken a combination of all three eventualities occurs.

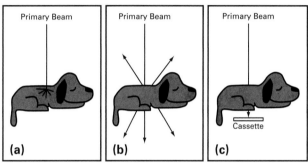

11.9 X-ray paths. **(a)** Absorption: photoelectric effect. **(b)** Compton effect, or Compton scatter. **(c)** Radiation through the patient to the cassette.

Absorption of X-rays

The degree to which X-rays are absorbed depends on the thickness of the tissue and the molecular density (atomic number) of the element(s) in the tissue. Tissues with a high atomic number, such as bone, absorb X-rays very well. Gases, with low atomic numbers, absorb X-rays much less readily than fluids or solids. As a result of this, five **radiographic opacities** are recognized according to the ability of tissues (and other materials) to absorb X-rays rather than allow them to pass through on to the X-ray cassette (Figure 11.10).

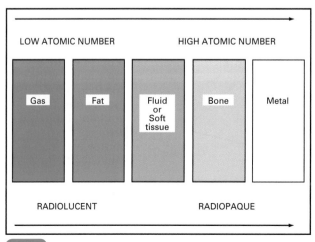

11.10 The five radiographic opacities.

- **Radiolucent** describes features that only slightly absorb X-rays (e.g. gas).
- **Radiopaque** (radiodense) describes those that absorb X-rays readily (e.g. bones).
- Differences between radiolucency and radiodensity produce X-ray film **contrast**.

Scatter of X-rays

Scattered radiation outside of the body is referred to as 'Compton effect' or 'Compton scatter' (see Figure 11.9b), where some X-ray photons collide with electrons in the tissue's atoms in such a way that they will go off in a completely different direction as 'scatter'. This scattered radiation has enough energy to emerge from the patient in a random pattern-less way. The Compton effect is *not* affected by the atomic density of the tissue but is affected by its *thickness*. Scattered radiation produces a poor image quality and is hazardous to personnel.

Control of scatter

Scatter production can be reduced by:

- Collimation of the primary beam by light-beam diaphragm or lead cylinder
- Compression of the patient (e.g. with a paddle or compression band) to make them 'thinner'
- *Increasing* kV to reduce the amount of scatter (however, this results in an increase in energy and therefore increased deleterious effects of the scatter).

The amount of scatter reaching the film can be reduced by:

- Use of a grid
- Air-gap technique – by leaving a space between patient and cassette, a large amount of scatter will miss the film. Because of the inverse square law (see below) this requires an increased exposure. The disadvantage of this technique is that there is loss of definition of the image
- Using lead backing for cassettes and table, or placing a lead rubber mat on the table – this results in absorption of the photons passing through the film and prevents 'backscatter' from the table or floor to the film.

Film focal distance

In a veterinary practice, the X-ray machine is usually positioned over an X-ray table on which the patient can be placed. An X-ray film in a cassette is place under the part of the animal to be radiographed. The distance between the target of the anode of the X-ray head and the X-ray film in the cassette is referred to as the film focal distance (**FFD**) and is critical to the image produced. Reducing the FFD will result in a greater 'penumbra effect' from the object being radiographed (Figure 11.11). **Penumbra** refers to an area in which distinction or resolution is difficult or uncertain. This can also occur when the **object-to-film distance** (**OFD**) is altered (Figure 11.12).

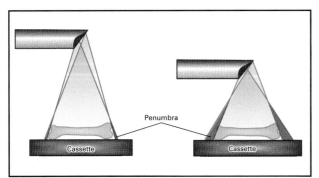

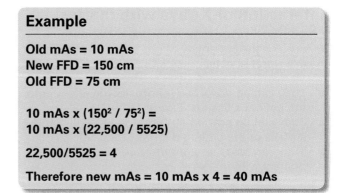

11.11 Increasing the film focal distance (FFD) decreases the amount of penumbra, increasing radiographic detail and divergence of the primary beam.

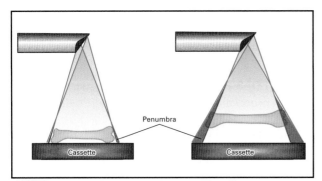

11.12 Increasing the object-to-film distance (OFD) increases the amount of penumbra, decreasing radiographic detail and thus increasing the magnification of the image.

The intensity of the X-ray beam varies with the FFD according to Newton's inverse square law (Figure 11.13). Therefore radiographic density is affected by a change in distance. When the distance is changed, the total number of X-rays must be decreased or increased to compensate. This can be done by changing the mAs. When a different distance is used, the adjustment of the mAs can be calculated as follows:

Old mAs x [(new FFD)^2 / (old FFD)^2] = new mAs

Example

Old mAs = 10 mAs
New FFD = 150 cm
Old FFD = 75 cm

10 mAs x (150^2 / 75^2) =
10 mAs x (22,500 / 5525)

22,500/5525 = 4

Therefore new mAs = 10 mAs x 4 = 40 mAs

The FFD should be kept constant, usually at 90–110 cm.

Radiographic film

Radiography is the creation of images by exposing a radiographic film to X-ray radiation. Because X-rays penetrate solid objects, but are weakened by them depending on the object's composition, the resulting image reveals the internal structure of the object. When X-rays are exposed directly to the film, this causes blackening; unexposed areas remain clear after development.

X-ray film is sensitive to visible (white) light and should therefore only be handled in conditions of special 'safe-lighting' until processed.

Structures found within film include a protective layer of emulsion known as the 'supercoat' followed by the silver halide crystal-containing layer of emulsion. This is then secured to the film base using a form of glue known as the substratum layer (Figure 11.14) (see 'Care of radiographic equipment', below).

Film speed

Radiographic film speed can be considered as being either 'slow' or 'fast'. Speed refers to the amount of exposure required to obtain an acceptable image. The speed of the film is determined by the size and number of silver halide crystals within the film emulsion layer. Different film speeds are used for different areas of the body in veterinary radiography.

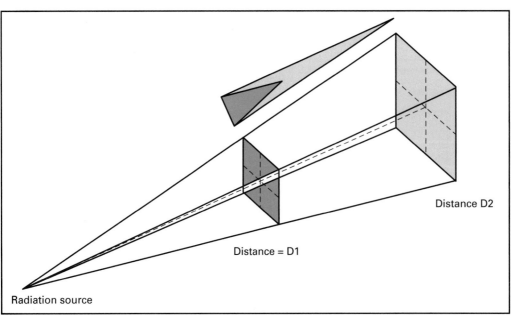

11.13 Newton's inverse square law states that the intensity of an effect is reduced in inverse proportion to the square of the distance from the source. Thus, doubling the distance from the source will reduce intensity by $\frac{1}{4}$.

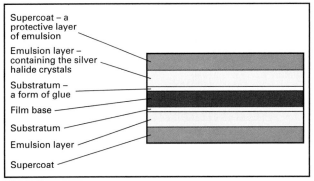

11.14 Film structure.

Slow *versus* fast film

Slow film	Fast film
Many tiny crystals	Fewer larger crystals
More X-rays required	Fewer X-rays required
Highly detailed image	Less detailed image
Sharp appearance	Grainier appearance

Types of film

- Screen film
  - Most commonly used in veterinary radiography
  - More sensitive to light
  - Available in green and blue sensitivities.
- Direct exposure/non-screen film
  - More sensitive to X-rays than light
  - Requires higher exposures
  - Packaged in a paper folder within a light-proof envelope
  - Used for intraoral and dental radiography.
- Mammography film
  - Only has emulsion on one side to produce finite detail and is used with a single intensifying screen
  - Can be recognized by having a small nick on its edge, allowing it to be orientated correctly
  - Used most commonly for orthopaedic radiographs of extremities.

Formation of the latent image

As the silver halide crystals absorb energy from the X-rays (i.e. are exposed) a physical change takes place and a latent (invisible) image is formed. Following processing, the latent image is converted into a visible one with the exposed silver halide crystals changing to metallic silver. The metallic silver appears black on the radiograph once developed.

How the latent image is formed

Film emulsion is gelatine containing silver halide microcrystals. Silver halide is a compound containing 90–99% silver bromide and 1–10% silver iodide.

- Light or X-rays liberate an electron from each halide ion, rendering it neutral.
- The liberated electrons are attracted to 'electron traps' or 'sensitivity specs' located at the edge of the microcrystals.
- Silver ions in the microcrystals are positively charged and therefore attracted to these electrons (opposites attract).
- When silver ions meet free electrons they become neutral atoms of silver.
- The end result is the formation of minute clumps of silver atoms, which form the latent image.
- The latent image is converted to a visible image by means of processing.

Intensifying screens

Intensifying screens absorb the energy of X-rays that have penetrated the patient and convert this energy into a light pattern. The more light a screen produces, the less X-ray exposure and thus shorter exposure time is needed to expose the film. In most film–screen systems, the film is sandwiched between two screens in a cassette so that the emulsion on each side is exposed to the light from its contiguous screen.

The use of intensifying screens has three major benefits:

- Reduction of patient radiation dose
- Reduction of tube and generator loading (exposure factors)
- Reduction of patient motion artefacts.

If X-ray film were used alone to produce images, exposure factors would always have to be very high (see below). Intensifying screens intensify the effects of X-rays on the film. This is done by using crystals of phosphorescent materials that emit light when exposed to X-rays that are found within the intensifying screen. It is important to note that 95% of the image is formed by visible light, and only 5% by X-rays. These crystals of **phosphor** are evenly distributed in a binder.

- **Calcium tungstate screens** emit blue light when exposed to X-rays and are therefore used with film that is sensitive to blue light.
- **Rare-earth screens** have been used more recently. They are more efficient at producing light and are required in thinner layers.

The two main rare-earth phosphors are gadalinium oxysulphide (emits green light) and lanthanum oxybromide (emits blue light). As they emit different coloured light, it is vital to ensure that the correct sensitivity screen is used with the correct film type.

Speed and detail in relation to intensifying screens

This is similar to the way in which X-ray film has been referred to above. Intensifying screens can be regular/high/fast, medium or detail/fine/slow. Their speed can be varied in many ways:

- Rare-earth screens emit more light than tungsten screens
- Volume of phosphor within screen can be varied

- Increase or decrease phosphor crystal size (larger crystals absorb more X-rays and emit more light)
- Presence of an absorptive or reflective layer
- Alter thickness of phosphor layer (a thicker layer emits more light but produces a less sharp image than a thin layer)
- Add dyes to the phosphor binder to help reduce blurring.

Grids

Anti-scatter grids improve the diagnostic quality of radiographs by trapping the greater part of scattered radiation. Scattered radiation is probably the biggest factor contributing to the poor diagnostic quality of radiographs. Its effect produces a general radiographic fog on the film, which reduces the contrast.

The anti-scatter grid is the best known way of effectively removing the greater part of scatter radiation that is not required for the creation of the final image. Lead strips within the grid absorb radiation that does not travel in the same direction as the primary beam. Dr Gustav Bucky first built the grid in 1913, and his original principle of lead foil strips standing on edge, separated by X-ray-transparent interspacers, has remained one of the best known techniques in trapping scatter radiation. All grids have a **grid ratio**, which is the ratio between the height of the lead strips and the width between them; for example, with interspacers 5 times as high as they are wide, the grid ratio is said to be 5:1. Generally speaking, the higher the ratio of a grid, the more scattered radiation is absorbed. On average, grids contain 20–28 strips of lead per centimetre.

Either of the following necessitates the use of a grid:

- Patient thickness being radiographed is >10 cm (Figure 11.15)
- Exposures >60kV are being used.

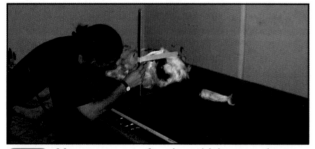

11.15 Measurement of patient thickness using callipers.

Stationary grids

X-ray grids are commercially available with either *focused* or *parallel* lead strips, which are produced in either a *linear* or a *crossed* grid configuration (Figure 11.16).

- Focused grid lead strips are angled to mimic the divergent primary beam from the tube head.
- Parallel grids have strips that are perpendicular to the surface of the grid, but this can lead to 'grid cut-off' when the diverging primary beam fails to make contact with the film due to the angle of the primary beam against the height of the strip.

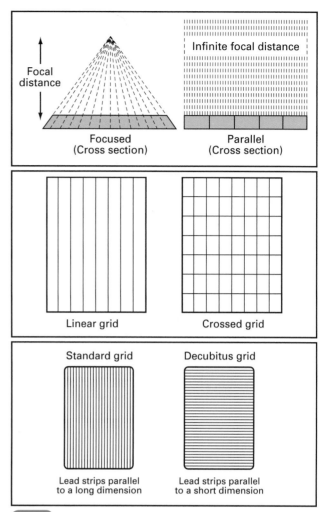

11.16 Different grid designs.

- A *pseudofocused* grid is designed to help to reduce this by having perpendicular strips that are reduced in height from the centre to the edges of the grid.
- *Decubitus* grids are designed to reduce grid cut-off by having the lead strips parallel to the short dimension of the grid, in line with the cathode–anode direction of the X-ray tube. This allows greater positioning latitude when aligning the X-ray tube with the grid, producing an improved image quality.

For all angled and pseudofocused grids, it is vital that they are placed the correct way up and placed between the patient and the cassette. Some grids are manually placed between the patient and cassette and are referred to as *stationary grids*; other types can be incorporated into the actual X-ray table and are referred to as *moving grids*, known as Potter–Bucky grids.

Moving grids

Stationary grids produce fine lines on the radiograph that can distract from the subject. To eliminate these lines a moving grid is used. In high-power X-ray machines there is an electrical connection to the grid. As the exposure is made, the grid is moved at high speed.

Grid factor

It must be noted that some of the primary beam will also be absorbed by the grid. To compensate for this, more X-rays will be needed, which means increasing the mAs.

> **All grids have a grid factor marked on them and this is the amount by which the mAs must be increased to compensate for using the grid. To calculate the new mAs, the old mAs is multiplied by the grid factor:**
>
> **New mAs = old mAs x grid factor**
>
> **The grid factor is usually 2.5–3.**

Disadvantages of using grids

- Need to increase exposure factors to compensate for absorption of part of primary beam.
- Longer exposure time (increases chance of blurring).
- Increased exposure leading to increased radiation hazard to patient and personnel.
- Grid lines and grid cut-off can detract from the image.
- Correct film focal distance must be used.
- Cannot be used for oblique views, as must be perpendicular to the X-ray beam.
- Expensive to purchase and must be looked after.
- Focused grids need to be used the right way up (potential for human error).

Cassette holders

Film cassette holders offer the opportunity for personnel to avoid being in the direct path of the primary beam and at increased distance from the radiation area, if not out of the Controlled Area altogether. Holders are available in portfolio, handheld or block designs.

Digital radiography

Digital radiography allows for more convenient image storage and image retrieval, better image display, improved educational experiences for teaching and training purposes, and faster and more convenient remote usage. This type of equipment therefore requires different cassettes/developer from the methods previously discussed. It is only due to the costs involved with digital radiography that it is not seen more commonly in practice, but it will in time replace current methods.

Fluoroscopy

Fluoroscopy is used during many diagnostic and therapeutic procedures where an image is obtained in a 'live' motion action. This allows continuous visualization of the patient, or observation of the action of instruments being used either to diagnose or to treat the patient.

The radiologist uses a switch to control a continuous low-frequency X-ray beam that is transmitted through the patient. The X-rays strike a fluorescent plate that is coupled to an image intensifier, which is coupled to a television camera. The images can then be watched live on the TV monitor.

Fluoroscopy is often used to observe the digestive tract (e.g. a barium swallow for upper gastrointestinal studies, or a barium enema for lower gastrointestinal studies).

Routine radiographic procedures

Exposure charts and choosing exposures

The choice of exposure factors may be based on past experience, may make use of exposure charts, or may be done by altering settings based on the developed film. Exposure charts help to provide consistently good-quality radiographs. No one exposure chart can be used for all X-ray machines as there will always be variation in equipment, materials and settings. Good exposure charts help to reduce repeated exposures, preventing time wasting and reducing the potential hazard to staff. Details that should be recorded are:

- Date
- Signalment and weight
- Depth of the area being radiographed (measured by ruler or callipers)
- Area radiographed
- View
- Film and cassette type used
- Whether grid used or not
- Film focal distance (if different from standard)
- Exposure factors (kV and mAs) used
- Persons involved
- Results (quality of exposure, any faults).

When previously taken exposure figures are not available (e.g. with a new X-ray machine), or when the area to be radiographed differs greatly from previously recorded figures, the guidelines set out in the box below can be useful.

> **From the settings of a basic good exposure, alter the settings according to the following:**
>
> - **For puppies and kittens: halve the mAs**
> - **For heavily muscled, fat dogs: double the mAs**
> - **For dry plaster cast material: double the mAs**
> - **For wet plaster cast material: multiply mAs by 3**
> - **If a grid is used: increase the mAs by 3 or the kV by 10–15**
> - **For positive contrast studies: increase the kV by 5–10**
> - **For areas consisting largely of bone: increase the kV by 5–10**
> - **For views involving the skull, vertebral column or pelvis: increase the kV by 5–10.**

To help to set up an exposure chart for a new machine the general rule is to keep mAs the same but, for every 1 cm increase in thickness, increase the kV by:

- 2 for up to 80 kV
- 3 for 80–100 kV
- 4 for above 100 kV.

Sante's rule:

2 x thickness (cm) + 40 = kV (without a grid or Bucky system)

Patient preparation

The patient must be appropriately presented for radiography, for which the following should be noted.

- Ensure that the coat is dry and clean (as dirt and sand may produce artefacts within the image).
- If using contrast agents, ensure that none is on the animal's coat.
- Groom beforehand if necessary.
- Ultrasound gel can produce artefacts and so should be removed.
- Remove any bandages or splints that may interfere with the results produced.
- Some casts are radiolucent and may be left in place. If using plaster of Paris, exposures should be altered to accommodate this (see above).
- Remove any choke chains, collars or leads.
- Avoid skin-fold artefacts by pulling the skin away from the area of interest.
- Positioning aids such as foam wedges should be moved away from the area of interest.

Patient positioning

Positioning of the patient is critical in ensuring optimal images suitable for diagnostic purposes. Appropriate immobilization of the patient prevents the need for repeat exposures and prevents movement blur occurring. Difficult positioning, such as that required for the BVA Hip Score radiograph, can be obtained using positioning aids alone with the anaesthetized patient (Figure 11.17); holding should **never** be used for this procedure as positioning *is* achievable. Practice with dummies can be helpful.

Positioning is not difficult and is never impossible, but it does require:

- Patience (most important!)
- An understanding of the anatomical structures involved
- Adequate immobilization of the patient
- Correct use of any positioning aids or restraint equipment
- Consideration of the patient's comfort and medical condition
- Consideration of scatter radiation and exposure to personnel.

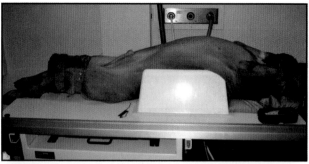

11.17 Positioning for BVA hip dysplasia scoring. A variety of restraint aids can be used to help prevent rotation of the patient and keep the femurs extended and parallel. In this case a trough, ties and sandbags stop rotation of the thorax, whilst a foam wedge and parcel tape help position the hindlimbs. (Courtesy of E Mullineaux)

Positioning aids

To position the animal correctly for radiography, special aids should be used to help to obtain and hold that perfect position. Different types of aids can be used for a variety of purposes (Figures 11.18 to 11.20).

Positioning aid	Description, purpose and comments
Adhesive tape, gauze bandages	Various types of tape and bandaging may be tied around, or placed over, an anatomical region to fix it into position for radiography. They can also remove an overlying anatomical region from the area of interest
Velcro straps	Velcro, stitched back to back, provides a useful tool for securing the position of the hindlimbs with the hips rotated inwards for BVA hip scoring, avoiding the necessity of holding the animal for this view
Sandbags	The sand should be contained within a sealed bag with an outer cover that can be removed for cleaning or replacing once soiled. Various sizes should be available; long sausage shapes allow greater versatility
Blocks	Foam, plastic, wood or sand-filled containers allow the propping of the animal into position. Wooden or sand-filled blocks provide a bit more weight to lean against
Positioning troughs	V-shaped and made of either timber, Perspex, foam or plastic; useful for maintaining an animal's position for ventrodorsal or dorsoventral projections
Radiolucent pads	Foam, plastic or rubber pads can be purchased (or made) in a variety of shapes and sizes to help position the animal correctly. Plastic bags filled with cotton wool also work well for propping
Cassette holders	Simple devices that allow cassettes to be held at a distance, helping to provide distance between source and personnel and allowing standing lateral radiographs to be taken
Mouth gags	Used to help keep the mouth positioned open for oral, skull or dental views
Artery forceps	Can be useful for holding areas away from the point of interest (e.g. the tail)

11.18 Positioning aids.

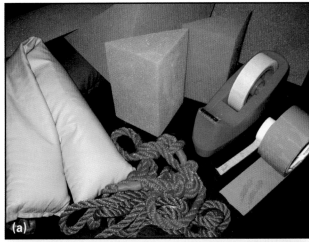

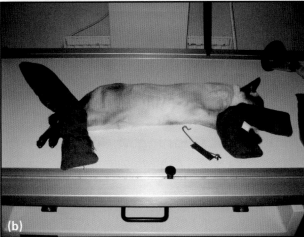

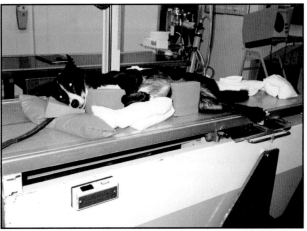

11.20 A chemically restrained patient along with a variety of positioning aids.

11.19 **(a)** A selection of positioning aids (from top left, clockwise): foam wedges in several shapes and sizes; various forms of semi-adhesive tape; rope ties (calving and lambing ropes are soft and suitable for this purpose); sandbags in assorted weights. **(b)** A sedated cat gently restrained using two lightweight sandbags. (Courtesy of E Mullineaux)

Beam adjustment

Centring

Adjustments of the primary beam can be achieved using the light-beam diaphragm that is found on most X-ray machines. The anatomical landmarks of the patient and palpation of specific bony prominences should be used to help to centralize the beam to the area of interest. Most light beams produce a cross that is central to the area of collimation and which can be positioned over the point of greatest interest.

Collimation

It is essential that the entire primary beam is kept within the perimeters of the X-ray cassette so that any scatter radiation or unused X-ray energy is absorbed by the lead backing of the cassette, reducing the potential for radiation exposure. Views will be scored with 25% per successful collimation along one side of the film; ideally 100% collimation should be achieved with all of the views used (Figure 11.21).

Physical restraint guidelines (Ionizing Radiation Regulations 1999):

- Avoid manually holding the patient unless it is *critically* ill
- If the patient is held, full protective equipment must be used
- Handle the patient carefully, gently and firmly
- Keep the patient calm and stress free
- Padding and support are essential.

Chemical restraint guidelines:

- General anaesthesia or sedation required
- Allows precise positioning
- Allows the position to be maintained
- Necessary for some contrast studies
- Padding and support are essential – consider the patient's comfort at all times (Figure 11.20).

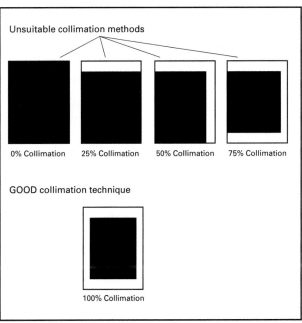

11.21 Collimation techniques: the unsuitable and the good.

Successful collimation requires:

- 100% collimation
- Inclusion of the area of concern only
- No part of any personnel included (even if wearing protective clothing)
- Reliable equipment and light source indicating the perimeter of the emerging primary beam.

Standardized nomenclature

A standardized system of nomenclature should be concise and understandable. This allows a person who is familiar with radiography to produce any given radiographic projection when directed, using familiar veterinary anatomical terms. Abbreviations that may be used are given in Figure 11.22.

Radiographic projections should be described in terms of the direction in which the central ray of the primary beam penetrates the body part of interest: *from point of entrance to point of exit*.

With many projections, it is necessary to use combinations of the basic directional terms to give an accurate description of the point of entrance and point of exit of the primary beam. It is recommended that these terms be combined in a consistent order to increase standardization of radiographic nomenclature.

- The terms 'right' and 'left' are not used in combination and should precede any other terms. (*Example*: right cranioventral)
- The terms 'medial' and 'lateral' should be subservient when used in combination with other terms. (*Example*: dorsomedial)

- On the head, neck, trunk and tail, the terms 'rostral', 'cranial' and 'caudal' should take precedence when used in combination with other terms. (*Example*: craniodorsal)
- On the limbs the terms 'dorsal', 'palmar', 'plantar', 'cranial' and 'caudal' should take precedence when used in combination with other terms. (*Example*: dorsoproximal)
- The term 'oblique' is added to the names of those projections in which the central ray passes obliquely (not parallel to one of the three major directional axes – medial/lateral, dorso/ventral or cranio/caudal) through the body part.
- The 'skyline' views require no special designation since the point of entry to point of exit method describes these views concisely.
- In those views requiring a combination of directional terms a hyphen should be inserted to separate the point of entry and point of exit. (*Example*: palmaroproximal-palmarodistal)

The recommendations above for standardized nomenclature at first appear very confusing. However, the rules are logical and will begin to make sense with continued use.

Standard positioning of dogs and cats

Figures 11.23 to 11.27 show positioning for some of the standard radiographic views used in dogs and cats (and other species). It is good practice to take more than one view of each area so as to ensure that abnormalities are not missed. For most areas this involves taking at least two perpendicular views (e.g. lateral and dorsoventral).

Term	Abbreviation	Term	Abbreviation	Term	Abbreviation
Standardized anatomical directional terms and abbreviations				*Terminology combinations*	
Left	Lt	Medial	M	Caudocranial	CdCr
Right	Rt	Lateral	L	Caudodorsal	CaD
				Craniocaudal	CrCd
Ventral	V	Proximal	Pr	Cranioventral	CrV
Dorsal	D	Distal	Di	Dorsopalmar (forelimb)	DPa
Cranial	Cr	Palmar	Pa	Dorsoplantar (hindlimb)	DPl
				Dorsoventral	D/V
Caudal	Ca	Plantar	Pl	Lateral	Lat
Rostral	R	Oblique	O	Ventrodorsal	V/D

11.22 Radiographic nomenclature.

Area to be radiographed	Beam centre	Positioning and collimation
Lateral view of the pelvis	Over greater femoral trochanter	Place into lateral recumbency with the side of interest closest to the cassette. Place foam wedge between patient's stifle joints to keep the femurs parallel to the cassette and to prevent rotation. The limb closest to the cassette should be pulled cranially, so that the femurs can be distinguished. The field of view should include entire pelvis and a portion of the lumbar spine and the femurs. Ensure the pelvis is centred to the middle of the cassette

11.23 Positioning chart for the pelvis and hindlimb. (Drawings reproduced from Lavin, 2003, with the permission of the publisher) (continues) ▶

Area to be radiographed	Beam centre	Positioning and collimation
Ventrodorsal view of the pelvis – frog leg projection	Over level of pubis and acetabulum	The 'frog leg' is suitable if pelvic trauma is suspected. Minimal stress and tension are placed on the pelvis and joints. Patient is in dorsal recumbency, placed in a trough. The femurs should be at a 45° angle; it is important for the femurs to be positioned identically to maintain symmetry
Ventrodorsal view of the pelvis – extended projection	Over level of pubis and acetabulum	Standard evaluation for hip dysplasia. Position as for frog-leg except that the hindlimbs are extended caudally, with the stifles 2.5–5 cm from each other. Secure the stifles with Velcro or ties, and secure metatarsals with sandbags. The following criteria must be met: ■ Femurs are parallel ■ Both patellas are centred between the femoral condyles ■ Pelvis is without rotation; obturator foramens, hip joints, hemipelvis and sacroiliac joints appear as a mirror image ■ Tail is secured with tape between the femurs ■ Field of view includes pelvis, femurs and stifle joints
Lateral view of the femur	Middle of femur	Place into lateral recumbency with the affected limb closest to the cassette. Opposite limb is abducted and rotated out of the line of the X-ray beam. Place foam pad under the proximal tibia to alleviate any rotation of the femur. Field of view includes hip joint, femur and stifle joint
Craniocaudal view of the femur	Middle of femur	Place into dorsal recumbency with limb of interest extended caudally. Slight abduction of affected limb will eliminate superimposition of the proximal femur over the tuber ischium. The opposite limb is flexed and rotated laterally to facilitate abduction. The patella should be between the two femoral condyles. Field of view includes hip joint, femur and stifle joint
Lateral view of the stifle	Over stifle joint	Place into lateral recumbency with the affected joint next to the cassette. The opposite limb is flexed and abducted from the line of the X-ray beam. The stifle joint should be in a natural, slightly flexed position. Place pad under the tarsus so that the tibia is parallel to cassette. Elevation of the tibia will ensure superimposition of the two femoral condyles and facilitate a true lateral projection
Caudocranial view of the stifle	Over stifle joint, distal end of the femur	Place into sternal recumbency with affected limb in maximum extension. Opposite limb is flexed and elevated with foam wedge. This will control the lateral rotation of the stifle joint. The patella should be centred between the femoral condyles (which can be palpated)
Craniocaudal view of the stifle	Over stifle joint, distal end of the femur	Place into dorsal recumbency with the affected limb extended as for the craniocaudal view of the femur. Although this view may be easier to position, it has the disadvantage of some magnification and distortion of the image due to increased object–film distance

11.23 (continued) Positioning chart for the pelvis and hindlimb. (Drawings reproduced from Lavin, 2003, with the permission of the publisher) (continues)

Area to be radiographed	Beam centre	Positioning and collimation
Skyline projection of patella – also known as sunrise view or sunshine view	Over patella	This view demonstrates changes that can occur to the patella and the femoral trochlear groove. Place into lateral recumbency with the opposite limb down on the table. The affected limb should be in a fully flexed position. Tape or roll gauze can be placed around the mid-tibia and femur to hold the stifle joint in this flexed position. The stifle should remain horizontal and can be supported on a foam pad. The cassette is placed behind the stifle joint vertically and a horizontal X-ray beam is centred to the patella and travels caudocranially
Lateral view of the tibia and fibula	Middle of the tibia and fibula	Place into lateral recumbency with the affected limb placed on the cassette. The stifle should be slightly flexed and maintained in a true lateral position. A sponge wedge can be placed under the metatarsus to eliminate any rotation of the tibia. The opposite limb is pulled cranially or caudally so that it is out of the line of the beam. Field of view includes stifle joint, tibia and fibula and tarsal joint
Caudocranial view of the tibia and fibula	Middle of the tibia and fibula	Place into sternal recumbency with the affected limb extended caudally. Support the body with foam blocks placed beneath the caudal abdomen and pelvic region. Elevating the hind end will minimize the weight placed on the stifle joint extended caudally and will facilitate positioning. The tibia/fibula should be in a true caudocranial position so that the patella is placed between the two femoral condyles. Opposite limb is flexed and placed on a pad to control rotation of the affected limb. Secure tail out of beam. Field of view includes the stifle joint, tibia/fibula and tarsal joint
Lateral view of the tarsus	Middle of tarsus	Place into lateral recumbency with affected limb next to cassette. Tarsus is placed in a natural slightly flexed position. The opposite limb should be pulled cranially out of line of the X-ray beam
Dorsoplantar view of the tarsus	Middle of the tarsal joint	Place into sternal recumbency with the affected limb extended cranially alongside the body. The limb should be slightly abducted from the body wall to prevent any superimposition over the tarsus. A true dorsoplantar position is ensured by rotating the stifle medially in order to centre the patella between the femoral condyles
Plantarodorsal view of the tarsus	Middle of the tarsal joint	Place into sternal recumbency with the affected limb extended as for the caudocranial view of the tibia/fibula. Place foam under the caudal abdomen and pelvic region to prevent tarsus rotation. Foam also under the stifle joint to achieve maximum extension of the tarsus. If stifle is in true caudocranial position the tarsus will naturally follow in a true plantarodorsal position
Lateral view of the metatarsus–phalanges	Midmetatarsal region	Place into lateral recumbency. The opposite limb can be pulled caudally or cranially out of view of the beam. The joint is positioned in a natural flexed position. A sponge pad can be placed under the stifle joint to maintain a true lateral position of the metatarsus. Field of view should include the tarsal joint, metatarsus and phalanges

11.23 (continued) Positioning chart for the pelvis and hindlimb. (Drawings reproduced from Lavin, 2003, with the permission of the publisher) (continues) ▶

Area to be radiographed	Beam centre	Positioning and collimation
Dorsoplantar and plantarodorsal view of the metatarsus–phalanges	Mid-metatarsal region	Place into sternal recumbency with limb of interest pulled cranially and slightly abducted from the body wall. To achieve a true dorsoplantar view, the stifle joint of the affected limb is rotated laterally and secured with tape. Field of view includes tarsus, metatarsus and phalanges. Positioned as for the plantarodorsal view of the tarsus

11.23 (continued) Positioning chart for the pelvis and hindlimb. (Drawings reproduced from Lavin, 2003, with the permission of the publisher)

Area to be radiographed	Beam centre	Positioning and collimation
Lateral view of the scapula positioned dorsal to the vertebral column	Middle of scapula. (midway between the greater tuberosity and the acromium process)	Place in lateral recumbency with affected limb closest to the cassette and perpendicular to spine. Opposite leg pulled ventrally. Thorax will be slightly rotated. Collimate C4 to T8
Lateral view of the scapula superimposed over the cranial thorax	Middle of scapula	Less traumatic than dorsal scapula but does not provide whole scapula. Affected limb is pulled caudally and ventrally. Upper limb extended cranially. Rotate sternum slightly away from table
Caudocranial view of the scapula	Middle of scapula	Place in dorsal recumbency with both forelimbs extended cranially. Sternum rotated away from the scapula (approx. 10–20°). This avoids superimposing ribs. Should be a clear, unobstructed view. Collimate proximal humerus to 11th rib
Lateral view of the shoulder	To shoulder joint	Affected limb lowermost, patient in lateral recumbency. Leg is extended cranial and ventral to sternum to prevent superimposition. Other leg is pulled in a CaD direction. The neck is extended dorsally. Sternum is rotated slightly. Collimate mid-scapula to mid-humerus
Caudocranial view of the shoulder	To shoulder joint	Place in dorsal recumbency with both forelimbs extended cranially until parallel with cassette. *Caution: do not rotate humerus.* Collimate mid-humerus, and two-thirds along scapula
Lateral view of the humerus	Centre of humerus	Place in lateral recumbency with affected limb lowermost. Extend in CrV direction with the opposite limb drawn in a CaD direction. Head and neck should be extended dorsally. Collimate mid-radius/ulna and distal end of scapula

11.24 Positioning chart for the forelimb. (Drawings reproduced from Lavin, 2003, with the permission of the publisher) (continues)

Area to be radiographed	Beam centre	Positioning and collimation
Craniocaudal view of the humerus	Middle of humerus	Place in dorsal recumbency. Pull affected leg caudally until the line of the humerus is parallel to the cassette. Abduct slightly from the thorax to alleviate superimposition of the ribs. Include shoulder, humerus and elbow. This view has object–film distance, which will cause slight magnification
Caudocranial view of the humerus	Middle of humerus	Place in dorsal recumbency with forelimbs extended cranially. Leg of interest parallel to cassette, to minimize distortion. Keep head and neck between forelimbs to eliminate superimposition and rotation of the body. Should include entire humerus and distal end of scapula and proximal end of radius/ulna
Flexed lateral view of the elbow	Middle of elbow	Place in lateral recumbency with affected limb lowermost. Carpus is pulled toward the neck region, flexing the elbow. Care should be taken to keep elbow in true lateral position during flexion. By keeping the carpus lateral, the elbow should also remain in a true lateral position
Lateral view of the elbow	Over elbow joint	Place in lateral recumbency with affected limb lowermost. Slightly extend the head and neck in a dorsal direction and the unaffected limb in a caudodorsal direction. Place foam wedge under the metacarpal region to maintain a true lateral of the elbow
Craniocaudal view of the elbow	Over elbow joint	Place in sternal recumbency with the affected limb extended cranially. Elevate patient's head and position away from affected side. Exact view will provide the olecranon between the medial and lateral humeral epicondyles. Place foam pad under point of elbow to prevent rolling or rotation
Lateral view of the radius and ulna	Middle of radius and ulna	Place in lateral recumbency with affected limb centred on cassette. The opposite limb is drawn caudally out of the way. The primary X-ray beam should include the elbow and carpal joints
Craniocaudal view of the radius and ulna	Middle of radius and ulna	Place in sternal recumbency with affected limb extended cranially. Elevate head and position away from affected side. Olecranon should be placed between the humeral condyles. Collimate to include the elbow and the carpus

11.24 (continued) Positioning chart for the forelimb. (Drawings reproduced from Lavin, 2003, with the permission of the publisher) (continues) ▶

Area to be radiographed	Beam centre	Positioning and collimation
Lateral view of the carpus	Over distal row of carpal bones	Place in lateral recumbency with affected limb in centre of cassette. Place foam wedge under elbow to prevent carpus moving away from cassette. Other leg is pulled caudally out of the way. Flexed lateral can be obtained in this position also. Collimate to include distal radius/ulna, whole of carpus and proximal end of metacarpals
Dorsopalmar view of the carpus	Middle of distal row of carpal bones	Place in sternal recumbency with affected limb extended cranially. Carpus is flat against cassette. Place foam wedge under elbow. Oblique views are obtained with 45° angle of the dorsopalmar view to provide DPaML and DPaLM views. Stress views are with the carpus in DPa position, with radius and ulna firmly held in place. Paw is pushed medially or laterally with a ruler or a wooden paddle. Do not apply *too* much stress. Collimate to include entire carpus with two-thirds of the metacarpals and the distal end of the radius/ulna
Dorsopalmar view of the metacarpus-phalanges	Middle of metacarpal bones	Place in sternal recumbency with limb of interest extended. Paw is placed flat on the cassette, with tape used to flatten the digits if necessary. Collimation should be large enough to include the carpal joint and the digits
Lateral view of the phalangeal isolation	Centre of digit	Place in lateral recumbency with affected side adjacent to cassette. Place a foam pad under the elbow to alleviate rotation. Superimposition is a problem here: if one digit is to be examined, isolate from the other digits by taping it cranially in a fixed position; a further band of tape can be used to hold the remaining digits back. Collimate distal ulna/radius and entire paw

11.24 (continued) Positioning chart for the forelimb. (Drawings reproduced from Lavin, 2003, with the permission of the publisher)

Area to be radiographed	Beam centre	Positioning and collimation
Lateral view of the skull	Lateral canthus of eye	Place into lateral recumbency with affected side next to cassette. Place a foam wedge under the ramus of the mandible to stop rotation. The nasal septum should be parallel to the cassette. Place another wedge under the CrV cervical region, pull the front limbs caudally. Field of view should include the tip of the nose to the base of the skull
Dorsoventral view of the skull	Lateral canthus of eye, over high point of cranium	Place into sternal recumbency with the head resting on the cassette. A sandbag should be gently placed over the cervical region to help gain a true D/V position. Keep the forelimbs in a natural position alongside the head, but out of the beam. The sagittal plane of the head should be perpendicular. Tape over the cranium can be used to secure this position. Field of view includes tip of nose to base of skull

11.25 Positioning chart for the skull. (Drawings reproduced from Lavin, 2003, with the permission of the publisher) (continues) ▶

Area to be radiographed	Beam centre	Positioning and collimation
Ventrodorsal view of the skull	Lateral canthus of eye, midline mandibular rami	Place into dorsal recumbency. A trough or sandbags can be used to keep animal in position. The front limbs are extended caudally and secured. A foam pad should be placed under the mid-cervical region to gain proper positioning of the skull on the cassette. The nose must remain parallel to the cassette, and the skull must be balanced in a true ventrodorsal position. Place a small pad under the cranium to prevent rotation, if needed. Field of view includes the tip of the nose to the base of skull
Rostrocaudal view of the frontal sinuses	Through centre of frontal sinuses between eyes	Place into dorsal recumbency with the nose pointing upwards. Pull forelimbs caudally alongside the body. Nose is positioned perpendicular to cassette. Apply a tie around the nose to stabilize. A tongue clamp may also be used to help secure, if needed. Field of view includes the entire forehead of the patient
Ventrodorsal open-mouth view of the nasal cavity	Through level of third upper premolar. To centre on nasal cavity	Place into dorsal recumbency, extending forelimbs caudally alongside the body. Keep the maxilla parallel to the cassette and secure with a tie or tape. Tie the endotracheal tube to the mandible. Apply a tie around the mandible and pull in a caudal direction to open the mouth (a tongue clamp may also be used, also being secured caudally). Angle the tube head to 10–15°, to direct into the mouth. Field of view should include the entire maxilla from the tip of the nose to the pharyngeal region
Open-mouth lateral oblique view of the lower dental arcade	Over site of interest	Place into lateral recumbency with affected mandible next to the cassette. Place a radiolucent gag into the mouth, to separate the upper and lower jaws. Rotate the cranium approx. 20° away from the tabletop and maintain this position with a foam wedge
Lateral intraoral view of the teeth	Over site of interest	An intraoral non-screen dental film is the best method for visualizing the tooth and tooth root. Place into lateral recumbency with non-affected side to the table. The area of interest is therefore uppermost. Insert the film into the mouth and place against the medial border of the maxilla or mandible behind the affected tooth. Maintain the film in position with a pair of forceps. Alter the angle of the X-ray tube or skull as necessary, so that the film is perpendicular to the X-ray beam
Ventrodorsal intraoral view of the mandible	Over site of interest	Place into dorsal recumbency. Extend the head cranially. Place a non-screen film into the mouth with the corner edge of the film introduced first. Advance until the lips allow no further. Pull the tongue cranially to eliminate uneven density over the mandibular area. Because the source–image distance is reduced (as the film is elevated from the table), the X-ray tube should be raised to compensate

11.25 (continued) Positioning chart for the skull. (Drawings reproduced from Lavin, 2003, with the permission of the publisher) (continues) ▶

Area to be radiographed	Beam centre	Positioning and collimation
Open-mouth ventrodorsal oblique view of the upper dental arcade	Over third premolar	Place the patient halfway on to its back with the maxillary arcade of interest closest to the cassette. Rotate the head approx. 45° to the cassette, and stabilize on a foam wedge. The rotation prevents superimposition. Maintain the mouth open with use of a radiolucent mouth gag or by securing the mandible back, with the tongue being pulled back by a tongue depressor
Dorsoventral intraoral view of the maxilla	Over site of interest	Place into sternal recumbency with the head kept in line with the spine. Place a non-screen film into the mouth, and advance caudally between the lips. The X-ray tube should be elevated to compensate for the reduction in source–image distance
Lateral oblique view of the tympanic bullae	Over centre of tympanic bullae	Place into lateral recumbency with unaffected tympanic bulla toward the cassette. The forelimbs are extended slightly caudally. The skull should lie naturally at 8–12° rotation from true lateral. This causes the tympanic bullae to lie separately, allowing visualization of a single bulla. This view can also be used to examine an oblique projection of the temporomandibular (TM) joints
Rostrocaudal open-mouth view of the tympanic bullae	At level of commissure of lips	Place into dorsal recumbency with nose pointing upwards and forelimbs pulled caudally, along the body. Secure the mouth open with ties and tongue clamp, and pull caudally. Pull the nose 5–10° cranially, pulling the mandible caudally. The bullae should be projected free from the mandible and the hard palate of the maxilla. Field of view includes the entire nasopharyngeal region of the skull
Rostrocaudal view of the cranium	Midpoint between eyes	Place into dorsal recumbency with the nose pointing upwards and forelimbs pulled caudally alongside the body. Angle the nose slightly caudally (approx. 10–15°). A tie around the nose (+/– tongue clamp) may be used to secure this position. Field of view includes the entire cranium. *Warning: ensure endotracheal tube does not kink*
Ventrodorsal oblique view of the TM joint	Over centre of TM joint	Place in lateral recumbency with affected side next to the cassette. Rotate the cranium 20° towards the cassette. Place a sponge wedge under the mandible to secure the skull into position. This rotation will help prevent superimposition. This view can be taken with or without the mouth open

11.25   (continued) Positioning chart for the skull. (Drawings reproduced from Lavin, 2003, with the permission of the publisher)

Area to be radiographed	Beam centre	Positioning and collimation
Flexed lateral view of the cervical spine	C3–4 intervertebral space	Place into lateral recumbency. Pull forelimbs in a caudal direction. Tie around the mandible and pull caudally (between the forelimbs). A small wedge should be placed along the spine, to prevent rotation. Field of view includes base of skull and first few thoracic vertebrae. *Warning: care must be taken not to bend the endotracheal tube causing a blockage, or further traumatize the spine (i.e. atlanto-axial subluxation)*
Extended lateral view of the cervical spine	Intervertebral space of C4 and C5	Place into lateral recumbency. Extend the head and neck, pull forelimbs caudally. Push the head in a cranial direction, and secure with a tie. Place a foam wedge under the mandible to prevent rotation. Another wedge under the mid-cervical region may be necessary. Field of view should include base of the skull, entire cervical spine and first few thoracic vertebrae. Larger patients (>27 kg) may require two views: (i) base of skull to C4, (centring on C2–3); (ii) C4 to T1 (centring on C5–6)
Hyperextended lateral view of the cervical spine	C3–4 intervertebral space	Place into lateral recumbency. Extend forelimbs caudally. Extend the head and neck dorsally until resistance is met. Place small wedges under the mandible and under the mid-cervical region to prevent rotation. Field of view includes base of skull to the first few thoracic vertebrae
Ventrodorsal view of the cervical spine	Over C4–5 intervertebral space	Place into dorsal recumbency. Extend the head cranially and pull forelimbs cranially along the body. Place a small wedge under the mid-cervical region to eliminate any distortion. Field of view includes the base of the skull, entire cervical spine and the first few thoracic vertebrae. Larger patients (>27 kg) may require two views: (i) base of skull to C4 (centring on C2–3); (ii) C4 to T1 (centring on C56)
Lateral view of the thoracic spine	Over 7th thoracic vertebral body	Place into lateral recumbency. Extend forelimbs cranially and hindlimbs caudally. Place a wedge under the sternum so that the sternum is at the same height as the thoracic vertebrae. Field of view includes the area from the 7th cervical vertebral body to the 1st lumbar vertebral body
Ventrodorsal view of the thoracic spine	Over level of caudal border of scapula	Place into dorsal recumbency. Extend forelimbs cranially. Allow hindlimbs to lie naturally. The sternum should superimpose the thoracic spine; a trough may be required. Field of view includes all the thoracic vertebrae from C7 to L1

11.26 Positioning chart for the spine. (Drawings reproduced from Lavin, 2003, with the permission of the publisher) (continues) ▶

Area to be radiographed	Beam centre	Positioning and collimation
Lateral view of the thoracolumbar spine	Over thoracolumbar junction	Place into lateral recumbency. Extend forelimbs cranially and hindlimbs caudally. Place a wedge under the sternum to bring it level to the spine. Field of view includes the entire thoracolumbar spine
Ventrodorsal view of the thoracolumbar spine	Over thoracolumbar junction	Place into dorsal recumbency. Extend forelimbs cranially. Hindlimbs can lie in their natural position. Superimpose the sternum with the thoracic vertebrae; a trough can be used. Field of view includes all the thoracic and lumbar vertebrae
Lateral view of the lumbar spine	Over level of 4th lumbar vertebral body	Place into lateral recumbency. Extend the forelimbs cranially and hindlimbs caudally. Place foam wedges under the sternum, mid-lumbar region and between the hindlimbs to prevent rotation. Field of view includes from the 13th thoracic vertebral body to 1st sacral vertebral body
Ventrodorsal view of the lumbar spine	Over 4th lumbar vertebral body	Place into dorsal recumbency with forelimbs extended cranially. Allow hindlimbs to lie in natural position; wedges may be placed under the stifles and use a trough to stabilize. Field of view includes the entire lumbar spine from the 13th thoracic vertebral body to the 1st sacral vertebral body
Ventrodorsal view of the sacrum	Over level of sacrum	Place into dorsal recumbency with hindlimbs in a natural frog-legged position. Use a trough to help stabilize. Angle the X-ray tube at 30° towards the sacrum. Field of view includes the area from the 6th lumbar vertebral body to the iliac crests. Positioning for the lateral sacrum is the same as for the lateral pelvic view
Lateral view of the coccygeal vertebrae	Over area of interest	Place into lateral recumbency. Extend the tail caudally. Raising the cassette with a foam wedge raises the cassette to the same level as the tail, keeping the tail parallel to the cassette
Ventrodorsal view of the coccygeal vertebrae	Over area of interest	Place into dorsal recumbency. Allow hindlimbs to lie in their natural frog-leg position. Use a trough to stabilize. The tail should be extended caudally. Tape can be used to secure the tail into position

11.26 (continued) Positioning chart for the spine. (Drawings reproduced from Lavin, 2003, with the permission of the publisher)

Area to be radiographed	Beam centre	Positioning and collimation
Lateral view of the pharynx	Over pharynx	Place into lateral recumbency. Extend forelimbs caudally. Extend head and neck cranially. Place a wedge under the mandible, to help prevent rotation. The upper respiratory tract passages act as a negative contrast agent allowing the structures of the pharynx to be visible. Field of view includes the entire area of the neck between the lateral canthus of the eye and the 3rd cervical vertebral body
Lateral view with horizontal beam of the thorax	Over caudal border of scapula	This view can be used to confirm the presence of fluid or free air in the thoracic cavity, and to help in the estimation of how much is present. Place into sternal recumbency on top of a 5–10 cm piece of foam. Extend the head and forelimbs cranially. Place cassette in a vertical position against the lateral side of the patient. Field of view includes the manubrium sterni caudally to the 1st lumbar vertebral body; including all ribs. This can be used for lateral abdomen also
Lateral view of the thorax	Over caudal border of scapula	Place into right lateral recumbency – this provides the most accurate view of the cardiac silhouette. If lung metastases are suspected, both right and left views should be obtained for any subtle changes. Extend forelimbs cranially; this helps reduce superimposition of the triceps and humeri over the cranial aspect of the thorax. Extend hindlimbs slightly caudally. Extend the head slightly. Place a wedge under the mandible and thorax, and between the hindlimbs, to prevent rotation. Field of view includes the entire thoracic cavity from the line of the manubrium sterni caudally to the 1st lumbar vertebral body. Exposure is taken at full inspiration
Lateral decubitus view (ventrodorsal view with horizontal beam) of the thorax	Over caudal border of scapula	Used to confirm presence and quantity of fluid or air within the thorax. Place into lateral recumbency on top of a 5–10 cm thick foam pad; this allows visualization of both sides of the thorax. Extend forelimbs and head cranially. Extend hindlimbs caudally as this helps keep good patient-to-cassette contact. Place the cassette behind the patient in a vertical posture. Field includes entire thorax
Ventrodorsal view of the thorax	Over caudal border of scapula	This view allows full visualization of the lung fields, providing better views of the accessory lung lobe and caudal mediastinum. Place into dorsal recumbency. Extend forelimbs cranially. Hindlimbs stay as normal. Superimpose the sternum with the spine. Use of a trough may help secure the position. Exposure is taken at full inspiration. _This view is contraindicated in patients with respiratory problems_
Dorsoventral view of the thorax	Over caudal border of scapula	D/V is best for the evaluation of the heart, because the heart is nearer the sternum and it sits in its normal position. This position is difficult for deep-chested breeds; use plenty of wedges and positioning aids; if unable to do, V/D will have to be taken. Place into sternal recumbency. Superimpose the sternum with the spine. Extend forelimbs slightly cranially to keep elbows out of view. Hindlimbs are as normal (difficult for hip dysplastic dogs). Lower the head and place between the two forelimbs. Field of view includes the entire thorax, including all ribs. The exposure should be taken at full inspiration, to allow complete visualization of the lung tissue

11.27 Positioning chart for soft tissue. (Drawings reproduced from Lavin, 2003, with the permission of the publisher) (continues) ▶

Area to be radiographed	Beam centre	Positioning and collimation
Lateral view of the abdomen	Over caudal aspect of 13th rib (for feline, measure 2–3 fingerbreadths caudally)	Place into right lateral recumbency. Extend hindlimbs caudally. The right view facilitates longitudinal separation of the kidneys. Extend the hindlimbs caudally to prevent superimposition of the femoral muscles over the caudal portion of the abdomen. Place a pad between the femurs to prevent rotation of the pelvis and caudal abdomen. A pad should also be placed under the sternum, to keep sternum at the same level as the spine. Field of view includes the diaphragm caudally to the femoral head. Take the exposure at the time of expiration so that the diaphragm is displaced cranially
Ventrodorsal view of the abdomen	Over caudal aspect of 13th rib (for feline measure 2–3 fingerbreadths caudally)	Place into dorsal recumbency. Use a trough or sandbags for positioning. Field of view includes the entire abdomen from the diaphragm to the level of the femoral head. Larger patients may require two views: one of the cranial abdomen and the other of the caudal abdomen. Take exposure during the expiratory phase so that the diaphragm is in a cranial position and not placing any compression on the abdominal contents

11.27 (continued) Positioning chart for soft tissue. (Drawings reproduced from Lavin, 2003, with the permission of the publisher)

Positioning of exotic species

Further details can be found in BSAVA Manuals of specific exotic groups.

Guinea pigs and rabbits

Guinea pigs and rabbits require careful positioning, avoiding any stress to the patient. Handling should be kept to a minimum and sedation or general anaesthesia should be considered in order to help to maintain struggle-free restraint.

A short exposure using a high definition is preferred that will not necessitate the use of a grid. Positioning aids for cats and dogs (see earlier) can be used, or alternatively radiolucent tapes, which are easily removed at the end of the procedure.

Mice, gerbils and hamsters

These patients may require restraint using either a Perspex or cardboard tube or box as a means of security and to reduce the likelihood of stress due to handling. If chemically restrained, tape as discussed for other small mammals could also be employed.

Birds

Dorsal or ventral recumbency views can be obtained by extending the wings away from the body and securing with tape. The legs need to be extended caudally and secured in extension.

Lateral views can be obtained with the bird secured in position using tapes or a material cover. The wings then need to be extended above the body and taped into position.

Reptiles

The patient should be allowed to cool to room temperature and their eyes should be covered to reduce their anxiety and increase their compliance. Dorsoventral body radiographs are often possible with no further restraint. Lateral recumbency is generally not possible; therefore this would require the use of a horizontal beam if needed.

Snakes may be radiographed while conscious inside a Perspex or cardboard tube.

Labelling radiographs

Radiographic images require appropriate and reliable labelling methods. To ensure that there is no mistake with clinical interpretation, correct identification of the patient to which the image belongs is essential. Mismatched results could lead to the patient receiving an inappropriate care or treatment regime.

Radiographs are considered part of an animal's medical record; therefore there is also a legal obligation to ensure that all documentation has been completed appropriately.

Labelling of the actual radiograph can be achieved by one of the following methods.

- *Peri-exposure* (allows labelling to occur at the time of exposure):
  - Lead letters and numbers can be used to form details of the patient being radiographed; these can be placed either on the cassette itself or into a translucent container that allows the letter tiles to be slotted into place so that they do not get displaced during the preparation for exposure
  - Sticker-strip of lead paste that can be cut to requirement and labelled with ballpoint pen.
- *Post exposure*:
  - White light markers can be used to further expose an area of the film that will have been protected by a lead rectangle, specifically designed to allow this type of labelling to be

performed. The details are written on a paper label and placed into a device that has the unexposed area of film positioned and then closed to be exposed to light, which then picks 'shadows' of the details from the paper label. This is performed entirely within the darkroom prior to the processing of the film
  – Sticky labels can be used and placed on a processed radiograph. This is considered a non-permanent method of labelling as it could be removed or altered or could fade in time. It would be considered an inadequate method to use if submitting for a BVA scoring scheme as this style of labelling potentially could be altered and details falsified.

Anatomical markers

Anatomical markers should be used at all times to indicate which side of the patient is left and which side of the patient is right. It is routine to take thoracic and abdominal lateral views with the animal placed into right lateral recumbency; therefore it is generally only required to use a 'left/right' marker when the patient is placed into left lateral recumbency. By convention, limb markers should be placed along the dorsal or lateral aspect of the limb. However, not everyone follows this convention, which can result in mistakes being made with some oblique views.

The most exact method of labelling is the use of markers that clearly indicate the radiographic projection. These are easy to obtain and are relatively inexpensive.

Radiographic identification for BVA Hip/Elbow Scoring Schemes

Each radiograph must be identified using a permanent form of labelling, which is achieved using either X-rite tape (or similar), or a darkroom imprinter. This label must include the following details:

■ Kennel Club number
■ Date of radiography
■ Left or right marker indicating which side is which.

Contrast techniques

Contrast media

■ There are two types of contrast media: **positive** and **negative**.
■ Positive + negative contrast = **double contrast**.

Positive contrast media

Positive contrast media are barium or iodine compounds that contain elements of a high atomic number. They absorb more X-rays than tissue or bone, thus appearing white.

Barium sulphate

■ Used exclusively for gastrointestinal (GI) tract studies.
■ Completely insoluble.

■ Not absorbed by intestine.
■ Available as liquid, paste or powder, or as capsules known as BIPS (barium-impregnated polyethylene spheres).
■ Liquid barium should be shaken before use to remix the solution.
■ Powdered barium should be used immediately once reconstituted.
■ Can cause abdominal adhesions if medium leaks into peritoneal cavity.
■ If inhaled, may result in aspiration pneumonia.

Water-soluble iodine-based preparations

■ Water soluble, low viscosity, low toxicity.
■ Used for intravenous work and myelography studies.
■ Low osmolar non-ionic preparations used for myelography (e.g. metrizamide, iopamidol and iohexol).
■ May produce side effects (vomiting, anaphylactic reaction).
■ Some may be used for GI studies (sodium/meglumine amidotrizoate; Gastrografin).
■ Some agents may crystallize; therefore gently warm by placing in a jug of warm water and shake bottle prior to use.

Care of contrast material

■ Keep away from any source of non-ionizing radiation, such as radio, microwave or sunlight.
■ Keep away from X-ray radiation.
■ Store below 25°C.

Negative contrast media

Negative contrast media consist of gases (e.g. air, oxygen, nitrous oxide or carbon dioxide). They have a low specific gravity, making the medium more radiolucent to X-rays and thus appear black.

Alimentary tract studies

Indications

■ Obstruction.
■ Distortion.
■ Lesion.
■ Displacement.
■ Normal or abnormal function.

Contrast agent

■ Barium sulphate.
■ Gastrografin.

Equipment required

■ Catheter-tip syringes (60 ml).
■ Orogastric tube or stomach tube (take care to prevent inhalation).
■ Plastic bottle with a nozzle.

Patient preparation

- Nil by mouth 24 hours pre-examination.
- Enema may be necessary 4 hours prior to the procedure.
- General anaesthetic or sedation contraindicated (slows peristalsis).
- Sedate only if necessary.

To view the oesophagus

- Barium sulphate paste.
- Barium sulphate powder mixed in food.
- *Contrast medium:*
  - 70–100% barium sulphate (liquid or paste) or iodinated oral contrast.
- *Equipment required:*
  - Optional canned or hard pet food.
- *Patient preparation:*
  - None necessary.

Procedure for an oesophogram

1. Expose survey radiographs.
2. Use 1 ml barium suspension (60% wt/vol) per 5 kg bodyweight.
3. Place patient in lateral recumbency on X-ray table.
4. Slowly infuse liquid contrast medium inside patient's cheek and allow patient to swallow.
5. Expose several radiographs of the thorax to monitor its passage. Field of view should include the entire oesophagus from the pharynx to the stomach. The first exposure should be within seconds of swallowing.
6. Repeat these views with the patient in dorsal recumbency.
7. Place the patient back into lateral recumbency.
8. Slowly administer barium paste and expose the radiograph during swallowing.
9. If abnormalities are still not detected, mix with tinned food and give orally.
10. Radiographs are repeated; right and left lateral views may be indicated. Ventrodorsal views are contraindicated for patients with dilated oesophagus that is full of contrast medium. Placing the patient on its back may result in aspiration.

Stomach and small intestine

Procedure

1. Take plain radiographs first, four views after contrast and then at intervals of 5–10 minutes. Fluoroscopy may be used.
2. Administer barium to distend the stomach with contrast:
   a. Route: orally by placing the positive contrast into the oral cavity and allowing the patient to swallow, or via orogastric tube. To ensure correct placement of the orogastric tube, infuse a small amount of water. If the tube is incorrectly placed and is located in the trachea, the patient should cough.
   b. Dose: 4–8 ml/kg bodyweight (20–100 ml of 100% barium sulphate).

3. Expose dorsoventral, ventrodorsal, right and left lateral radiographs immediately after contrast administration.
4. Expose right lateral ventrodorsal or dorsoventral radiographs at intervals until contrast reaches the large bowel (suggested times: 15, 30, 60 and 90 minutes).

Large intestine

- Pre-examination enema necessary 2–4 hours prior to procedure.
- 20% barium sulphate at 10 ml/kg by enema.
- May be under general anaesthetic or sedation.
- Double contrast gives better mucosal detail using barium suspension at 13 ml/kg and air at 6 ml/kg.

Urogenital tract studies

Kidneys and ureters: intravenous (excretion) urography (IVU)

Indications

- Evaluation of size, shape and position.
- Urinary incontinence.
- Haematuria.

Patient preparation

- Starve for 24 hours.
- Enema 2–4 hours before procedure.
- General anaesthetic.

Doses and techniques

There are two techniques: low volume, rapid injection; and high volume, drip infusion:

- 2 ml/kg of a 300–400 mg/ml contrast medium injected rapidly i.v. Take films immediately
- 8 ml/kg of a 150 mg/ml contrast medium infused over 10–15 minutes i.v. Take films at 5, 10 and 15 minutes after start of infusion.

Bladder studies: cystography

Indications

- Persistent haematuria.
- Dysuria.
- Urinary retention.
- Urinary incontinence.
- Identification and integrity of the bladder.
- Presence of lesions/calculi.

Patient preparation

- Pre-enema.
- General anaesthetic or deep sedation.
- Catheterize and empty bladder after plain films.

Pneumocystography (negative contrast)

1. Fill bladder with a gas.
2. Take ventrodorsal and lateral views.

Positive contrast cystography

- Gives slightly better mucosal detail.
- Dilute (20–30%) water-soluble contrast medium.
- Use 50–300 ml (depending on size).

Double contrast cystography

- Optimal mucosal detail.
- 5–15 ml contrast medium.
- Then inflate bladder (do not over-inflate).

Intravenous cystography

- As for IVU but take films after 30 minutes.

Urethral studies: retrograde urethrography, vagino-urethrography

Indications

- Haematuria.
- Dysuria.
- Urinary incontinence.
- Lesions/neoplasia.
- Calculi.

Technique

Dog

1. Plain radiograph is taken first.
2. Catheterize, passing only 2.5–5 cm into the urethra.
3. Use dilute water-soluble contrast medium (150–200 mg iodine/ml) at 1 ml/kg, mixed 50:50 with sterile K-Y jelly.
4. Introduce contrast medium mixed with the K-Y jelly; pinch end of penis to reduce any leakage of the contrast.
5. Take lateral view with hindlegs pulled cranially.

(Note that prostatic enlargement repositions urethra)

Bitch

1. Introduce water-soluble dilute iodine (150–200 mg iodine/ml) at 1 ml/kg into the vagina via a Foley catheter, then inflate the bulb.
2. Take lateral view.

Contrast radiography of the spine: myelography

This is a routine procedure for the presenting neurological patient, where a positive contrast agent is injected via a cisternal puncture or lumbar puncture to assess for possible spinal cord trauma or vertebral disorders, neoplasia or infection. The contrast medium is injected by a trained veterinary surgeon into an area that contains cerebrospinal fluid (CSF). Analysis of a CSF sample taken at the time of puncture may assist with the diagnosis for the patient.

Myelography technique

Because of the area that is to be assessed, strict asepsis must be maintained: an infection introduced directly into the meninges could have disastrous consequences.

The skin is prepared as it would be for a surgical procedure and the patient is anaesthetized and intubated in order to control the patient and their rate of ventilation.

One person must be responsible for the patient's anaesthetic whilst another person is responsible for positioning and holding the patient securely in the appropriate position.

The anaesthetist must pay careful attention to the endotracheal (ET) tube, which may be compromised due to the positioning of the patient's neck. To avoid kinking of the tube it is recommended either to use a specially reinforced ET tube, or to deflate the cuff of the tube so that the patient may at least breathe around the tube if kinking should occur. For this reason also it is important to ensure that the maximum size of ET tube is used in the first instance. The anaesthetist must ensure that the patient is at a moderate to deep plane of anaesthesia, due to the stimulation that may occur on penetration of the dura mater. This can be observed by an increase in respiratory and cardiac rates. The patient must be kept extremely still while the needle is placed, but if increasing the volatile agent care must be taken that the patient does not become too deep due to the increased respiratory breaths. It should be anticipated that a short period of apnoea can occur following cisternal puncture.

It is essential therefore to achieve a good level of anaesthesia prior to the start of the procedure.

Equipment required

- Low-osmolar non-ionic water-soluble warmed iohexol contrast agent at 240 or 300 mg/ml with a dose rate of 0.25–0.5 ml/kg.
- Sterile 5 ml plain containers and an EDTA container.
- 22–19 gauge x 1–3.5 inches spinal needle.
- Skin preparation solutions.
- Sterile gloves for sample collector.
- Surgical drape.
- Special reinforced endotracheal tube of a suitable size for the patient, with a syringe to deflate and inflate the cuff of the tube as necessary.
- Suitable depth of anaesthesia before the procedure is performed.

Anatomical landmarks for cisternal puncture

1. Position the patient into left lateral recumbency for right-handed operators, and right lateral for left-handed operators. The contrast agent is to be injected between cervical vertebrae 1 (atlas) and 2 (axis) via the cisterna magna. It is essential that the patient's collar is removed and the nose remains parallel to the table, therefore take a position that can be maintained comfortably for the next few minutes. Use of the elbows as a form of anchorage and security may be helpful but this will differ from person to person.

2. The animal's head is flexed to make an angle of 90 degrees with the vertebral column so that the sample can be collected from the cisterna magna at the atlanto-occipital articulation.
3. The clinician, once scrubbed, gowned and gloved, prepares the area and slowly inserts the spinal needle within the centre of the triangle. Care must be taken as insertion of the needle beyond the subarachnoid space may result in temporary or permanent paralysis of the patient.

Method for needle insertion

1. The needle is slowly advanced through the skin.
2. The stylet is removed.
3. The needle is advanced slowly by the operator until CSF appears.
4. The operator can usually detect a 'pop' sensation as the needle penetrates the dura mater (no twitch should be observed as would be seen with the lumbar puncture technique).
5. CSF is allowed to drip slowly into the plain and EDTA collection pots without altering the needle's position.
6. The needle must be kept still and parallel to the table at all times.
7. Negative pressure should not be used to withdraw the CSF.
8. Once the CSF sample has been obtained, the contrast agent is introduced carefully and slowly, taking care that the needle remains still.
9. The needle is removed carefully in the exact position that it was introduced.

Myelography using lumbar puncture

The dye is to be injected at the L5–L6 lumbar space in the dog, or L6–L7 in the cat. CSF is collected from the anaesthetized animal by percutaneous insertion of a spinal needle into the lumbar area and into the subarachnoid space of the spinal column, prior to the injection of the contrast agent. A free-flow sample is collected with the animal in either lateral or sternal recumbency. The position must be comfortable as it will be necessary to keep hold of the patient securely until the end of the procedure, without allowing any movement of the patient.

Method

1. General anaesthesia and lateral or sternal recumbency.
2. Clip and surgically prepare the area.
3. If in lateral recumbency, the hindlimbs are pulled cranially under the abdomen; if in sternal, the legs are either side of the animal, pulled forward and lifted up towards the ceiling to open the spaces between the lumbar vertebrae.
4. For dogs the site is between L5 and L6; the needle is inserted alongside the spinous process of L6. In the cat L6–L7 is used.
5. The needle must penetrate through the ligamentum flavum, which can be quite tough.
6. A 'pop' sensation is felt by the operator, but less so than when using the cisternal puncture technique.

7. The stylet is removed intermittently to check progress as the needle is slowly inserted.
8. The needle is inserted until the needle end touches the ventral surface of the vertebral canal, then withdrawn about 1 mm to be located within the subarachnoid space.
9. When the needle penetrates through the cauda equina the patient will 'twitch', which is an excellent indicator that the needle is in the correct place.
10. Collection of CSF from the lumbar region is slower than that from a cisternal puncture.
11. Blood contamination may occur and the puncture must be repeated to avoid impairing the results.
12. Respiratory and cardiac rates may increase. The patient must be stable before the procedure commences.
13. Once the CSF sample has been obtained, the contrast agent is introduced carefully and slowly, taking care that the needle remains still.

Other contrast techniques

Other contrast techniques are described in Figure 11.28.

Term	Description
Angiography	Shows up the vascular system
Angiocardiography	Demonstrates congenital or acquired lesions of the heart ■ Non-selective – inject contrast via jugular ■ Selective – catheterize heart via femoral artery under fluoroscopy
Arthrography	Shows joint irregularities, e.g. shoulder osteochondrosis dissecans (OCD)
Bronchography	Propyliodine is administered to the base of the trachea via the ET tube. Demonstrates bronchial obstruction or lesions. Less used now that bronchoscopy has been introduced
Cholecystography	Shows up liver irregularities via i.v. injection
Dachryocystorhinography	Outlines nasolacrimal duct (inject via cannulation of the puncta of the eye)
Hysterosalpingography	Uterus = hysterogram Fallopian tubes = salpingography
Lymphangiography	Outlines lymphatic system (methylene blue dye is injected into intestinal veins)
Portal venography	For diagnosis of congenital or acquired portosystemic shunts (inject via jejunal vein via a laparotomy)
Sialography	Outlines the glands and ducts (salivary) via cannulation of the salivary duct (sublingual, submandibular, parotid)

11.28 Other contrast techniques.

Film processing

Processing systems

Film processing systems include:

- Manual with tanks (large tanks with solutions)
- Dish processing (cheaper – less solution required)
- Automatic processing (quicker and produces a dry film)
- Polaroid system (expensive, but portable, and useful for large animal practice).

Manual processing

Darkroom design

A darkroom is required for manual processing and should include:

- Separate, partitioned wet and dry areas with non-static (not black) work surfaces
- Timing devices and thermostats
- Film drying area: dry film hangers (channel or clip); drying cabinet or area with drip catcher
- Safelights.

The darkroom should:

- Ideally be of an area >2.6 x 2 m (8 x 6 ft)
- Be completely light-proof (prevents fogging)
- Have water and electricity supply
- Have a locking door and a notice 'IN USE' (to prevent accidental opening)
- Have a darkroom entrance with rotational or double-door action, or around a bend (as light cannot go around corners)
- Have doors that close properly (no cracks)
- Be used exclusively as a darkroom
- Be kept clean and tidy
- Be compact, but big enough to work in comfortably
- Have adequate ventilation, which must be light proof
- Have a non-slip floor that can be washed easily
- Have white or cream walls and ceiling to reflect available light
- Not be subject to extremes of temperature (guide 18–20°C) or high humidity
- Have tiles on the walls by the developing tanks.

Safelights

A safelight provides a suitable light source that allows visibility for the operator in the darkroom without affecting the film exposure during processing. Generally safelights meet the following criteria:

- Constructed within a box fixed to the wall
- Light produced does not affect film *over a short time period*
- Prolonged time may cause fogging of the film
- 15-watt bulb
- Filter fitted to eliminate green and blue light
- Brown filter for blue-sensitive film (calcium tungstate)
- Red filter for green-sensitive film (rare earth)
- Red acceptable for both types of film
- Minimum of 1.2 metres above work surface
- Indirect: directs light upwards
- Direct: directs light downwards.

If two safelights are used, the light must *not* overlap as twice the light density may cause fogging.

To check safelight:

1. Place underexposed film 1 metre from the safelight under black cardboard or paper.
2. Uncover a small portion for periods of 10, 20, 30 and 60 seconds and then process the film.

Once developed there should be *no* evidence of blackening.

Manual processing procedure

The first rule is to standardize all procedures.

1. Check that levels of fixer and developer are correct.
2. Check that developer is at the right temperature.
3. Agitate both solutions.
4. Ensure that hands are clean and dry.
5. Lock the room.
6. Switch on the safelight and load the film hanger. Types include channel hangers (Figure 11.29) and clip hangers (Figure 11.30).
7. Place the film hanger and film into the developer, agitate to remove any surface air bubbles and replace the lid.
8. Develop for the appropriate time (Figure 11.31).
9. Drain, then rinse for a least 10 seconds.
10. Place the film hanger and film into the fixer.
11. After 30 seconds the light can be switched on and the film viewed, though it will need fixing for a total of 10 minutes.
12. Rinse for 10–20 minutes under running water.
13. Allow to dry.

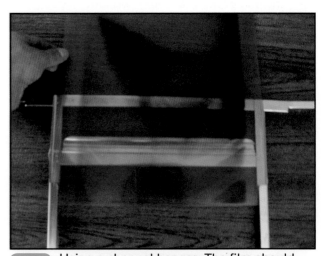

11.29 Using a channel hanger. The film should sit within the channels. At the top of the channel hanger there is a strip of metal that folds down to help secure the film in place.

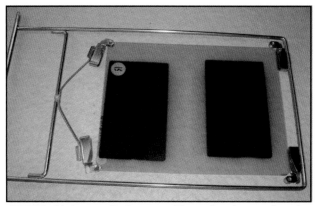

11.30 Using a clip hanger. Two clips located at the top and two at the bottom help to hold the film in a secure manner.

Temperature		Time (minutes)
°C	**°F**	
15.5	60	8.5
18.5	65	6
20	68	5
21	70	4.5
24	75	3.5

11.31 Optimum developing temperature and time guidelines.

Figure 11.32 illustrates the manual processing procedure. This is a suggested guideline, which can be adjusted to standardize the practice's own methods depending upon equipment, chemicals and environmental conditions. Note that oxidizing increases as the temperature rises, and also if there are no lids on the chemicals (i.e. floating lids within the fixer and developer tanks).

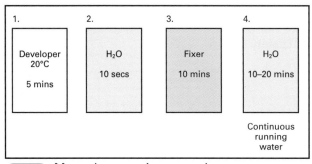

11.32 Manual processing procedure. Exact timings will vary – follow the manufacturer's recommendation.

- *Developer*: enhances the latent (hidden) image on the film emulsion by the process of a chemical reaction with the silver ions. If using a non-screen film, due to the thicker emulsion this will need 1 minute longer in the solution.
- *Rinsing*: running water/fresh tank for 10–20 seconds
  - Halts the development process
  - Removes surplus developing chemicals
  - Prevents contamination of the fixer solution.

- *Fixing*: prevents further development and fixes the images. Any undeveloped silver salts are removed ('clearing') and the emulsion is hardened ('tanning'). Non-screen films require several minutes more fixing time, due to the thicker emulsion layer.
- *Washing*: running water for at least 10–20 minutes (but in hard-water areas this may produce a scum on the film, which may affect results).
- *Drying*: remove from the channel hanger and clip to a line or dry in a drying cabinet.
- *Reducer solution*: can be used to improve over-developed films by removing the silver from the image, giving better image detail; this simply requires the film to be left in the solution until the correct development has been achieved, before being rinsed, fixed and washed as normal.

Making up the chemicals

- *Developer*: either powder and water (cheaper and easier) or liquid and water.
- *Replenishment*: makes up for lost volume, maintains even activity, able to replenish equal volume (e.g. 9 litre tank can take 9 litres of replenishment 'top-up'). Solutions must be changed at least every 3 months.
- *Fixer*: either powder and water (cheaper and non-staining) or liquid (and hardener) and water.

Used chemicals are hazardous healthcare waste and must be disposed of accordingly (see below).

Automatic processors

An automatic processor (Figure 11.33) is convenient and cost effective for practices with a high radiographic workload. It can produce a dry radiograph from within 90 seconds up to 8 minutes (depending on the model). One type of automatic processor removes the need for a darkroom altogether; it is commonly used in dental radiography. Stand-alone units with arm holes allow the removal and insertion of film from the cassette and into the processor without coming into contact with light. Without careful maintenance, however, such processors can experience problems.

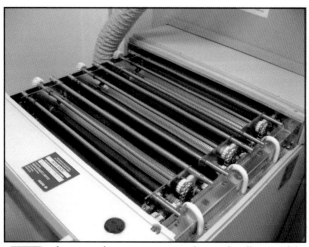

11.33 Automatic processor tanks and rollers, with lid removed. (Courtesy of R Dennis)

Automatic processors can come in a variety of sizes and may be bench-top operated or free standing. The processor consists of two tanks and a drying chamber; the films are passed though a roller transport system operated by a motor that drives a chain passing around cogs fitted to the ends of the rollers.

- To enable quicker processing times the *developer* temperature is higher, usually around 27–35°C (it may take 15–20 minutes to reach the correct temperature when first switched on).
- The *rinsing* phase is omitted, because the squeezing effect of the rollers removes all chemical residue from the film.
- The *fixer* is essential for its hardening properties, to protect the emulsion at warmer temperatures. The fixer solution may become warmed due to its proximity to the heated developer tank.
- *Washing* time is reduced by an increased water flow rate (of at least 6 litres/minute). The squeezing action of the rollers again reduces washing time by reducing the amount of fixer left on the film.
- The *dryer* works by blowing hot air on to both sides of the film as it is conveyed through the chamber by rollers.

The chemicals of the processor are continually replenished. Developer and fixer are stored in reservoir tanks close to the machine, and measured quantities are pumped into the appropriate tanks each time a film is processed. First thing in the morning it is advisable to put one old film through, to clean any residue from the rollers, and to replenish the solution that has been sitting in the tanks overnight. This replenishment rate can be adjusted to suit film throughput.

Adequate drainage for the overflow of excess 'spent' chemicals must be provided and should comply with COSHH regulations. For practices with a low radiographic load, an unwanted film should be passed through the processor on a regular basis to help to prevent oxidization of the developer chemicals.

The rollers of an automatic processor should be cleaned weekly. Use of abrasive substances must be avoided.

Reading X-ray films

How to view and assess a radiograph

- Have the main lighting dimmed or completely switched off.
- Place the radiograph into the centre of the viewer.
- Ensure that the viewer is clean and dry.
- Ensure that the viewer is evenly lit.
- Check that all light bulbs are in working order.
- Right and left lateral views should be placed with the head to the left and spine to the top.
- Ventrodorsal or dorsoventral views should be placed with the head at the top and the patient's right on the viewer's left.

In summary, when assessing a radiograph the following points should be appraised:

- *Labelling* – identification is present and correct
- *Centring* – correct area has been included
- *Positioning* – correct positioning
- *Exposure* – adequate contrast, density and detail
- *Processing* – any faults identified
- *Collimation* – 100%
- *Extraneous marks* – scratches, dust or static
- *Quality* – is it a good-quality image?
  - Density – blackness
  - Contrast – density differences between different areas
  - Sharpness – any evidence of blurring?

Film faults

There are numerous causes of film faults (Figures 11.34 to 11.36), which in a worst-case scenario could result in the image being so poor that it is deemed non-diagnostic.

Non-diagnostic images should be avoided at all costs in order to reduce the necessity of repeating any radiographic exposure, which ultimately exposes both the patient and personnel to additional health and safety risks.

Fault	Causes
Background too light	Probably underdeveloped Possibly underexposed (exposure too low) Low line voltage
Poorly penetrated 'silhouette' image	Underexposed or underdeveloped
Penetrated image with a thin background	Overexposed and underdeveloped (Underdevelopment leads to overexposure)
Background correct but image too dark	Overexposed (exposure factors too high) Fogged (chemicals, light, wrong safelight filter or bulb) White light leakage into darkroom or cassette Old film or film exposed to scatter/chemicals, pressure Over-development

11.34   Film faults and their causes. (continues)   ▶

Fault	Causes
Blurred image	Movement of the patient, tube head or cassette during exposure Poor screen–film contact Incorrect screen Scatter Film fogging
Film discoloured after storage	Poorly washed or poorly fixed film
White marks on the film	Dirt or scratch on the screen Scratch on film before exposure or after processing Splash of fixer on to film or greasy fingerprints before developing
Black marks on the film	Scratch on film between exposure and processing Splash of developer before processing Water splash after developing Bending or pressure after exposure ('crimp marks')
High contrast	Low kV technique used
Low contrast	High kV Scatter (no grid used) Poor processing (e.g. exhausted developer)
Uneven processing	Poorly mixed chemicals Films touching during processing Poor agitation of films during processing
Black spots or lightning-like lines	Static electricity

11.34 (continued) Film faults and their causes.

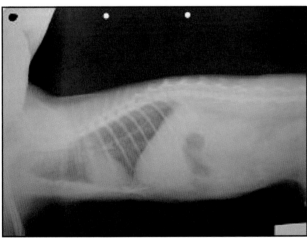

11.35 Lateral view of the thorax and abdomen of a cat. The positioning is adequate, although the forelimbs could have been extended more cranially and the thorax is slightly rotated (a foam wedge would have decreased this rotation). It is unclear whether the desired view was of the lateral thorax or the lateral abdomen, since the radiograph is centred on the diaphragm. The thoracic inlet and thoracic vertebrae are missing from the image. The film is too pale overall, indicating underexposure. The anatomical structures are not clearly visible, especially caudal to the diaphragm. Collimation is not evident (0%) as the primary beam is off the film edges. There is no L/R marker or label. Brown coloration at the edges of the film suggests insufficient rinsing or fixer splashes. There is damage in the corners from clip hangers and water marks are evident.

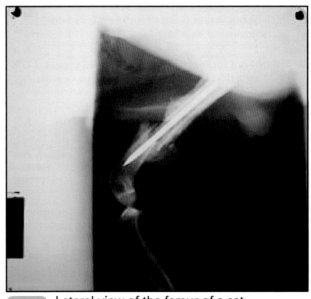

11.36 Lateral view of the femur of a cat. Positioning is poor, as the abdomen is overlying the proximal end of the femur and obscuring the bone. Exposure is good enough to enable a diagnosis to be made. Centring is poor -- it should be on the mid-shaft of the femur. The radiograph is labelled but there is no L/R marker. Collimation is not evident, as the primary beam went beyond the edges of the film. The white areas on the left and at the top are due to light leakage, as a result of the cassette not being properly closed or incorrect storage of film prior to exposure. A brown tinge indicates poor or inadequate rinsing during processing.

Causes of potential film faults include :

■ Poor patient positioning (see Figure 11.36)
■ Operator error
■ Faulty equipment
■ Inappropriate handling of the film
■ Poor care and maintenance of film, screens or cassettes
■ Chemical contamination
■ Poor development technique.

Poor patient positioning and operator error

Incorrect positioning or immobilization of the patient can alter the quality of a radiograph significantly.
Try to avoid:

■ Patient movement
■ Superimposition from other structures
■ Artefacts from an animal's collar or lead obscuring the view
■ Artefacts from spilt contrast material or dirt found on the animal or the equipment
■ Positioning aids placed in the field of interest
■ Exposure taken at the wrong time (e.g. a thoracic radiograph should be taken on inspiration and an abdominal radiograph should be taken on expiration to help to provide better definition of the structures)
■ Incorrect film/cassette combination used
■ Poor film/screen contact
■ Poor positioning (see Figure 11.36)
■ Incorrect exposures chosen (see Figure 11.35)
■ Incorrect use of a grid (e.g. upside-down)
■ Lack of collimation (see Figures 11.35 and 11.36)
■ No anatomical markers (see Figures 11.35 and 11.36)
■ No patient identification or date (see Figure 11.35)
■ Poor centring resulting in elongation, distorting the image (see Figure 11.36)
■ Incorrect film focal distance (FFD) chosen, resulting in a penumbra effect (see Figure 11.12) that is a distortion of the image giving a fuzzy outline rather than a sharp image
■ Incorrect object-to-film distance (OFD) chosen, resulting in a penumbra effect (see Figure 11.13) giving magnification of the image
■ Incorrect positioning, e.g. the area of interest not being parallel to the cassette, causing distortion of the image known as foreshortening.

It is absolutely essential that the following should *never* happen:

■ The wrong area has been radiographed
■ The wrong patient has been radiographed
■ The radiographer is found within the image.

Faulty equipment

■ Damaged cassette.
■ Damaged film.
■ Faulty safelight.
■ Out-of-date film.
■ Poorly maintained or non-serviced equipment (may not be functioning appropriately).

Inappropriate handling of the film
Emulsion damage
Subtle defects can be detected by inspecting the film surface while holding it horizontally at eye level. Emulsion damage can be caused by contact with rough worktops, floors, hanger clips and human fingernails, especially when it is wet.

Larger areas of emulsion can be destroyed if films are allowed to come into contact with each other or with the walls of tanks during any of the stages of developing. Rollers of automatic processors can 'handle' films and cause scratching, either as a result of contamination with insoluble chemical salts or by incorrect alignment. Overlapping of films within the processor can also damage the emulsion. After processing, if the film becomes wet again this can lead to damage.

Crescent marks
Bending or creasing of the film can result in small curvilinear defects, either light or black, due to mishandling of the film. These marks will be white if the damage occurred before exposure, or black when they occur between exposure and development.

Fingerprints
When the film is viewed horizontally, fingerprints from wet or greasy hands show as silver stains. Black prints show as black marks when the film has been handled prior to exposure.

Static marks
Films drawn rapidly across smooth worktops may generate static electricity. This occurs more in dry weather with low humidity. A distinct black 'forked lightning' effect appears on the film. Static can also be caused by black plastic benches; ideally bench surfaces should consist of Formica with a slightly textured surface.

Poor care and maintenance of equipment
Dust, dirt and hair
Bright, white unexposed shadows appear on the processed radiograph if any of these were inside the cassette at the time of exposure. The shape will be of the same shape as the hair etc.

Surface defects on screens
Fluid, chemical splashes, scratches, folds (see Figure 11.37) or prolonged exposure to water can damage the screen surfaces. Horizontal inspection of the screens can usually detect the fault, though some defects will not prevent light emission completely. These faults will result in lighter patches on exposed screens

Light leaks
These result from accidental opening of the cassette in the light. Causes include faulty screen hinges or hooks, preventing complete closure of the cassette (see Figure 11.36), and incorrect fitting of automatic processor lids or manual processing tanks. Light may also be passing into the darkroom around the door if incorrectly designed.

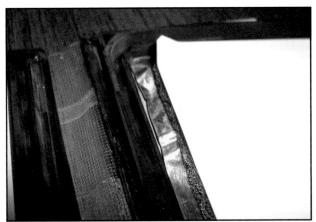

11.37 A damaged screen will affect the screen/film contact.

Light leakage produces blackening of the film (either patchy or as a distinct line). The source can be determined by determining whether this blackening is affecting the whole film or is along one or more sides.

Chemical contamination

Dichroic fog

This may be apparent as a pinkish staining of the film when viewed through transmitted light, or as a yellowish-green colour when viewed along the film surface. It is seen when the pH of the fixer becomes alkaline (it is normally acidic). The use of buffers in the fixer helps to prevent this.

Fixer stains

Yellowing of stored films is due to insufficient washing following the fixing of the film at the time of processing. Improperly washed films may also have a tacky or gritty feeling.

Splashes

Developer splashes on unprocessed films cause black marks (over-development). Fixer splashes on films will prevent any development and will therefore appear as white marks.

Hanger marks

If films are left inside the hangers, any leftover chemical may cause yellow stains. This can also result from incorrect immersion within the tank, incorrect washing or the use of incorrect amounts of solution.

Drying marks

These come from uneven drying and are usually caused by buckling of the film in its hanger, which causes longitudinal shading stains on the film.

Retention of emulsion

If the level of fixer is too low, the top part of the film will retain its emulsion and will keep the greenish-grey appearance that it had when first removed from the film box.

Poor development technique

Over-development

If the developer is too hot, or the development time is extended, this will result in blackening of the film. It will also reduce film contrast.

Under-development

This results in a pale processed radiograph. The background, which should be an even black colour, is grey and often has a cloudy, streaky appearance. This effect can be produced by exhausted oxidized solution, too low a temperature or too short a development time. Lack of solution agitation or uneven heating increases the patchy background effect. The temptation to increase the exposure to compensate for under-development is *bad practice* and should not be done.

Low developer level

If the top portion of the film is not immersed because the level is too low, it will not be developed. This will appear as a transparent smooth upper border once cleared by the fixer solution.

Environmental problems

Film faults may also be caused by environmental factors, such as:

- *Dirty wash water* – a roughened feel will occur on dry films; black spotting may also be seen, especially if the film is left in the dirty wash tank too long
- *Dust in the drying environment* – very similar to the effect of dirty wash water
- *Light leaks into the darkroom* from safelight bulbs or filters, or improper door seals
- *Overheating of dry radiographs* – resulting in brittle films where the emulsion may crack and craze.

Care of radiographic equipment

Careful preparation, maintenance and usage of the equipment is vital in ensuring optimal performance and standardization of the expected radiographic quality and results. Maintenance procedures for specific items of radiographic equipment are as follows.

Dosemeters
Storage

- Free from X-ray radiation.
- Free from chemicals.
- Free from excessive heat (e.g. hot pipes).
- Away from any source of non-ionizing radiation, such as radio, microwave or sunlight.
- Film badges: same storage requirements as for film, below.

Maintenance

- Return used dosemeters in packaging clearly identifying that it contains radiation-sensitive materials.
- Maintain current and accurate records of the dosemeters issued to personnel and the dosages recorded.
- Identify any late, lost, damaged or contaminated dosemeters immediately.
- Follow up any missing or late-return dosemeters promptly.

Radiographic film

Storage

Radiographic film is extremely sensitive; therefore it is important to store it correctly to prevent fogging or damage. The environmental requirements are:

- Free from light
- Free from heat (temperature 20°C or less)
- Free from chemicals
- Free from X-ray radiation
- Humidity 40–60%.

The following rules should be born in mind.

- Store films end on.
- Store in date order.
- Do not place any weight on stored films.
- Use within shelf-life.
- Rotate stock to ensure that the oldest film is used first.
- When loading into a cassette, be careful not to trap the film within the cassette edges.

In-house film storage

- Light-tight.
- Temperature 20°C or less.
- Keep dry.
- Away from radiation and chemical fumes.
- Not stored flat (film hoppers are available).

Light-beam diaphragm

- Careful rotation of the aluminium box helps to maintain the position of the LBD components.
- Check for leakage by closing the LBD fully (thereby preventing the electrons from leaving the tube head) and taking an exposure. Process the film for any evidence of radiation exposure (blackening) once processed.

Intensifying screens and cassettes

General inspection of the intensifying screen or cassette must be performed every time it is used, checking for damage or faults that may alter the radiographic quality. Any damage will usually result in a poor screen/film contact, which inevitably will affect the overall results (see Figure 11.37). Routine cleaning should be performed every two weeks as a minimum, or more frequently depending on how often the equipment is being used.

Storage

- Do not place any weight on the cassette or screen.
- Keep environment dust-free.
- Avoid exposure to extreme environmental conditions such as temperature or humidity.
- Storage area should be free from any X-ray radiation or chemical fumes.

Cleaning

Routine cleaning of screen and cassette ensures high image quality. Never put excess cleaner on screen surface.

1. Moisten a cellulose cloth (non-fluffy) with a proprietary antistatic cleaning agent or a mild soap solution (Figure 11.38).
2. Wipe the proprietary cleaner or dilute detergent softly and evenly over the whole surface of the screen in a circular motion, working from side to side down the screen or cassette.
3. Remove dust and any other debris from corners of cassette.
4. Leave the cassette open and on a flat surface for approximately 10 minutes to enable the solvent to evaporate completely.
5. Once the screen surface has dried completely, close the cassette immediately. Never put the cassette on end for drying, as this may lead to distortion of the screen. If the cassette will not close perfectly it needs to be replaced.

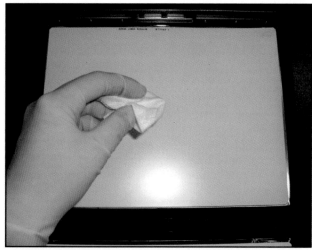

11.38 Cleaning the cassette. The cassette should be kept on a flat surface at all times, even for drying.

Grids

A general inspection should be performed to check for any obvious damage and to ensure that the grid is free of any dirt or contrast agent, which may appear as extraneous marks on the film.

- Clean down after every use, using a damp swab.
- Never store end on, always flat.
- Take precautions against damage and store away carefully.

Protective clothing

Storage

- Store under conditions of constant room temperature and normal humidity.
- Use heavy-duty hangers or a hanger system for storing all protective garments.
- Never fold this type of material as it may crack or the lead may be damaged.
- Hang as directed by the manufacturer.
- Avoid exposing to high temperatures and never hang over a radiator.

General inspection

- Check for any visible damage.
- Thoroughly examine every 3 months for potential underlying cracks by placing on top of a cassette, taking a 100 kV 4 mAs exposure at an FFD of 110 cm and then examining the film for any signs of exposure (black fissures).
- Constantly check for faults such as tears, places of unevenness or visible fold lines.
- A lead equivalency test can be performed to determine the lead thickness of protective clothing and ensure that it does meet legal requirements.

Cleaning

- Use a soft cloth with lukewarm water and liquid soap or proprietary cleansing agent.
- Allow to dry.
- Do not use any solution containing alcohol as this may damage the material.

X-ray machine

Before an X-ray machine can be brought into use, a practice principal must first obtain approval from the Health and Safety Executive (HSE) and complete a radiation safety assessment as part of the notification process. An initial risk assessment must be carried out in consultation with the RPA and then reviewed at least annually or when changes are observed.

Maintenance of the machine involves appropriate care of the tube, appropriate storage to avoid being knocked unnecessarily and regular servicing by an approved professional.

Guidelines for general use

- Avoid high exposures as this will cause the cathode filament to overheat and subsequently fail.
- If it is necessary to use a high exposure, gradually warm up the tube with increasing exposure factors to the level required.
- High exposures may cause deposits of tungsten within the tube, which may cause 'arcing' by attracting the electrons, reducing the number of electrons in the primary beam and therefore giving poor film density.
- Poor film density may indicate another problem within the tube head: air gets into the oil and acts as an attractant to the electrons, reducing the number of electrons within the primary beam.

- To avoid the danger of overheating, switch off when not in use.
- If the machine has a standby button that pre-heats the filament (and rotates the anode), do not keep this depressed for a long period of time before the exposure is taken, for the reasons discussed above.
- Observe the mA meter on the console. If it does not move, this may indicate filament failure.
- Unnecessary use of the pre-exposure button may overheat the rotating anode, so that the bearings wear down over time and subsequently fail.
- Changes in the noise of a rotating anode may indicate failing bearings.
- Excessive heat exposure due to failing bearings may lead to anode target failure, presenting as varying degrees of film density and exposures.
- Select high kV peak and low mAs techniques to help to preserve the anode.

General inspection

- Check the tube house for any evidence of oil leakage (which would cause overheating and destruction of the tube as the heat would not be effectively dissipated).
- Avoid rough handling of the tube head as this may damage the cathode filament.
- Record radiograph qualities to monitor for any unexpected variations or abnormal outcomes.
- Listen for any abnormalities.
- Check that mA needle movement corresponds to selected settings.

Automatic processors

Automatic processors require routine cleaning and maintenance. Units are usually designed to give easy access to the chemical/water baths and removal of the rollers for cleaning. The processor's performance and developer temperature should be monitored regularly whilst observing for any mechanical faults. The manufacturer's guidelines must be followed for each model.

Chemical checks

These should include:

- Measurement of pH values for developer and replenisher, fixer and replenisher
- Measurement of specific gravity and fixer silver levels.

Ideally pH values for developer and fixer should be measured daily and it is important to record these measurements, as regular logging provides very useful information. The daily measurements can be plotted to observe the trend of variations in these values compared with normal pH operating levels to identify any problems.

Silver trap

Hazardous waste from the film, containing silver, lead foil and silver/mercury amalgam, collects in the fixer.

Silver, lead and mercury can be dangerous to human health and can pollute the environment if not properly handled and disposed of.

A 'silver trap' consists of a clear housing with a cartridge, which is connected to the fixer's waste outlet and attracts these dangerous metals like a magnet. It traps residual fixer and then allows the resultant overflow to drain safely through the waste outlet. Once the trap is full the cartridge is disposed of by an authorized waste disposal company.

Untreated fixer waste is a hazardous material and cannot be placed down the sink or disposed of via the drains. Failure to comply with the appropriate waste disposal acts and regulations (Figure 11.39) could result in a fine, an order to pay costs and/or imprisonment.

- The Control of Pollution Act 1974
- The Control of Pollution (Special Waste) Regulations 1980
- Collection and Disposal of Waste Regulations 1988
- Controlled Waste Regulations 1992
- Special Waste Regulations 1996
- Chemicals (Hazard Information and Packaging for Supply) Regulations 2002
- COSHH 2002 (Control of Substances Hazardous to Health)
- Hazardous Waste Regulations 2005 (England and Wales)

11.39 Current waste disposal Acts and Regulations.

Other diagnostic imaging techniques

The following section provides an overview of advanced diagnostic imaging techniques. Further information will be found in the *BSAVA Manual of Advanced Veterinary Nursing*. These techniques are often used in conjunction with conventional radiography rather than instead of it.

Ultrasonography

Ultrasonography utilizes the inherent properties of piezoelectric crystals (transducers). When an electrical current is applied to these crystals a sound wave, above human hearing range, is emitted. Individual crystals produce a particular frequency: higher frequencies are useful for viewing superficial structures, lower frequencies for deeper structures. It is possible to view superficial and deep anatomical structures simultaneously due to the ultrasound machine's time-compensation mechanism. When sound waves are directed into the body they are reflected back towards the transducer and are referred to as 'echoes'. Sound waves are most commonly converted into a two-dimensional grey-scale image, visible on the ultrasound machine monitor.

Body tissues reflect and absorb sound waves differently, allowing distinctions to be made between anatomical structures. Bone appears white; soft tissues appear as various shades of grey; and fluids appear black. Air scatters sound, making visualization of air-filled structures impossible.

Veterinary patients generally tolerate ultrasound well. It is important to ensure that patients are comfortable; minimal restraint is often more effective than a heavy-handed approach. Hair removal and use of coupling gel reduces the amount of air between the transducer and the patient's skin and therefore helps to produce a clearer image.

Advantages of ultrasonography

- General anaesthetic rarely required.
- No confirmed health risks to patient or personnel.
- Radiolucent objects visible.
- Interior of fluid-filled structures visible.
- Earlier diagnosis of pregnancy and fetal death.

Disadvantages of ultrasonography

- No use for diagnosis of bone disease.
- Cannot be used to image lung tissue.
- Specialist interpretation skills required.
- Artefacts common.
- Definitive diagnosis rarely achieved.

Endoscopy

This technique allows visualization of internal body structures by using bundles of tiny glass fibres known as fibreoptics. Flexible endoscopes are used for examination of the gastrointestinal and respiratory tracts whereas rigid endoscopes are more commonly used for arthroscopy. Endoscopes require careful maintenance, and manufacturers' guidelines regarding disinfection and sterilization should be followed closely.

Advanced imaging techniques

Computer-aided tomography (CT/CAT scan)

This technique uses radiation, in common with conventional radiography. A tube head housed in a 360-degree circular gantry is rotated around the patient as they are advanced through the centre. Multiple transverse images are produced, allowing visualization of structures without superimposition of adjacent structures. Differentiation between fluid and soft tissue is also possible.

Magnetic resonance imaging (MRI)

Patients are placed at the centre of a magnet. Hydrogen ions within the body align with the magnetic field. They are then briefly bombarded with a radio frequency that knocks the ions out of alignment. As they realign, an energy signal (referred to as 'resonance') is released that allows tissue differentiation.

Nuclear imaging (scintigraphy)

Unstable radioactive chemicals (radionuclides) are administered intravenously to the patient. A gamma camera is used to detect nuclear emissions and translate them into a visible image. Radionuclide uptake is increased in tissues where there is increased blood flow, metabolism or tissue turnover. Patients must be housed in specialized units for up to 72 hours following administration.

Further reading

Dennis R and Williams A (2007) Diagnostic imaging. In: *BSAVA Textbook of Veterinary Nursing, 4th edn*, ed. DR Lane *et al.*, pp. 412–456. BSAVA Publications, Gloucester

Easton S (2002) *Practical Radiography for Veterinary Nurses.* Butterworth-Heinemann, Oxford

Gorrel C (2005) *Veterinary Dentistry for the Nurse and Technician.* Butterworth-Heinemann, Oxford

Han C and Hurd C (2004) *Practical Diagnostic Imaging for the Veterinary Technician, 3rd edn*, Mosby, St Louis

Lavin LM (2003) *Radiography in Veterinary Technology, 3rd edn.* WB Saunders, Philadelphia

Orpet H and Welsh P (2002) *Handbook of Veterinary Nursing.* Blackwell Science, Oxford

Acknowledgements

College of Animal Welfare, Edinburgh; Derek Copland; Katie Dargan (Head Nurse) at Veterinary Specialist Services, Brisbane, Australia; Nicola Forrest BSc, DipAVN (Surgical) VN, Edinburgh.

12

Anaesthesia and analgesia

Garry Stanway and Annaliese Magee

This chapter is designed to give information on:

- How to prepare anaesthetic equipment
- How to prepare an animal prior to anaesthesia
- How to assist the veterinary surgeon during anaesthesia
- How to care for the animal at the end of anaesthesia
- How to anaesthetize exotic pets

Introduction

What is general anaesthesia?

General anaesthesia is defined as reversible insensitivity to pain. The patient should be insensible to noxious stimuli and unable to recall them. It is common to talk about the 'triad of anaesthesia'. This refers to the three components that make up a general anaesthetic:

- Narcosis – the loss of consciousness
- Muscle relaxation
- Analgesia or the loss of reflex responses to the stimuli of surgery.

Narcosis and muscle relaxation are self-explanatory but analgesia can initially appear confusing when applied to an anaesthetized animal. In the case of an anaesthetized bitch being spayed, who starts to pant and whose heart rate goes up when tension is applied to the ovarian ligament, the animal is responding to the surgical stimuli but is not conscious and cannot perceive pain. But these responses *can* be suppressed with analgesics (opiates, NSAIDs or local analgesics) and so this component of anaesthesia is often referred to as analgesia in the triad. An alternative definition of analgesia in this case would be 'suppression of the reflex responses to surgical stimulation'.

When is general anaesthesia used?

General anaesthesia is used to perform surgery humanely and painlessly on animals. It is also commonly used to facilitate the humane handling of animals. The Protection of Animals Act 1964 (and its amendments) makes the use of anaesthesia a legal requirement for almost all operations performed on animals. The exceptions include castration and docking of lambs under 5 days old using rubber rings.

How is anaesthesia produced?

The exact mechanism of most anaesthetic agents on the brain is poorly understood. However, there is a variety of drugs available that, when inhaled or injected, induce a state of anaesthesia along with a variety of undesirable side effects. It is the role of the anaesthetist to administer these drugs in such a way as to induce anaesthesia whilst at the same time minimizing the adverse side effects.

Anaesthetic equipment

In order to induce and maintain anaesthesia safely, a wide variety of special equipment has been developed.

The anaesthetic machine

The anaesthetic machine provides a supply of anaesthetic gases and volatile anaesthetic agents to the patient during anaesthesia. It also:

- Includes facilities to mix anaesthetic gases and volatile anaesthetic agents together accurately and to deliver them at the correct flow rate
- Incorporates safety devices to prevent a toxic or harmful mixture of gases from being delivered to the patient
- Provides facilities to enable the anaesthetist to deal with anaesthetic emergencies
- Can collect and safely dispose of waste anaesthetic gases without contaminating the operating theatre.

It consists of (Figure 12.1):

- A supply of oxygen provided either by cylinders fitted directly to the machine or through a system of piped gas
- Regulators to control the pressure of the gas within the machine
- Needle valves and rotameters to control the flow rates of the anaesthetic gases
- An emergency oxygen flush valve to provide a high flow of oxygen to the patient should it be required
- One or more vaporizers
- A low-oxygen alarm
- Facilities for scavenging waste anaesthetic gases.

Some anaesthetic machines also include a supply of nitrous oxide and safety devices that prevent the anaesthetist from accidentally administering a hypoxic gas mixture (a mixture of anaesthetic gases containing <30% oxygen).

Gas supply

Anaesthetic gases are stored in cylinders.

- Oxygen cylinders have a black cylinder body and white top.
- Nitrous oxide cylinders are blue.

These cylinders are either fitted directly to the anaesthetic machine or stored some distance from the machine and gas piped to it using a system of rigid and flexible pipes and connectors.

Using a piped gas system

- **The pressure gauges on the machines only show the pressure in the pipeline and not the pressure in the cylinders. In order to estimate the contents of the cylinders, the pressure gauges on top of the cylinders must be consulted.**
- **At the end of the day the anaesthetic machine should be disconnected from the gas supply. This is usually achieved by twisting the metal collar on the supply coupling.**
- **When disconnecting the gas supply, the nitrous oxide should be disconnected first, followed by the oxygen supply.**
- **When connecting the piped gas supply, the oxygen should be connected first, followed by the nitrous oxide.**

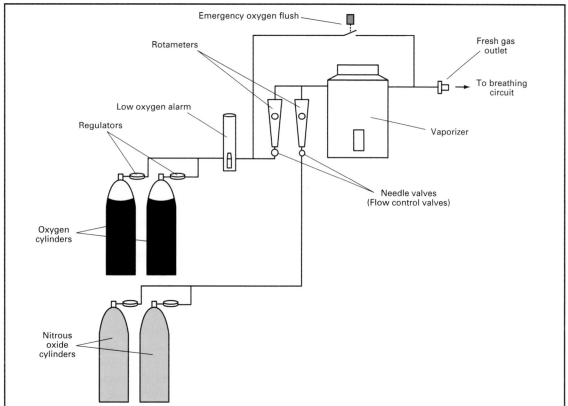

12.1 The anaesthetic machine.

Figure 12.2 shows how to change a pin index cylinder; and Figure 12.3 explains how to estimate the contents of a cylinder.

Oxygen can now also be manufactured relatively cheaply using mains-powered oxygen generators. These machines use a pair of membranes to remove the nitrogen from compressed air and are able to provide a constant flow of 100% oxygen for veterinary use. Oxygen generators are rare at the moment but may become a popular alternative to oxygen cylinders.

The machine

Figure 12.4 sets out how to set up and check the anaesthetic machine and circuits.

---

1. Make sure that the cylinder valve is fully closed.
2. Undo the screw that holds the cylinder to the yoke and lift up the connecting bar.
3. Pull the cylinder off the index pins (be prepared to take the weight of the cylinder).
4. Make sure that the Bodok washer has not come away with the old cylinder.
5. Remove the plastic seal that protects the new cylinder.
6. Offer the cylinder up to the yoke and engage it on to the index pins. Use your foot to help to support the weight of the cylinder.
7. Close the connecting bar and tighten up the retaining screw.
8. Open up the cylinder valve and listen for any leaks. If there is a leak, try tightening the cylinder retaining screw. If this does not work, the leak is most commonly due to a missing Bodok washer or dirt on the washer. Remove the cylinder, check the washer and refit the cylinder. Sometimes turning the washer around can cure the problem.
9. Once the cylinder is fitted, open the valve fully and then back it off half a turn. This reduces wear on the valve.
10. Check the cylinder pressure gauge to ensure that the cylinder is full.
11. Label the cylinder with either a FULL or IN USE label, as appropriate.

12.2 How to change a pin index cylinder.

Oxygen

- The pressure in the oxygen cylinder falls proportionally as the gas is used up.
- Use the pressure gauge to estimate the amount of oxygen left.
- A full oxygen cylinder is at a pressure of 137 bar (13.7×10^3 kPa = 2000 psi).
- A half-full oxygen cylinder is at a pressure of 68 bar (6.8×10^3 kPa = 1000 psi).

Nitrous oxide

When nitrous oxide is compressed in the cylinder, it condenses into a liquid. The pressure above the liquid is constant until all of the liquid has evaporated.

To estimate the contents of a nitrous oxide cylinder:

1. Weigh the cylinder.
2. Subtract the weight of the empty cylinder (which is stamped on the valve block).
3. This gives the weight of the liquid nitrous oxide inside.
4. Multiply the weight (kg) of the liquid nitrous oxide by 534 to get the number of litres of nitrous oxide left in the cylinder.

12.3 How to estimate the contents of a cylinder.

---

1. (i) If fitted, *turn on the spare oxygen cylinder* and check the pressure gauge. A full cylinder should read 137 bar (13.7×10^3 kPa = 2000 psi).
   (ii) Turn off the spare oxygen cylinder. (If the spare cylinder is left turned on at the same time as the in-use cylinder, both cylinders will empty together.)
2. *Turn on the in-use oxygen cylinder* and note the pressure. If the pressure reading is in the red, change the cylinder.
3. (i) If fitted, *turn on the spare nitrous oxide cylinder* and note the pressure reading. It should be 44 bar (4.4×10^3 kPa = 640 psi).
   (ii) *Turn off the spare nitrous oxide cylinder.*
4. *Turn on the in-use nitrous oxide cylinder* and note the reading on the pressure gauge. Again it should be 4.4×10^3 kPa. If it is lower than this, the cylinder is nearly empty and should be replaced.
   Note: Whilst checking the cylinders, listen for any leaking gas. Leaks are most commonly due to a faulty Bodok washer.
5. (i) Check the low oxygen alarm: *turn off the in-use oxygen cylinder* and operate the oxygen flush valve. The alarm should sound once the pressure falls to a dangerously low level.
   (ii) *Turn on the in-use oxygen cylinder.*
6. (i) Connect the scavenging receiver to the fresh gas outlet.
   (ii) Open each rotameter valve, starting with the nitrous oxide, and check that the bobbin or ball rises smoothly and rotates inside the tube.
   (iii) Ensure that a good fresh gas flow rate can be produced, by opening the rotameter valves until the rotameters are at their maximum reading.
7. Operate the oxygen flush valve and check that you get a good flow of oxygen out of the common gas outlet.
8. Check that the vaporizer is connected properly and that it is full. Check that the control valve will operate correctly. If there are several vaporizers on the machine, check each in turn, making sure that you never have more than one vaporizer switched on at one time.
9. Check that the circuit you have selected fits your machine. Check the circuit for signs of damage. Pay particular attention to the inside tube in coaxial circuits. Check the reservoir bag for leaks and damage.
10. Check that the endotracheal tube you have selected fits your circuit and that it is undamaged. If it is a cuffed tube, inflate the cuff and check for any leaks.

12.4 How to set up and check the anaesthetic machine and circuit.

Low-oxygen warning devices

These devices give an audible warning (and in some cases a visual warning) when the oxygen pressure falls to a dangerously low level. Common devices are the Ritchie Whistle, the Bosun Whistle and the Howison Oxygen Failure Alarm.

■ The *Bosun whistle* is the oldest of the three devices. It is unreliable and machines fitted with it should be used with extreme caution. It relies on a supply of nitrous oxide to drive the whistle and if the nitrous oxide supply fails or is not connected the device does not sound. Its operation also contaminates the theatre with potentially harmful nitrous oxide.

■ The *Ritchie whistle* and the *Howison oxygen failure alarm* use the oxygen left in the emptying cylinder to blow a whistle when the pressure falls below a predetermined level. They sound regardless of the state of the nitrous oxide supply. They also sound briefly when the oxygen supply is first turned on, providing a frequent and automatic check of the alarm's proper operation. The Howison oxygen failure alarm sounds an alarm *and* turns off the other gas supplies to prevent a hypoxic gas mixture being supplied to the patient.

Needle valves and rotameters

The flow rate is read off the top of the bobbin or through the centre line of the ball (Figure 12.5).

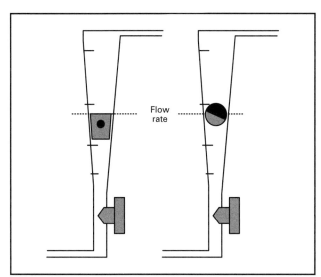

12.5 Reading gas flow rates on rotameters.

■ Do not over-tighten the control knob, as the valve seat is easily damaged.
■ The bobbin or ball must rotate freely in the tube. If it does not, the reading will be inaccurate and the machine should be checked by a service engineer.

Emergency oxygen flush valve

This valve is used to deliver a high flow of pure oxygen to the breathing circuit (the oxygen bypasses the vaporizer), flushing the anaesthetic agents out of the circuit and providing the patient with 100% oxygen. Oxygen is delivered at around 30–35 litres/minute when the oxygen flush valve is operated.

Vaporizers

Vaporizers are classified as either calibrated or uncalibrated.

■ *Uncalibrated vaporizers* include Boyle's bottle (Figure 12.6) and basic draw-over types:
  – The output of the vaporizer cannot be predicted. It can be varied, using the control, but it also varies with temperature and the flow of fresh gas through the vaporizer
  – Draw-over vaporizers are included in some circle circuits (e.g. Goldman and Komesaroff vaporizers).

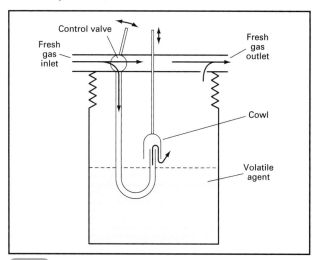

12.6 Boyle's bottle vaporizer.

■ *Calibrated vaporizers* include the 'Tec' and 'Penlon' types (Figure 12.7):
  – They are designed to produce a known concentration of anaesthetic vapour regardless of temperature and fresh gas flow
  – To remain accurate, they must be serviced annually
  – They are anaesthetic-agent specific – isoflurane vaporizers should only be filled with isoflurane.

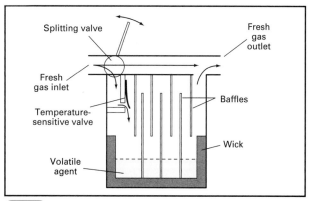

12.7 Tec and Penlon type vaporizers.

Anaesthetic circuits

The pipework that is used to connect the patient to the anaesthetic machine is called the anaesthetic breathing circuit (often abbreviated to 'anaesthetic circuit'). Its function is to:

■ Deliver oxygen-rich carrier gas (and anaesthetic vapour) to the patient
■ Carry carbon dioxide-rich gas away from the patient

■ Deliver potentially harmful waste anaesthetic agents to the scavenging system, which carries them away from the operating theatre.

Figure 12.8 defines some of the respiratory terms used in this section and gives some of the relevant values.

Adjustable pressure-limiting or pop-off valve

The APL valve allows gas out of the circuit without letting air from the atmosphere back in. In order to carry out intermittent positive pressure ventilation (IPPV; see later), it is sometimes necessary to use the control knob to increase the pressure at which the valve opens to let gas out.

Circuit classification

The older classification of anaesthetic circuits was confusing: the same circuit was classified differently, depending on the way it was used. The following simpler classification (Davey *et al.*, 1997) is much more useful:

Circuit classification and examples

Non-rebreathing systems (use a valve to control gas flow): 'Ambu bag' (used for resuscitation in situations where a source of compressed gas is not available)

Systems where rebreathing of alveolar gas is possible though not always intended (with bidirectional flow within the system): T-piece; Magill; Lack; Bain; Humphrey ADE circuit without the soda lime canister fitted

Circuits containing soda lime: Circle; to-and-fro; Humphrey ADE with soda lime canister fitted

Figure 12.9 compares some of the advantages and disadvantages of the rebreathing and carbon dioxide absorption systems. Figure 12.10 will help in the choice of a suitable circuit for a patient.

Term	Definition	Values
Tidal volume	The volume of gas an animal breathes in during a normal breath	Dog, cat: 10–15 ml/kg
Respiratory rate	The number of breaths an animal takes each minute	Dog: 10–30; cat: 20–30 breaths/min
Minute volume	The total volume of gas breathed in by an animal in 1 minute (= tidal volume x respiratory rate)	Dog, cat: 200 ml/kg/min
Oxygen consumption	The volume of oxygen metabolized by an animal in 1 minute	5–10 ml/kg/min
Dead-space gas	Gas that has been breathed in by the animal but has not reached the alveoli and so has not been used in gas exchange. In anaesthesia, this is taken to include the gas in the endotracheal tube as well as any gas within the dead space of the breathing circuit	

12.8 Definitions of some respiratory terms and their values.

Magill, Lack, T-piece, Bain, ADE without soda lime	Circle, to-and-fro, ADE with soda lime
Need high fresh gas flow rates and use relatively large amounts of volatile agent. (The ADE circuit without soda lime is more efficient than the others.)	Very efficient use of volatile anaesthetic agents and oxygen
Very low resistance to breathing and so more suitable for small animals	Not suitable for animals weighing less than 10 kg
Cheap lightweight construction	Expensive to buy
The large volumes of cold dry anaesthetic gases used with these circuits results in greater cooling of the patient, especially during long procedures. (The Humphrey ADE without soda lime conserves the warmed and humidified dead-space gas so patient cooling is significantly reduced)	During long procedures, the patient loses less heat and moisture, as warm and moist exhaled gas is re-breathed
The concentration of anaesthetic vapour delivered to the patient is the same as the vaporizer setting	The concentration of anaesthetic vapour being delivered to the patient differs slightly from the vaporizer setting
Changes to the vaporizer setting are almost immediately followed by changes in the concentration of anaesthetic vapour delivered to the patient	Changes to the vaporizer setting are only slowly reflected in changes in the concentration of anaesthetic vapour delivered to the patient
Can use trichloroethylene, carbon dioxide or nitrous oxide with these circuits	Cannot use trichloroethylene, carbon dioxide or nitrous oxide (unless respiratory gas monitoring is available) with these circuits

12.9 Advantages and disadvantages of circuits.

Circuit	Description	Used for continuous IPPV	Fresh gas flow rate	Circuit factor	Patient weight range	Can be used with nitrous oxide?	Advantages	Disadvantages	Comments
T-piece		Yes	400–500 ml/kg/min	2–2.5	<8 kg	Yes	Lightweight, cheap, semi-disposable	Difficult to scavenge from	Circuit often now sold with a plastic APL and closed reservoir bag that, although not technically a T-Piece, can be used in the same way and is easier to scavenge from
Bain		Yes	400–500 ml/kg/min	2–2.5	8–15 kg	Yes	Lightweight, cheap, semi-disposable. Can be used for continuous IPPV	High fresh gas flow rates preclude its use in larger animals	Can be used with a ventilator to provide continuous mechanical IPPV. Inner pipe can become disconnected or leak at the anaesthetic machine end, resulting in re-breathing
Lack		No	140–200 ml/kg/min	0.7–1	>12 kg	Yes	Lightweight, cheap, semi-disposable. Lower flow rates than the Bain	Not suitable for continuous IPPV	Inner pipe can become disconnected or leak at the anaesthetic machine end, resulting in re-breathing
Parallel Lack		No	140–200 ml/kg/min	0.7–1	>12 kg	Yes	Lightweight, cheap, semi-disposable. Lower flow rates than the Bain	Parallel breathing pipes increase the drag on the endotracheal tube	Identical in function to the Lack. Leaks or damage more easily identified
Humphrey ADE without soda lime cannister		Yes	70–100 ml/kg/min	0.35–0.5	<10 kg	Yes	Lower flow rates than a standard parallel Lack	Suitable for continuous IPPV (and can be configured to work with a mechanical ventilator)	The special APL valve fitted to these circuits maximizes dead-space gas conservation, allowing lower flow rates to be used. The APL valve design might also reduce alveolar collapse during anaesthesia
Magill		No	140–200 ml/kg/min	0.70–1	>12 kg	Yes	None	Valve at the patient end of the circuit is difficult to scavenge	The Humphrey ADE and parallel Lack have now replaced the Magill and should be preferred

12.10 How to choose an anaesthetic breathing circuit. (continues)

Circuit	Description	Used for *continuous* IPPV	Fresh gas flow rate	Circuit factor	Patient weight range	Can be used with nitrous oxide?	Advantages	Disadvantages	Comments
Circle		Yes	Initially: 2–4 l/min After 5 minutes: 1–2 l/min	N/A	>15 kg	No, unless respiratory gas monitoring is available	Low flow rates reduce costs and environmental pollution	Large resistance to breathing Not suitable for short procedures	Do not use with nitrous oxide (unless respiratory gas monitoring is available) The relative positions of the fresh gas inlet, the reservoir bag and the APL valve vary between manufacturers. The reservoir bag is best placed on the inspiratory limb. Circle circuits with the inspiratory bag on the expiratory limb offer a much greater resistance to inspiration.
Humphrey ADE with soda lime canister		Yes	Initially: 30 ml/kg/min After 5 minutes: 10 ml/ kg/min (minimum flow 300 ml/min)	N/A	>7 kg	No, unless respiratory gas monitoring is available	Very low flow rates achievable (a 30 kg dog requires only 300 ml/min) reducing costs and environmental pollution Lightweight valves allow it to be used on patients that would not be able to use a normal circle Made of non-ferrous metals so can be used in an MRI scanner The unique APL valve ensures that gas is conserved within the circuit even during rapid respiration.	Initial purchase price is high	Do not use with nitrous oxide (unless respiratory gas monitoring is available)
To-and-fro		Yes	Initially: 2–4 l/min After 5 minutes: 1–2 l/min	N/A	>12 kg	No, unless respiratory gas monitoring is available	None	Circuit dead space increases rapidly, causing the patient to rebreathe CO_2 Soda lime dust from canister often inhaled by patient Not suitable for short procedures	Do not use with nitrous oxide (unless respiratory gas monitoring is available) Circuit should not be used in modern practice It is only of historical interest now

12.10 (continued) How to choose an anaesthetic breathing circuit.

Systems where rebreathing is possible

With these there is bidirectional flow within the system. The carbon dioxide-rich alveolar gas is removed from the circuit by the flow of fresh gas coming in from the anaesthetic machine. The flow rate needed for the circuit to function properly is calculated from the patient's weight using the breathing circuit's circuit factor (Figure 12.11).

Jackson Rees modified T-piece

Gas flow in this circuit is illustrated in Figure 12.12.

- The absence of an APL valve means that this circuit offers little resistance to breathing, making it especially suitable for small patients.
- It is difficult to scavenge from, because of the open-ended bag.

Circuits that do not contain soda lime rely on the flow of fresh gas coming into the circuit from the anaesthetic machine to wash away the carbon dioxide-rich alveolar gas that the patient exhales. The flow rate needed to achieve this is a multiple of the patient's minute volume (see Figure 12.8).

It is common to see the flow rate needed by a circuit expressed either as an absolute figure (the **circuit flow rate**) or as the **circuit factor**. The circuit factor multiplied by the minute volume gives the circuit flow rate.

- The T-piece needs a fresh gas flow rate equal to 2–2$^1/_2$ times the patient's minute volume. This is a **circuit flow rate** of 400–500 ml/kg/minute (the minute volume for dogs and cats is 200 ml/kg/min).The Bain requires twice the patient's minute volume and so has a circuit flow rate of 400 ml/kg/minute. The Lack circuits need one times the patient's minute volume and so have a circuit flow rate of 200 ml/kg/minute.
- Alternatively, the T-piece has a circuit factor of 2 to 2.5, the Bain has a **circuit factor** of 2 and the Lacks have a circuit factor of 1.

Thus the fresh gas flow rate needed can be calculated using the following equations.

Fresh gas flow rate = circuit flow rate x patient's weight
Fresh gas flow rate = minute volume x circuit factor x patient's weight

---

Examples:

1. Calculate the flow needed to use a Lack circuit with a 20 kg Staffordshire Bull Terrier.
The Lack circuits require 200 ml/kg/min, so the fresh gas flow rate needed in this case is:

200 x 20 = 4000 ml/min (4 litres/min)

2. Calculate the flow rate needed to use a Bain circuit with a 8 kg Jack Russell Terrier.
The T-piece has a circuit factor of 2 and the minute volume of dogs and cats is 200 ml/kg/min, so the fresh gas flow rate needed in this case is:

2 x 200 x 8 = 3200 ml/kg (3.2 litres/min)

Fresh gas flow rates and nitrous oxide
The fresh gas flow rate calculated above is the total fresh gas flow, not just the oxygen flow. If you are using 100% oxygen these are the same but when nitrous oxide is used as part of the anaesthetic protocol, you need to calculate the rates of both gases.

Example:

Calculate the fresh gas flow rates for a 30 kg Labrador that is being anaesthetized using a parallel Lack circuit. You want to use nitrous oxide along with the oxygen.

Knowing that the Lack circuits need a fresh gas flow of 200 ml/kg/min you can calculate the total fresh gas flow as follows:

200 x 30 = 6000 ml/min (6 litres/min)

Thus the total fresh gas flow is 6 litres/minute. When using nitrous oxide it is usual to administer it with oxygen at a ratio of two-thirds to one-third (i.e. 66% nitrous oxide and 33% oxygen). In this example, to achieve the correct flow rate and ratio it is necessary to administer:

Nitrous oxide at 4 litres/minute (two-thirds of 6 litres)
Oxygen at 2 litres/minute (one-third of 6 litres)

12.11 Calculating the fresh gas flow rate.

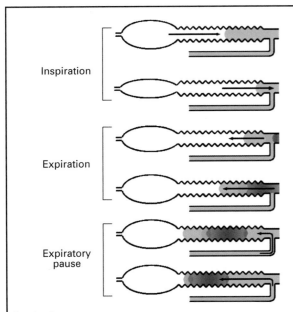

Inspiration
When the patient breathes in, fresh gas is drawn partly from the fresh gas entering the circuit and partly from the gas within the corrugated tube.

Expiration
During expiration, the exhaled gas cannot flow back up the narrow fresh gas tube because of the flow of fresh gas coming into the circuit. All of the exhaled gas must flow into the relatively wide corrugated tube. The first gas to be exhaled is the patient's dead-space gas. This is immediately followed by the carbon dioxide-rich alveolar gas.

Expiratory pause
If the exhaled gases were not flushed away by the fresh gas entering the circuit during the expiratory pause, the animal would inhale stale alveolar gas. To ensure that this does not occur, the fresh gas flow rate needs to be 400 ml/kg/min (a circuit factor of 2). The open-ended bag gives a visual indication of the patient's respiratory work and facilitates IPPV.

In some T-piece circuits the open-ended bag has been replaced with an APL valve and a closed bag. The circuit works in the same way (except that the gases escape through the valve and not through the open-ended reservoir bag) and has the same circuit factor. This configuration is sometimes known as a Mini-Bain.

12.12   Gas flow within the Jackson Rees modified T-piece circuit. ▨ Fresh gas; ▩ dead-space gas; ■ alveolar gas.

- Fresh gas flow rate should be 400–500 ml/kg bodyweight per minute (giving the T-piece a circuit factor of 2–2.5).
- Suitable for continuous IPPV.

Bain

Gas flow in this circuit is illustrated in Figure 12.13.

- The fresh gas flow rate should be 400–500 ml/kg/min (a circuit factor of 2–2.5).
- This circuit is suitable for continuous IPPV (and can be used in conjunction with a mechanical ventilator for this purpose).

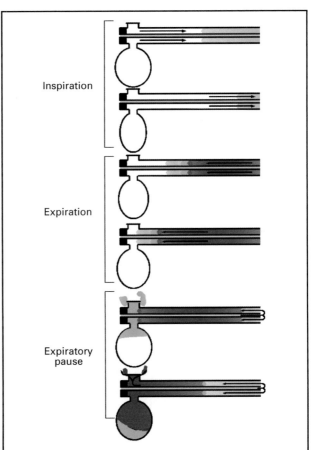

Inspiration
Fresh gas is drawn partly from the fresh gas coming into the circuit through the inner pipe and partly from the outer pipe, causing the reservoir bag to collapse slightly.

Expiration
The exhaled gases pass up the outer tube towards the APL valve. The first gas to be exhaled is the carbon dioxide-free dead-space gas. This is followed by the carbon dioxide-rich alveolar gas.

Expiratory pause
Fresh gas from the anaesthetic machine drives the exhaled gases up the outer pipe and either into the reservoir bag or out of the APL valve. The volume of fresh gas coming into the circuit during the expiratory pause must exceed the patient's tidal volume if rebreathing of carbon dioxide-rich alveolar gas is not to occur. (This is similar to the situation in the T-piece.) This necessitates a fresh gas flow of 400 ml/kg/min (twice the patient's minute volume), giving the Bain a circuit factor of 2.

12.13   Gas flow within the Bain circuit. ▨ Fresh gas; ▩ dead-space gas; ■ alveolar gas.

- The circuit must be carefully checked prior to use as a leak in the inner pipe close to the anaesthetic machine results in total rebreathing, with no fresh gas reaching the anaesthetized animal.

Magill

Gas flow in this circuit is illustrated in Figure 12.14.

- Fresh gas flow rate should be 200 ml/kg/min to avoid rebreathing (a circuit factor of 1).
- Suitable for continuous IPPV.

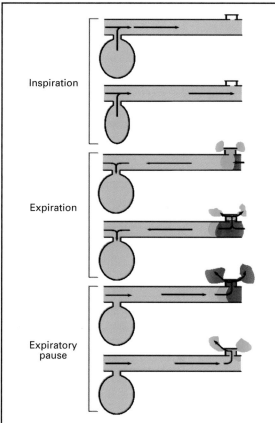

Inspiration
As the animal breathes in, gas is drawn from fresh gas coming into the circuit from both the anaesthetic machine and the reservoir bag.

Expiration
The exhaled gases pass both back down the circuit towards the reservoir bag and out of the APL. Before the end of expiration the reservoir bag will become full (because throughout the respiratory cycle fresh gas continues to enter the circuit) and the last of the alveolar gas is expelled from the circuit through the APL valve.

Expiratory pause
During the expiratory pause fresh gas coming into the circuit drives more of the alveolar gas out of the APL. Finally, the carbon dioxide-free dead-space gas is driven out of the APL. This is very similar to the situation with the Lack circuits and, like the Lack circuits, the fresh gas flow needed to ensure that rebreathing does not occur is 200 ml/kg/min, giving the Magill a circuit factor of 1.

Intentional rebreathing of the dead-space gases
Like the Lack circuits, some rebreathing can be tolerated because the gas rebreathed will be the carbon dioxide-free dead-space gas. Partial rebreathing can be achieved with a circuit factor of 0.7, equivalent to 140 ml/kg/min.

12.14 Gas flow within the Magill circuit. ▦ Fresh gas; ▦ dead-space gas; ■ alveolar gas.

▦ The position of the APL valve makes the circuit difficult to scavenge from and it has, to all intents and purposes, been replaced by the Lack circuits.

Lack and parallel Lack
The Lack circuit (Figure 12.15) is similar to the Magill but the APL valve has been moved away from the patient connector and placed near the anaesthetic

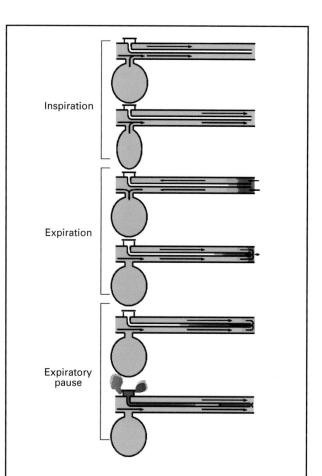

Inspiration
The animal breathes gas from the circuit, collapsing the reservoir bag.

Expiration
Some of the exhaled gases pass back down the larger outer tube towards the reservoir bag, refilling it, whilst some escape down the inner tube towards the APL valve. (The APL valve opens during early expiration.) The reservoir bag is also partially refilled by fresh gas coming from the anaesthetic machine. Towards the end of expiration the reservoir bag becomes full and the last of the exhaled gases (the carbon dioxide-rich alveolar gas) is forced down the inner pipe towards the pop-off valve.

Expiratory pause
Fresh gas continues to enter the circuit from the anaesthetic machine, pushing ahead of it the exhaled gases still remaining in the outer tube. These gases pass into the inner tube and back towards the pop-off valve. The last gas to be pushed up the inner tube is the carbon dioxide-free dead-space gas.

Intentional rebreathing of the dead-space gases
If the fresh gas flow rate is reduced, not all of the exhaled gases are expelled out of the APL valve during the expiratory pause. Some remain in the circuit and are rebreathed. This may seem undesirable but, as the last of the gas to be expelled from the circuit is the carbon dioxide-free dead-space gas, it does not matter if this is inhaled during the next respiratory cycle. In fact, rebreathing this dead-space gas is both *economical* (reducing the amount of volatile anaesthetic agent used) and *desirable*: the dead-space gas is warm and wet, having already been humidified the first time it entered the animal, and this conserves the animal's heat.

Rebreathing of the dead-space gas in a Lack circuit can be achieved with fresh gas flows of 140 ml/kg/min, equivalent to a circuit factor of 0.7

12.15 Gas flow within the Lack circuit. ▦ Fresh gas; ▦ dead-space gas; ■ alveolar gas.

machine. The parallel Lack (Figure 12.16) is the same as the Lack but with parallel rather than coaxial tubes.

■ Fresh gas flow rate should be 200 ml/kg/min (a circuit factor of 1).
■ Not suitable for continuous IPPV.
■ The fresh gas flow can be reduced to 140 ml/kg/min. This makes the patient rebreathe carbon dioxide-free dead-space gas, saving some volatile agent and reducing pollution.

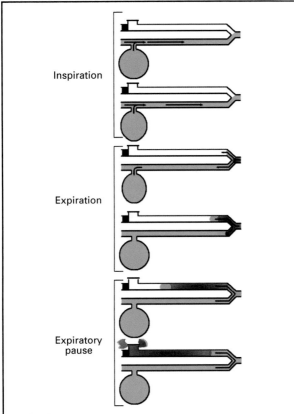

Inspiration
The animal breathes gas from the circuit, collapsing the reservoir bag.

Expiration
As with the Lack, some of the exhaled gases pass down the inspiratory limb towards the reservoir bag and some down the expiratory limb towards the APL valve.

Expiratory pause
During the expiratory pause fresh gas pushes the exhaled gases still remaining in the inspiratory limb out towards the APL valve. The last gas to be pushed up the expiratory limb is the carbon dioxide-free dead-space gas exhaled in early expiration. The fresh gas flow needed to achieve this is around 200 ml/kg/min, giving the parallel Lack a circuit factor of 1.

Intentional rebreathing of dead-space gases
Like the Lack circuit, intentional rebreathing can be used to conserve the dead-space gas.
   Rebreathing of the dead-space gas in a parallel Lack circuit can be achieved with fresh gas flows of 140 ml/kg/min, equivalent to a circuit factor of 0.7.

12.16 Gas flow within the Parallel Lack circuit. ■ Fresh gas; ■ dead-space gas; ■ alveolar gas.

Humphrey ADE circuit without soda lime canister
This is a miniature parallel Lack circuit with a redesigned APL valve and works in a very similar way (Figure 12.17).

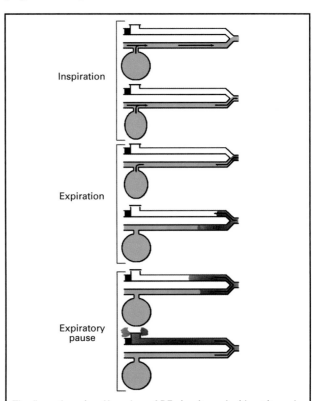

The flow of gas in a Humphrey ADE circuit used without its soda lime canister differs from its nearest relative, the parallel Lack, because of the unique design of its APL valve (see Figure 12.18). The valve helps to conserve *all* of the dead-space gas within the expiratory limb, making the circuit very efficient.

Inspiration
The animal breathes gas from the circuit, collapsing the reservoir bag.

Expiration
The exhaled gases pass back down inspiratory limb towards the reservoir bag, refilling it. The reservoir bag is also partially refilled by fresh gas coming from the anaesthetic machine. Towards the end of expiration the reservoir bag becomes full and the last of the exhaled gases (the carbon dioxide-rich alveolar gas) is forced down the expiratory limb towards the APL valve.

Expiratory pause
During the expiratory pause fresh gas continues to enter the circuit from the anaesthetic machine, pushing ahead of it the exhaled gases in the inspiratory limb. These gases pass into the expiratory limb and back towards the APL valve. The last gas to be pushed up the inspiratory limb is the carbon dioxide-free dead-space gas. At the correct flow rate, this carbon dioxide-free dead-space gas is not expelled up the expiratory limb but is conserved in the inspiratory limb to be rebreathed during the next inspiration.

Intentional rebreathing of the dead-space gases
This intentional rebreathing of dead-space gas is achieved at flow rates of 70–100 ml/kg/min, giving the Humphrey ADE a circuit factor of 0.35–0.5.

12.17 Gas flow within the Humphrey ADE circuit without soda lime. ■ Fresh gas; ■ dead-space gas; ■ alveolar gas.

- The design of this circuit's APL valve allows it to be used with even lower fresh gas flow rates than its close relative, the parallel Lack.
- Fresh gas flow rates should be 70–100 ml/kg/min (a circuit factor of 0.35–0.5).
- Not suitable for continuous *manual* IPPV.

Humphrey ADE circuit

The Humphrey ADE circuit is a relatively new innovation in veterinary anaesthesia but it has been used in medical practice for the last two decades. It was invented by Dr Humphrey in the 1980s. Because of some of its unique design features, it can be used in animals varying in size from a cat to a Great Dane. The circuit can be used in two basic configurations: with or without soda lime.

Humphrey ADE circuit with soda lime

- **The Humphrey ADE circuit can be fitted with a soda lime canister, making it into a small circle circuit. This can be used for animals weighing more than 7 kg.**

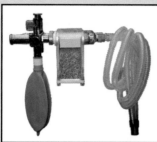

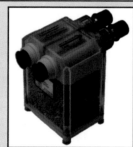

Humphrey ADE circuit without soda lime

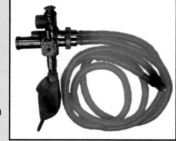

- **Without soda lime, the circuit works like a Lack with a proportion of the dead-space gas being rebreathed.**
- **The narrow smooth-bore tubing means that it can be used on cats, larger birds and reptiles as well as dogs.**
- **The modified pop-off valve improves on the efficiency of the normal Lack circuit, allowing lower flow rates than those recommended for a normal Lack circuit to be used safely (Figure 12.18).**

'Lever' on the Humphrey ADE circuit

- **The lever on the side of the Humphrey ADE circuit changes its configuration so that it can be used with a mechanical ventilator either with or without the soda lime canister.**
- **The lever *must* be left up, unless the circuit is connected to a ventilator (Figure 12.19).**

The Humphrey ADE circuit is fitted with a special APL valve that contributes to the circuit's efficiency. Like a parallel Lack, it is possible to reduce the fresh gas flow used until the animal starts to rebreathe the dead-space gas from the previous breath. Of the gas exhaled by an animal, 30–40% is dead-space gas and, as it is free of carbon dioxide, it can be conserved in the breathing circuit and delivered to the patient during the next breath. In theory, the exhaled dead-space gases in a Lack and parallel Lack pass back down the inspiratory limb of the circuit until the reservoir bag is full. Then the alveolar gases pass down the expiratory limb towards the APL valve. In practice, the APL valve opens before the reservoir bag is full and some of the dead-space gas is lost.

The Humphrey APL valve is designed not to open until the reservoir bag is full, conserving more of the dead-space gas in the inspiratory limb of the circuit.

The Humphrey APL valve has another benefit. During anaesthesia, the alveoli in the dependent (lower) lung lobes collapse and do not fill with anaesthetic gases. This reduces gas exchange and can contribute to hypoxia in patients with compromised pulmonary function. The APL valve on the Humphrey ADE circuit closes earlier in the breathing cycle, maintaining a slight positive pressure (1 cm H_2O) in the circuit and the patient's lungs. In children this has been demonstrated to prevent alveolar collapse and it is likely that the same benefit exists in small animals.

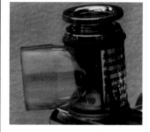

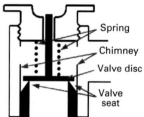

Spring
Chimney
Valve disc
Valve seat

Phase 1 – early expiration
The pressure in the circuit rises and the valve disc lifts off the valve seat, but the valve effectively remains closed as the valve disc does not get pushed completely out of the valve chimney. This prevents the dead-space gas from leaving the circuit and it must all flow into the *inspiratory* limb, where it is conserved.

Phase 2 – late expiration
Once the reservoir bag is full the pressure in the circuit rises still further, lifting the valve disc beyond the valve chimney and allowing the alveolar gases to escape into the scavenging system.

Phase 3 – Expiratory pause
At the end of expiration the valve closes again but the valve disc falls back into the chimney at a pressure of 1 cm H_2O, preventing the last few millilitres of gas from escaping and maintaining a slight positive pressure in the circuit *and* in the patient's lungs during the expiratory pause. In children at least, this prevents alveolar collapse.

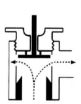

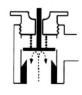 **12.18** The Humphrey APL valve. (Photo courtesy of Dr D Humphrey) (continues) ▶

Phase 4 – Inspiration
The valve disc is held against the valve seat by the spring, preventing gas from being drawn back in from the atmosphere. This prevents carbon dioxide-rich alveolar gas now sitting in the expiratory limb from being drawn back towards the patient. The patient must breathe carbon dioxide-free dead-space gas and fresh gas from the inspiratory limb.

12.18 (continued) The Humphrey APL valve.

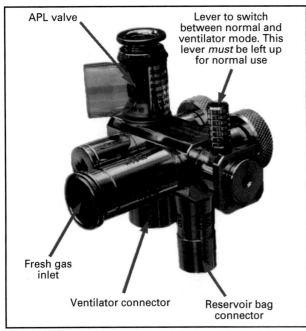

12.19 Humphrey ADE circuit connections.

APL valve

Lever to switch between normal and ventilator mode. This lever *must* be left up for normal use

Fresh gas inlet

Ventilator connector

Reservoir bag connector

Non-rebreathing systems utilizing carbon dioxide absorption

For larger dogs and large animals, it is more efficient to absorb the carbon dioxide chemically than rely on the fresh gas flow to remove the waste gas from the circuit.

The three circuits in which the carbon dioxide is removed chemically are:

- Circle circuit
- To-and-fro circuit
- Humphrey ADE circuit when used with the soda lime canister.

All three contain soda lime (NaOH), which reacts with the carbon dioxide, removing it from the circuit:

$$CO_2 + 2NaOH = Na_2CO_3 + H_2O$$
$$Na_2CO_3 + Ca(OH)_2 = 2NaOH + CaCO_3$$

Soda lime also contains a chemical indicator that changes colour as the ability of the soda lime to absorb carbon dioxide becomes exhausted. There are two indicators in common use:

- One in which pink soda lime changes to white
- One in which white soda lime changes to purple.

The expected colour change is indicated on the manufacturer's packaging. This colour change is most pronounced immediately following use. Soda lime that appears to be exhausted at the end of anaesthesia should be replaced. If left to stand the colour regenerates, so the next person who uses the circuit could be fooled into thinking that the soda lime is still fresh. Figure 12.20 gives some hints on using circuits containing soda lime. Figure 12.21 explains how to change a used canister.

Oxygen flow	Vaporizer setting (isoflurane)	Result
Immediately post induction		
2–4 litres/min (1 litre/min)[a]	2–3%	Washes the nitrogen out of the circuit and the patient
Once anaesthesia is stable		
1–2 litres/min (0.5 litres/min)[a]	1–2%	Low oxygen flow rates produce a stable anaesthetic because the concentration of the inspired anaesthetic vapour will only change very slowly
End of anaesthesia		
2–4 litres/min (1 litre/min)[a]	0%	Oxygen flow rate is increased to wash the volatile anaesthetic agent out of the circuit, allowing the patient to recover

12.20 Hints on using a circle circuit, a Humphrey ADE circuit with the soda lime canister fitted and a to-and-fro circuit. When using a circle, Humphrey circle or to-and-fro circuit, it is important to note that changes in the inspired vapour concentration only slowly follow changes in the vaporizer setting. The lower the oxygen flow rate, the more slowly the inspired concentration changes. Therefore, if the inspired concentration needs to be changed quickly (either up or down), the oxygen flow rate must be increased. [a] Because of its small volume, the Humphrey ADE circuit with soda lime canister fitted needs lower flow rates than most circle circuits.

 Remember that soda lime is caustic. Handle it with care.

Circle circuits

- The soda lime canister in circle circuits should be filled according to the manufacturer's instructions.
- Do not partly fill a canister in order to save soda lime. The reaction between the expired gas and the soda lime is not instant. The gas must stay in contact with the granules for a short time. This occurs during the expiratory pause when the exhaled breath is held within the canister. If the canister is not filled, some of the expired gas may only pass through the granules and so have insufficient time to react with the soda lime.

12.21 Replacing the soda lime. (continues) ▶

> **To-and-fro circuits**
>
> - When filling the Waters' canister from a to-and-fro circuit it is important that the canister is packed tightly. If it is not, the exhaled gas may be able to pass over the top of the granules and bypass the soda lime.
> - It is possible to place a pan scourer in the end of the canister in order to hold the soda lime in place.

12.21 (continued) Replacing the soda lime.

Circle circuit

Gas flow in this circuit is illustrated in Figure 12.22.

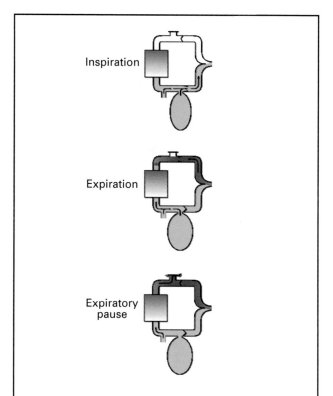

Inspiration
When the patient breathes in, gas is drawn from the circuit, collapsing the reservoir bag. The one-way valves ensure that only fresh gas or gas that has passed through the soda lime and is therefore free of CO_2 is inhaled.

Expiration
Gas exhaled by the patient cannot go directly back into the reservoir bag because of the one-way valves in the circuit. Instead, it is directed around the circuit and through the soda lime canister before refilling the reservoir bag.

Expiratory pause
Throughout the respiratory cycle fresh gas constantly enters the circuit. At the end of expiration and during the expiratory pause, any excess gas escapes through the pop-off valve. In larger dogs it is sometimes necessary to close the APL valve partially as some gas escapes through it during expiration, causing the reservoir bag to collapse.

12.22 Gas flow inside the circle circuit. ■ Fresh gas; ■ dead-space gas; ■ alveolar gas; ■ soda lime.

- Unidirectional valves direct the gas around the circuit and through the soda lime.
- The circuit's weight is supported by the anaesthetic machine.
- There is a large resistance to breathing and so circles are generally not suitable for use with patients under 20 kg.

To-and-fro

Gas flow in this circuit is illustrated in Figure 12.23.

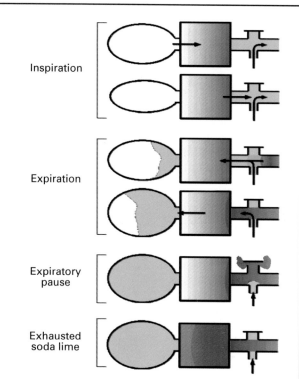

Inspiration
During inspiration, gas is drawn mainly from the reservoir bag and partly from fresh gas coming in from the anaesthetic machine.

Expiration
Expired gases must pass through the soda lime canister and into the reservoir bag. Carbon dioxide is removed from the alveolar gas as it passes through the soda lime.

Expiratory pause
At the end of expiration and during the expiratory pause, excess gas is expelled out of the pop-off valve.

Exhausted soda lime
The soda lime nearest the patient becomes exhausted first (as it is this soda lime that has the first opportunity to react with the patient's expired carbon dioxide). This exhausted soda lime cannot remove the carbon dioxide from the last portion of alveolar gas exhaled by the patient and this carbon dioxide-rich gas is then rebreathed with the next breath. The volume of carbon dioxide-rich alveolar gas rebreathed with each breath increases as more and more soda lime is exhausted. This steady increase in rebreathing is one of the to-and-fro circuit's major limitations.

12.23 Gas flow inside the to-and-fro circuit. ■ Fresh gas; ■ dead-space gas; ■ alveolar gas; ■ soda lime.

- Gas passes backwards and forwards through the soda lime as the patient breathes.
- As the soda lime is exhausted, the active face moves away from the patient, increasing the circuit dead space. The patient will rebreathe ever larger volumes of carbon dioxide-rich gas until its own level of carbon dioxide reaches dangerous levels. The volume of dead space could eventually exceed the patient's own tidal volume.
- The close proximity of the soda lime to the patient can result in irritant dust being inhaled by the patient.
- Because of these faults, the to-and-fro circuit should not be used.

Humphrey ADE circuit with soda lime canister fitted

- The function of this circuit (Figure 12.24) is identical to that of a normal circuit (the slightly different positions of the fresh gas inlet and the APL valve do not affect the circuit's operation).

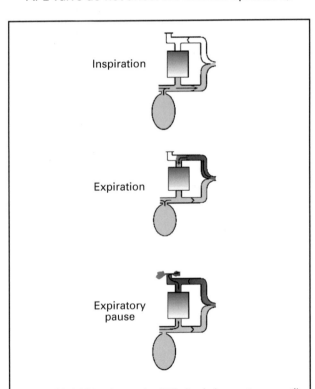

The modified APL valve on the ADE circuit does not open until the reservoir bag is full, causing more of the exhaled gases to be recycled through the soda lime and thus increasing the circuit's efficiency.

The position of the reservoir bag on the inspiratory limb conserves fresh gas and reduces the circuit resistance – the animal does not have to suck the gases through the soda lime canister during inspiration. The gases are driven through the soda lime by the passive elastic recoil of the chest during expiration. (The exact reverse happens in circuits where the reservoir bag is on the expiratory limb, making them unsuitable for smaller animals.)

12.24 Gas flow inside the Humphrey ADE circle circuit with soda lime canister fitted.
Fresh gas; ■ dead-space gas; ■ alveolar gas; ■ soda lime.

- The small canister volume and the small diameter of breathing tubes make this circuit more responsive to changes in the vaporizer setting than larger circles and so it is more suitable for short procedures.
- The smooth inner wall of the breathing tubes and the lightweight one-way valves allow this circuit to be used in smaller animals than most circle circuits (the ADE can be used with its soda lime canister in animals weighing >7 kg).

Reservoir bags and circuits containing soda lime

The reservoir bag in a circuit containing soda lime should be of a greater volume than the tidal volume of the patient to which it is connected. In general, for dogs between 15 and 30 kg, a 1 litre reservoir bag is suitable. A 2 litre bag should be used for dogs between 31 and 70 kg.

Circle circuits and vaporizers

It is possible to include a basic uncalibrated draw-over vaporizer within a circle circuit (Figure 12.25).

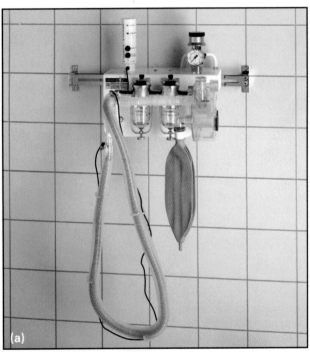

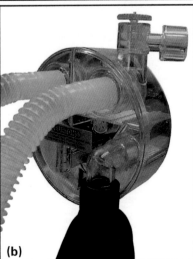

12.25 Circle circuit machines. **(a)** With in-circuit vaporizer. **(b)** With out-of-circuit vaporizer.

- The vaporizer is fitted between the reservoir bag and the inspiratory valve.
- Komesaroff vaporizers are often used.
- The incorporation of a vaporizer within the circuit removes the need to have an expensive calibrated vaporizer on the anaesthetic machine and many veterinary practices have used this type of machine as a cost-effective way of using isoflurane.
- These circuits are often sold as part of a complete machine.
- The resistance to breathing offered by this type of circle circuit is quite large and they are not suitable for animals weighing <20 kg.

Nitrous oxide and soda lime

- **Nitrous oxide should not be used routinely with circuits that contain soda lime.**
- **Unlike oxygen, nitrous oxide is not removed from the circuit.**
- **Its concentration will slowly increase as the circuit is used.**

Consider a situation where nitrous oxide and oxygen are both being introduced into a circuit at a rate of 1 litre/min. A 40 kg dog will use 200 ml oxygen/min. However, none of the nitrous oxide will be metabolized. This means that, at the end of 1 minute, the ratio of oxygen to nitrous oxide will be only 0.8:1. Eventually, the oxygen concentration can become dangerously low. Nitrous oxide can be used if respiratory gas monitoring is available.

Manual IPPV

Intermittent positive pressure ventilation (IPPV) is often used to maintain oxygenation and reduce carbon dioxide levels in animals that either are not breathing for themselves (e.g. animals given opiate analgesics often do not breathe adequately) or cannot breathe for themselves (e.g. animals that are undergoing thoracotomies or have been given neuromuscular blocking agents). The breathing circuit is used to force anaesthetic gases into the patient's lungs and the animal is then allowed to exhale. This can be achieved by repeatedly squeezing and releasing the reservoir bag or using a mechanical ventilator connected to the circuit.

The Lack, parallel Lack and Magill circuits are not suitable for continuous IPPV because they are likely to cause the animal to rebreathe carbon dioxide-rich alveolar gas. However, the circuits can be used for short periods of IPPV when, for instance, an animal is not breathing after the induction of anaesthesia.

The Bain, T-piece, Humphrey ADE with or without soda lime and circle circuits (including the Humphrey ADE with soda lime) are more suited to continuous IPPV and these should be used in cases where continuous IPPV is envisaged (e.g. the repair of a ruptured diaphragm in a cat).

IPPV techniques

T-piece with open-ended bag

1. The reservoir bag is held closed and the bag is allowed to fill a little.

2. The bag is gently squeezed, inflating the patient's lungs.
3. The end of the bag is released, allowing the patient to exhale.

T-piece with APL valve, Bain and circle

Either:

1. Close the APL valve.
2. Squeeze the bag to inflate the animal's lung.
3. Then open the valve to allow the animal to exhale.

Or:

1. Partially close the APL valve.
2. Squeeze the bag. This will inflate the patient's lungs and force some gas out of the APL valve.
3. Release the bag to allow the animal to exhale.
4. Adjust the amount of 'leak' from the APL valve until the reservoir bag becomes neither too full nor too empty.

Humphrey APL

The specially designed APL valve on the Humphrey ADE circuit can be closed by simply applying pressure to the orange plastic button in the top of the exhaust valve (Figure 12.26). This means that the 'close valve, squeeze, open valve' technique is particularly easy on this circuit. Alternatively, the APL valve can be partially closed by turning the knurled ring on top of the valve and then employing the 'leaky APL' technique.

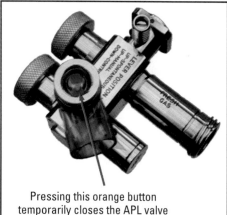

12.26 Detail of the APL valve on a Humphrey ADE circuit.

Pressing this orange button temporarily closes the APL valve so the patient can be ventilated

---

Anaesthetic techniques and commonly used anaesthetic drugs

It is easiest to consider drugs in the order in which they are used during a typical anaesthetic. However, because some drugs (such as isoflurane and propofol) can be used as both induction and maintenance agents, drugs will be defined according to their most common usage. For example, isoflurane will be considered to be a maintenance anaesthetic agent and propofol will be classed as an induction agent.

Analgesics will also be considered in this section as they are used both as premedicants and for postsurgical analgesia.

Premedication

Drugs used for premedication are listed in Figure 12.27. Most anaesthetic premedicants for dogs and cats consist of sedatives and an analgesic (Figure 12.28). Premedicant combinations for small mammals, reptiles and birds often simply consist of analgesics on their own or are not given at all.

Sedatives

Sedatives calm the induction of and recovery from anaesthesia. They reduce the amount of anaesthetic induction agent needed to induce anaesthesia, especially if alpha-2 agonists are used as part of the premedicant combination. Sedatives are often classified according to their pharmacological grouping (Figure 12.29).

Drug family	Typical use	Drug names
Anticholinergics	Drying agents. Traditional use (required when ether was used as a maintenance agent). No real justification for routine use with modern inhalation agents. Used to treat bradycardia during anaesthesia	Atropine, glycopyrrolate
Sedatives (see Figure 12.29)	Used to calm patient prior to the induction of anaesthesia. Synergistic effect with opiates (neuroleptanalgesia)	Acepromazine, diazepam, alpha-2 agonists (xylazine, medetomidine)
Analgesics (see Figure 12.37)	Provide pain relief. Prevent reflex responses to surgical stimuli. Three major classes: non-steroidal anti-inflammatory drugs (NSAIDs); opiates; and local analgesics. Should be given prior to surgery for maximum effect. Should try to use combinations of NSAIDs, opiates and local analgesics where possible	**NSAIDs:** carprofen, meloxicam **Opiates:** morphine, pethidine, methadone, buprenorphine, butorphanol, papaveretum, fentanyl **Local analgesics:** lidocaine, bupivacaine

12.27 Drugs used for premedication.

Species	Sedative	Dose	Analgesic	Dose
Dog	**Acepromazine**	0.03–0.05 mg/kg	**Pethidine** *or* **Morphine** *or* **Methadone** *or* **Papaveretum** *or* **Buprenorphine** *or* **Butorphanol**	1–2 mg/kg 0.1–0.5 mg/kg 0.1–0.5 mg/kg 0.2–1.0 mg/kg 0.01–0.02 mg/kg 0.1 mg/kg
	Diazepam	0.1–0.25 mg/kg	Pethidine *or* Morphine	1–2 mg/kg 0.1–0.5 mg/kg
	Medetomidine	10–40 µg/kg 10 µg/kg	On its own *or* Butorphanol	0.1 mg/kg
Cat	**Acepromazine**	0.03–0.05 mg/kg	**Pethidine** *or* **Morphine** *or* **Buprenorphine** *or* **Methadone**	1–3 mg/kg 0.1 mg/kg 0.01–0.02 mg/kg 0.1 mg/kg
Rabbit	**Fluanisone** [a]	3 mg/kg [b]	**Fentanyl** [a]	95 µg/kg [b]

12.28 Premedicant combinations. The combinations in bold are neuroleptanalgesics. [a] Fentanyl with fluanisone is a neuroleptanalgesic combination made commercially for sedation in rabbits (Hypnorm) that is often used as a premedicant prior to the induction of anaesthesia with diazepam. [b] These doses are the same as giving Hypnorm at 0.3 ml/kg.

Group/drug	Usage and effects	Contraindications and warnings
Phenothiazine derivatives: Acepromazine	Perhaps the most commonly used sedative premedicant in veterinary anaesthesia	Has been associated with causing seizures. Should be avoided in patients with epilepsy or undergoing anaesthesia for myelography Boxers particularly sensitive to effects of acepromazine – should be used with caution and at greatly reduced dose in this breed
Benzodiazepines: Diazepam	Used as premedicant for sick patients and to treat seizures. Most useful as premedicant when combined with morphine or pethidine	Does not always cause sedation in veterinary species; more likely to cause excitement than sedation in fit dogs, especially when used on its own

12.29 Sedatives. (continues) ▶

Group/drug	Usage and effects	Contraindications and warnings
Alpha-2 agonists: Xylazine, medetomidine	Newer sedatives used on their own or in combination with opiates for sedation for simple procedures or as premedicants. Medetomidine has specifically licensed 'reversal agent' (atipamezole) which can be used to reverse its effects at end of a procedure, or during anaesthetic emergency	Alpha-2 agonist drugs have profound effects on cardio-vascular system of dogs and cats Produce extreme bradycardia (heart rate in dogs may fall to below 40 beats/min). Useful but drugs should be used with caution, and avoided in sick or debilitated patients Alpha-2 agonists reduce required dose of intravenous induction agents by *up to 80%*. (They also increase delay between intravenous injection of an anaesthetic induction agent and its effects being seen) ⚠ **Great care should be taken when using alpha-2 agonists prior to induction of anaesthesia with intravenous induction agents**

12.29 (continued) Sedatives.

Analgesics

Analgesics provide relief from pain and reduce distress and excitement during the recovery period.

Using analgesics routinely prior to surgery is a good habit. It should be remembered that the effects of some analgesics are fairly short lived (e.g. pethidine only provides analgesia for 1–2 hours, butorphanol is beneficial for less than an hour, and the effects of morphine last for about 4 hours in dogs). Analgesics are most effective if given before surgery and it is often necessary to give repeat doses of analgesic throughout the postsurgical period.

For maximum effect analgesics from different classes should be combined (opiates and NSAIDs, for example). Analgesics will be discussed more fully later in this chapter.

Neuroleptanalgesia

The combination of a phenothiazine or benzodiazepine sedative with a strong opioid analgesic is called neuroleptanalgesia. At low doses, this combination is useful for premedication. At higher doses, the central depression produced is sufficient to carry out minor surgical procedures. Premedicant combinations that can be considered to be neuroleptanalgesics are shown in Figure 12.28.

Routes of administration of premedication

Subcutaneous:

- Slow uptake of drugs
- Not reliable in patients that are dehydrated or in physiological shock
- Easy to administer
- Not usually painful.

Intramuscular:

- Can be painful, particularly with some drugs and when large volumes are used
- More reliable uptake of drug
- Most failures due to inadvertent injection into fat
- Difficult in some dogs.

Intravenous:

- Technically quite difficult
- Some drugs not suitable for intravenous injection.

Induction of anaesthesia

The induction techniques of intravenous injection, intramuscular injection and mask induction are compared in Figure 12.30. Induction agents are listed in Figures 12.31 and 12.32.

Intravenous injection
Produces a smooth induction of anaesthesia. Dose of induction agent can be titrated so that the patient gets just enough to induce anaesthesia and no more. Must have good patient restraint
Intramuscular injection
Technically easier than intravenous injection. Must give the induction agents according to the patient's weight – cannot titrate dose according to the patient's need. More suitable for very fractious patients or small creatures where intravenous injection is not possible
Intraperitoneal injection
Sometimes used where large volumes of drugs need to be given to small animals (e.g. hamsters, mice). Can be very painful
Mask induction
Can be very distressing for the patient. Significant pollution hazard (ventilate the room well to reduce this). Induction in anaesthetic chamber useful for small animals and exotics. Sevoflurane induces anaesthesia more rapidly than isoflurane and may be less stressful (but many animals still seem to find its smell objectionable)

12.30 Induction techniques.

Drug	Usage and effects	Contraindications and warnings
Barbiturates		
Pentobarbital	A medium-acting barbiturate anaesthetic agent. Only commonly used at high doses for humane euthanasia	Extravascular injection is painful
Thiopental	Short-acting: a single intravenous dose induces around 20 minutes of anaesthesia in the dog Recovery from anaesthesia is mainly through redistribution into the patient's fat and not through metabolism Available in a number of concentrations: 2.5% (25 mg/ml) concentration should be used in small animals; 1.25% (12.5 mg/ml) is more suitable for use in very small dogs and cats	Unstable in solution. Made up from crystalline form with sterile water. Made-up solutions should be kept refrigerated and any unused portion should be discarded after 24 hours Prolonged recoveries seen in Greyhounds and other sight hounds; thiopental should be avoided in these breeds Not suitable for use in puppies and kittens under 3 months of age Thiopental is cumulative and so is not suitable for use as a maintenance agent Extravascular injections of thiopental, especially at concentrations of 5% and above, are painful and can cause severe injury including skin sloughing if not treated; dilute extravascular thiopental by injecting 2–10 ml of sterile water or 2% lidocaine around the vein and massage well
Steroids		
Alfaxalone and alfadalone	A combination of these two steroids is marketed as Saffan When given intravenously it produces around 10 min anaesthesia Saffan can be administered by the intramuscular route but the volume needed can be very large. The combination is non-irritant if given extravascularly Saffan is licensed for the induction of anaesthesia in cats, ferrets and goats. It is suitable for use in a variety of exotic species	The two steroids are not soluble in water and the preparation contains the solvent Cremophor EL, which causes severe anaphylaxis in dogs, making the drug *unsuitable* for use in this species Cremophor EL also causes histamine release in cats which can cause swollen paws and ears Laryngeal oedema may occur in some cats anaesthetized with Saffan
Alfaxalone	Alfaxan contains 10 mg/ml of alfaxalone. It is available in Australia, New Zealand and the UK. Because it does not contain Cremophor EL it can be used in dogs as well as cats for the induction and maintenance of anaesthesia	It must be injected slowly to avoid respiratory depression and resultant apnoea
Dissociative anaesthetic agents: *Produce a light plane of anaesthesia along with profound analgesia. The animal appears dissociated from its surroundings and procedures being carried out*		
Ketamine	Used on its own and in various combinations with alpha-2 agonists, opiate analgesics and benzodiazepines to produce anaesthesia in dogs, cats, rabbits and other exotics Used with alpha-2 agonists for the induction of anaesthesia in horses.	Not suitable for use in animals with impaired renal function or hepatic function
Tiletamine	Similar to ketamine Available premixed with zolazepam (a benzodiazepine) in USA and Australia	
Substituted phenols		
Propofol	Marketed as a milky white emulsion in soya bean oil, egg phosphatide and glycerol Intravenous injection results in a rapid induction of anaesthesia which, if not maintained with an inhalation agent or further boluses of propofol, lasts about 15–20 minutes Rapidly metabolized in the liver and elsewhere in the body. Animals with impaired liver function are less likely to experience prolonged recoveries when given propofol Because of its rapid metabolism, it is non-cumulative and can be used as a maintenance anaesthetic agent. When used for this purpose, it is often delivered as a constant-rate infusion using a syringe driver Does not produce prolonged anaesthesia in Greyhounds and other sight hounds	Some individuals develop severe muscle twitches after prolonged use Following intravenous injection, a transient fall in blood pressure and cardiac output is seen along with a brief period of apnoea The cardiovascular effects of propofol are at least as profound as those seen with thiopental Propofol's main advantage over thiopental is its short duration of action and extra-hepatic metabolism. It is not a 'safer' anaesthetic even though it is often sold to owners as such Propofol does not contain any preservative and part-used vials should be disposed of after use

12.31 Intravenous anaesthetic agents.

Species	Combination	Dose
Cat	Medetomidine with ketamine and butorphanol	40 µg/kg i.v. 2.5 mg/kg i.v. 0.1 mg/kg i.v.
	Medetomidine with ketamine and butorphanol	80 µg/kg i.m. 5 mg/kg i.m. 0.4 mg/kg i.m.
	Medetomidine with ketamine	80 µg/kg i.m. 2.5–5 mg/kg i.m
	Diazepam with ketamine	0.25 mg/kg i.m 5 mg/kg i.m.
Dog	Medetomidine with butorphanol *followed 15 minutes later by* ketamine	25 µg/kg i.m. 0.1 mg/kg i.m. 5 mg/kg i.m.
	Xylazine *followed 10 minutes later by* ketamine	1–2 mg/kg i.m. 5 mg/kg i.m.
Rabbit	Fentanyl/fluanisone (Hypnorm) *followed 5 minutes later by* diazepam	0.3 ml/kg i.m. 1–2 mg/kg i.v. or i.p.
	Fentanyl/fluanisone (Hypnorm) *followed 5 minutes later by* diazepam	0.3 ml/kg i.v. or i.p. 1–2 mg/kg i.v.

12.32 Intravenous and intramuscular combinations for inducing anaesthesia.

Induction is one of the most dangerous periods of anaesthesia. Cardiac arrest may occur in the immediate post-induction period.

There is a lot going on in the theatre following the induction of anaesthesia and an arrest can easily be missed. By carrying out the following 'ABC', any problems will be quickly noticed.

Airway
Intubate the patient and check that the endotracheal tube is correctly positioned.

Breathing
Watch the patient's chest and the reservoir bag of the breathing circuit to see whether the patient is breathing or not. There is often a short period of apnoea following the induction of anaesthesia with thiopental or propofol. If this occurs, ventilate the patient until spontaneous respiration returns.

Circulation
Check that the patient has a pulse. The femoral and lingual pulses are easy to check but remember to check more peripheral pulses such as the carpal or dorsal pedal artery. These give a much better idea of the adequacy of the peripheral perfusion.

Placing an intravenous catheter in a suitable vein prior to the induction of anaesthesia is good practice, because:

- In the event of an anaesthetic emergency, drugs can be easily administered
- The animal has time to relax after the 'painful bit' of catheter placement before it feels the effects of the anaesthetic agent, producing smoother inductions.

Intubation

Before intubation is possible, the patient must be sufficiently deeply anaesthetized to abolish any gag reflex. Intubation should be possible if:

- The patient's jaw tone is relaxed
- The patient's tongue can be pulled out of the mouth without any resistance
- Attempts to introduce the endotracheal tube into the patient's oropharyngeal region do not result in swallowing or gagging movements.

Steps in the intubation and extubation of dogs and cats are set out in Figure 12.33.

Intubation

Dogs

1. The dog is positioned in sternal or lateral recumbency.
2. The assistant holds the dog's head, supporting it behind the ears with the left hand and pointing the dog's nose upwards.
3. The tongue should be gently pulled rostrally until it is fully extended and the larynx can be visualized (ensuring that the tongue lies between the two lower canine teeth) and the mouth opened by pulling down gently on the tongue.
4. Use a suitably sized and lubricated endotracheal tube to push the soft palate dorsally, away from the epiglottis. (This is not always necessary.) The epiglottis is then pushed down with the end of the tube, which is gently inserted between the vocal folds.

A laryngoscope is useful for brachycephalic dogs.

12.33 Steps in intubation and extubation of dogs and cats. (continues) ▶

Intubation

Cats

A laryngoscope makes intubation in cats much easier.

1. The cat is positioned in sternal or lateral recumbency.
2. An assistant holds the cat's head, extending its neck and supporting it behind its ears.
3. The cat's tongue should be gently pulled rostrally until it is fully extended and the larynx can be visualized (ensuring that the tongue lies between the two lower canine teeth). Be very careful not to damage the delicate frenulum whilst doing this.
4. Hold the cat's tongue between the thumb and first finger and hold the laryngoscope with the other fingers. This leaves the other hand free to manipulate the endotracheal tube.
5. At this point the cat's larynx must be desensitized with local anaesthetic spray. It may be necessary to dislocate the epiglottis from the soft palate by pushing the soft palate dorsally with the anaesthetic spray nozzle before the larynx can be seen. After spraying the larynx, wait for a minute before proceeding, to allow the local anaesthetic to work.
6. The tip of the laryngoscope blade should be used to press down on the cat's tongue just rostral to the epiglottis. It should not be used to push down on the epiglottis itself.
7. A lubricated tube is gently passed between the laryngeal folds. This is made easier by observing the movement of the laryngeal folds as the cat breathes. The tube should be inserted during inspiration, whilst the vocal folds are open.

The author prefers to use uncuffed endotracheal tubes in cats whenever possible, so that the cat's delicate trachea cannot be traumatized by an over-inflated cuff.

Checking the position of the tube and inflating the cuff

1. Ventilate the patient with 100% oxygen, using the breathing circuit, whilst observing the chest wall. If the endotracheal tube has been correctly placed in the animal's trachea, the chest should be seen to expand as the reservoir bag is compressed.
2. If the tube is correctly positioned, the cuff can be inflated. Only inflate it sufficiently to prevent oxygen from escaping around the cuff. Over-inflation can damage the tracheal mucosa or occlude the tube.

Tying the tube in place

- In order to reduce the risk of accidental extubation, the endotracheal tube can be tied in place with a bandage.
- The tie should be fastened around the end of the tube, over the plastic connector. The connector supports the wall of the tube and ensures that the tube does not collapse as the tie is pulled tight.
- The material is then fastened behind the patient's head or around its muzzle or lower jaw to secure the tube in place.
- Ensure that any knot used to fasten the tube in place is easily released in the event of an emergency. A simple bow is best, because people are familiar with it and know how to release it quickly in an emergency.

Extubation

- The cuff should be left inflated until just before the tube is removed.
- During oral surgery some fluid may go around the endotracheal tube and down the trachea. In dogs, the endotracheal tube can be removed with the cuff partially inflated. This removes a lot of debris from the proximal trachea.
- Dogs should be extubated once their gag reflex has returned.
- Cats should be extubated before their gag reflex returns (if a cat gags on an endotracheal tube, the trauma to the laryngeal mucosa can cause laryngeal oedema).
- The endotracheal tube should always be removed gently in a downward arc, so as to avoid damage to the larynx or trachea.

12.33 (continued) Steps in intubation and extubation of dogs and cats.

Maintenance of anaesthesia

Most of the modern anaesthetic induction agents only produce a short period of anaesthesia. If the procedure is going to require a longer anaesthetic, a maintenance agent is used. Most of these are inhalational anaesthetic agents but some intravenous anaesthetic agents can be used for maintenance; each type has advantages and disadvantages.

With an intravenous agent:

- No special equipment is needed (but catheters should be used to provide good venous access and oxygen supplied)
- There is no pollution hazard
- Once given, it cannot be taken back (risk of overdose)

- The use of intravenous agents to maintain anaesthesia is often known as TIVA (total intravenous anaesthesia)
- TIVA is becoming common in medical practice (where computers record the patient's electroencephalogram and adjust the anaesthetic dose accordingly) and is often used for field anaesthesia in horses for short procedures.

With an inhalation agent:

- An anaesthetic machine is required
- There is a potential pollution hazard (see below)
- The anaesthetic vapour can be taken back by ventilating the patient with 100% oxygen (overdose potentially reversible).

Intravenous anaesthetic maintenance agents

Almost all intravenous anaesthetic agents (see Figure 12.31) can be used as maintenance agents with more or less success, but only propofol can be used to prolong anaesthesia for a long time without affecting the patient's recovery. Extending anaesthesia with many of the other intravenous anaesthetic agents leads to problems with drug accumulation and prolonged recoveries or with other side effects.

Long-acting induction agents not requiring a maintenance agent

Some anaesthetic combinations induce surgical anaesthesia that lasts long enough to perform short procedures such as a spay or castration without resorting to a maintenance agent. These are typically combinations of alpha-2 agonist sedatives (medetomidine or xylazine), opiates and ketamine. The use of these agents does not remove the need to intubate the patient's trachea or provide an oxygen supply. All anaesthetized animals should be intubated where possible – this allows them to breathe 100% oxygen and allows the anaesthetist to perform IPPV should it be required in an emergency.

Inhalation anaesthetic maintenance agents

With the exception of nitrous oxide, the inhalation anaesthetic agents are all volatile liquids, the vapours of which induce anaesthesia when inhaled. Volatile anaesthetic agents (Figure 12.34) have two properties that are often talked about: their solubility and their minimum alveolar concentration (MAC).

Solubility

Anaesthetic agents are inhaled into the lungs. They cross the alveolar membranes, dissolve into the blood and are carried to the brain, where they cross the blood–brain barrier and exert their effect. The concentration in the brain determines the depth of anaesthesia, and the rate at which the concentration can be changed determines how quickly the animal will succumb to or recover from the drug's effects.

- Very *soluble* volatile anaesthetic agents (methoxyflurane, halothane)
  - These have a high solubility coefficient and are easily absorbed into the blood but, once dissolved, tend not to come out again. When the blood reaches the brain, the concentration of anaesthetic in the brain rises slowly.
  - The reverse happens at the end of anaesthesia, when the agents are only slowly released into the alveoli and exhaled, resulting in a slow recovery.
- Very *insoluble* anaesthetic agents (sevoflurane, desflurane)
  - These have a low solubility coefficient and are still absorbed into the blood but are very readily released into the brain, resulting in rapid anaesthetic inductions.
  - The reverse happens at the end of anaesthesia and the agents are quickly eliminated via the lungs, allowing the animal to recover.

In summary:

> **Soluble anaesthetic agent = slow induction of and recovery from anaesthesia (e.g. halothane and methoxyflurane)**
>
> **Insoluble anaesthetic agent = rapid induction of and recovery from anaesthesia (e.g. sevoflurane and desflurane)**

The blood/gas solubility coefficient for the various anaesthetic agents is given in Figure 12.34.

Minimum alveolar concentration (MAC)

This is a measure of the volatile anaesthetic agent's potency. It is defined as the minimum alveolar concentration of an anaesthetic that produces immobility in 50% of subjects exposed to a supramaximal (i.e. painful) stimulus. This means that, for example, if no other drugs are given, 50% of all dogs will not respond to stimuli when their alveolar concentration of halothane is 0.87% (the MAC of halothane is 0.87% in dogs).

MAC is used to compare volatile anaesthetic agents and is measured experimentally. It can be thought of as a guide to the concentration of anaesthetic that must be given to an animal to keep it anaesthetized during surgery. It must be emphasized that it is only a guide. Animals given opiate analgesics and older animals tend to require lower concentrations of volatile anaesthetic agents. The time of day (the animal's circadian rhythm) and whether the animal is pregnant or not will also affect the concentration of volatile anaesthetic agent needed.

MAC is measured for each species and varies between them (the MAC of most anaesthetic agents is higher for cats than dogs). MAC values for dogs, cats and rabbits are given in Figure 12.34.

The concentration of anaesthetic vapour needed to maintain anaesthesia is often higher than the agent's MAC (usually around 1.5 x MAC).

Anaesthetic gases

Anaesthetic gases include oxygen, nitrous oxide and carbon dioxide. Their roles in anaesthesia vary but they are considered together as they are all gases at room temperature and pressure. The anaesthetic gases do not include agents such as halothane, isoflurane and sevoflurane – these are known as volatile anaesthetic agents or anaesthetic vapours.

The difference between a gas and a vapour

The terms vapour and gas are often used interchangeably but there is a difference.

- Technically, a *vapour* is an element or compound in the gas phase under conditions (temperature and pressure) when it would normally be a liquid.
- Conversely, a *gas* is an element or compound in the gas phase under conditions (temperature and pressure) when it would normally be a gas. ▶

Inhalation agent	Usage and effects	Contraindications and warnings	Minimum alveolar concentration %	Solubility coefficient (blood/gas)	Maximum legal occupational exposure limits (ppm)	Global warming potential
Methoxyflurane (of historical interest only)	Very soluble – recoveries from anaesthesia are very prolonged Not very volatile: vapour concentrations sufficient to induce anaesthesia cannot be achieved, so cannot be used as an induction agent Good analgesic: high solubility means the analgesic properties last well into the recovery period	Do not use with patients with renal impairment: its metabolites have been implicated in renal toxicity Do not use in patients that have been given flunixin – this will lead to severe kidney damage Produces less cardiovascular depression than halothane	Dog 0.23 Cat 0.23	15.0	–	–
Halothane	Relatively low solubility produces more rapid recovery from anaesthesia compared with methoxyflurane	Produces a dose-dependent fall in cardiac output and blood pressure as well as depressing respiration Sensitizes heart to arrhythmic effects of adrenaline High levels of adrenaline often occur following *stressful* anaesthetic inductions, in which circumstances fatal cardiac arrhythmias may be seen. The situation is made even worse if thiopental has been used as the anaesthetic induction agent	Dog 0.87 Cat 1.14 Rabbit 0.82	2.5	10	–
Isoflurane	Less soluble than halothane and therefore produces even more rapid induction of and recovery from anaesthesia Can be used as both induction and maintenance agent Very useful for induction of anaesthesia in small mammals Does not sensitize heart to adrenaline as much as halothane and so causes fewer cardiac arrhythmias More potent respiratory depressant than halothane	Produces less severe myocardial depression than halothane (but overall fall in blood pressure is similar, due to more profound peripheral vasodilation)	Dog 1.28 Cat 1.63 Rabbit 2.05	1.5	50	1100
Sevoflurane	Less soluble still than isoflurane so rapid induction of and recovery from anaesthesia as well as rapid changes in anaesthetic depth Depresses myocardial contractility (strength of heart's contractions) – similar to isoflurane, as is degree of peripheral vasodilation produced Does not sensitize heart to adrenaline so causes fewer arrhythmias	Rapid recoveries from anaesthesia can expose poor analgesic techniques – animals can wake up quickly and vocalize in pain. This must not be dismissed as dysphoria or 'a reaction to the anaesthetic' Reacts with dry soda lime to produce 'Compound A' – a chemical known to be toxic to rats. It is not toxic to dogs in concentrations found during clinical use and sevoflurane can be used with circuits containing soda lime in dogs	Dog 2.1–2.36 Cat 2.58 Rabbit 3.7	0.68	60	1600
Desflurane	Very volatile (is nearly boiling at room temperature) and must be delivered using special electronically controlled vaporizer/blender The least soluble of all the volatile agents and so produces the most rapid induction and recovery	Not yet in common use in veterinary practice	Dog 7.2 Cat 9.8 Rabbit 5.7–7.1	0.42	–	–

12.34 The volatile anaesthetic agents.

For example, water is a liquid at room temperature and pressure and so gaseous water in the atmosphere at room temperature and pressure is known as water *vapour.* Oxygen, on the other hand, is a gas at room temperature and pressure and so gaseous oxygen in the atmosphere at room temperature and pressure is a *gas.*

This is why volatile anaesthetic agents are referred to as *vapours* (they are all liquids at room temperature and pressure) whereas nitrous oxide is an anaesthetic *gas* (it is a gas at room temperature).

Oxygen

- Oxygen is essential for supporting life. It is administered at concentrations of between 33 and 100%.
- Oxygen strongly supports combustion. It forms an explosive mixture with some flammable anaesthetic agents, especially ether.

Carbon dioxide

- Carbon dioxide is rarely used in veterinary anaesthesia.
- Over-enthusiastic IPPV can cause hypocapnia (low carbon dioxide in the blood). This can have negative effects on the patient. The addition of 5% carbon dioxide to the carrier gas will prevent this from occurring but nowadays it is more usual to measure the patient's end tidal carbon dioxide concentration and adjust the ventilator accordingly.

Nitrous oxide

- Nitrous oxide is a weak anaesthetic agent but has very good analgesic properties.
- Synergy with volatile anaesthetic agents reduces the amount of volatile agent needed to maintain anaesthesia.
- Nitrous oxide diffuses into gas-filled spaces within the body more quickly than nitrogen diffuses out of them. This means that these spaces can become very distended with gas. For this reason, nitrous oxide should not be used in cases of:
  - Gastric dilatation and volvulus (GDV)
  - Uncorrected pneumothorax
  - Any other case where there might be a potential gas-filled space.
- Because nitrous oxide is not removed by soda lime, it is not suitable for use in circle circuits or the Waters' to-and-fro canister (unless respiratory gas monitoring is available).
- The uptake of a volatile anaesthetic agent at the beginning of anaesthesia is more rapid if nitrous oxide is included in the carrier gas. This is known as the second gas effect (see *BSAVA Manual of Advanced Veterinary Nursing* for more information).

- At the end of anaesthesia, nitrous oxide leaving the circulation can displace enough air from the patient's lungs to produce a condition known as diffusion hypoxia. To avoid it, the patient should be allowed to breathe 100% oxygen for 2–5 minutes after the nitrous oxide has been turned off.
- Nitrous oxide is a significant contributor to both operating theatre and environmental pollution (see below).

Pollution

The volatile anaesthetic agents and nitrous oxide pollute both the operating theatre and the general environment.

Operating theatre pollution

It has been known for some time that chronic exposure to low levels of volatile anaesthetic agents and nitrous oxide carries health risks. For example, exposure to halothane is known to change the ratio of male to female babies born to medical workers. When using these agents care must be taken to minimize theatre pollution.

- Refill vaporizers away from the operating theatre in a well ventilated area or at the end of the day so that any spilled vapour has time to disperse.
- Use scavenging religiously – either charcoal canisters or scavenging systems.
- Charcoal canisters get heavier as they absorb volatile anaesthetics – weigh them regularly and change them when they reach their maximum weight.
- Charcoal canisters do not absorb nitrous oxide – if nitrous oxide is used, a scavenging system must be used.
- Use the correct size of endotracheal tube and inflate the cuff.
- Turn the vaporizer and nitrous oxide on *after* the circuit has been connected to the patient.
- Turn the vaporizer and nitrous oxide off, 'dump' the contents of the reservoir bag into the scavenging and flush the circuit with 100% oxygen *before* disconnecting the patient.
- Avoid mask and chamber inductions wherever possible.
- Monitor levels of exposure to volatile anaesthetics and nitrous oxide by using commercially available personal dosemeters. These perform a similar job to radiation badges but measure anaesthetic exposure instead of X-ray exposure.

Environmental pollution

The volatile anaesthetic agents and nitrous oxide are potent greenhouse gases – they contribute to global warming. For example, 1 kg of sevoflurane warms the atmosphere as much as 1600 kg of carbon dioxide. Put another way, using 250 ml of isoflurane warms the environment as much as driving 1200 miles in a family car. Environmental pollution can be reduced by using efficient breathing circuits (e.g. the circle or Humphrey ADE circuit), by accurately calculating the fresh gas flow rate needed by each patient or by using total intravenous anaesthetic techniques.

End of anaesthesia

- Do not allow the depth of anaesthesia to lighten before the end of surgery. It is not ethical to allow a patient to come round as the last skin suture is being placed.
- Switch off the vaporizer and the nitrous oxide once the surgery is *finished*. If nitrous oxide has been used, allow the patient to breathe 100% oxygen for a couple of minutes to prevent diffusion hypoxia. (Do not forget to increase the flow of oxygen in order to compensate for the reduction in total fresh gas flow being delivered to the circuit.)
- Before disconnecting the patient from the breathing circuit, flush the circuit with oxygen to wash any trace of anaesthetic vapour or nitrous oxide into the scavenging system.
- Monitor the patient carefully during the recovery period. Animals are often neglected at this time as everyone is busy with the next patient. (For more details, see section on monitoring.)
- After the last anaesthetic of the day, switch off the gas supply to the machine, clean and put away the circuits and endotracheal tubes and wipe down the anaesthetic machine surfaces with a suitable disinfectant.

Special techniques in anaesthesia

Local anaesthesia

In large animals local anaesthetics are used for a variety of surgical procedures. In small animal practice they tend to be used to complement general anaesthesia – either as the analgesic component of balanced anaesthesia or to provide analgesia in the postsurgical period – rather than as the sole agents for surgery. Local anaesthetic techniques and their common uses are described in Figure 12.35.

Local anaesthetic drugs used include:

- Lidocaine
  - Rapid onset
  - Short duration of action (45 minutes without adrenaline, 90 minutes with)
  - Good for regional nerve blocks and general surgery
- Bupivacaine
  - Much longer duration of action than lidocaine (6–8 hours)
  - Very useful for postoperative analgesia and epidural analgesia
- Proxymetacaine
  - Used for topical analgesia of the eye
  - Less initial sting than other agents.

Technique	Description	Common use
Topical	Local anaesthetic can be applied directly to moist mucous membranes Absorbable gel containing local anaesthetic is available for use on skin	Applied to the eye to facilitate ocular examination Local anaesthetic cream can be placed over site of intended venous puncture (such as the marginal ear vein of a rabbit) making procedure much less traumatic for patient
Regional nerve blocks	Nerves innervating region where surgery is to be performed are blocked by injecting local anaesthetic into tissues surrounding them as they run close to surface or at some other anatomically convenient site	Cornual nerve block used to desensitize horn buds of calves prior to disbudding Paravertebral nerve block used to desensitize flanks of cows prior to Caesarean section. Local anaesthetic solution is infiltrated into the tissues surrounding the spinal nerves as they emerge from the vertebral canal Intercostal nerves are infiltrated with local anaesthetic solution as they run down the caudal border of each rib to provide postsurgical analgesia following lateral thoracotomies
Intravenous regional analgesia	Tourniquet is placed around animal's limb and local anaesthetic is introduced into one of distended veins distal to it; local anaesthetic blocks conduction of nerves running in close proximity to veins; this results in extremely good analgesia of distal portion of limb for as long as tourniquet remains in place	Used for performing surgery on feet of cattle and occasionally limb surgery in dogs
Epidural analgesia	Local anaesthetic can be introduced into liquid fat surrounding spinal cord; this blocks the nerves as they leave the spinal canal, resulting in loss of sensation and motor activity in region of body supplied by affected nerves	Very useful for providing analgesia to the anus, perineum and hindlimbs of animals undergoing surgery
Local infiltration	Local anaesthetic is injected into tissues at surgical site	Useful for small surgical procedures in conscious animals

12.35 Local anaesthetic techniques.

Neuromuscular blocking agents

Although volatile agents all produce a degree of muscle relaxation at normal concentrations, it may not be enough for certain procedures. If a greater degree of muscle relaxation is required, specific neuromuscular blocking agents are used. These act directly on the neuromuscular junction to stop the transmission of motor nerve impulses to striated muscle. The drugs are classified as either depolarizing or non-depolarizing agents (Figure 12.36).

Group/drug	Usage and effects	Contraindications and warnings
Depolarizing agents		
Suxamethonium	Very short-acting Only of historical interest now	Associated with muscle pain on recovery
Non-depolarizing agents		
Pancuronium	Only of historical interest now	Long duration of action and cumulative, so top-up doses cannot be used
Vecuronium	Intermediate duration of action (30 min in dog and cat) Non-cumulative Very popular agent but being replaced in most situations by atracurium	May produce tachycardia in dogs and cats
Atracurium	Intermediate duration of action (30–40 min in dog and cat) Major advantage: breaks down spontaneously inside body Can be used in animals with poor kidney and liver function	Inactivated by contact with thiopental and other alkaline solutions Ensure any intravenous catheters flushed thoroughly before using them to administer

12.36 Common neuromuscular blocking agents.

Neuromuscular blocking agents are useful in the following situations.

- High-risk cases
  - Using neuromuscular blocking agents reduces the amount of volatile anaesthetic agent required to produce surgical anaesthesia. This reduces the degree of cardiovascular depression produced by the volatile anaesthetic agents.
- Oesophageal foreign bodies
  - The oesophagus in the dog contains some striated muscle. Neuromuscular blocking agents can make the removal of an oesophageal foreign body easier.

- Corneal surgery
  - During surgical anaesthesia the eye is rotated ventrally, making corneal surgery impossible. Neuromuscular blocking agents bring the eye back to a central position.
- Orthopaedic surgery
  - Some dislocations can be easier to reduce following the administration of neuromuscular blocking agents. However, these agents do not make the reduction of fractures any easier.
- Thoracic surgery
  - By reducing the muscle tone of the intercostal muscles, access to the thorax is made easier. The intercostal muscles are less severely damaged by the rib retractors, resulting in less postsurgical pain.

Analgesia

Analgesia was mentioned earlier in the section on Premedication. Types of analgesic are described in Figure 12.37.

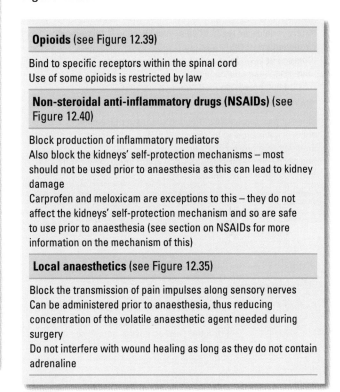

Opioids (see Figure 12.39)

Bind to specific receptors within the spinal cord
Use of some opioids is restricted by law

Non-steroidal anti-inflammatory drugs (NSAIDs) (see Figure 12.40)

Block production of inflammatory mediators
Also block the kidneys' self-protection mechanisms – most should not be used prior to anaesthesia as this can lead to kidney damage
Carprofen and meloxicam are exceptions to this – they do not affect the kidneys' self-protection mechanism and so are safe to use prior to anaesthesia (see section on NSAIDs for more information on the mechanism of this)

Local anaesthetics (see Figure 12.35)

Block the transmission of pain impulses along sensory nerves
Can be administered prior to anaesthesia, thus reducing concentration of the volatile anaesthetic agent needed during surgery
Do not interfere with wound healing as long as they do not contain adrenaline

12.37 Types of analgesic.

Using an analgesic pre-emptively (before surgery or a painful procedure) will produce better analgesia than using it after the event. This is because of a phenomenon known as '**wind-up**', or sensitization. 'Wind-up' refers to the brain's *increased* sensitivity to stimuli following injury. This means that if analgesics are given after surgery they are much less effective and the animal experiences greater pain. Analgesics should be given pre-emptively wherever possible.

Analgesia is very important in veterinary anaesthesia:

- It is more humane to use analgesics than not to use them

- The dose (and hence the adverse effects) of anaesthetic agents needed are significantly reduced
- Animals eat sooner and recover more quickly if given analgesics following surgery
- Animals cannot express pain in the same way that humans can and sometimes deliberately hide evidence of pain (particularly prey animals, such as rabbits and rodents). It is best to assume that they are in pain, rather than wait for signs of distress (Figure 12.38).

Opioid analgesics

Opioid analgesics are subject to abuse and are physically addictive. Because of this, their purchase, storage and use are strictly controlled and detailed records must be kept (see Chapter 3).

Opioid analgesics bind to specific receptors in the spinal cord. These receptors have been classified into types according to the effects seen when they are occupied. Some are associated with excitement and euphoria (hence their abuse by humans); others are associated with analgesia.

The pain-relieving receptors are called the mu (μ) receptors. Opioid analgesics bind to these receptors and produce analgesia, and are themselves classified as either pure or partial mu agonists, according to the way in which they interact with these receptors (Figure 12.39):

- Pure mu agonists occupy the mu receptor and produce analgesia
- Partial mu agonists occupy the mu receptor but do not stimulate it fully.

The degree of analgesia varies with dose and can even be less when higher doses are used.

- Partial mu agonists tend to be poorer analgesics than pure mu agonists.
- They also tend to have a greater affinity for the mu receptor than the pure mu agonist opioids (they stick more firmly to receptors).
- If they are given after pure mu agonists, they will 'knock' some of the pure mu agonists off the receptors. This can result in less analgesia for the patient.

Partial mu agonists should be used in patients where the postsurgical pain is expected to be mild. In cases where moderate to severe postsurgical pain is likely, pure mu agonist opioids should be used.

Dogs
Spontaneous vocalization – whining, growling
Biting at wound
Fear – hiding at back of kennel
High heart rate
Rapid shallow breathing rate

Cats
Rarely vocalize as result of pain – vocalization in this species often indicates severe pain
Hiding at back of cage
Cowering when approached
Hissing and growling when wound is touched

Rabbits and rodents
Signs of pain extremely difficult to assess in these species – prey animals have evolved to hide signs of pain and illness as defence against being picked off by predators
Immobility, anorexia and a reduced water intake may be the only outward signs of discomfort

12.38 Signs of pain.

Drug	Usage and effects	Contraindications and warnings
Pure mu agonists		
Pethidine	Short acting; only 1–2 hours in the dog Very good analgesic but needs relatively frequent top-up dosing, sometimes as often as every hour Occasional histamine release	Should not be given by intravenous route Can cause vomiting, though less so than morphine
Morphine	Longer acting than pethidine: 4–5 hours in the dog, 6–8 hours in the cat	Will cause vomiting in some dogs if they are not in pain when it is given. Incidence of vomiting can be reduced by administering it along with acepromazine Produces pupil constriction, peripheral vasodilation and (rarely in veterinary species) respiratory depression
Methadone	Very similar to morphine but less likely to cause vomiting	Produces less sedation than morphine
Papaveretum	Mixture of opiate alkaloids Very good sedative, especially when combined with acepromazine	Similar side effects to morphine
Fentanyl	Very potent short-acting pure mu agonist Used as the analgesic component of the neuroleptanalgesic combination Hypnorm® Used during surgery to provide the analgesic component of the triad of anaesthesia	Causes profound respiratory depression When given by intravenous route, produces several minutes of apnoea during which time patient must be ventilated

12.39 Opioids: pure and partial mu agonists. (continued) ▶

Drug	Usage and effects	Contraindications and warnings
Pure mu agonists continued		
Fentanyl patches	Fentanyl can be administered by transdermal route using slow-release patches Produce excellent analgesia but take up to 24 hours to reach maximum effect so must be placed in good time Very useful for animals in chronic pain or undergoing elective surgery Patches available in 25, 50, 75 and 100 µg/hour sizes Dose is 2.5–5 µg/hour/kg	Patches should *not* be cut to reduce their dose – if 'half' a patch is needed, the whole patch should be used but only half of the active surface exposed Cutting the patch in half actually *increases* rate at which fentanyl is absorbed by animal Patch must be placed on an area of clipped skin on back of animal's neck and covered with dressing to stop animal removing it
Partial mu agonists		
Buprenorphine	Provides 8–12 hours of analgesia	Has bell-shaped dose–response curve, i.e. peak analgesic effect is achieved, after which giving more drug will produce less analgesia Giving 15–20 µg/kg every 8 hours will not produce this effect Onset of action is slow (45 minutes) so must be given in good time
Butorphanol	Used in combination with alpha-2 agonists ± ketamine for sedation and anaesthesia Used as cough suppressant Useful as analgesic in birds	Poor analgesic and very short acting (30–40 minutes) *Butorphanol is not an adequate postoperative analgesic in dogs and cats – other opiates such as buprenorphine or morphine should be used instead*

12.39 (continued) Opioids: pure and partial mu agonists.

Non-steroidal anti-inflammatory drugs

NSAIDs (Figure 12.40) inhibit the synthesis of prostaglandins (inflammatory mediators) by blocking the action of cyclooxygenase, the enzyme that converts arachidonic acid into prostaglandin. By blocking the production of these inflammatory prostaglandins, NSAIDs reduce pain and inflammation. There are two types of cyclooxygenase (COX1 and COX2) that act slightly differently.

Drugs	Usage and effects	Contraindications and warning
Aspirin Paracetamol Phenylbutazone Flunixin Tolfenamic acid Ketoprofen	Longer acting than many opioid analgesics Ineffective against severe pain	Many toxic, especially to cats Should be avoided in patients with cardiac, renal or hepatic disease Should not be used prior to or during anaesthetics; may cause kidney damage Interval between doses should be increased in neonates and geriatrics to avoid toxicity. Ketoprofen is licensed for up to 5 days orally in cats
Carprofen	Very potent analgesic COX2 selective: ■ Less likely to cause gastric ulceration than other NSAIDs ■ Does not block kidneys' self-protection mechanism so can be used prior to anaesthesia	Should be avoided in patients with hepatic, renal or cardiac disease Licensed for preoperative use in cats (single dose) with *one* follow-up half dose
Meloxicam	Postoperative analgesia COX2 selective Can be given prior to anaesthesia Very good analgesic	Not for use in animals less than 6 weeks of age or cats under 2 kg Available in oral form for long-term management of pain in dogs Only licensed for single use in cats (so cannot be used orally to provide follow-up analgesia)
Tepoxalin	New NSAID that inhibits lipoxygenase (LOX) activity along with cyclooxygenase activity LOX activity produces powerful inflammatory mediators and by preventing this LOX inhibitors have analgesic properties Available for control of arthritic pain in dogs	*Not for perioperative use* Inhibits both COX1 and COX2 activity like the older NSAIDs *but* is less likely to cause gastric ulceration because of its effect on LOX activity See main text for more details

12.40 Non-steroidal anti-inflammatory drugs (NSAIDs).

COX1, COX2 and LOX

Arachidonic acid is converted into inflammatory and non-inflammatory prostaglandins by the action of the cyclooxygenase enzymes.

- Cyclooxygenase 1 (*COX1*) produces regulatory and protective prostaglandins and it is the inhibition of this enzyme that is responsible for the side effects of NSAIDs (namely gastric ulceration and renal damage during anaesthesia).
- Cyclooxygenase 2 (*COX2*) produces prostaglandins at sites of cell injury and these inflammatory mediators cause pain, oedema and fever. It is the inhibition of COX2 that is responsible for the beneficial effects of NSAIDs.

Older NSAIDs (aspirin, flunixin, etc.) are very non-selective and inhibit both COX1 and COX2 activity, reducing pain and swelling but also reducing the production of regulatory and protective prostaglandins.

Newer NSAIDs (carprofen and meloxicam) are much more COX2 selective.

Lipoxygenase (*LOX*) acts on arachidonic acid to produce other inflammatory mediators and LOX inhibitors also have anti-inflammatory properties. The newest NSAIDs (tepoxalin) inhibit LOX, COX1 and COX2 activities and thus have potent anti-inflammatory and analgesic properties. Their safety under anaesthesia has not yet been proven so they are currently only licensed for the management of chronic pain in dogs.

Local anaesthetics

Local anaesthetics can be useful for postsurgical analgesia. The techniques described in Figure 12.35 are used to desensitize the surgical site. If they are used, they should be administered prior to surgery to get the best effects. Bupivacaine is the most suitable because it is the longest acting (6–8 hours).

Some local anaesthetic preparations contain adrenaline to increase the drug's duration of action. The adrenaline causes peripheral vasoconstriction that slows down the drug's dispersal and so prolongs its effect. This vasoconstriction can also affect wound healing and so only preparations free from adrenaline should be used for local infiltration into surgical wounds.

Combinations of analgesic drugs

Where possible, analgesics from two or more different classes of drug can be used. For example, following thoracic surgery, infiltration of the intercostal nerves with local anaesthetic can be combined with the use of a pure mu agonist opioid and an NSAID to produce excellent analgesia.

Stages of anaesthesia

In order to judge the depth of anaesthesia, it is important to understand the stages of anaesthesia and the signs a patient will show while undergoing the journey to unconsciousness. There are four stages. It is important to remember that these stages merge together. The aim of the information below is to enable recognition of when the animal is too deeply anaesthetized.

Stage I: voluntary excitement

Stage I begins with induction of the patient and finishes when unconsciousness is reached.
The signs of Stage I are:

- Fear/stress/apprehension
- Pulse/heart rate and respiratory rate increased
- Disorientation
- Muscle activity may be prominent
- May urinate/defecate.

Stage II: involuntary excitement

Stage II begins at the start of unconsciousness. It finishes when the patient is no longer excited and respiration is stable.
The signs of Stage II are:

- Howling
- Excessive movement/struggling
- All reflexes present
- The eye remains open and central
- Pupils are dilated
- Respiration may be irregular but should stabilize
- Vomiting may occur.

Stages I and II can both be made more pleasant for the animal by administration of a premedicant and by giving the correct amount of induction agent. This enables these two stages to pass very quickly; thus they are not seen that often.

Stage III: surgical anaesthesia

Stage III is divided into three planes (Figure 12.41). Minor procedures such as radiography can be performed at plane I. Surgical procedures should be performed at plane II.

Stage IV: overdose

Stage IV ends with paralysis of all the respiratory muscles.
The signs of Stage IV are:

- Respiration rate greatly reduced, the pattern is irregular and shallow/jerky, leading to apnoea
- Heart rate reduced along with capillary refill time and blood pressure
- Pulse weak and slow, will eventually diminish
- Reflexes all absent, including corneal reflex
- Eye position centrally fixed with pupil fully dilated and unresponsive to light
- Muscle tone flaccid.

Plane	Heart rate	Pulse	Respiration	Reflexes	Eye position	Muscle tone
Plane I (Light)	Reduced slightly Regular	Rate is reduced slightly Strong and regular	Regular, smooth, deep Rate increases with painful stimuli	Movement of head and limbs is absent All others present but not as prominent	Nystagmus often seen Eyeball rotates ventrally Third eyelid moves across the eye	Present and responsive, some resistance may occur (e.g. jaw tone)
Plane II (Medium)	Reduced slightly Regular Blood pressure also slightly reduced	Strong and regular	Tidal volume decreased but will increase with stimuli Rate may increase or decrease	Palpebral reflex slow or absent Pedal reflex increasingly slow then absent Corneal reflex present	Nystagmus no longer present Eye has slight ventral rotation Pupil may be constricted	Relaxed Some resistance may be seen in very muscular dogs
Plane III (Deep)	Rate is further reduced along with blood pressure	Weak due to low blood pressure	Tidal volume decreased Rate usually decreased and shallow	All absent except corneal reflex	Eye is central are fixed Third eyelid returns to correct position	Greatly reduced or absent

12.41 Planes in Stage III surgical anaesthesia.

Monitoring the anaesthetized patient

Monitoring anaesthesia is a very important role for the veterinary nurse. It is essential that all aspects of monitoring are understood.

Monitoring can be divided into three categories:

- Pre-anaesthesia
- Intra-anaesthesia
- Post-anaesthesia.

Pre-anaesthesia

The veterinary nurse should take certain steps when the patient first arrives. General information on patient admission procedures is given in Chapter 2. Any animal that requires an anaesthetic or sedation needs a full physical examination and an account of its previous history to determine its health status. The findings from this examination will influence the type and quantity of the drugs used for premedication and for anaesthetizing the animal, or whether in fact the procedure should take place at all.

Questions to ask the client

- **Has the patient urinated or defecated this morning?**
- **Is the patient well in itself? For example, is there any coughing, exercise intolerance, excessive drinking or urinating, vomiting or diarrhoea?**
- **Has the patient had any reactions to an anaesthetic before?**
- **Has the patient been starved overnight (cats and dogs only)?**
- **Is the patient suffering from any illness (e.g. diabetes mellitus, epilepsy, cardiac disease)?**
- **Is the patient taking any medications? If so, which drugs and how often?**
- **Are the patient's vaccinations up to date?**

The examination is carried out by the veterinary surgeon, who assesses the cardiovascular and respiratory systems, the central nervous system and hepatic and renal function, all of which are affected by anaesthesia. If there is a concern regarding any of these systems, further investigation should be carried out (e.g. electrocardiography, radiography, or further blood tests). All the normal 'resting' parameters (e.g. pulse, respiratory rate and temperature) should be recorded on the anaesthetic monitoring chart. Remember: it is impossible to know what is abnormal if the normal is not known.

Once the health status has been determined, the premedication may be given to the patient to produce sedation or tranquillity. This is achieved by giving a combination of drugs usually selected by the veterinary surgeon.

The veterinary surgeon may ask the nurse to give the premedication. If so:

- Double-check the drug, the dose and the route via which it is to be administered (this will depend on how quickly it is required to act)
- Record all drugs given and watch for any reactions.

Intra-anaesthesia

After the premedication has taken effect, anaesthesia can be induced. This will be achieved either by an injectable anaesthetic agent (e.g. barbiturate, phenol) or by using one of the volatile anaesthetic agents and a mask (e.g. sevoflurane).

The anaesthetic should be monitored using a 'hands-on' approach. Monitoring aids (see below) are a useful adjunct but do not replace the veterinary nurse's hands, eyes and ears.

Throughout anaesthesia, the following parameters should be measured and recorded, ideally on an anaesthetic monitoring sheet (Figure 12.42), and the findings compared with the 'resting' parameters.

- Respiration (rate and pattern)
- Heart rate
- Pulse (rate and pattern)
- Mucous membranes (colour and capillary refill time – CRT)

- All reflexes
- Temperature
- Blood loss
- Salivary and lachrymal secretions
- Fluid administration and intravenous catheter placement
- Gas flow rates.

Each parameter should be checked every 5 minutes. Higher-risk cases may need more frequent monitoring. It is important to check *all* the parameters and not to rely or make decisions on just one of them.

Respiration

The rate, rhythm and depth should be noted. The respiratory rate can be measured by counting the number of inspirations *or* expirations over 30 seconds and multiplying by two. Abnormal respiratory rates are described in Figure 12.43.

12.42 Example of a form for recording details of anaesthesia (reproduced courtesy of The University of Liverpool).

Term	Definition	Causes
Bradypnoea	Respiratory rate lower than normal	Anaesthesia too deep Effects of drugs
Tachypnoea	Respiratory rate higher than normal	Insufficiently anaesthetized Aware of pain
Dyspnoea	Difficulty in breathing	Obstruction in the circuit Obstruction in thorax (e.g. secondary tumours, fluid, stenosis of bronchial tree)
Apnoea	Cessation of breathing	Effects of drugs such as propofol, methohexital and thiopental Respiratory arrest

12.43 Abnormal respiration.

Abnormal respiratory patterns are:

- Hypoventilation
  - Slow and shallow breathing
  - End tidal carbon dioxide above 50 mmHg (**hypercapnia**)
- Hyperventilation
  - Rapid breathing
  - End tidal carbon dioxide below 30 mmHg (**hypocapnia**).

Respiration should be smooth and regular. Ketamine can cause a distinctive respiration pattern in which there is a prolonged pause between inspiration and expiration; this is known as **apneustic** respiration.

- Ensure that both the thorax and the reservoir bag are inflating and deflating.
- If there is no movement in the reservoir bag, check that:
  - The circuit is connected correctly and there are no leaks
  - The endotracheal tube has been placed in the trachea and not the oesophagus
  - The endotracheal tube is not blocked or kinked
  - The respiratory tract is not obstructed.

Heart rate

Normal heart rates for a range of small pets are given in Chapter 9. Abnormal heart rates are described in Figure 12.44.

The heart rate can be measured by:

- Auscultation of the heart sounds
- Palpation of the apex heart beat on the left side of the patient's chest
- Counting the number of complexes seen on an ECG trace
- Use of a cardiac monitor with an audible bleep.

Heart rate must be analysed along with the pulse, mucous membrane colour and capillary refill time, as the presence of a heartbeat does not mean that the circulatory system is functioning correctly.

Pulse

Peripheral pulses can be felt in the following arteries:

- Lingual pulse (found on the ventral aspect of the tongue)
- Femoral pulse (found on the medial aspect of the femurs)
- Digital pulse (found on the palmar/plantar aspect of the carpus/tarsus)
- Coccygeal pulse (found on the ventral aspect of the base of the tail).

A peripheral pulse may also be monitored by a pulse oximeter (see later).

The pulse rate should be:

- Regular
- Of a consistent quality
- Reasonably strong.

Term	Definition	Causes
Bradycardia	Heart rate lower (slower) than normal	Increasing depth of anaesthesia Effects of drugs (e.g. acepromazine, medetomidine) Illness
Tachycardia	Heart rate higher (faster) than normal	Insufficiently anaesthetized Decreasing depth Drugs (e.g. atropine, ketamine)
No heart beat		Cardiac arrest

12.44 Abnormal heart rates.

Abnormal pulse rates and their causes are listed in Figure 12.45.

- There should be no pulse deficit (pulse rate lower than the heart rate, denoting a cardiac arrhythmia).
- Sinus arrhythmia (the rate increasing on inspiration and decreasing on expiration) is normal in the dog.

Pulse	Causes
Lowered rate	Myocardial depression caused by anaesthetic drug, e.g. medetomidine; systemic illness; anaesthesia too deep
Increased rate	Anaesthesia too light; stress; pain; pyrexia; hypoxia; hypercapnia
Weak	Poor circulation, possibly due to hypovolaemic shock; peripheral venous constriction, possibly due to hypothermia; alpha-2 agonists
Strong and jerky (known as 'water hammer' pulse)	Heart valves performing incorrectly; congenital heart defects, e.g. patent ductus arteriosis, pulmonary/aortic stenosis

12.45   Causes of abnormal pulse rates.

Mucous membranes

The mucous membranes can be observed by looking at:

- The gingiva
- The conjunctiva
- The anus
- The vagina or penis.

The mucous membranes should be salmon pink in colour. Abnormal colours are described in Chapter 7.

Capillary refill time (CRT) is the time it takes a mucous membrane to return to its original colour after it has been blanched by the application of light pressure. The time taken should be <2 seconds. If it takes any longer, this may indicate hypovolaemic shock or cardiovascular depression.

Reflexes

General anaesthesia affects the animal's reflexes, its jaw tone and its eye position. These changes are used to assess anaesthetic depth.

Palpebral reflex

Gently stroking the eyelashes or touching the medial canthus of the eye results in a slow blink. This reflex disappears as the animal enters stage III of anaesthesia. (Take care not to touch the animal's cornea as this will also produce a blink – the corneal reflex – and this reflex persists to a much greater anaesthetic depth – see below.)

Eye position

The eye is ventrally rotated during surgical anaesthesia. As the depth of anaesthesia increases further, the eye starts to move back to a central position. This means that the eye is centrally positioned when the patient is either too lightly or too deeply anaesthetized. If the patient is too deeply anaesthetized, the palpebral reflex will be absent.

The pupil gradually dilates as anaesthetic depth increases but should be responsive to light at all times. A lack of response indicates an anaesthetic overdose. Remember that the pupil will also be dilated if an anticholinergic drug or an opioid has been given.

Pedal reflex

The reflex caused by pinching in between the digits will gradually diminish as the depth of anaesthesia increases. It is usually lost by Stage III, Plane II.

Jaw tone

This is assessed by stretching apart the mandible and maxilla. Jaw tone will gradually diminish as the depth of anaesthesia increases and is usually lost by Stage III, Plane II.

Corneal reflex

This reflex should only be tested as a last resort, as the cornea is extremely sensitive and easily damaged. The reflex should always be present. Its absence indicates an anaesthetic overdose.

Temperature

Normal rectal (core) temperatures for a range of small pets are given in Chapter 9. The core temperature can be measured using a mercury thermometer or a flexible thermistor probe (in either the rectum or the oesophagus).

The peripheral temperature may be monitored by feeling the patient's extremities (ears, paws), which will give adequate information regarding the peripheral circulation. If the extremities are cold or becoming cold, this can be an early sign of hypothermia.

Hypothermia

Hypothermia (35°C or below) is common during surgery. Common reasons for hypothermia include:

- Excessive shaving (keep the surgical clip to a feasible minimum)
- Excessive use of skin preparation (do not soak the skin while preparing it)
- Anaesthetized animals unable to create heat by shivering or movement
- Administration of cold intravenous fluids (warm to blood temperature, 38°C)
- Lavage with cold fluids (warm to blood temperature, 38°C, prior to lavage)
- Administration of cold anaesthetic gases (use a thermovent between the endotracheal tube and the circuit, to warm the inspired gases)
- Low ambient room temperature in the preparation room, theatre and the kennel/ recovery area. The theatre should ideally be maintained above 24°C. When very small animals are being anaesthetized, the temperature of the operating theatre should be much higher than this; alternatively use a warm-air blanket (e.g. BairHugger, Figure 12.46) to surround the patient with warm air.

Small pets, such as rabbits and hamsters, have a high body surface area in relation to their body mass and therefore lose heat more rapidly than animals with a relatively smaller body surface area, such as cats and dogs. They are especially susceptible to the effects of excessive clipping and use of wet scrub preparations. It is imperative that small pets have their core temperature maintained, to avoid further increasing the risk of anaesthesia for these creatures. Items such as wheat heat-pads, bubblewrap, mini foil blankets or even latex gloves filled with warm water can be used to maintain temperature throughout surgery and recovery.

An increasing gap between the peripheral temperature and the core temperature indicates a poor peripheral circulation. Undetected hypothermia increases the recovery time as the liver is slower to metabolize the anaesthetic drugs. Death can occur if hypothermia is not detected.

Heat and moisture exchangers (thermovents)

Heat and moisture exchangers sit between the anaesthetic circuit and the endotracheal tube. They consist of a matrix of plastic through which the animal breathes. The plastic traps heat and moisture as the animal breathes out and this then warms and humidifies the animal's next breath.

They help to reduce heat loss from the animal partly by warming the anaesthetic gases breathed by the patient but mainly by humidifying the inspired gases – a lot of heat is lost through evaporation when the animal continually has to humidify dry inspired anaesthetic gases.

Warm air blankets

These devices (Figure 12.46) blow warm air around the anaesthetized patient, keeping them warm. They are electronically controlled and very safe. The air is pumped through a disposable paper blanket with holes in it, placed over the patient. They greatly reduce heat loss during prolonged procedures.

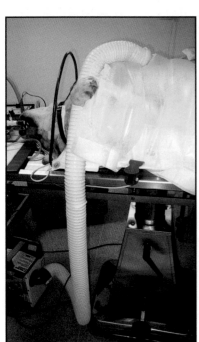

12.46

A BairHugger warm-air blanket in use. A heater unit blows warm air into a special blanket placed over the patient. It is thermostatically controlled and therefore unable to overheat the patient. (Photograph courtesy of Northwest Surgeons, Cheshire)

Blood loss

Haemorrhage from the surgical site will result in a drop in the blood pressure (hypotension). If not treated, this will develop into hypovolaemic shock, producing:

- Weak and rapid pulse
- Tachycardia
- Slow capillary refill time
- Pale mucous membranes.

These signs will be seen when the following amounts of blood are lost:

- Dog: 8–18 ml/kg
- Cat: 6–12 ml/kg.

Figure 12.47 describes how to measure blood loss on to swabs. Additional blood loss on to drapes and gowns and into the environment (e.g. table, floor) should be approximated. If surgical suction is used, the

---

The volume of blood lost can be measured accurately using the following technique:

1. Calculate the weight of a dry swab
2. Multiply this by the number of swabs used during the surgery (in order to calculate their dry weight)
3. Subtract this dry weight from the weight of the blood-soaked swabs to calculate the weight of the blood lost during the surgery
4. Divide this weight by 1.3 to convert it into millilitres of blood (1 ml blood weighs 1.3 g).

Example:
100 dry swabs weigh 230 g. Hence, one dry swab weighs 2.3 g (230/100).

During an operation, the 20 blood-soaked swabs used are found to weigh 100 g. When dry, the 20 swabs would weigh 46 g (2.3 x 20). Therefore the blood must weigh 64 g (110 – 46). Hence the swabs contained 49 ml of blood (64/1.3).

Alternatively, a good estimate of the patient's blood loss can be calculated using the following technique:

1. Find out the volume of water needed to saturate 10 swabs
2. Divide this by 10 for the volume of water needed to saturate one swab
3. This is roughly equivalent to the volume of blood that will be contained in one swab
4. Multiply the volume of blood contained in one saturated swab by the number of swabs used in the surgery to estimate the volume of blood lost.

Example:
If 10 swabs will absorb 50 ml of water, one swab will absorb 5 ml. During an operation, 14 swabs become saturated in blood. An estimate of the volume of blood soaked into these swabs is 70 ml (14 x 5).

When using either technique, remember to subtract the volume of any lavage fluids that have been used and that have also been soaked up by the swabs.

12.47   How to measure blood loss.

volumes of blood in the canister can be measured (but subtracting any fluids used to lavage the surgical site as these will also have been collected by the suction machine).

Fluids should be given to compensate for the blood loss (see Chapter 8). Ideally, whole blood should be given, or colloidal plasma expanders. Crystalloids may be used if plasma expanders are not available.

Further information on dealing with surgical blood loss is given in Chapter 13.

Salivary and lachrymal secretions

Salivation and tear production can help to indicate the depth of anaesthesia: production of these secretions becomes less as anaesthetic depth increases, and they are absent during deep anaesthesia.

Artificial tear solutions can be used to prevent the cornea drying out. These solutions are most important during ketamine anaesthesia, when eyes are most prone to drying.

Fluid administration

It is necessary to monitor the rate at which fluids are being administered and to ensure that the animal receives the correct amount and type of fluid (see Chapter 8). The intravenous catheter through which the fluids are being administered should also be checked periodically to ensure that:

■ It is still in the vein
■ It is not blocked.

The catheter should be flushed with heparin saline (5–10 IU/ml), not plain saline or other crystalloid fluid. Using anything other than heparin saline to flush a catheter can potentially push any clots further into the circulatory system. In extreme circumstances, should a clot reach the heart, death could occur.

Gas flow rates

The concentration of anaesthetic gas being delivered to the patient should always be checked. Oxygen and nitrous oxide flow meters should be checked at the same time. In the absence of alarms, falling fresh gas flow rates indicate that the anaesthetic gas (oxygen or nitrous oxide) is running out.

For information on gas alarms, see the section on anaesthetic equipment, above.

Post-anaesthesia

This is the period during which the patient is allowed to regain consciousness and the stages of anaesthesia are seen in reverse.

The recovery period is one of high risk, as patients are often poorly observed. Monitoring and recording of all parameters should continue until the patient is fully conscious. The endotracheal tube should be removed as described in Figure 12.33.

The following should be monitored until the patient is standing or fully recovered:

■ Return to consciousness, sternal recumbency and standing
■ Heart rate and pulse rate
■ Respiratory rate
■ Mucous membrane colour and capillary refill time
■ Reflex responses
■ Temperature
■ Pain (give appropriate analgesic and TLC)
■ Urine output (normal values for the cat and dog are 1–2 ml/kg/hour).

The patient should be allowed to recover in a quiet warm room where there is easy access to emergency equipment (Figure 12.48). The length of time taken to recover depends on:

■ The type of anaesthetic given and the route of administration
■ How long the patient was anaesthetized
■ The patient's health status
■ The patient's age
■ The patient's body temperature
■ Environmental temperature.

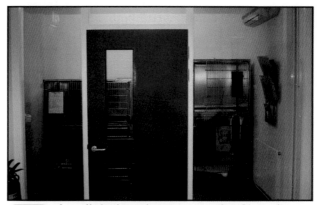

12.48 A well designed recovery suite. Note the large windows that allow staff to watch recovering patients from the adjacent preparation room. (Photograph courtesy of Northwest Surgeons, Cheshire)

Monitoring equipment

A number of anaesthetic monitoring aids are available for use in practice (Figure 12.49).

Equipment	Function
Oesophageal stethoscope	Simple device that allows the patient's heart sounds to be monitored constantly without disturbing surgical drapes. Closed end of stethoscope is positioned in patient's oesophagus next to heart. Cheap and disposable
Electrocardiogram	Monitors electrical activity of heart. Produces continuous trace or simple beep when heartbeat is detected. Existence of electrical activity in heart does not mean heart is producing good cardiac output

12.49 Anaesthetic monitoring aids. (continues) ▶

Equipment	Function
Respiratory monitor	Measures only the rate. Functions on temperature difference between inspired and expired gas. Prone to false alarms or, worse, interpreting slight fluctuations in temperature caused by beating heart moving air up and down trachea as respiration – animal may have stopped breathing but machine does not notice. Too temperamental to be of any use
Pulse oximeter (Figure 12.50)	Measures oxygen saturation of blood and patient's pulse rate. Probes are placed on tongue or ear or into rectum or cloaca. Normal oxygen saturation is 97% or more. Oxygen saturations of 90% or less represent serious hypoxia. Some pulse oximeters are prone to frequent false alarms and this can detract from their usefulness
Capnograph (Figure 12.51)	Measures carbon dioxide concentration of exhaled gas and displays it as trace on monitor. End tidal carbon dioxide ($ETCO_2$) is maximum CO_2 reading registered by the machine. Normal $ETCO_2$ is 30–50 mmHg. Variations in CO_2 concentration result from variations in respiratory rate (either spontaneous ventilation or mechanical ventilation)
	Hypoventilation results in a high $ETCO_2$
	▪ Hypoventilation often seen when opiate analgesics used
	▪ Also caused by relative anaesthetic overdose
	▪ Underlying cause should be treated and IPPV started to bring $ETCO_2$ back to normal
	Hyperventilation results in a low $ETCO_2$
	▪ Hyperventilation is often because patient is insufficiently anaesthetized and is panting
	▪ Sudden drop in $ETCO_2$ (particularly in animals on mechanical IPPV) can indicate animal's heart has stopped beating – no blood flow to return CO_2 to lungs so no longer detected in exhaled gas
	If the CO_2 does not return to zero at the beginning of inspiration:
	▪ Either soda lime in a circuit containing soda lime has become exhausted
	▪ Or fresh gas flow in a circuit that does not contain soda lime is inadequate for patient
	Low CO_2 often seen in small dogs and cats because exhaled gas is diluted by fresh gas before machine is able to measure it
Blood pressure monitors	Variations in blood pressure provide anaesthetist with a lot of information about patient's cardiovascular system
	Low blood pressure under anaesthesia is caused by:
	▪ Relative anaesthetic overdose
	▪ Haemorrhage
	High blood pressure results from:
	▪ Relative anaesthetic underdose
	▪ Overhydration
	Blood pressure can be measured directly:
	▪ A catheter is placed into a suitable superficial artery (the dorsal pedal artery in the dog, the femoral artery in the cat or the middle auricular artery in the rabbit)
	▪ The catheter is connected to a mechanical or electronic transducer which displays the patient's blood pressure
	▪ Direct blood pressure monitors provide a continuous pressure readout
	Or blood pressure can be measured indirectly (provides intermittent readings only):
	▪ A cuff is placed around a limb, inflated to above arterial blood pressure and then slowly deflated. The return of blood flow through an artery distal to the cuff is detected using an ultrasonic blood flow detector
	▪ Automatic blood pressure monitor detects changes in the limb volume beneath an inflated cuff as the heart beats

12.49 (continued) Anaesthetic monitoring aids.

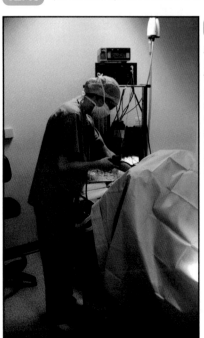

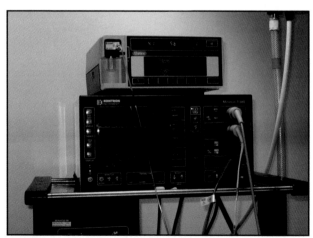

12.50 A veterinary nurse measuring the blood pressure of an anaesthetized dog. (Photograph courtesy of Northwest Surgeons, Cheshire)

12.51 Anaesthetic monitoring aids. A capnograph sits on top of a multi-function device that includes an ECG machine, a pulse oximeter, an indirect blood pressure monitor and a thermometer; a direct blood pressure transducer can also be attached. (Photograph courtesy of Northwest Surgeons, Cheshire)

Anaesthetic accidents and emergencies

There are many things that can go wrong during anaesthesia. Most can be prevented by forethought and good preparation. The outcome of emergencies depends very much on their early detection, quick and accurate diagnosis and swift treatment.

Monitoring of the patient is essential if emergencies are to be detected quickly. It is one thing to notice that an anaesthetized animal has stopped breathing, but good monitoring will detect the early warning signs of slowed respiratory rate and reduced depth of respiration, allowing the problem to be corrected before respiratory arrest occurs. Good anaesthetic practices, such as intubation and the placement of a intravenous catheter, make anaesthetic emergencies easier to deal with.

An anaesthetic emergency is anything that poses an immediate threat to the patient's life. The signs of some of these emergencies, along with the action to be taken, are given in Figure 12.52. Drugs used in emergencies are listed in Figure 12.53.

Emergency	Signs	Action
Respiratory obstruction	Patient will make extreme respiratory efforts that do not result in any movement of reservoir bag; cyanosis; eventually cardiac arrest	Find and remove obstruction (make sure patient's mouth is safely gagged before trying to remove foreign bodies). Intubate and ventilate with 100% oxygen. If obstruction cannot be removed but involves laryngeal/oropharyngeal region perform emergency tracheotomy
Bradycardia	Very slow heart rate	Commonly due to anaesthetic overdose, so ventilate with 100% oxygen. Use vagolytic agents such as atropine and glycopyrrolate
Apnoea/ respiratory arrest	Reservoir bag stops moving; no respiratory effort from patient; cyanosed mucous membranes; dilated pupils	Most commonly due to anaesthetic overdose, so ventilate with 100% oxygen. Respiratory stimulants may be useful but can have severe side effects
Cardiac arrest	Lack of femoral pulse; dilated pupils; usually (but not always) accompanied by respiratory arrest; pupillary dilation; agonal breathing	Start aggressive CPR

12.52 Anaesthetic emergencies.

Drug	Effect	Indication	Dose
Adrenaline (epinephrine)	Stimulates heart and increases systolic blood pressure	Cardiac arrest Unresponsive hypotension	0.02–0.2 mg/kg 1 ml of 1:1000 solution per 10 kg i.v., intratracheal or intracardiac
Atropine	Vagolytic	Bradycardia	0.02–0.04 mg/kg 1 ml of a 0.6 mg/ml solution per 15 kg i.v.
Glycopyrrolate	Vagolytic	Bradycardia	10 µg/kg 1 ml of a 200 µg/ml solution per 20 kg i.v.
Dobutamine	Increases cardiac output	Hypotension	1–5 µg/ml/kg/min
Lidocaine	Stabilizes the myocardium	Used to treat ventricular premature contractions and ventricular tachycardia	*Dogs* 2–4 mg/kg intravenous bolus 1 ml of a 2% solution per 10 kg i.v. *Cats* 0.25–1.0 mg/kg intravenous bolus 0.1 ml of a 2% solution per 4 kg cat
Dexamethasone	Anti-inflammatory	Often used after successful CPR	0.25–1 mg/kg i.v.
Atipamezole	Alpha-2 antagonist	Used to reverse effects of alpha-2 agonist sedatives	*Dogs* 0.05–0.2 mg/kg i.m. *Cats* 0.5 mg/cat i.m.
Naloxone	Opiate antagonist	Used to treat opiate overdose (but also reverses analgesic effects of opiates, possibly exposing animals to pain)	0.05–1 mg/kg i.m., i.v., s.c.
Doxapram	Respiratory stimulant	Used to treat respiratory arrest. Often used to stimulate respiration in newborn kittens and puppies Can be used during anaesthesia but *if the animal is intubated it is better to ventilate and treat the underlying cause of the respiratory arrest* Many side effects, including cardiac arrhythmias, hyperventilation leading to cerebral vasoconstriction and cerebral hypoxia More commonly used as a treatment of delayed recovery in reptiles	1–2 mg/kg i.v. or orally 1 ml of a 2 mg/ml solution i.v.

12.53 Drugs used in anaesthetic emergencies. (continues) ▶

Drug	Effect	Indication	Dose
Crystalloid fluids	Restore circulating volume and help maintain blood pressure	Circulatory collapse, shock	10–90 ml/kg/hour depending on animal's need
Colloid fluids	Restore circulating volume, particularly following haemorrhage	Haemorrhage, burns	5–20 ml/kg over 30 minutes to make up the blood or plasma loss

12.53 (continued) Drugs used in anaesthetic emergencies.

Anaesthetic accidents often occur due to human error. Drug overdose is quite a common mistake. The most important thing is to realize that a mistake has been made and set about correcting it. When a drug overdose is accidentally given, it may be possible to administer another drug that acts as an antidote.

Cardiac arrest

Anaesthetic emergencies and some accidents can ultimately lead to cardiac arrest. The heart stops pumping blood to the essential organs and the patient is brain dead within 4 minutes in dogs and cats, or much sooner in small mammals. Cardiopulmonary resuscitation (CPR) (Figure 12.54) is aimed at maintaining a flow of oxygenated blood to the brain in order to keep the animal alive whilst the cause of the arrest is identified and treated. Further information on dealing with cardiac and respiratory arrest is given in Chapter 7.

Anaesthesia for small mammals
Anatomical and physiological considerations
Drug administration

There are fewer routes available for the administration of drugs in small animals. Venous access is often difficult or impossible and so most drugs have to be administered via the intramuscular, subcutaneous or intraperitoneal routes. Oral or intraosseous routes can also be used for some drugs. Venous access in medium and large rabbits can be easily achieved via the marginal ear vein (see below).

Fluid administration

Intravenous fluid administration is difficult in many small mammals; alternatives include the subcutaneous, intraperitoneal or intraosseous routes (see Chapter 8).

⚠️ Switch off any anaesthetic agents that are being administered to the patient. Turn off the vaporizer and the nitrous oxide, and increase the flow of the oxygen. Purge the circuit of anaesthetic by flushing it, using the oxygen flush valve.

Use the mnemonic ABCD to remember the correct approach to CPR.

Airway
- Check to see that the patient's airway is patent.
- Do not presume that an endotracheal tube coming from the patient's mouth means that it has a patent airway. Check the tube to make sure it is not blocked and that it is correctly positioned within the trachea.
- If the patient is not intubated, intubate it if possible.
- In some circumstances an endotracheal tube may not be available. It is possible to ventilate a patient adequately using a snug-fitting face mask or mouth-to-muzzle 'kiss of life'.

Breathing
- The animal must be ventilated with 100% oxygen at a rate of 20–30 breaths per minute.

Circulation
- Check the patient's pulse. Note its quality and rate.
- If pulse is absent, thoracic massage must be started at a rate of 60–80 compressions per minute.
- When performing thoracic massage, the aim is to compress the whole of the chest. Press down on the chest at its widest point, not over the heart.
- If possible, place a compression bandage around the dog's abdomen to increase the return of blood to the heart, resulting in a greater cardiac output.
- If thoracic massage is working, it should be possible to feel a reasonable femoral or sublingual pulse.

Drugs
- Drugs are administered once a good cardiac output is being generated by the thoracic massage. A list of drugs used in CPR is given in Figure 12.53.
- Provided that the thoracic massage is producing a good cardiac output, intravenous injection is the best route for the administration of emergency drugs.
- If venous access is not available, many drugs can be given by the intratracheal or intracardiac routes.

12.54 How to perform cardiopulmonary resuscitation (CPR).

Heat loss

The large ratio of surface area to bodyweight in small mammals makes them very prone to hypothermia under anaesthesia. The techniques discussed above should be used to minimize heat loss in small mammals.

Blood loss

Small mammals can have a surprisingly small circulating volume. A 60 g hamster might have only 4 ml of blood, which means that the loss of only 0.4 ml represents a serious haemorrhage. Blood transfusions in small animals are not possible in a clinical situation and so the only approach is to minimize blood loss where possible and to administer crystalloid fluids (or colloids where intravenous or intraosseous access is available) to support the circulatory system.

Pre-anaesthetic management

Withholding food and water

Starvation for long periods is not required as rodents and rabbits are unable to vomit.

- Withholding food and water for a short time can reduce the volume of the gut contents and so reduce pressure on the animal's diaphragm, improving respiration.
- Food and water should be withheld for 1 hour (small mammals) to 2 hours (rabbits) in healthy animals.
- If possible, animals that are dehydrated should not be anaesthetized until their water deficit has been corrected.
  - This can be achieved with subcutaneous, intraperitoneal or intravenous administration.
  - Note that subcutaneous administration is not as effective as intraperitoneal administration in animals already dehydrated (the reduced peripheral circulation of dehydrated animals

is often not able to absorb the depot of fluid under the skin).
- Do not dismiss the option of oral fluid administration as well as parenteral fluid in dehydrated animals. This can be particularly effective in rats and rabbits.

Premedication and analgesia

Sedatives are not usually included in the premedicants given to small mammals. The premedicant is often just an analgesic and it is not unusual for small mammals not be given any premedication prior to anaesthesia. Special care must be taken when using injectable anaesthetic induction agents. Prior administration of opiate analgesics can significantly reduce the dose of induction agent required and, as this reduction is difficult to predict, it is probably best not to use opiate analgesics preoperatively in small mammals.

Analgesic drugs for small pets

Small animals have a high metabolic rate and need to eat frequently during their waking periods to maintain blood glucose. Postsurgical anorexia is often related to inadequate analgesia and can be very detrimental. All small pets undergoing surgery should receive adequate analgesia (Figure 12.55).

NSAIDs

These can be used in many species. Meloxicam and carprofen both provide good analgesia particularly if given prior to surgery and especially when used in combination with an opioid analgesic.

Opioid analgesics

Morphine, buprenorphine and butorphanol can all be used to provide analgesia for small pets. The doses required are often much higher than those used in dogs and cats. Buprenorphine provides good analgesia and has a much longer duration of action than butorphanol.

Species	Analgesic dose		
	Buprenorphine	*Butorphanol*	*Carprofen*
Ferret	0.05 mg/kg s.c. every 6–12 h	0.4 mg/kg i.m. every 4–6 h	4 mg/kg s.c. daily
Rabbit	0.05–0.1 mg/kg sc., i.m. every 6–12 h	0.1–0.5 mg/kg s.c. every 4 h	1.5 mg/kg orally bid 1–3 mg/kg s.c. daily
Chinchilla	0.05 mg/kg s.c. every 8 h	1–2 mg/kg s.c. every 2–4 h	4 mg/kg s.c. daily
Guinea pig	0.05 mg/kg s.c. every 8 h	1–2 mg/kg s.c. every 2–4 h	5 mg/kg s.c. daily
Gerbil	0.05 mg/kg s.c. every 8 h	1–2 mg/kg s.c. every 4 h	4 mg/kg s.c. daily
Hamster	0.05 mg/kg s.c. every 8 h	1–2 mg/kg s.c. every 4 h	4 mg/kg s.c. daily
Rat	0.05 mg/kg s.c. every 8 h	1–2 mg/kg s.c. every 2–4 h	5 mg/kg s.c. daily
Mouse	0.05 mg/kg s.c. every 8 h	1–5 mg/kg s.c. every 2–4 h	5 mg/kg s.c. daily

12.55 Analgesic drugs for small mammals. (Adapted from Flecknell, 1999)

Local analgesics

As with larger mammals, local analgesics such as bupivacaine can be used to great effect in small mammals but the dose must be carefully calculated. The toxic dose of lidocaine is approximately 10 mg/kg and so 0.05 ml of a 2% solution of lidocaine would be toxic to a 100 g hamster.

Local anaesthetics may need diluting before being given to small mammals.

Induction

For most small mammals (except rabbits) inhalational anaesthetics make excellent induction agents. There are also a number of injectable anaesthetic drug combinations that are very effective.

Ketamine combinations

- Ketamine is often combined with midazolam, diazepam, acepromazine, xylazine or medetomidine to produce anaesthesia in small pets.
- Ketamine combinations are probably the most popular injectable anaesthetic mixtures used in small pets.
- They are relatively safe, and if ketamine is combined with an alpha-2 agonist (xylazine or medetomidine) atipamezole can be given at the end of anaesthesia to reverse the alpha-2 agonist's effects.
- Ketamine in combination with diazepam or acepromazine produces heavy sedation/light anaesthesia whereas ketamine and alpha-2 agonist combinations produce surgical anaesthesia.
- The duration of anaesthesia induced with these combinations varies between species and also between individuals.
- Anaesthesia can be extended or supplemented with volatile anaesthetic agents.

Fentanyl and fluanisone followed by midazolam or diazepam

- The commercially available neuroleptanalgesic combination Hypnorm, containing fentanyl and fluanisone, is given to rabbits by intramuscular injection to produce sedation.
- Anaesthesia can then be induced with midazolam or diazepam given intravenously (marginal ear vein).
- Hypnorm can also be combined with midazolam and water and given by intraperitoneal injection in other species.
- The combination induces surgical anaesthesia that lasts for about 15 minutes and can be prolonged with volatile anaesthetic agents.
- At the end of anaesthesia the effects of Hypnorm can be partially reversed using buprenorphine (see below).

Propofol

- Propofol has been used to induce anaesthesia in mice, rats and rabbits. It is of most use in rabbits.

- The doses required are large and the effects short lived, in the rabbit at least.
- Propofol is mainly used as an anaesthetic induction agent. Anaesthesia is usually maintained with a volatile anaesthetic agent.

Volatile anaesthetic agents

- Halothane, isoflurane and sevoflurane are all used to induce (and maintain) anaesthesia in small mammals.
- They are administered via a facemask or using an induction chamber (see below).
- Sevoflurane is the least soluble of the three and therefore the most rapid acting.
- Halothane is the most soluble and therefore takes longest to work.
- These agents are suitable for most species, but rabbits will hold their breath for several minutes rather than inhale volatile anaesthetic agents and so mask or chamber inductions in rabbits should be avoided.
- Sevoflurane reacts with soda lime to produce the haloalkene compound A, which is known to be toxic to rats. This should not be a problem in practice as it is not necessary to use circuits containing soda lime in such small animals.

Maintenance

Where it is necessary to prolong anaesthesia after induction, halothane, isoflurane or sevoflurane can be used. They are administered in oxygen using a facemask or endotracheal tube connected to a suitable breathing circuit.

- Simple facemasks are never a good fit on the animal's muzzle and result in a lot of operating theatre pollution. Good theatre ventilation is important.
- Coaxial facemasks are available for those involved in a lot of small mammal anaesthesia. They are used in conjunction with an active scavenging system and any volatile anaesthetic agent escaping from the facemask is carried away down the outer portion of the mask into the scavenging system (Figure 12.56).

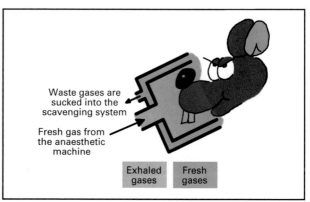

Waste gases are sucked into the scavenging system

Fresh gas from the anaesthetic machine

Exhaled gases | Fresh gases

12.56 Coaxial facemask specifically designed for small mammals. There is a loose seal around the animal's head, but any anaesthetic gas that escapes is sucked into the scavenging system, thus avoiding theatre pollution.

Anaesthetic recovery

- The patient should be placed back in its normal environment as soon as practicably possible so that its recovery from anaesthesia is stress free.
- It should also be monitored closely during the recovery period. Watch for prolonged recoveries which might be a sign of hypothermia.
- Small mammals continue to be susceptible to hypothermia until their normal activity returns and so recovery areas must be kept warm (>26°C).
- Food and water should be provided as soon as the animal has recovered from anaesthesia. Small mammals are more likely to eat and drink if they have been provided with adequate analgesia.
- Many authors recommend giving subcutaneous or intraperitoneal fluids to all small mammals that have undergone anaesthesia.

Signs and stages of anaesthesia

The assessment of the depth of anaesthesia in small mammals is difficult because there are significant species variations.

- The eyelid aperture of rabbits and ferrets increases with increasing anaesthetic depth but the same is not true in rats.
- The strength of the corneal reflex is a very poor guide to anaesthetic depth in ferrets and rodents.

In all species, a fixed dilated pupil and the absence of a corneal reflex indicate a relative anaesthetic overdose.

In practice the anaesthetist must judge anaesthetic depth based on changes in the animal's reflexes, the animal's response to surgical stimuli and the vaporizer setting.

Monitoring

Because of their size, it can very difficult to monitor small mammals when they are anaesthetized.

Respiration

Chest movements should be watched but can be difficult to see. Attaching a piece of brightly coloured tape to the animal's chest can make small chest movements more visible. If the animal is intubated, the reservoir bag can be watched; again, a small piece of tape can make the movement of the bag more obvious.

Heart rate

Simple chest auscultation with a stethoscope is a reliable way of monitoring the heart. This often involves furtling under the surgical drapes periodically during the surgery to listen to the animal's chest. Oesophageal stethoscopes can be very useful in larger small mammals.

Blood pressure

Measurement of blood pressure is possible in rabbits but much harder in smaller animals. Indirect blood pressure measurement can be performed in rabbits if suitably small cuffs are used but is often quite inaccurate. Arterial catheters can be placed in the auricular artery of larger rabbits to allow direct measurement of blood pressure.

Temperature

This is one of the most important parameters to be measured in small mammals. Small rectal probes connected to electronic thermometers can be used in almost all small mammals.

Oxygen saturation

Special pulse oximeter probes are available for use around the feet of small mammals but their use tends to be limited to specialist practice.

Doppler blood flow detectors

Ultrasonic Doppler blood flow detectors use the change in frequency of ultrasound waves reflected off moving blood cells to identify blood flow in superficial arteries or in the heart itself. The probe is placed over a suitably superficial artery or directly over the heart and blood flow can be heard as a whooshing noise. Suitable sites include the ventral aspect of the tail base, the carotid, femoral and auricular arteries and the heart. The site must be clipped and ultrasound contact gel used.

Special techniques in small mammal anaesthesia

Intubation of rabbits

Rabbits are one of the few small mammals that can be routinely intubated. There are two techniques: direct visualization with a laryngoscope or otoscope; or blind intubation. In small rabbits (2 kg or less), endotracheal tubes with an outside diameter of 2.5 mm should be used. Larger rabbits can be intubated with a 3–3.5 mm tube.

Direct visualization

The rabbit's larynx can be visualized using a Wisconsin blade on a laryngoscope or an otoscope.

1. A thin stiff introducer is passed into the larynx (dog urinary catheters with the leur connector removed make good introducers).
2. The endotracheal tube is threaded over the introducer and through the larynx.
3. The introducer is then removed.

Blind intubation

1. The rabbit is held with its head and neck extended and the endotracheal tube is slowly advanced towards the rabbit's pharynx.
2. The anaesthetist listens to the breath sounds at the end of the endotracheal tube.
3. The breath sounds slowly increase as the tube approaches the larynx.
4. The tube is gently moved towards and (hopefully) through the larynx. If the breath sounds cease, the tube has entered the oesophagus.
5. If tracheal intubation is successful, the anaesthetist will hear a soft cough from the rabbit and the persistence of breath sounds.

Anaesthetic chamber inductions

It is common to use volatile anaesthetic agents as anaesthetic induction agents for small pets. The animal is placed in an induction chamber and a mixture of oxygen and volatile anaesthetic agent is introduced. There are a number of good design features that are desirable in an induction chamber:

■ Clear sides so that the patient can be observed during the induction process
■ Variable volume so that patients of different sizes can be accommodated (this is usually achieved with a divider that can be moved up and down the box)
■ The facility to scavenge the gases – the exhaust aperture should be connected to the scavenging system
■ The exhaust aperture should be at the top of the box – volatile anaesthetic agents are denser than air and will sink to the bottom of the chamber. If the exhaust aperture is at the bottom of the box, the animal could easily hold its head in the 'clean' air above the vapour and avoid inhaling it (Figure 12.57)
■ Easily cleaned.

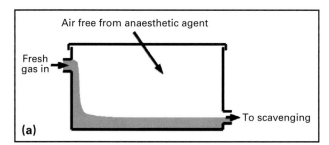

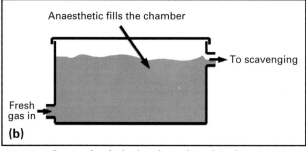

12.57 Anaesthetic induction chamber layouts. **(a)** Induction chamber with the exhaust at the bottom. If the exhaust is low down, the heavy volatile anaesthetic vapour sinks to the bottom and an area of anaesthetic-free gas is left at the top of the chamber. An animal can then hold its head in this 'clean' air and avoid breathing the anaesthetic vapour. **(b)** Induction chamber with the exhaust at the top. Placing the exhaust higher up on the chamber fills the entire chamber with volatile anaesthetic vapour and the animal has no choice but to breathe the gas mixture.

Using an anaesthetic induction chamber

1. Place the animal in the chamber and allow it to settle for a few minutes. Soft bedding or a fluffy blanket can be placed in the box so that the patient does not slide around on the bottom and become distressed.
2. Make sure that the chamber is sealed and that the fresh gas and exhaust pipes are connected.
3. Introduce 100% oxygen initially – the fresh gas flow rate should be between 2 and 5 litres per minute, depending on the size of the chamber.
4. Introduce the volatile agent slowly. Increasing the concentration too quickly can make the animal in the chamber breath-hold; rabbits will often breath-hold for >2 minutes and volatile anaesthetic agents should not be used to induce anaesthesia in rabbits.
5. Watch the animal as it loses consciousness (gently move the chamber to stimulate the patient in order to assess its level of consciousness).
6. Once the animal is anaesthetized, flush the chamber through with 100% oxygen to wash the anaesthetic vapour into the scavenging system before removing the patient (washing the chamber with oxygen reduces theatre pollution).
7. Anaesthesia can be maintained with the volatile anaesthetic agent and oxygen delivered via an endotracheal tube or a facemask.

Sequential analgesia in small mammals given Hypnorm

One popular drug combination used to induce anaesthesia in small mammals is Hypnorm with either diazepam or midazolam (see above). Hypnorm contains fentanyl and fluanisone which, when given with midazolam or diazepam, provides 15 minutes or so of surgical anaesthesia.

Fentanyl is a potent mu agonist opiate that provides good analgesia but also causes moderate respiratory depression. At the end of the anaesthetic the effects of the fentanyl can be reversed with a mu receptor antagonist such as naloxone, but this also reverses the fentanyl's analgesic effects. An alternative is to administer a partial mu agonist such as buprenorphine. Buprenorphine has a high affinity for mu receptors and displaces a lot of the fentanyl but, because buprenorphine is itself an analgesic, the animal is not at risk of being exposed to postsurgical pain. This technique is known as sequential analgesia.

Drawing up and mixing drugs for small pets

The smallest syringe that will hold the volume of drug intended to be given should be used. For example, it is impossible to accurately draw up 0.24 ml of drug in a 2 ml syringe; a 0.5 ml insulin syringe should be used instead.

Mixing drugs

It is common to mix small volumes of anaesthetic drugs together in the same syringe prior to administering them to the patient, but care should be taken. If this is done in a normal syringe, the volumes of drugs given will not be the volumes intended because of the dead space in the needle hub. For example:

■ Imagine mixing ketamine and medetomidine for a ferret. When 0.1 ml of ketamine is drawn up, actually 0.2 ml is drawn up (0.1 ml in the syringe and 0.1 ml in the needle hub)

- If 0.1 ml of medetomidine is then added, the actual mixture is 0.1 ml of medetomidine with 0.2 ml of ketamine – not what was intended.

To mix drugs in the same syringe, insulin syringes with swaged-on needles should be used as these have very little dead space in the needle hub. It would be better still not to mix small volumes of drugs but instead administer them individually.

Marginal ear vein in rabbits

Rabbits have a large marginal ear vein that can be used to gain venous access either for direct intravenous injection or for venous catheterization.

The peripheral vein must *not* be confused with the more central auricular artery. Injection into the latter vessel is painful and can destroy the blood supply to the distal pinnae.

1. To facilitate pain-free injection or catheterization, the hair is clipped from over the peripheral ear vein and EMLA (local anaesthetic) cream is applied to the skin.
2. The cream is then covered with cling-film and protected with a bandage.
3. After 45 minutes the skin under the cream is desensitized, allowing a pain-free catheter placement or injection.
4. If a catheter is placed in the vein it is easier to tape it in place if a splint is placed on the inside of the ear. Rolls of bandage still in their plastic wrappers or plastic syringe barrels make good splints.

Anaesthesia for reptiles

There is a lot of variation between different species of reptile and it is important that the anaesthetist correctly identifies a patient's species and recognizes any species characteristics that might adversely affect the anaesthetic. It is also important to be comfortable with the basic handling and restraint techniques that can be applied to these animals (see *BSAVA Manual of Exotic Pets*).

Anatomical and physiological considerations

Body temperature

Reptiles are incapable of generating their own body heat (ectothermic, often referred to as 'cold-blooded') and so there is a narrow range of temperature at which these creatures function normally, both behaviourally and physiologically. Each species has a preferred optimal temperature zone (POTZ). It is possible to check whether the animal is within its POTZ by measuring its heart rate and comparing it with the following calculation:

$$\text{Heart rate} = 34 \times (\text{reptile's weight in kg})^{-0.25}$$

If the reptile's heart rate is not close to this calculated rate, it is likely that it is too cold or too hot

and will not respond to anaesthetic and analgesic drugs in a predictable way. Adjustment and monitoring of environmental temperature is therefore an essential part of anaesthetizing these species.

Respiratory system

- Reptiles do not have a muscular diaphragm.
- Air is drawn into the lungs by the action of intercostal and intrapulmonary muscles in the case of snakes and lizards. Chelonians use the muscles of the pelvic and pectoral girdles (they breathe by pulling their legs into and out of their shells).
- Because of this, the muscle relaxation caused by anaesthesia severely impairs the respiratory function of lizards, snakes and chelonians and IPPV should be used to maintain respiration in these animals.
- Because the large central space found in the lungs of reptiles (along with the air sac in snakes) acts as a reservoir for anaesthetic gas, recovery may be prolonged if the patient is not ventilated on oxygen or oxygen/carbon dioxide at the end of anaesthesia.
- In tortoises and turtles, the trachea is very short and divides into two mainstream bronchi almost immediately behind the glottis. This means that it is easy to intubate one bronchus inadvertently if care is not taken over species identification.

Cardiovascular system

Reptiles can endure anaerobic metabolism and so can breath-hold for a long time, making chamber or mask inductions with volatile anaesthetic agents difficult.

Drug administration

Reptiles are very susceptible to infection and their skin must be thoroughly scrubbed to ensure asepsis prior to injection.

It is possible to gain venous access in many lizards using the ventral tail vein. This can be accessed both laterally and ventrally and can be used either to give intravenous anaesthetic drugs or to collect blood samples.

The intraosseous route can also be for drug and fluid administration. The tibia is usually used for this purpose.

Pre-anaesthetic fasting

Where possible reptiles should be fasted prior to anaesthesia – chelonians and lizards for 18 hours, snakes for 72–98 hours. This is mainly to prevent the ingesta compressing the lungs.

Premedication

Where surgery is planned, analgesia should be administered prior to anaesthesia. The NSAIDs carprofen and meloxicam are useful for this purpose, as are the opiates buprenorphine and butorphanol (Figure 12.58).

Drug	Indication	Dose
Diazepam	Sedation/premedication	0.22–0.62 mg/kg i.m.
Carprofen	Analgesia (premedication and post surgery)	2–4 mg/kg i.m., s.c., i.v., initially (can be followed by 2 mg/kg every 24–72 hours)
Meloxicam	Analgesia	0.1–0.2 mg/kg orally for chronic pain
Butorphanol	Analgesia (premedication and post surgery)	Tortoises: 25 mg/kg i.m.
Buprenorphine	Analgesia (premedication and post surgery)	0.01 mg/kg i.m.
Pethidine	Analgesia (premedication and post surgery)	20 mg/kg i.m. every 12–24 hours
Alfaxalone/alfadalone	Induction of general anaesthesia	Lizards: 6.6 mg/kg i.v. Chelonians: 9 mg/kg i.v. Snakes: 6–9 mg/kg i.v.
Propofol	Induction of general anaesthesia	Lizards: 13 mg/kg i.v. Chelonians: 3–15 mg/kg i.v. Snakes: 10 mg/kg i.v.

12.58 Drugs used in anaesthesia and analgesia for reptiles. (Adapted from Malley, 1999)

Anaesthetic induction

Intravenous injection of either propofol or alfaxalone/alfadalone (see Figure 12.58) is the induction technique of choice where venous access is possible. Alternatively mask induction with volatile anaesthetic agents is possible (although difficult in aquatic species due to breath-holding – see above) and it is even possible to intubate conscious snakes and induce anaesthesia using volatile anaesthetic agents in conjunction with IPPV.

Maintenance

IPPV is essential in reptiles and can be achieved using a mechanical ventilator or manually. The lungs (and air sac if present) are inflated until the cranial two-fifths of the coelomic cavity (the reptile equivalent to the mammalian abdomen) is seen to rise.

In chelonians, where there is no movement of the abdominal wall, care must be taken not to over-inflate the lungs, causing damage to tissues and subsequent oedema. The use of a pulse oximeter and monitoring of heart rate will indicate when adequate oxygenation is being achieved.

Ideally, reptiles should not be positioned in dorsal recumbency as the viscera compress the lung, compromising ventilation. If this position is unavoidable, the table can be tilted slightly to reduce some of the compression.

Recovery

IPPV should be continued into the recovery period to wash any volatile anaesthetic agent out of the reptilian central lung chamber (and air sac if present). The patient should be ventilated on 100% oxygen, or a mixture of 90% oxygen and 10% carbon dioxide. This should be continued until spontaneous respiration returns. Doxapram at 5 mg/kg can be given by intracardiac injection in cases of prolonged recovery.

The patient must also be observed closely until its righting reflex has returned.

The vivarium must be ventilated to remove any exhaled volatile anaesthetic agents.

Signs and stages of anaesthesia

The signs and stages of reptile anaesthesia differ from those in mammalian anaesthesia. A brief summary is given in Figure 12.59.

Stage	Signs
Stage 1	Slow movements Odd placement of limbs Positive righting reflex Muscles not relaxed Painful stimuli registered Serpentine (slithering) movements in snakes persist
Stage 2	Few spontaneous movements Poor righting reflex Tongue withdrawal reflex almost abolished Response to painful stimuli reduced or absent Light muscle relaxation Serpentine movements almost abolished in snakes
Stage 3	No movements No righting reflex No response to painful stimuli Good muscle relaxation Retention of corneal reflex
Stage 4	Loss of corneal reflex (not all reptiles have an eyelid) Death

12.59 Signs and stages of anaesthesia in reptiles. (Adapted from Malley, 1999)

Monitoring

- The heart rate can be monitored by observing the carotid pulse and palpation of the apex beat of the heart.
- Auscultation of the heart is also possible in snakes and lizards. Simple auscultation is harder in chelonians because of the noise produced

by the stethoscope scraping on the animal's shell. This noise can be reduced by placing a towel between the shell and the stethoscope diaphragm. An oesophageal stethoscope makes a good monitoring tool in all reptiles.

- In larger lizards the electrocardiograph can be recorded using limb leads connected with crocodile clips or needle electrodes.
- Pulse oximeters can be used with tongue probes in lizards and tortoises, or a rectal probe may be placed in a snake's vent.
- Doppler blood flow detectors can be used to detect blood flow in the heart and peripheral vessels of reptiles and chelonians.

Anaesthesia for birds

Avian anaesthesia can be challenging, because birds often hide signs of ill health. Although outwardly healthy, they may be suffering from significant respiratory disease that might adversely affect the anaesthetic.

Anatomical and physiological considerations

Respiratory system

The avian pulmonary respiratory system differs dramatically from the mammalian system.

- Avian lungs are rigidly fixed to the roof of the thorax and do not expand.
- Birds do not have a muscular diaphragm. Gas is drawn into and expelled from the lungs and air sacs by ventral movement of the sternum.
- They have several air sacs, which do not take part in gas exchange but act as air reservoirs.
- Fresh air passes into the gas exchange tissues (the parabronchi) on both inspiration and expiration (Figure 12.60), effectively doubling the time available for gas exchange (compared with a mammalian lung). This is reflected in the high partial pressures of oxygen found in avian blood compared with mammalian blood.
- The presence of air sacs in the abdominal cavity means that abdominal masses or ascites have an adverse effect on respiration.
- The presence of abdominal air sacs allows a novel route of ventilation in birds: an opening can be made into the air sacs and anaesthetic gases insufflated through the lung. This can be used as an alternative to tracheal ventilation when access to the head or trachea is required.
- Care must be taken when placing birds in sternal recumbency as this can restrict sternal movement and compromise respiration. Care must also be taken not to restrict the bird's sternal excursions by using drapes or bandages.

Body temperature

Birds are very susceptible to hypothermia, partly because of their small size and high ratio of surface area to bodyweight.

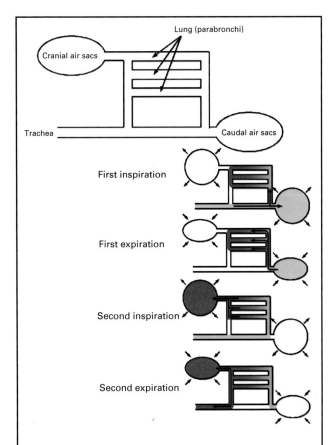

The unique anatomy of the avian respiratory system means that fresh air is drawn into the parabronchi (the gas exchange tissue of birds) on both inspiration and expiration. It is this dual cycle that makes the avian respiratory system so efficient, allowing the high metabolic rates needed during flight.

First inspiration
Air is drawn through the nares and down the trachea. Some of it passes into the parabronchi and some into the caudal air sacs.

First expiration
Air from the caudal air sacs passes into the parabronchi.

Second inspiration
Air passes from the parabronchi into the cranial air sacs.

Second expiration
Air passes from the cranial air sacs and out of the trachea.

 Air flow through the avian respiratory system. ▨ Fresh gas; ▧ exhaled gas.

Pre-anaesthetic fasting

The high metabolic rate of birds means that they should not be starved for a prolonged period before anaesthesia. In general, they need only be starved for long enough for the crop to be empty. They should not be starved for >3 hours at the most (except waterfowl and carnivorous birds) and small birds should not be starved at all. Waterfowl and carnivorous birds can be starved for between 4 and 10 hours, depending on their size.

Premedication

Analgesia is essential in birds. They do not show outward signs of pain but, without analgesics, the time to recovery is prolonged. Opiates and NSAIDs can both be used to good effect. Interestingly, unlike in mammals, butorphanol is more effective than some of the other opiates. This is because kappa receptors predominate over mu receptors in birds and butorphanol is a kappa agonist.

Anaesthetic induction

Alfaxalone/alfadalone (not all species), alpha-2 agonists with ketamine, benzodiazepines with ketamine, and volatile anaesthetics are all used to induce anaesthesia in birds.

Ketamine and alpha-2 agonists

- Ketamine and xylazine – *not* recommended, because of complications.
- Ketamine and medetomidine – the combination of choice
  - Provides 20 minutes or so of anaesthesia
  - Anaesthesia can be extended using volatile anaesthetics or shortened using alpha-2 antagonists
  - Use with care in patients with renal or cardiac disease or suffering from obesity.

Ketamine and benzodiazepines

- Ketamine can be combined with diazepam or midazolam.
- Can be used for short medical examinations.

Alfaxalone/alfadalone

- Can be used by intravenous or intramuscular route.
- Produces about 10 minutes of anaesthesia that can be prolonged with volatile anaesthetic agents.
- Not safe in all species (notably red-tailed hawks and psittacine birds) and so must only be used in species in which it is known to be safe.

Propofol

This is too short acting in birds to be of any real use.

Volatile anaesthetic agents

- Halothane, isoflurane and sevoflurane have all been used to induce anaesthesia in birds, but halothane has been associated with unexpected anaesthetic deaths and the newer volatile anaesthetic agents should be used instead.
- The highly efficient lung tissue of birds results in rapid uptake of volatile anaesthetic agents and consequently rapid induction of anaesthesia.
- Apnoea can occur with isoflurane and so it is recommended that the patient be intubated to facilitate IPPV.

- Sevoflurane reacts with soda lime to produce the haloalkene compound A that is toxic to rats. It is not known if this is toxic to birds but sevoflurane should not be used in circuits containing soda lime with birds until more information is available.

Maintenance

Intubation

Intubation is fairly straight forward in birds because the rima glottidis (the avian equivalent of the mammalian larynx) is easily visible in many species. In psittacines it can be visualized by pulling the tongue forward.

It is sometimes necessary to manufacture suitably small endotracheal tubes but wide-bore long intravenous catheters such as 12 or 14 gauge 125 mm over-the-needle catheters are very useful. The needle is discarded and the catheter is used as an endotracheal tube. The connector from a 3.5–4 mm endotracheal tube will fit nicely into the leur connector of the catheter, allowing it to be connected to the breathing circuit.

Most birds can be anaesthetized using an Ayre's T-piece or a mini-Bain circuit. Small mechanical ventilators are available for use on birds and these are useful if large numbers of birds are to be anaesthetized.

Recovery

Like all anaesthetized patients, birds should be monitored closely whilst they recover from anaesthesia, but they should also be allowed to recover quietly and without disturbance. Startling birds can cause them to flap around and potentially injure themselves in their container. To prevent wing flapping and damage to wings or feathers while the bird is not yet fully conscious, many veterinary surgeons like to wrap birds lightly in paper towels or cloth (according to size of bird) during recovery.

Like reptiles, it can be useful to ventilate birds on 100% oxygen for a few breaths at the end of anaesthesia to help to wash the volatile anaesthetic agent out of the air sacs.

Signs and stages of anaesthesia

There are few good indicators of depth of anaesthesia in birds.

- Unlike mammals, their eye position does not vary with anaesthetic depth.
- Unlike mammals, the presence or absence of the palpebral reflex is an unreliable indicator of anaesthetic depth.
- Breathing rate does not vary consistently with anaesthetic depth.

The most reliable indicator is the bird's corneal reflex. This is stimulated by gently touching the cornea. At a surgical plane of anaesthesia, the corneal reflex should be slow but still present. The bird should also not respond to painful stimuli.

Monitoring

Cloacal probes are available to enable pulse oximeters to be used in birds. In larger birds an oesophageal stethoscope makes an excellent cheap monitoring tool. A bird's tidal volume is usually too small to register on thermistor-based respiratory monitors (electronic devices that measure the time between breaths by monitoring the temperature of the gas in the endotracheal tube).

Special techniques used in birds

Air sac insufflation

Because of the unique avian respiratory anatomy, it is possible to introduce anaesthetic gas into a bird's respiratory system via the caudal air sacs instead of the trachea and this is useful for certain procedures, such as:

- Head and beak surgery
- Endoscopic examination of the trachea and crop.

The caudal air sacs are close to the skin surface and anaesthetic gas can be introduced into them via a small tube placed percutaneously (Figure 12.61).

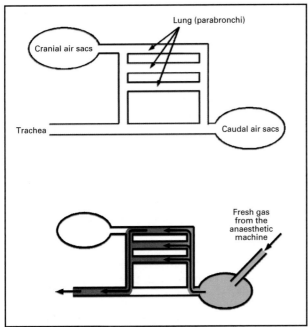

12.61 Using caudal air sac insufflation to ventilate birds during anaesthesia. When air sac insufflation is used to maintain anaesthesia in birds, oxygen and volatile anaesthetic agent is introduced into the caudal air sac via a small tube inserted percutaneously. The fresh gas flows out of the air sacs, through the parabronchi and out of the bird's trachea. When a bird is being anaesthetized in this way, it does not breathe: the flow of gas through the parabronchi delivers oxygen and removes carbon dioxide. ■ Fresh gas; ■ exhaled gas.

A mixture of volatile anaesthetic gas and oxygen is insufflated into the air sac through this tube. The anaesthetic mixture passes through the parabronchi (the bird's lungs) and out through the trachea. This flow of gas oxygenates the blood and removes carbon dioxide. Initially the anaesthetic mixture is introduced at a low flow rate (0.5–1.0 litres/minute) and then the flow rate is slowly increased. The flow rate is set when the bird stops breathing (because the bird's arterial CO_2 has fallen, reducing the bird's respiratory drive). If the flow rate is too high, the arterial CO_2 will fall too low, making the bird alkalotic.

The concentration of volatile anaesthetic agent is adjusted to maintain surgical anaesthesia.

The waste anaesthetic gases flow out of the trachea and so, if possible, the trachea should still be intubated to enable these waste gases to be scavenged.

Further reading

Brodbelt DC and Girling SJ (2007) Anaesthesia and analgesia. In: *BSAVA Textbook of Veterinary Nursing, 4th edn*, ed. DR Lane *et al.*, pp. 507–560. BSAVA Publications, Gloucester

Clutton E (1993) Management of perioperative cardiac arrest in companion animals, Part 1. *In Practice* **15**, 267–270

Clutton E (1994) Management of perioperative cardiac arrest in companion animals, Part 2. *In Practice* **16**, 3–6

Clutton E (1995) The right anaesthetic machine for you? *In Practice* **17**, 83–88

Davey A, Moyle JTB and Ward CS (eds) (1997) *Ward's Anaesthetic Equipment, 3rd edn*. WB Saunders, London

Flecknell P (1999) Rabbits, rodents and ferrets. In: *BSAVA Manual of Small Animal Anaesthesia and Analgesia*, ed. C Seymour and R Gleed, pp. 295–304. BSAVA Publications, Cheltenham

Flecknell P and Waterman Pearson A (2000) *Pain Management in Animals*. Saunders, Philadelphia

Hall LW and Clarke KW (eds) (1991) *Veterinary Anaesthesia, 9th edn*. Baillière Tindall, London

Hall LW and Taylor PM (eds) (1994) *Anaesthesia of the Cat*. Baillière Tindall, London

Mader DR (ed.) (2006) *Reptile Medicine and Surgery, 2nd edn*. Elsevier, Philadelphia

Malley D (1999) Reptiles. In: *BSAVA Manual of Small Animal Anaesthesia and Analgesia*, ed. C Seymour and R Gleed, pp. 295–304. BSAVA Publications, Cheltenham

Meredith A and Redrobe S (eds) *Manual of Exotic Pets, 4th edn*. BSAVA Publications, Gloucester

Quesenbery K and Carpenter JW (2004) *Ferrets, Rabbits and Rodents: Clinical Medicine and Surgery, 2nd edn*. WB Saunders, Philadelphia

Rosenthal KL (ed) (1997) *Practical Exotic Medicine*. Veterinary Learning Systems, Trenton, New Jersey

Seymour C and Duke-Novakovski T (eds) (1999) *Manual of Canine and Feline Anaesthesia and Analgesia, 2nd edn*. BSAVA Publications, Gloucester

Short CE (1987) *Principles and Practice of Veterinary Anaesthesia*. Williams and Wilkins, Baltimore

13

Surgical nursing

Karen Scott and Alasdair Hotston Moore

This chapter is designed to give information on:

- Preparation of the surgical environment and surgical equipment
- Theatre clothing and drapes
- Asepsis and sterilization, including methods of packing
- Instrument cleaning and maintenance
- Preparation of small animals for surgery
- Providing the veterinary surgeon with general intraoperative assistance
- Providing postoperative care to promote rapid recovery
- Recognition and management of pre-, peri- and postoperative problems
- Common surgical conditions of small animals and their nursing

---

Introduction

The care and maintenance of the surgical environment and the instruments and equipment within it is vitally important for the smooth running of all the procedures performed within the operating room. Whether there is a purpose-built theatre with all the latest equipment, or rooms converted into an operating theatre with minimal equipment, there are basic rules that should be followed.

Preparation of the surgical environment

In order to achieve an aseptic technique within the operating theatre, the surgical environment itself must be maintained to a high standard of cleanliness. All efforts to practise aseptic techniques will be wasted if the environment itself is not clean.

It is advisable to have a routine preparation for surgery that is followed strictly whenever surgery is performed. Work schedules should be set out for daily and weekly cleaning routines; this helps to maintain the operating theatre at the appropriate standard.

The following is a guide – some of the points may not be appropriate for all situations, but they can be adapted to particular circumstances in order to achieve the best results of cleanliness.

Theatre design and layout

Very few veterinary nurses will be able to design their own operating facilities, but an awareness of the ideal requirements will assist in the adaptation of existing facilities if appropriate. The following points should be considered in the design and layout of the patient preparation and surgery areas.

All areas of the surgical suite should be clearly marked, ideally with coloured floor tape and door signs. This marks areas of restricted access to all members of staff and warns that the appropriate theatre clothing should be worn before proceeding into these areas. The theatre suite can be made up of several rooms, including the preparation room and theatre.

Preparation room

This is where the induction of anaesthesia takes place and where any preoperative procedures such as clipping, bathing or catheterization are performed before the patient is moved into the operating room. The preparation room should lead into the operating room.

The function and hygiene standards of the preparation room are described in Chapter 4. The room must have suitable work surfaces, storage facilities, anaesthetic induction and clipping-up equipment, lighting, ventilation and sound insulation. The necessary cleaning and equipment preparation procedures are also described in Chapter 4.

- It is sensible to have an anaesthetic emergency box or crash kit in the preparation room (the contents of this are described in Chapter 7).
- The clippers (with surgical blades) and vacuum cleaner to remove loose hair after clipping should be positioned by the table.
- Preparation tables incorporating sinks are ideal for cleaning the patient or emptying its bladder prior to surgery.
- There should be a sink for cleaning anaesthetic equipment.

Theatre

If facilities permit, there may be more than one room for operating, so that each theatre may be designated for a specific type of surgery – for example, orthopaedic surgery, soft tissue surgery and dirty procedures such as dentistry.

- Ideally, the operating room should have only one doorway so that it does not become an area for through-traffic. This doorway must be large enough to allow trolleys or pieces of large equipment into or out of the theatre.
- The room should have good natural lighting with additional ceiling lighting, preferably flush mounted.
  - Operating lights, usually ceiling mounted, should have maximum manoeuvrability.
  - Two lights pointed at the surgical site from different angles give ideal lighting.
- The room should be easy to clean, and if possible constructed of impervious materials, with no seams where dust could collect and make cleaning difficult.
  - There should be minimal furniture and shelving, as these will also collect dust.
- Areas of storage should be located in the preparation or scrub area.
  - If storage cupboards are necessary they should be recessed in the wall or built from the floor to ceiling to prevent dust collection. Trolleys are preferred.
- Room temperature is important to maintain the patient's body temperature under anaesthesia and create a pleasant working environment.
  - A room temperature of 15–20°C is acceptable.
  - Methods of heating vary but fan heaters create dust movement and so should be avoided.
- Ideally ventilation should be achieved by using air conditioning; it should not be provided by open windows.

- The room should have plenty of splash-proof electrical sockets in appropriate places.
- An X-ray viewer, preferably flush mounted, should be available in the theatre.
- Near the theatre there should be a room where patients can recover after surgery, with all the necessary equipment to deal with any postsurgical emergencies (see Chapters 4 and 12).
- Scrub sinks should not be located in the theatre itself; ideally they should be in a separate room or in the preparation room.

Preparation of the operating theatre

Daily cleaning

All horizontal surfaces, lights, furniture and equipment should be damp-dusted daily with a suitable disinfectant that is bactericidal, fungicidal, sporicidal and viricidal (see Figure 4.1). The disinfectant should be diluted according to the manufacturer's instructions and handled only when wearing disposable plastic apron, gloves and mask.

As soon as the patient has been removed from theatre and before the next one arrives in the anaesthetic room:

- Remove dirty instruments and place in cool water and cleaning solution for later cleaning and re-sterilization
- Wipe over all flat surfaces, anaesthetic equipment, operating table and other equipment that may have become dirty, using a suitable disinfectant as described above for damp-dusting
- Clean the floor only if necessary (usually this applies only to the soiled areas around the operating table)
- Reposition the table, heating pad and diathermy plate
- Restock if necessary
- Prepare the instruments and equipment for the next surgery
- Place waste materials in the appropriate receptacles.

Immediately after surgery finishes at the end of the day, the operating room should be cleaned thoroughly. This is best done at the end of the day when no further operations are scheduled. This gives any airborne particles, disturbed during cleaning, time to settle before the next procedure begins. At the end of the day the operating room should be ready for use again, either for the following day or in case of any emergencies.

- Clean and re-sterilize all instruments that have been used during the day, ready for use again when needed.
- Thoroughly clean all surfaces, equipment and the floor within theatre, including the scrub sink area.
- Restock and refill supplies and drugs as necessary.
- Empty and clean all bins and vacuum cleaners.
- Wash all drapes and theatre clothing, including boots and shoes worn in theatre.

Weekly cleaning

Weekly cleaning is important to maintain the standards of cleanliness and reach all areas not cleaned in the daily routine. This cleaning should include the preparation rooms and changing rooms associated with the theatre.

- The operating room should be emptied of movable equipment, which should be cleaned (including the castors, where appropriate) before it is returned to theatre.
- Working from ceiling to floor, all fixed structures should be cleaned – including all walls, floors, scrub sinks and drains – using a disinfectant as described above for damp-dusting.
- Although cupboards are not recommended in theatre, they are necessary in the preparation and scrub area; all of them should be emptied, cleaned and restocked during the weekly clean.

Preparation of the operating table

After cleaning, the table should be put into position for surgery. Any heat pads, supports and other equipment should be put in place. The operating table is very important to the procedures taking place within the surgery and the positioning of it may be crucial to the success of the surgery.

There are many different types of operating table and they can vary hugely, so it is impossible to describe how to set out a table for each procedure. However, the following points should be considered when preparing the table for surgery.

- The table should be adapted for the correct position of the patient according to the surgical procedure that is to be used.
- The table should be of a suitable size for the size of patient.
- The height of the table should be easy to adjust to enable it to be positioned correctly for the height of the surgeon.
- To make the table more comfortable there should be some sort of padding (preferably anti-static) available for the area where the patient will be recumbent. This will reduce the risk of muscle damage through ischaemia and reduce heat loss from the patient.
- Theatre lighting should always be checked prior to the start of surgery.

Preparation of diathermy and anaesthetic equipment

A safety check should be carried out on anaesthetic machines at the beginning of each day.

There are two types of diathermy: bipolar and monopolar. If monopolar diathermy is to be used during surgery, the patient must be 'earthed'. This is done by means of a contact plate, which should be placed in a suitable position (usually on hairless or clipped skin), and contact gel should be placed on the plate (this is not necessary for machines that use disposable adhesive plates). Bipolar diathermy requires no contact plate.

Preparation of other equipment

- Have ready scrub solutions and brushes, towels, gowns and gloves suitable for the surgical team.
- Set out skin preparation materials for the patient.
- Lay out the instrument trolley and prepare any spare instruments, drapes and swabs that may be required during the surgery. It is always better to have them close at hand in case of an emergency.
- Prepare suction equipment prior to surgery if required.
- Check that any other electrical equipment (e.g. orthopaedic drills) has the batteries charged if necessary and check that the equipment is working.

Instrument trolley

The laying out of the instruments on the trolley is one of the duties performed by the nurse in the immediate preparation for surgery (Figure 13.1). It should be done in an area of the operating room that is away from the preparation of the surgeon and the patient, and it should be performed in a sterile manner, using a pair of Cheatle forceps. Alternatively, it may be carried out by the surgeon or scrubbed assistant once they are gowned and gloved.

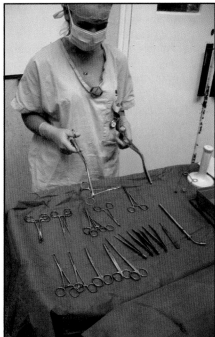

13.1 A veterinary nurse using Cheatle forceps to lay out sterile surgical instruments on a trolley in an aseptic manner.

Preparation of surgical equipment

Asepsis

Asepsis is described as freedom from infection. Therefore 'aseptic technique' is the term used to describe all precautions taken to prevent infection arising from contamination of the wound during surgery, which would cause a delay in postoperative wound healing.

The rules of aseptic technique are as follows.

- Only scrubbed personnel should touch sterile items.
- Non-scrubbed personnel should touch only non-sterile items.
- Only sterile items should touch patient tissue.
- Only sterile items should touch other sterile items.
- Any sterile item touching anything non-sterile becomes non-sterile itself.
- If the sterility of any item is in doubt, it should be considered non-sterile.

Sterilization

- **Disinfection** is defined as the destruction of vegetative forms of bacteria, but not necessarily spores.
- **Sterilization** is the process of destroying all microorganisms, including spores.

Sterilization can be achieved by several different methods, usually divided into:

- Cold or chemical sterilization
- Heat sterilization.

Heat sterilization can be further divided into wet or dry heat: the addition of moisture destroys the bacteria at a lower temperature and in a shorter time. Hence the most common method of sterilization is the autoclave, which provides moist heat in the form of saturated steam under pressure.

Boiling water does not reach high enough temperatures to destroy bacterial spores and should therefore only be considered as a method of disinfection.

Methods of heat sterilization

Hot-air oven

Sterilization is achieved by exposure to a very high temperature for a long period of time. This is a slow method of sterilization but is useful for items that cannot tolerate moist heat, such as oils and powders. It is also suggested that sharp cutting instruments may be sterilized by this method so as not to damage the cutting edge, with the possibility of rusting; however, a long cooling period is needed before use and the very high temperatures may cause damage to the metal.

Autoclave

This method is commonly used in veterinary practice. The destruction of microorganisms is achieved through applying a higher temperature, by producing steam under pressure. The steam comes into direct contact with the items to be sterilized, penetrating or heating each one to the desired temperature. Figure 13.2 gives temperature, time and pressure combinations.

Routine servicing should be carried out as directed by the Pressure Systems Safety Regulations (2000).

Methods of cold sterilization

Ethylene oxide (EO)

Items to be sterilized are exposed to ethylene oxide gas in adequate concentrations at an appropriate temperature and humidity for a sufficient time. The gas

Pressure (psi)	Temperature (°C)	Time (minutes)
0	100	360
15	121	9–15
20	125	6.5
25	130	2.5
35	133	1

13.2 Autoclave temperature, time and pressure combinations.

diffuses and penetrates items rapidly; after sterilization it diffuses away; therefore objects sterilized with this method should have a suitable time for 'airing' before use.

- EO is a very efficient method of sterilization but the gas is highly flammable, explosive and toxic to body tissues.
- It can be used for the sterilization of objects that would be damaged by heat sterilization, such as reusable plastic items.
- It should always be used with the correct equipment (a plastic container with an attached ventilation system) provided by the manufacturers and with strict adherence to their instructions, so as to comply with COSHH regulations.
- Items sterilized by this method must be aired after exposure to the gas, as suggested by the manufacturer.

Chemical solutions (cold soaking)

This refers to the soaking of items in liquid to kill the bacteria. It should really only be regarded as a method of disinfection rather than sterilization. It is commonly used for disinfecting older endoscopes that cannot be sterilized by other means. The types of solution that may be used are based on glutaraldehyde or chlorhexidine. Such solutions must be prepared strictly to the dilutions suggested by the manufacturer and the equipment may need to be rinsed with sterile water after soaking.

Radiation

This method is used for items that cannot be sterilized by heat or chemicals. It is not used within veterinary practice, although many items used will have been sterilized by this method prior to their supply, such as suture materials.

Method of packing for sterilization

Many different methods are available for packing instruments and equipment before sterilization. Choice will be affected by a variety of factors, the most important of which is probably the method of sterilization to be used. For example, some packing materials suitable for use with an autoclave may not be suitable for use with gas sterilization. Figure 13.3 gives some examples of different packing materials with an appropriate method of sterilization.

Packing materials	Advantages	Disadvantages	Type of sterilization method
Linen drapes	Readily available; conforming; can be used to pack difficult items	Porous; liable to wear; time spent laundering and folding	Autoclave with drying cycle or ethylene oxide if not too tightly packed
Paper drapes	Water-resistant so useful as outer layer to package surgical kits	Non-conforming; can be easily torn	Autoclave with drying cycle or ethylene oxide
Self-seal sterilization bags	Easy to pack; clear front so able to see contents	Heavier or sharp instruments may puncture bag (to prevent punctures double packing may be necessary, which increases cost)	Autoclave with ethylene oxide
Nylon films	Cheap; long-lasting; readily available	Punctures easily – punctures not easily seen so may be missed	Autoclave
Metal tins	Easy to pack; very long lasting after initial expense; cannot be punctured by sharp or heavy instruments	Expensive to buy; bulky to store; need a large autoclave with a drying cycle	Autoclave or hot-air oven
Special polythene bags supplied by manufacturers of ethylene oxide	Easy to use, strong bags	Must use specific polythene bags with correct equipment; can over pack so gas cannot circulate	Ethylene oxide
Cardboard cartons	Sturdy and not easily punctured by sharp objects; regular shape makes them neat to store	Expensive to buy; can be bulky to store	Autoclave with drying cycle

13.3 Sterilization and packing methods.

Whatever the method used for packing, each pack should be labelled with the following information before sterilization:

- Contents of the pack (e.g. 'large gown', 'general kit')
- Full date on which the pack was sterilized (e.g. '30.5.07')
- Name of the person who prepared the pack for sterilization.

Efficacy of sterilization methods

It is advisable to check the method of sterilization regularly, to ensure that the correct conditions have been met. Different types of indicator are available for this purpose (Figures 13.4 and 13.5). Ideally, a combination of easily visible surface indicators (demonstrating exposure to the method of sterilization) together with indicators placed in the centre of the pack (demonstrating that sterilization has taken place throughout the pack) is used.

Method	Comments	Use with
Chemical indicator strips	Show a colour change when exposed to the correct conditions. Should be placed in centre of pack before sterilization ■ Chemical indicator strips: paper strips that change colour when exposed to correct conditions of temperature, pressure and time; also available for ethylene oxide ■ Browne's tube: small glass tube filled with orange liquid that changes to green when correct temperature is reached and maintained for correct length of time. Available for different temperatures	Autoclave, ethylene oxide Autoclave, hot-air oven
Indicator tape	Often used as method of securing other packing methods. Both of these tapes only indicate exposure, not that correct time or pressure has been achieved; therefore cannot be considered as reliable method for checking sterilization ■ Bowie Dick tape: beige with series of lines on it that change to black after exposure to temperature of 121°C ■ Ethylene oxide tape: green with series of lines that change to red after exposure to EO gas	Autoclave Ethylene oxide
Spore strips	Paper strips that contain a controlled-count spore population. After sterilization, strips are cultured for 72 hours to see if all spores destroyed. Main disadvantage is delay in obtaining results	Autoclave, hot-air oven, ethylene oxide

13.4 Indicators of sterilization. (See also Figure 13.5.)

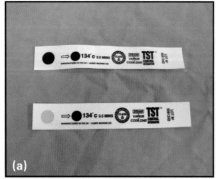
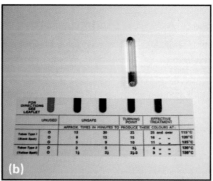
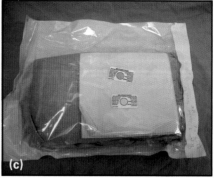
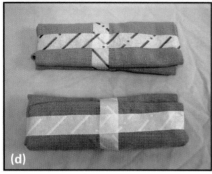
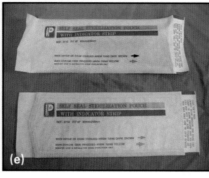

13.5 Indicators of sterilization in common use. **(a)** Chemical indicator strip for steam autoclave (TST strip). Blue = sterile; yellow = not sterile. **(b)** Browne's tube. **(c)** Indicator adhesive label for ethylene oxide (yellow; turning blue on exposure). **(d)** Autoclave (Bowie Dick) tape after (top) and before (bottom) exposure to steam. **(e)** Peel-and-seal bags after (top) and before (bottom) exposure to steam.

Storage after sterilization

- If possible, sterile packs should be stored in closed cabinets rather than on open shelves. In closed cabinets, storage times are generally longer and there is less chance that the packs will come into contact with water.
- The packing method may also affect the length of time the pack can be safely stored before re-sterilization should be considered.
- Any pack that is damaged or becomes wet during storage should be considered non-sterile.
- If there is any doubt regarding the sterility of a pack it is safer to consider it non-sterile and to re-sterilize it before use.
- As a general rule, any item that has not been used by 3 months after sterilization within the clinic (rather than industrially) should be re-sterilized before use.

Surgical gowns

Surgical gowns are worn by the surgeon and surgical assistant to provide a barrier to the transmission of microorganisms from the surgeon to the surgical site or instruments. Studies have shown that the use of disposable non-woven materials during surgery dramatically reduces the number of microorganisms isolated from the surgical environment compared with the use of cloth material.

Ideally all gowns should:

- Have an overlapping back, to ensure complete sterility
- Have wide sleeves, to allow comfortable movement during surgery
- Be available in a range of sizes to fit all.

Long-sleeved gowns, preferably with knitted cuffs or 'wristlets', are preferred to short-sleeved gowns, except for some ophthalmic procedures. The cuffed part of the sleeves of any gown can act as a wick, so these should be covered by the surgical gloves.

Gowns that tie at the back or side are available. Side-tying gowns are preferred since they wrap around the surgeon and cover all areas of the scrub suit. Side-tying gowns are generally made of non-woven material and are disposable.

Sterilization of reusable gowns

After use, reusable gowns need to be folded ready for sterilization. There are several variations in the method for folding, one of which is described in Figure 13.6. The most important point is that the gown is folded with its outside surface on the inside, to ensure that only the inside surface will be touched when the gown is being put on (gowning is described later).

---

1. Lay the gown on a flat surface with the outside facing up.
2. Position the sleeves and ties so that they will be folded within the gown.
3. Fold one edge to the middle.
4. Fold the remaining edge right over to the other side.
5. Concertina the gown from the bottom upwards, leaving the collar on the top.
6. The folded gown is ready to be packed for sterilization. For convenience, a hand towel is often packed with the gown (placed so that it is uppermost when the package is opened).

13.6 One method of packing a gown for sterilization.

Gowns are usually sterilized by autoclaving, as this is the most practical method. It is also possible to sterilize gowns with ethylene oxide. Autoclaves used for sterilizing gowns or other materials must include a drying cycle in the sterilization process. Items that are wet at the end of the sterilization cycle and then left to dry cannot be considered sterile.

Disposable gowns

Disposable non-woven gowns are pre-packed, sterile and folded. Although these gowns are considered sterile when opened, areas that are subjected to more friction (such as the elbows) may become permeable. It should also be remembered that, during particularly lengthy surgical procedures, the gown will be subjected to more pressure and stretching and will have an increased risk of contamination through moisture strike. Any surgical gown should be only considered as sterile from the surgeon's shoulder to waist, including the sleeves.

Surgical drapes

Surgical drapes are used to maintain an aseptic technique by reducing the risk of contamination to the wound from the hair of the patient and the immediate surrounding area. Most drapes are made of cloth (reusable) or are paper-based (disposable). Figure 13.7 gives some of the advantages and disadvantages of each type. Some drapes are self-adhesive or have adhesive areas around the incision site.

Type of drape	Advantages	Disadvantages
Disposable	Water-resistant; impermeable to microorganisms; pre-packed and folded; guaranteed sterility; lint-free	More expensive; often less conforming; large stock needed in a variety of sizes and patterns; less adaptable to size of fenestration; adverse environmental impact of production and disposal
Reusable	Conforming and soft; readily available; fenestration can be easily adapted; cheaper	Not water-resistant; become poor quality with repeated use; time spent washing and folding; sterility not guaranteed after autoclaving in bench-top model with no drying cycle; adverse environmental impact of cleaning and resterilizing

13.7 Reusable and disposable drapes: advantages and disadvantages.

Drapes should:

- Be readily available, conforming, water-resistant and lint-free
- Cover the whole of the patient
- Have a suitably sized fenestration for the surgery being performed.

Types of drapes

There are basically two different patterns of drapes, but as these are available in different forms the final choice is more extensive. The two main types are plain and fenestrated:

- **Plain**: rectangular drapes, placed one at a time at right angles around the surgical site. Four drapes are used to create a 'window' around the incision site.
- **Fenestrated**: a single drape that already has a 'window' prepared in it.

Instruments

Surgical instruments may be made of either chromium-plated carbon steel or stainless steel.

- **Chromium-plated carbon steel** instruments are lower in price and are commonly used in practice. However, the surface is susceptible to attack by solutions with a low pH. This makes the instruments prone to pitting, rusting and blistering and they may need replacing more frequently.
- **Stainless steel** instruments are of better quality and are usually more durable, with better resistance to corrosion.

Some stainless steel instruments, such as scissors and needle holders, have tungsten carbide inserts added to the tips of cutting or gripping surfaces. This makes the instruments tougher, with better resistance to wear, but they are more expensive. Such instruments can usually be identified by their gold-coloured handles.

There are many different types of surgical instrument available. It is not necessary to know every different one; it is more important to know the commonly used instruments (Figure 13.8) and it is useful to know the instruments used in the practice.

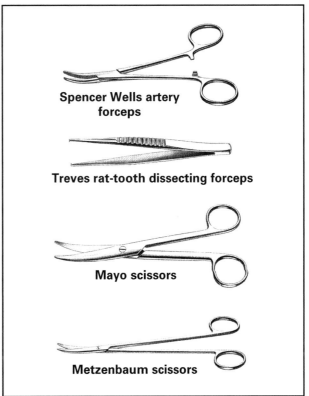

Spencer Wells artery forceps

Treves rat-tooth dissecting forceps

Mayo scissors

Metzenbaum scissors

13.8 Examples of commonly used instruments. (Courtesy of Veterinary Instrumentation.) (continues) ▶

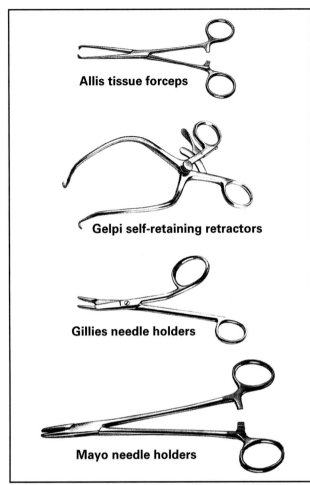

Allis tissue forceps

Gelpi self-retaining retractors

Gillies needle holders

Mayo needle holders

13.8 (continued) Examples of commonly used instruments. (Courtesy of Veterinary Instrumentation.)

Surgical kits

It is often helpful to have some surgical kits made up ready for use. The contents of these will vary, depending on the type of surgery they are intended to be used with and personal preference.

When making up surgical kits, it is important to remember the general purpose of the kit and the size of the animal that the kit will be used with and then to assemble instruments for each function (Figure 13.9). The addition of swabs, bowls of a suitable size and drapes may also be appropriate. In some circumstances it will be necessary to make up more specialized kits. Figure 13.10 gives examples of a general surgical kit and some more specialized ones.

Function	Example
Cutting	Scalpel handle and blade
Dissection	Dissecting forceps, Mayo or Metzenbaum scissors
Haemostasis	Artery forceps
Tissue-holding	Allis forceps
Retraction	Gelpi or Langenback retractors
Suturing	Needle holders and suture scissors

13.9 Surgical function and instrument examples.

General surgical kit
Scalpel handle (No. 3)
Dissecting forceps – rat-toothed fine and plain fine
Scissors:
   Mayo – straight
   Metzenbaum
Artery forceps x 8
Allis tissue forceps x 2
Retractors:
   Gelpi
   Langenbeck
Probe
Backhaus towel clips x 6
Needle holders
Suture scissors

General eye kit
Eyelid speculum
Small scalpel handle (beaver handle) + blade
Fine dissecting forceps
Fine scissors
Corneal scissors
Capsular forceps
Irrigating cannula
Vectis
Iris repository
Castroviejo needle holders

Abdominal kit
General set +
Self-retaining retractors
Long-handled artery forceps x 6
Long dissecting forceps x 2
Bowel clamps x 4

Thoracic kit
General set +
Periosteal elevator
Rib cutters
Rib retractors
Long-handled artery forceps x 6
Long dissecting forceps x 2
Lobectomy clamps

Orthopaedic set
Periosteal elevator
Osteotome
Chisel
Mallet
Curette
Hohmann retractor x 2
Rongeurs
Bone-cutting forceps

Bitch spay kit
General set +
Spencer Wells haemostats
Ovariohysterectomy hook

Cat spay kit
General set +
Ovariohysterectomy hook
Halstead Mosquito haemostats (curved and straight)

13.10 Examples of instrument kits.

Instrument care and maintenance

There are three stages in the cleaning of a surgical instrument:

- Manual cleaning
- Ultrasonic cleaning
- Lubrication.

Manual cleaning

1. Gross visible debris should be removed immediately, so that blood and tissue debris do not have a chance to dry in the joints and serrations.
2. The instruments may then be soaked for a short time in cool water (preferably deionized) containing a mild, non-corrosive instrument cleaning agent.
3. Next, each instrument should be carefully scrubbed with a small hand brush, paying particular attention to the areas where debris may become trapped.
4. Finally, the instruments should be rinsed in water – preferably distilled or deionized as this gives a neutral pH and will not leave deposits on the surface of the instrument that might promote corrosion.

Ultrasonic cleaners

Ultrasonic cleaners are very efficient and remove debris from areas that are not accessible to manual cleaning. They work by a process called **cavitation**, in which minute bubbles form on the surface of the instruments. The bubbles expand until they implode (burst inwards), releasing energy which dislodges debris from the surface of the instrument. After being cleaned in the ultrasonic cleaner, the instruments should be rinsed thoroughly. Instruments cleaned by this method must be lubricated.

Lubrication

Lubrication is essential to maintain the working life of instruments. Without proper lubrication, all instruments (especially those with box joints) will become stiff and difficult to use. However, unsuitable types of lubricant (such as mineral oil) can leave a film coating on the surface of the instrument, which may prevent adequate contact between steam and any organisms during sterilization.

There are many different types of instrument lubricant available and these are special preparations that do not interfere with steam sterilization. Many also contain anti-rusting agents and antimicrobial agents to inhibit the growth of organisms.

Instrument identification

The marking of instruments is often used as a method of identification for a specific surgical pack. The most suitable method is to use thin strips of a coloured plastic autoclave tape. Engraving the surface of the instrument should be avoided as this causes damage and predisposes the instrument to corrosion.

Routine instrument checking

After cleaning and before sterilizing, all instruments should be inspected to ensure that they are functioning properly. A few simple tests to ascertain condition and function may save time during surgery.

- Check hinged joints for stiffness.
- Check the alignment of jaws and teeth.
- Check sharp instruments carefully for nicks or burrs.
- Check instruments with screws or pins for tightness of the screw or pin.
- Check forceps by lightly closing the jaws to see that the tips meet and that there is no overlap.
- Check that needle holders will hold a needle without it rotating easily.
- Check that ratchets do not easily spring when lightly tapped against a solid object.
- Check the tips of towel clips for damage. If the tips are bent out of position they will not hold the drapes in place.

Specialized instrument care

Compressed air machines

These machines should never be immersed in water or cleaned in an ultrasonic bath.

The machine and air hose should be wiped carefully as soon as possible after use and then dried. The hose can be wiped with anti-static cleaner to prevent hairs from sticking to it.

The machine should be oiled before sterilization, using the oil recommended by the manufacturer of the machine.

1. Several drops of oil should be put down the air coupling and around the quick coupling and the triggers.
2. The machine should then be reconnected to the air supply and run for approximately 30 seconds.
3. Any excess oil should be wiped off before packing the machine for sterilization.

Motorized equipment

The care of these machines is very similar to that of compressed air machines. Special attention should be paid to the manufacturer's instructions, as these machines may seize up after repeated autoclaving.

Dental instruments

A good standard of dentistry work relies on good quality, well maintained instruments and equipment. There are two types of dental instrument: hand-held and mechanical.

- **Hand-held** instruments (such as scalers, picks, luxators and curettes) may have delicate points or tips and should be very carefully washed and dried. Many of these instruments then require sharpening with an Arkansas stone and oil. Autoclaving may then be carried out as normal, though care should be taken to protect delicate tips and points.

■ **Mechanical** instruments (such as ultrasonic cleaners and polishers) need regular maintenance. The manufacturer's instructions will give the best guidance for each specific type of equipment but the following points may be useful:
  – Oil the hand-piece after each use and before cleaning, by putting two drops in the inlet port
  – Regularly remove the turbine from the high-speed hand-piece and clean with an aerosol lubricant
  – Check filters according to the manufacturer's instructions
  – Check compressor and air line for leaks.

Suction equipment

Surgical suction appliances are frequently used in less routine surgical procedures where they contribute to good surgical practice. They must be cleaned after each use.

■ The containers on the suction unit (usually plastic or glass jars) should be emptied, cleaned, disinfected and dried as soon as possible after use, or replaced if the units are designed to be disposable.

■ An anti-foaming agent is available to put in the jars to prevent foam getting into the mechanics of the machine.
■ The filters should be changed regularly; the frequency depends on usage, but monthly (at least) is recommended.
■ The filters must be changed if wet.
■ Regular servicing by the manufacturing company is also recommended.

Sutures

Suture materials

There are two main categories of suture materials: absorbable and non-absorbable (Figures 13.11 and 13.12). (These were previously referred to as dissolving and permanent, respectively, but since no suture truly retains its strength permanently, this classification is not appropriate.) The two categories can be further divided into:

■ Natural or synthetic
■ Monofilament or multifilament
■ Coated or uncoated.

Suture material	Trade name	Mono/multifilament	Synthetic/natural	Coated	Duration of strength	Absorption	Comments/uses
Polyglactin 910	Vicryl (Ethicon) Polysorb (USSC)	Multi (braided)	Synthetic	Yes (calcium stearate)	Retains 50% of tensile strength at 14 days, 20% at 21 days	Absorption 60–90 days by hydrolysis	Dyed or undyed Low tissue reactivity Uses: subcutis, muscle, eyes, hollow viscera
Polydioxanone	PDS II (Ethicon)	Mono	Synthetic	No	Retains 70% tensile strength at 14 days, 14% at 56 days	Only minimal absorption by 90 days, absorbed by 180 days Absorbed by hydrolysis	Good for infected sites as monofilament Very strong but springy Minimal tissue reaction Uses: subcutis, muscle, sometimes eyes
Polyglycolic acid	Dexon (USSC)	Multi	Synthetic	Can be coated with polymers	Retains 20% at 14 days	Complete absorption by 100–120 days Absorbed by hydrolysis	Similar to polyglactin but has considerable tissue drag Uses: as for polyglactin.
Poliglecaprone 25	Monocryl (Ethicon) Caprosyn (USSC)	Mono	Synthetic	No	Retains approximately 60% at 7 days, 30% at 14 days Wound support maintained for 20 days	Complete absorption between 90 and 120 days Absorbed by hydrolysis	New synthetic suture material Less springy than other monofilament absorbables with minimal tissue reaction and drag Available dyed or undyed

13.11 Absorbable suture materials.

Suture material	Trade name	Mono- or multifilament	Synthetic/ natural	Coated	Knot security	Duration	Comments
Polyamide (nylon)	Ethilon (Ethicon), Monosof (USSC)	Mono	Synthetic	No	Fair	Permanent	Causes minimal tissue reaction and has little tissue drag
Polybutester	Novafil (Davis & Geck)	Mono	Synthetic	No	Fair	Permanent	Very similar to Ethilon, with similar properties
Polypropylene	Prolene (Ethicon), Surgipro (USSC)	Mono	Synthetic	No	Fair, can produce bulky knots that untie easily	Permanent	Very inert, produces only minimal tissue reaction. Very strong but also very springy. Little tissue drag
Braided silk	Mersilk (Ethicon)	Multi	Natural	Wax coat	Excellent	Eventually may fragment and break down	Natural material with good handling properties but high tissue reactivity and should not be used in infected sites
Braided polyamide	Supramid or Nurolon (Ethicon)	Multi	Synthetic	Encased in outer sheath	Good	Outer sheath can be broken	Better handling characteristics than monofilament polyamide. Can be used in the skin but should not be used as buried suture
Surgical stainless steel wire		Available as either mono or multi	Synthetic	No	Excellent but knots may be difficult to tie	Permanent	Not commonly used now but can be useful in bone or tendon. Difficult to handle, may break

13.12 Non-absorbable suture materials.

The choice of suture material will depend on:

- Personal preference
- Type of tissue in which the material is to be used
- Risk of contamination
- Length of time the sutured tissues will require support.

As a general rule:

- **Absorbable** sutures are used to close internal layers where initial strength is required while tissue healing takes place.
- **Non-absorbable** sutures are used in the skin, from which they can be removed once sufficient healing of the wound has occurred. They are also used in areas where tissues may be slow to heal and so long-term support of the tissues is required.

Alternatives to sutures

There are several alternatives to suture that are becoming used more routinely, including staples, glue and adhesive tape (see later and Figure 13.28).

Staples

There are several different types of metal staple designed for use in different situations. Packed in a gun-type applicator, they are quick to insert. Skin staples are commonly used and are easily removed with the correct staple-removing forceps. Specialized staples can be used for procedures such as intestinal anastomosis and ligation.

Tissue glue (cyanoacrylate)

These glues, used for skin closure, are designed to give rapid healing. They are usually applied to small superficial wounds.

Adhesive tapes

These are designed for skin closure in humans. The tapes do not adhere well to animal skin and are therefore of limited use in veterinary practice.

Suture needles

Suture needles vary in design and shape (Figures 13.13 and 13.14). They are available with eyes, through which suture materials are threaded, or with the suture material already swaged on (Figure 13.15). Choice of needle is dependent on:

- Type of wound to be sutured
- Tissue to be sutured
- Characteristics of available needles.

Fully curved	Entire length of needle is curved into an arc Various degrees of curvature are available Half-circle is most common
Curved on straight/half curved	Sharp end of needle is curved but eye end is straight
Straight	Entire needle is straight

13.13 Suture needle shapes.

Type	Features	Suggested uses
Cutting	Point and sides of needle are sharp Triangular in cross-section with apex on inside of curve	Skin (other dense tissue)
Reverse cutting	Point and sides of needle are sharp Triangular in cross-section with apex on outside of curve Design used with small needles	Skin (other dense tissues)
Round-bodied	Round in cross-section with no sharp edges	Delicate tissues (e.g. fat; walled viscera)
Taper cut	Similar to cutting needle at tip As needle widens, becomes round-bodied in design	Dense tissues other than skin (e.g. fascia; thick-walled viscera; mucous membranes)

13.14 Needle point and shaft designs.

Swaged-on	Eyed
Lengths of suture bonded by manufacturer to a disposable needle Passes through tissue with less drag than eyed needle As a new needle is used each time, it is sharp Suture is secured to needle Relatively expensive Useful for delicate tissues as less traumatic	Surgeon threads needle at time of surgery Greater bulk of suture at eye increases drag (needle should not be double-threaded since this worsens drag further) Needles are commonly reused and therefore cheaper Care must be taken to keep needle joined to suture

13.15 Attachment of needle to suture.

Preparation of the patient

Patient preparation can vary greatly from case to case. Healthy patients undergoing elective (planned) surgery may require only routine preparation (see later). Other patients require longer periods to allow them to be optimally prepared for surgery. Some may require extended dietary control or medical treatment (e.g. diabetics) before they are ready for surgery. Other patients may need immediate surgical attention and preparation time may be limited.

Preoperative problems

The degree of preoperative care required in a particular case depends on the type of patient, the effect the disease has had on the patient and the presence and effect of other diseases. Young, fit and healthy animals presented for elective surgery require the minimum of special care. Older animals are more likely to have concurrent disease and, before surgery, require closer assessment to identify such diseases and their effect. Preoperative treatment can then be arranged if necessary to minimize the potential morbidity and mortality associated with anaesthesia and surgery. Figure 13.16 lists some typical preoperative patient problems and their implications.

The impact of the indication for surgery must be considered during preparation. For most elective surgeries (neutering, cosmetic procedures, chronic orthopaedic conditions), by definition, the indication has little effect on the patient's physiology. However, for emergency procedures, the animal can be severely affected by the disease (Figure 13.17).

Preoperative restriction of food and water

Food is normally withheld from adult dogs and cats for approximately 8 hours prior to surgery; this ensures an empty stomach and avoids vomiting in the perioperative period (which may be detrimental to the patient and to the surgical incision). Most owners can be instructed not to offer any food after midnight on the day before surgery. Surgery on certain parts of the alimentary tract may require dietary restriction for longer.

Immature animals of all types are prone to deleterious effects of starvation (notably hypoglycaemia) and food restriction should be limited to no more than a few hours, depending on their age and the procedure planned. The same can be said of many of the small species of mammals that have high metabolic rates and minimal risk of vomiting. Food should be withheld in birds for just long enough for the crop to be empty. Excessive withholding of food in these species may predispose to postoperative problems, with gut stasis in addition to hypoglycaemia, and starvation is therefore not used.

In most cases, water need not be withheld until after premedication. Owners often expect to withhold water for longer but this is rarely necessary and can be deleterious, for example in animals with compensated kidney failure.

Preoperative problem	Associated surgical complications	Steps in prevention
Advanced age	Exacerbation of pre-existing problems (e.g. organ failure)	Preoperative assessment and appropriate therapy
Obesity	Anaesthetic mortality; reduced surgical exposure	Normalize body condition prior to surgery
Emaciation	Delayed healing; reduced immunocompetence	Normalize body condition prior to surgery. Modify surgical technique to allow for reduction in rate of healing. Perioperative antibiotic use
Hypoproteinaemia	Delayed healing; reduced immunocompetence	Modify surgical technique to allow for reduction in rate of healing. Perioperative antibiotic use. Plasma or blood transfusion
Therapeutic corticosteroids Cushing's disease (hyperadrenocorticism)	Delayed healing; reduced immunocompetence	Withdraw corticosteroid therapy prior to surgery. Stabilize disease prior to surgery. Modify surgical technique to allow for reduction in rate of healing. Perioperative antibiotic use
Clotting or bleeding defects	Increased intra- and postoperative haemorrhage	Assess and treat before surgery. Minimize bleeding during surgery by careful attention to haemostasis. Fresh blood or plasma transfusion. Postoperative monitoring
Organ failure	Exacerbation by hospitalization, anaesthesia and surgery	Assess and treat before surgery. Tailor peri- and postoperative care appropriately
Skin infection Infections remote from surgical site (e.g. dental disease)	Infection of surgical site	Assess and treat before surgery. Perioperative antibiotic use

13.16 Preoperative patient factors and treatment.

Complicating factor	Causes	Associated problems	Steps in prevention
Hypoventilation	Many, including: respiratory tract obstruction; thoracic disease; abdominal distension; depression of central nervous system	Hypoxia; hypercapnia; respiratory acidosis	Avoid worsening by stressing patient or inappropriate use of drugs. Oxygen supplementation before, during and after surgery if necessary
Dehydration	Inability or unwillingness to drink; increased fluid losses	Hypovolaemia; delayed recovery	Reverse before surgery if possible. Use fluid therapy to expand blood volume (see Chapter 8)
Hypovolaemia	Dehydration; haemorrhage; septicaemia	Increased anaesthetic morbidity and mortality; delayed recovery	Reverse before surgery if possible. Use fluid therapy to expand blood volume (see Chapter 8)
Septicaemia	Trauma; organ rupture; migration of bacteria from gastrointestinal tract due to mucosal ischaemia	Increased anaesthetic morbidity and mortality; surgical infection	Aggressive pre- and intraoperative antibiotic and fluid therapy
Cardiovascular dysfunction	Many, including: shock; septicaemia; toxaemia; gastric-dilatation/volvulus; splenic diseases	Increased anaesthetic morbidity and mortality	Assess and treat underlying causes. Specific treatment with drugs to suppress arrhythmias (e.g. lidocaine) or increase force or rate of contraction (e.g. dopamine) may be required
Electrolyte or acid–base disturbances	Severe systemic disease of all types	Increased anaesthetic morbidity and mortality; delayed recovery	Reversal of hypovolaemia to allow homeostatic mechanisms to function. Specific treatment may be needed, e.g. with potassium (for hypokalaemia), glucose and insulin (for hyperkalaemia) and bicarbonate or lactate (for acidosis)

13.17 Factors to be considered and treated before, during and after emergency surgery.

Bowel and bladder evacuation

Patients should be given the chance to urinate and defecate immediately prior to surgery. For most cases it is sufficient to allow them access to a litter tray or to walk them before taking them into the surgery suite. This also reduces the chance of environmental contamination during anaesthesia. However, in some cases a more extensive preparation is required and this might include the use of enemas or urinary catheterization.

Enemas

In cases of rectal or colonic surgery it may be necessary to be more certain that the patient has defecated. These cases will require an enema before surgery. A soap-and-warm-water or phosphate (Fletcher's) enema is usually adequate for this. The patient may need bathing after administration of an enema. Enema administration is covered in more depth in Chapter 9. A purse-string suture in the anus is useful, particularly when the surgical site is close to the perineum or if an epidural anaesthetic technique is used (which abolishes all anal tone).

Urinary catheterization

Some patients may need an empty bladder before surgery is undertaken. Gentle manual expression under general anaesthesia may be adequate, or catheterization of the bladder may be required. An indwelling catheter can also be useful for measuring the production of urine during surgery and in the immediate postoperative period. In addition, for certain surgical procedures of the urinary tract, the surgeon may request that a urethral catheter is placed. All such catheters should be capped or connected to a closed collection system. Urinary catheterization is covered in more depth in Chapter 9.

Bathing

To remove loose hair and skin particles and so reduce the risk of contamination of the surgical site, it would be helpful to bath every patient prior to surgery but this is not always practical. It should be considered for patients that are excessively soiled or patients undergoing elective orthopaedic surgery with the use of implants (e.g. hip replacement). Enough time should be allowed to dry the patient thoroughly before surgery.

Clipping

Before clipping, the nurse must check that the correct patient is being prepared, which surgical procedure is to be performed, on which side of the patient and by which approach (e.g. dorsal or lateral).

There are advantages and disadvantages to clipping before or after the induction of anaesthesia and each patient should be considered individually depending on the area to be clipped, the type of surgery and the temperament of the patient. Clipping before surgery, or clipping that causes damage to the skin, increases the skin bacterial numbers at the time of surgery and the incidence of incisional infection.

For routine elective surgery the best time to remove the hair is after the induction of anaesthesia. This should be done in a preparation area outside of the theatre. Patients at greater anaesthetic risk may be clipped before induction to reduce the anaesthetic time, if this can be done without causing distress, but this increases the risk of postoperative wound infection.

Loose hair and debris caused by clipping should be removed by vacuuming before the patient enters theatre, so reducing the risk of contamination.

Points to consider when clipping prior to surgery include the following.

- Clipping against the hair is most effective, although it may be necessary to clip with the grain of the hair first to remove a thick coat.
- Be neat – owners will not be impressed by untidy clipping.
- Be gentle – avoid clipper rash and skin irritation.
- Be thorough – clip a large enough area and consider the possibility of an extended incision if the surgery does not go as planned. The area clipped should extend 5–15 cm beyond the anticipated incision site.
- If clipping near the eyes, make sure they are appropriately protected before starting (e.g. by application of a bland ointment).
- Areas close to the surgical site that are not to be clipped (e.g. tail, feet) can be covered by a cohesive bandage, clean plastic bag or glove.
- To avoid the transmission of skin organisms (e.g. *Staphylococcus aureus*) between patients, the clipper blades should be disinfected after each use. If used on patients known to be infected, or on grossly soiled areas, the blades should be removed, cleaned and sterilized.
- Clipping must be done with particular care in small mammals, because of their delicate skin and to avoid postoperative hypothermia. Depilatory creams are an alternative.
- For birds, parting the feathers is an alternative to removal (which could cause long-term disability). Feathers that need removal for surgery should be plucked, not cut, so that they will grow back rapidly (cut feathers will not grow back until the next moult).
- To prevent damage to the skin, clipper blades must be kept sharp and should be discarded if damaged.

Skin preparation

This is essential to remove dirt and organic debris from the skin of the patient and to disinfect the skin.

Initial preparation

This is carried out in the preparation room, outside the theatre itself.

- Wear gloves to prevent cross-contamination and protect the hands from sensitization to antiseptic solution.
- Use either chlorhexidine or povidone–iodine. Do not change between the two during one procedure.

- Mechanical scrubbing of the skin is important as it reduces the number of bacteria on the skin, but avoid abrading the skin surface – use lint-free swabs.
- Start scrubbing at the incision site in the centre of the clipped area, work out towards the edges, discard the swab and start at the centre again with a clean swab. Be careful not to return a swab from the edges to the centre of the area to be scrubbed.
- Include the hair at the edge of the clipped area to remove debris but be careful not to make the patient too wet.
- Remove the soap with sterile water or alcohol and swabs, then repeat the scrubbing process.
- Although it may occasionally be appropriate simply to spray the area with skin preparation solution if there is no gross debris, this will not remove organic debris and so the effectiveness of disinfection will be reduced.
- In small mammals and other 'exotic' species, take particular care to avoid hypothermia. Do not use excessive volumes of either scrub solution or spirit: damp swabs are more suitable than direct wetting of the skin.

Skin preparation in the theatre

Once the initial preparation of the skin is complete, the patient can be positioned on the operating table ready for surgery. Contamination of the skin is likely to occur during positioning and so a secondary scrub should be carried out in theatre immediately before surgery.

- Use sterile gloves and swabs for scrubbing.
- Repeat the procedure described for the initial preparation.
- Mop up any pools of fluid caused by preparing the skin.
- The final skin preparation should be performed in a sterile manner by a member of the surgical team. This usually consists of aseptic application of skin disinfectant in alcohol that is left to dry on the skin (Figure 13.18).

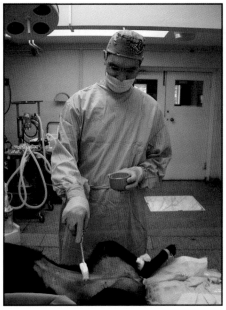

13.18 Final skin scrub of a patient in theatre.

Positioning of the patient

It is important to be familiar with the surgical procedure being undertaken to ensure that the animal is positioned correctly.

Although the initial positioning of the patient is usually a task for the veterinary nurse, it is wise to check on the final positioning with the surgeon or assistant before they begin to scrub up. Once surgery has started it is very difficult to alter the position of the patient without contaminating the sterile field.

Points to consider during patient positioning are as follows.

- Position the patient with the surgical site best presented to the surgeon.
- Check that the positioning will not interfere with respiratory function or peripheral circulation, or cause muscular damage.
- Use positioning aids to make the patient comfortable and avoid ischaemic damage.
- If using a heat pad underneath the patient, remember that the patient will not be able to move away from the heat and so make sure that it is not too hot. Use a thermostatically controlled electric heat pad, water blanket or circulating hot-air mattress.
- Place the return electrode or patient plate against the skin under the patient if monopolar diathermy is to be used. The plate should be in close contact with the skin in an area of good vascular supply and any hair should be clipped. Some plates are used with contact provided by a saline-soaked cloth (check with the equipment manufacturer) and others use self-adhesive disposable plates.
- Make sure that everything is in place before the sterile preparation of the skin begins and the drapes are placed on the patient.
- If sterile light handles are not available for the surgeon, move the operating lights to illuminate the site.

Draping the patient

Sterile surgical drapes are placed over the patient around the surgical site. The drapes separate the surgical field from surrounding areas that would otherwise contaminate the tissues during surgery. The exact method of draping a patient depends on the available materials, the type of surgery to be performed and the size of the patient.

Draping (Figure 13.19) begins once the patient is correctly positioned and the final skin preparation is complete.

Points to consider during patient draping are as follows.

- Drapes are applied by a scrubbed member of the surgical team once they are gloved and gowned and skin preparation is complete.
- Cover as much of the patient and table as possible, leaving only the surgical site exposed. The drapes must cover the area between the surgical field and the instrument trolley or tray.

Draping with four plain drapes

1. Pick up the first drape, still folded, from the trolley. Step back and unfold it away from the trolley and table so that it does not touch non-sterile areas.
2. One quarter of the drape is folded back underneath itself to produce a double layer at the edge of the draped area.
3. The drape is held along the folded edge, with the hands inside the drape so that they do not touch the patient as the drape is placed. Each subsequent drape is handled in the same way.
4. The first drape is placed on the side of the surgical field nearest the surgeon. This is so that the surgeon can later move close to the table and lean over to place the other drapes without contacting undraped areas.
5. The second drape is placed on the opposite side of the surgical area (assistant's side) by the surgeon, who can approach the table, which is covered by the first drape, or by the assistant in the same way as the surgeon placed the first drape.
6. The third and fourth drapes are placed at either end of the surgical field (the order of these is not important).
7. Any remaining areas of the table or patient that remain exposed are covered by additional sterile drapes.
8. Drapes are secured with towel clips: one towel clip is used at each corner of the surgical field.
9. The clip is placed diagonally across the edges of the two drapes, with one tip on each. The tips are pushed down on to the skin and the clip is closed to pick up the drapes and a small fold of skin.
10. The clip is then placed under one drape at the corner.

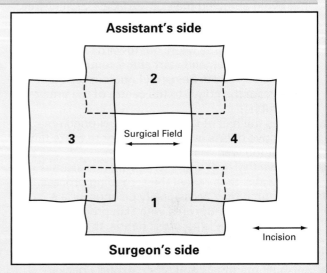

Draping with one fenestrated drape

1. The drape is picked up, still folded, from the trolley and is unfolded away from the trolley and table (as in step 1 above).
2. The drape is held along the top edge, with the hands inside the drape so that they cannot touch non-sterile areas as the drape is placed.
3. Look through the fenestration and place the fenestration over the surgical field.
   - The size of the fenestration should approximate the area required – it is unsatisfactory to fold the drape to reduce the size of the fenestration if it is too large
   - The preferred alternative, if necessary, is to place further plain drapes over the fenestration to reduce its size.
4. Secure the drape with towel clips at each corner of the fenestration (see steps 8 and 9 above). The clips cannot be concealed beneath the drapes and are more likely to interfere with the instruments during surgery.

Other draping techniques

- Plastic drapes secured with adhesive spray or self-adhesive drapes can be usefully combined with conventional drapes to reduce strike-through in the presence of excessive fluids or as a form of subdraping (see below)
- Fenestrated and plain drapes can be used together to cover the patient and table effectively without leaving gaps where drapes overlap. For example, a large fenestrated drape with large fenestration can be placed as a second layer over a field surrounded by four plain drapes
- Some surgical sites require special techniques to drape effectively. For example:
  - On the limb, the foot may be covered by a sterile foot bag or surgical glove, or sterile cohesive bandage can be used to wrap the limb
  - Draping of the oral cavity requires additional towel clips or staples to secure the drapes to the lips
- *Subdraping* is the practice of placing additional drapes close to or against the incised skin edge to limit further the surgical field and reduce contamination from the surrounding skin. It is not routine in veterinary surgery but should be considered for procedures at particular risk of infection (placement of orthopaedic implants is one example)
  - Use of an adhesive plastic drape over the field that is incised with the skin is one such technique, but these types of drapes often peel away, particularly on concave surfaces and in the presence of fluids
  - Alternatively, small cloth drapes or towels can be secured to the skin edge with towel clips or skin clips (Michel clips), or disposable drapes can be sutured to the skin edges, following the initial skin incision

13.19 How to drape a patient with four plain drapes.

- Water-resistant drapes are selected for procedures when irrigation or other fluids are likely to be present. Alternatively a waterproof drape may be placed under cloth drapes to prevent strikethrough.

- Transparent plastic drapes are useful to allow the patient to be more closely observed during anaesthesia. This is particularly important with very small animals (e.g. small mammals and reptiles).

- Conventional paper and cloth drapes are secured to the skin using towel clips. In some cases, skin staples are an alternative (useful around the lips, for example).
- Some disposable drapes have self-adhesive strips to secure them to the patient (Figure 13.20). These are particularly effective for hairless patients (e.g. reptiles) but work less reliably with clipped skin.

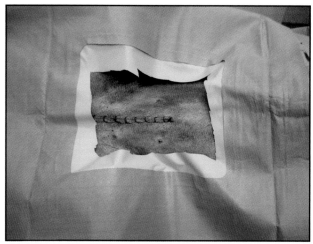

13.20 A patient draped with a disposable adhesive fenestrated drape.

- Plastic drapes can be fixed to the skin with an adhesive skin preparation spray, but this only works effectively if the skin has been closely clipped or is hairless and has been allowed to dry thoroughly.
- Once in position, drapes should not be moved since this would contaminate the surgical field. If positioned incorrectly, they should be removed and discarded.
- Some drapes have a pre-prepared opening for the surgical field (fenestration); for other surgeries the fenestration can be cut (if using paper drapes) or made to the required size using four plain drapes.
- When applying individual drapes, the edges of each drape at the incision should be folded under before the drapes are placed on the patient.
- Further asepsis can be provided by sub-draping: additional small drapes or towels are clipped to the edges of the skin incision once it is completed. A similar effect is achieved by using a thin adhesive drape on the skin exposed by the fenestration and incising through it.

Preparation of personnel for surgery

Theatre clothing

Theatre clothing cannot be considered as sterile, but as a permeable barrier to microorganisms. It should be worn in the operating room even when surgery is not in progress. The material should be lint-free, hard wearing and comfortable.

Scrub suits

Most scrub suits consist of top and trousers. Ideally, to reduce the shedding of microorganisms from the skin into the environment, the top should be worn tucked inside the trousers, which should have cuffed legs or be worn inside surgical boots.

To reduce the risk of contamination of the surgical site by organisms on the scrub suit, all scrub suits (particularly those of the surgeon) should be:

- Worn only within the operating room
- Covered with a clean laboratory coat if worn outside the operating room
- Not worn outside with the intention of returning to the operating room in the same scrub suit
- Changed at least daily, or more frequently if soiled
- Periodically autoclaved (in a steam autoclave with a drying cycle).

Footwear

Theatre footwear should only be worn within the operating room. Areas of access should be clearly marked with coloured floor tape and appropriate signs, as described earlier. This helps to prevent theatre shoes being worn outside the restricted area and also helps to make others aware that outside shoes should not be worn within the operating room.

- Shoes or boots should be anti-static, comfortable and easily cleaned. Ideally, they should be autoclaved periodically.
- Shoe covers can also be used; they should be lightweight, waterproof and durable.

Theatre hats

It is recommended that head covers are worn by all personnel in theatre, as hair sheds particles that may contain bacteria. There are several different types of head cover that can be worn in theatre.

Theatre hats are made of many different materials. They should be lint-free, durable and comfortable and should cover all hair easily. Hats may be disposable or reusable; the latter should be treated in the same way as scrub suits.

Facemasks

Facemasks only cover the nose and mouth. Although studies have shown that the wearing of facemasks does not significantly reduce the levels of environmental bacteria, they still have a role in the prevention of contamination in the surgical wound.

Most masks give effective filtration of organisms shed from the nose and oropharynx, but it should be noted that these organisms can reach the surgical environment via the sides and bottom of the mask. This can be prevented by wearing a hood-type theatre hat with the sides of the mask incorporated under the edges of the hat.

Facemasks can be made of cloth or, more commonly, disposable materials. Disposable masks are made of synthetic and natural materials; they usually have, across the nose, a section that can be shaped for comfort and they have pleats that give greater efficacy.

Aseptic preparation of surgical personnel

In addition to following the guidelines for theatre clothing above, the surgeon and any assistants must take extra precautions. In particular, they must aseptically prepare the skin of their hands and forearms, wear sterile clothing (surgical gowns) over their arms and front and put on sterile gloves.

Skin preparation ('scrubbing up')

The aim of scrubbing the skin before putting on a gown and gloves is to remove any gross dirt and to reduce as much as possible the number of microorganisms on the skin. Finally the scrub solution should have a prolonged effect in suppressing the levels of organisms on the skin once underneath surgical gloves.

There are variations in the methods for scrubbing up, mostly in the area of the hands and arms that are scrubbed using a brush. Studies have shown that there is no difference between using reusable or disposable brushes, but frequent autoclaving of reusable brushes will eventually make them hard and harsh on the skin. If the skin does become dry and damaged through repeated scrubbing procedures, there will be greater numbers of bacteria on the skin and effectiveness of the scrubbing procedure will be greatly reduced.

Whichever method of scrubbing is used, the basic principles are the same.

- The procedure should be a routine.
- It should not take an excessive amount of time.
- The antiseptic solution and technique should not be irritant to the skin.

A standard scrub routine is outlined in Figure 13.21.

Gowning

A sterile surgical gown is put on after scrubbing up and should cover the scrub suit from knee to neck and all of the arms. This provides protection to the surgical site from contamination by the theatre clothing during surgery. The gown is put on (Figure 13.22) after aseptic preparation of the hands and forearms that have been scrubbed up and dried on a sterile towel.

Surgical gloves

Surgical gloves are worn as a barrier between the surgeon's hands and the tissues of the patient. They come pre-packed in specific sizes with sterility guaranteed, unless the packet is damaged or out of date. They should be chosen to fit snugly but not too tightly. Sterile gloves should be worn for all operative procedures.

Some gloves are lubricated with a fine starch powder that is put on to assist the wearer in the gloving procedure. However, the powder can cause a foreign body inflammatory response that may interfere with wound healing and possibly cause adhesions during the healing process. When using these gloves it is advisable to wash off the powder with sterile water and wipe over with a sterile towel before commencing surgery.

1. Remove any jewellery or watches.
2. Fingernails should be short and any varnish removed.
3. Stand at the sink with arms held forward away from the body and with hands higher than the elbows. This allows the water to run away from the scrubbed area and prevents possible recontamination.
4. The scrubbing procedure should take a minimum of 5 minutes, so allow at least 1 minute for each of the washing procedures.
5. Remove all organic matter from the skin by washing hands and arms (up to and including the elbows) with a plain soap. Rinse, remembering to let the water flow down towards the elbows.
6. Repeat this procedure using surgical scrub solution and rinse in the same way.
7. Use a sterile brush to scrub the palm of each hand and each finger, paying particular attention to the nail area. Either rinse the brush or discard and use another one.
8. Repeat this procedure on the other hand. Always use the same system for this procedure to prevent missing out some areas. Rinse again.
9. Repeat the procedure in step 6. Wash hands and arms again using surgical scrub, but this time do not include the elbows so that the hands do not touch areas that have not been scrubbed. Rinse.
10. Use a sterile hand towel to dry one hand in one quarter of the towel and one hand in another quarter. Dry the arms to elbows on the two remaining quarters of the towel that have not been used.

This full routine should be used at the beginning of each surgical session. Between subsequent procedures, unless the hands have become grossly contaminated, an abbreviated 2-minute scrub, without the use of the brush, is adequate and helps prevent trauma to the skin.

13.21 How to scrub up.

1. Pick up the gown at the shoulders, hold it out in front of you and allow it to fall open.
2. Locate the sleeves. Insert each hand into the sleeve opening; push your hands forward into the sleeves, opening out your arms. Do not try to pull the gown up over your shoulders as this is a potential contamination risk.
3. An unscrubbed assistant should be available to adjust the gown as necessary, touching the inside of the gown only, and secure the gown at the back.
4. If the gown has front ties, these should be held out to the sides. The assistant should take the ties at the ends to avoid accidentally touching the gown and contaminating it. The ties should be secured at the back of the gown. For a side-tying gown, the scrubbed person then passes one of the side ties, attached to a paper tape, to an assistant. The assistant takes the paper tape and takes it with the tie around the gown. The scrubbed person can then pull the tie away, leaving the assistant holding the paper tape and the scrubbed person able to tie the two ties together at the side of the gown.

13.22 How to put on a sterile gown.

Alternatively, gloves without the addition of powder can be used and should be considered as the gloves of choice particularly when surgery involves delicate tissues (such as ophthalmic procedures).

Even the most rigorous hand-scrubbing procedure does not remove all the bacteria. Therefore, if a glove is punctured during a surgical procedure, it should be changed as soon as possible, or another glove should be applied over the top of the first one.

When changing gloves during a surgical procedure, the contaminated glove can be removed by the wearer and replaced by the open gloving method or removed by an assistant and replaced by the closed gloving method.

Open gloving and closed gloving are the two main methods of gloving that are practised and both are widely used. Closed gloving is preferred, since it minimizes the risk of contamination as the hands stay within the sleeves of the gown until they go straight into the glove. Only this method is covered here (Figure 13.23).

---

1. Keep hands within the sleeves of the gown throughout.
2. Turn the open glove packet so that the fingers point towards you.
3. With your right hand, pick up the right glove (now positioned on the left of the packet) by the rim of the cuff.
4. Turn your hand over. The fingers of the glove should now be pointing down towards your elbow.
5. With your left hand, pick up the other side of the rim of the cuff and pull it up and over your right hand.

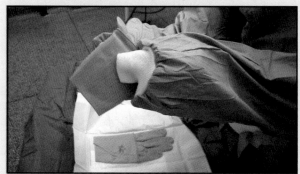

6. Push the fingers of your right hand into the glove.

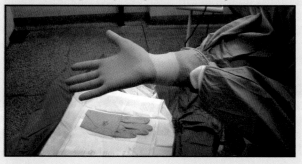

7. Keeping your left hand within the sleeve of the gown, you can move the glove into a comfortable position.
8. With your left hand, pick up the left glove and repeat exactly the same process.
9. The cuffs of the gloves should entirely cover the wristlets of the gown.

13.23 How to put on sterile gloves – closed gloving method.

The critical point to remember during gloving is not to touch the outside of the glove with an uncovered hand. During closed gloving the gloves are only handled through the sleeves of the gown; during open gloving only the inside of the gloves is touched by the scrubbed hands.

Intraoperative assistance

It is often the role of the nurse to provide the veterinary surgeon with help during the surgical procedure. This can be either as a circulating nurse or as a scrubbed assistant.

Circulating nurse

A nurse present during the surgery who does not assist as a scrub nurse or a surgical assistant is described as a circulating nurse, prep-nurse or non-scrub nurse. This person should be in attendance at all times during the surgery and performs the following tasks:

- Helping with final skin preparation
- Ensuring correct positioning of the patient
- Assisting with gowning
- Connecting apparatus such as diathermy or suction machines
- Fetching and unwrapping extra instruments or apparatus if they are needed during surgery
- Providing extra swabs or sutures and keeping account of used swabs or sutures removed from the trolley
- Cleaning the surgical site at the end of surgery and applying a dressing or bandage
- Preparing the surgical suite for the next procedure.

Scrub nurse or surgical assistant

The efficiency of the surgeon can be greatly increased with a competent surgical assistant. This is often the role of the veterinary nurse (Figure 13.24). Duties of the scrub nurse include:

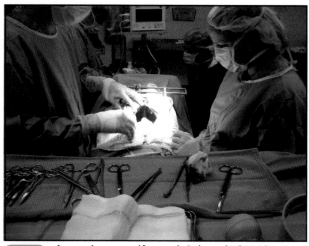

13.24 A scrub nurse (front right) assisting the surgeon and managing the instrument trolley. The trolley is raised over the patient, allowing the nurse to access the trolley and assist without moving around the table.

- Preparation of the instrument trolley for surgery. To ensure easy use of the trolley:
  - It should be set out in the same way each time
  - Instruments should be returned to the same place after use after being wiped of blood
  - Instrument handles should be placed towards the person in charge of the trolley
- Discarding contaminated instruments from the trolley
- Keeping the operating field neat and free of unnecessary instruments (those instruments not currently being used by the surgeons should be returned to the trolley)
- Anticipating the needs of the surgeon and having instruments at hand to pass as necessary
- Passing instruments to the surgeon
- Removing soiled swabs from the surgical field
- Counting swabs, needles and sutures before surgery begins (the nurse should keep a close watch on the whereabouts of these items)
- Counting disposables again before the end of surgery to ensure that nothing is accidentally left in the wound
- After surgery, identifying and separating instruments that require sharpening or other maintenance.

How to handle and pass instruments

The surgical nurse must have an understanding of the procedure to be performed so that the required instruments can be selected easily from the trolley when requested.

Instruments should be:

- Passed in a positive manner so that the surgeon can grasp them securely without looking away from the surgical field
- Placed in the surgeon's hand in the correct position to be used immediately
  - If curved, the tips should point away from the palm
- Removed from the surgical site after use
- Cleaned with a damp swab if necessary and replaced on the trolley.

Intraoperative problems

General surgical problems may include intraoperative contamination of tissues, haemorrhage and hypothermia. Additional complications may relate to the specific surgical procedure (see later) or to anaesthesia (see Chapter 12).

Intraoperative contamination of tissues

This results from incisions into already infected tissues, spillage from incisions into the gastrointestinal, urogenital or respiratory tract or breaks in the aseptic technique (such as movement of drapes and other accidents). Such contamination is minimized by careful technique and the use of swabs or towels to isolate organs prior to incision.

If contamination occurs, irrigation of the area with isotonic fluids is recommended. If parenteral antibiotics have not been given, immediate administration is helpful in most cases, with further doses of antibiotics given at the direction of the surgeon.

MRSA

Intraoperative contamination with certain organisms presents particular difficulties because of antibiotic resistance and must be avoided by particular care with asepsis. One such organism is a strain of the common bacterium *Staphylococcus aureus*. The strain that is resistant to the antibiotic methicillin is known as methicillin-resistant *Staphylococcus aureus*, abbreviated to MRSA. MRSA is carried by many people and some normal pets (e.g. in the nasal passages) and in this situation is considered to be a harmless commensal. However, when introduced into surgical wounds or catheter sites for example, MRSA can cause serious infection that is difficult to treat because the organism is resistant to many commonly used antibiotics. MRSA is a rare cause of postoperative infection in veterinary patients but is of particular concern because of the difficulty in treating the bacterium and its potential for transmission between inpatients and staff. Bacteria develop antibiotic resistance following prolonged and inappropriate exposure to antibiotics, which is one reason that antibiotics should only be used when indicated.

Haemorrhage

Blood loss is almost inevitable at the time of surgery. Careful technique and knowledge of anatomy will minimize the amount lost, as will control of bleeding points with instruments, ligatures, diathermy or pressure during surgery.

Catastrophic haemorrhage during surgery is not always readily controlled but in most cases even profuse arterial bleeding can be arrested by packing with swabs until definitive control can be established. After a measured 5 minutes of firm pressure, most sources of haemorrhage will be slowed enough for the surgeon to treat definitively.

The techniques for estimation of blood loss and decision making in blood replacement are covered in Chapter 8. In the context of surgery, blood loss can be estimated by the quantity absorbed on the surgical swabs or accumulating in the surgical suction jar. The quantity of blood absorbed by each surgical swab depends on the size and type of swab. The practice should experiment to discover how much the swabs they use absorb. In addition, during surgery the weight of used swabs can be compared with the weight of the same number of clean swabs. Unfortunately, both weighing swabs and measuring the volume collected in surgical suction will be confused by any lavage fluid used.

Small patients, such as small mammals, are at particular risk of complications due to haemorrhage and the surgeon must take particular care with haemostasis.

Hypothermia

Anaesthetized animals tend to cool because of their reduced metabolic rate and loss of homeostatic function. This can be exacerbated during surgery by exposure of viscera, with increased heat loss by convection and evaporation. Warming the fluids used during surgery and preventing the animal becoming excessively wet will also help to reduce unnecessary heat loss. Core temperature should be monitored periodically to assess the development of hypothermia and its response to corrective measures.

Severe hypothermia is life threatening, in addition to prolonging recovery from anaesthesia. Smaller patients have a relatively high surface area and low energy reserves and are at particular risk of hypothermia and failure to recover from anaesthesia. To avoid this, care is taken to avoid unnecessary cooling through all routes. Further information is given in Chapter 12.

Retained swabs

A key function of the surgical nurse is to ensure that no surgical supplies (notably swabs, instruments and needles) are left in the surgical wound. This is particularly likely during laparotomy or thoracotomy but can occur even during minor surgery. The number of swabs, instruments and needles opened for each procedure must be counted and during closure checked to ensure that all are accounted for. The use of swabs containing radio-opaque markers is recommended, particularly for surgery in the thorax and abdomen. This will make detection of retained swabs more straightforward postoperatively but does not prevent the problem. The problem can also be avoided by using only large swabs (laparotomy swabs), rather than conventional 10 cm square swabs, during abdominal or thoracic surgery. Large swabs are easier to count and less likely to be lost in a body cavity and they are equipped with tails of gauze that can be retained on the drapes when the swab is placed within the abdomen.

Surgical drains

Drains are devices implanted to remove fluids or gases from a surgical site, body cavity or wound. Drains can be considered in two groups: passive and active (Figure 13.25).

- **Passive drains**: exudate passes along or through the drain by gravity and capillary action. The commonest example of a passive drain is the Penrose (Figure 13.26). This is a soft tube, commonly of latex rubber, which acts as a conduit for fluid to exit a surgical or traumatic wound. Penrose drains are commercially available or can be fashioned from a latex surgeon's glove, for example. Less common examples of passive drains are the sump and corrugated drain, but these are rarely used in veterinary patients. A less satisfactory type of passive drain is the Seton, which is simply a piece of surgical gauze placed as a wick: there is an undesirable amount of tissue reaction to this material.

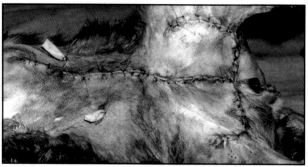

13.26 Two Penrose drains placed to manage a seroma after skin reconstruction in the groin of a cat.

- **Active drains**: a source of negative pressure is used to pull fluid (or air) out through the lumen of a tube. The most common type of active drain is the Jackson–Pratt, or grenade drain (Figure 13.27). These are available commercially and consist of a tube, whose end has multiple perforations to collect wound fluid, and a collapsible plastic chamber that generates the vacuum and acts as a reservoir for the fluid collected.

Type	Description	Advantages	Disadvantages
Passive	Tube drains by gravity and capillary action	Simply managed	Effectiveness limited by action of gravity; open to ascending infection
Penrose (Figure 13.26)	Flat tube of soft rubber	Cheap; low tissue irritation	May become folded or displaced, limiting effectiveness
Corrugated	Length of stiff ridged plastic	Resistant to folding	Greater tissue irritation
Sump drain	Double-lumen tube drain. Commonly made by modifying a Foley catheter	Greater efficiency due to ingress of air	Stiffer than Penrose, therefore greater tissue reaction
Active	Tube connected to source of vacuum	Wide variety of applications; less open to ascending infection	Greater cost and more nursing time required
Thoracic (chest) drain	Tube placed intercostally. Drained intermittently with syringe, or drained continuously by connecting to water trap or Heimlich valve	Suitable for draining pleural effusions or pneumothorax (see *BSAVA Manual of Advanced Veterinary Nursing* for more details)	
Active wound drain (Figure 13.27)	Tube placed within wound and attached to collapsible plastic reservoir	Action not limited by gravity	Greater cost than passive drain

13.25 Types of surgical drain.

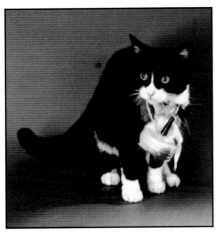

13.27 Active suction drain placed to manage a large subcutaneous abscess in the neck of a kitten.

Applications of drains

- Surgical wounds with large dead spaces – Penrose or active wound drain usually chosen.
- Localized peritonitis (e.g. associated with pancreatitis) – Penrose usually chosen, but efficacy is doubtful.
- Contaminated or infected wounds that have been closed.
- Abscesses.
- Thoracic surgery or trauma – thoracic drain used.

Care of drains

- Cover skin exit with a sterile dressing if possible, to prevent ascending infection. Dressing should be changed as necessary to prevent strikethrough of wound fluid to the outer dressing layer.
- Prevent the patient from interfering with the drain.
- Empty the reservoir of active drains as necessary in an aseptic fashion.
- Keep in place as long as necessary, i.e. until drainage has practically ceased (the drain itself will provoke some exudate formation).

- Typically drains are maintained for 3–5 days, but this is highly variable depending on the circumstances.
- Drains should not be used for longer than necessary, because of the risk of ascending infection and the requirement for increased patient care (often animals are hospitalized whilst drains are in place).
- Care of chest drains is a specialized procedure that is covered in more detail in the *BSAVA Manual of Advanced Veterinary Nursing*.

Further information on the use of drains in wound management is given in Chapter 14.

Skin closure

The skin incision is closed at the end of surgery. This task may be delegated to a veterinary nurse, under Schedule 3 of the Veterinary Surgeons Act (see Chapter 1), and the techniques are covered in more detail in the *BSAVA Manual of Advanced Veterinary Nursing*. The aim of skin closure is to appose the incised edges so that a seal quickly forms and the wound heals promptly. This is most commonly achieved by placing sutures but other methods can be used, as discussed earlier (Figure 13.28).

Sutures are placed in different patterns to achieve a variation in the way in which tissue edges are apposed. In most cases the aim is simply to appose the edges, i.e. to bring the tissue together so that the layers are aligned. In other instances suture patterns that tend to **invert** (fold the edges inwards) or **evert** (roll the edges out) are chosen. The trend in modern small animal surgery has been away from inverting and everting patterns and towards appositional patterns, with the recognition that the outcome (seal achieved, reduced scarring on healing) is generally better with an appositional pattern.

Suture patterns may be **continuous**, in which all of the length of a wound is closed by a single length of suture with a knot at either end, or **interrupted**, where the wound is closed by a number of separate stitches with individual knots (Figure 13.29). Common examples of skin suture patterns are summarized in Figure 13.30.

Method	Description	Advantages	Disadvantages
Skin sutures	Suture placed to appose the incised skin edges	Secure; flexible in application; familiar technique	Relatively time-consuming to place
Skin staples	Metal staples applied to bridge and appose the wound	Secure; rapid; well tolerated	More expensive than sutures
Skin adhesive	Cyanoacrylate glue placed over the skin surface to appose the edges	Rapid; painless; does not require removal; well tolerated	Less reliable, especially on long incisions; can cause tissue reaction if placed into wound
Adhesive strips	Self-adhesive strips placed across the wound	Well tolerated; rapid; painless	Unreliable on haired skin; insecure

13.28 Skin closure methods.

Type	Advantages	Disadvantages
Continuous	Placed more rapidly; less suture material used; allows spread of tension along suture line; produces better seal	Perceived to be less secure; potentially causes purse-string effect due to shortening of the wound
Interrupted	Perceived to be more secure, since one stitch may be lost without the incision disrupting	Slower to place; more suture material required; more material left if used in buried position

13.29 Interrupted and continuous sutures: advantages and disadvantages.

Type	Description	Particular features	Typical application
Continuous			
Simple continuous (SC)	Running stitch	Rapidly placed; prone to patient interference if used in skin; theoretically insecure	Fascia, including midline; muscle; viscera
Ford interlocking	'Blanket stitch'	Rapidly placed; better apposition than SC; slightly more secure than SC; effective seal	Long skin wounds
Intradermal/ subcuticular	Buried continuous stitch to close skin	Slower than other skin patterns; resists tension; avoids patient interference; does not require removal	Skin; presence of tension; sites prone to interference (e.g. castration)
Interrupted			
Simple interrupted appositional (SIA)	Individual stitches placed as simple loops across wound	The standard pattern; produces good apposition	Skin closure; midline closure; viscera closure
Horizontal mattress	Placed as loops with a bite on each side of wound parallel to wound edge	Produces some eversion; resists effects of tension more than SIA	Skin, especially in presence of tension
Cruciate mattress	Similar to horizontal mattress but strands cross over wound	Less eversion than above; resists effects of tension more than SIA; faster than above	Skin, especially in presence of tension
Vertical mattress	Placed as loops with a bite on each side of wound perpendicular to wound edge	Produces some eversion; resists effects of tension more than SIA; interferes with blood supply less than horizontal mattress	Skin, especially in presence of tension; most commonly used interspersed with SIA to resist effects of tension

13.30 Suture patterns summarized.

Postoperative care

Postoperative monitoring

Postoperative care begins when the last suture is placed and anaesthesia is stopped. Further detail is presented in Chapter 12, but to summarize here:

- The patient should not be left unattended until it is conscious (able to raise its head)
- Brachycephalic patients require particularly close attention, until able to stand
- The recovery area should be kept warm: an ambient temperature of 20–24°C should be adequate in most cases
- A warmer area (e.g. an incubator) should be provided for recovery of small and immature patients
- In the recovery area there should be easy access to facilities and equipment such as suction and anaesthetic machines
- Fluid therapy, as prescribed by the veterinary surgeon, should be monitored
- Urine output should be monitored, as requested by the veterinary surgeon
- The patient should be observed for signs of pain, and analgesia should be arranged as required
- The wound should be inspected periodically for signs of haemorrhage or other complications.

Postoperative problems

Postoperative problems are often specific to certain procedures and are discussed later; those related to anaesthesia are included in Chapter 12.

General postoperative problems include:

- Delayed wound healing, wound infection and patient interference with the wound (see Chapter 14)
- Prolonged recovery from anaesthesia (see Chapter 12)
- Pain (see Chapter 12)
- Anorexia
- Haemorrhage
- Inflammation.

Anorexia and ileus

Patients are expected to show an interest in food within a few hours at most after elective surgery. Recovery after emergency surgery is expected to be more prolonged, but anorexia of more than 12 hours is a serious cause of concern. It may indicate a significant surgical complication, the continuing effect of concurrent disease, pain or ileus. Whatever the cause, failure of food intake will further delay recovery, slow wound healing and prolong ileus.

Anorexia should be managed by treating the underlying cause and by providing assisted feeding as required (see Chapter 9).

Ileus is defined as loss of gastrointestinal movement. It is caused by disruption to food intake, pain, abdominal inflammation (following laparotomy), or disturbance to gastrointestinal flora in herbivores. Although it is a rare complication in dogs and cats, it is common in small herbivores, such as rabbits, in which it may prove fatal. In these species, the causes of ileus must be carefully avoided and if anorexia is observed it must be managed aggressively. Important components of prevention are avoiding food restriction, giving adequate analgesia and appropriate use of antibiotics. If ileus is diagnosed, oral intake must be encouraged, together with assisted feeding and the use of drugs to promote intestinal motility (e.g. metoclopramide).

Haemorrhage as a complication of recovery

Shock can occur during recovery as a complication of surgery or be due to a pre-existing condition. The most common cause of postoperative shock is hypovolaemia; other causes may be respiratory or cardiac insufficiency.

Hypovolaemic shock may be due to pre-existing conditions (e.g. preoperative dehydration that has not been corrected) or haemorrhage. The signs are:

- Tachycardia (rapid heart rate)
- Weak, rapid pulse
- Shallow, rapid respiration
- Pale or cyanotic mucous membranes
- Cold extremities
- Slow capillary refill time
- Delayed recovery from anaesthesia.

Haemorrhage from the wound can be an indication that hypovolaemia is developing but can be misleading: internal haemorrhage may not be evident at the incision and trivial wound haemorrhage is common. Internal haemorrhage after abdominal surgery may manifest as abdominal distension or abdominal pain. The production of large volumes of sanguinous wound fluid from drains also suggests that haemorrhage is occurring: measuring the volume and PCV of this fluid can be a useful guide to the severity of haemorrhage.

Inflammation

Inflammation is the way in which tissues react to injury, which may be chemical, thermal, infectious, or physical. The signs and processes of inflammation are covered in Chapter 14. Key features of inflammation of the surgical wound are:

- Erythema (redness)
- Oedema (swelling)
- Local pain
- Interference with function (e.g. lameness).

The inflammatory process is in general beneficial to the individual and results in an attempt to overcome the effects of the initial injury. For example, the inflammatory fluid contains cells of the immune system that help to overcome infection. However, the inflammatory processes can result in further tissue damage and unnecessary pain; therefore inflammation is often treated to overcome these adverse effects. Ideally treatment should remove the inciting cause – for example, antibiotic therapy to eliminate wound infection, or replacement of excessively tight skin sutures. Treatment to reduce the degree of inflammation is also used:

- Drug therapy – non-steroidal anti-inflammatory drugs (NSAIDs)
- Corticosteroid therapy – only used in extreme cases, because of potentially deleterious effects on wound healing and potentiation of infection
- Cold compresses – used in the first 1–2 days after surgery
- Warm compresses – used thereafter.

Patient interference with wounds

The causes of patient interference and some methods to prevent it are shown in Figures 13.31 to 13.34 (see also Chapter 14).

Cause	Avoidance/prevention
Infection	Appropriate initial wound management and antibiotic therapy
Contamination or presence of foreign body	Appropriate initial wound management
Tissue trauma during surgery	Careful surgical technique
Skin suture irritation	Place skin sutures loosely. Use non-irritating suture material
Pain	Analgesia
Dermatitis (clipper rash)	Careful skin preparation with clean sharp clipper blades. Avoid shaving the skin. Avoid scrubbing area with abrasive materials. Treat pre-existing dermatitis prior to surgery

13.31 Causes of patient interference with a wound.

Method	Application
Attention to factors in Figure 13.16	All surgical procedures
Bandaging	All accessible sites (areas such as the perineum, groin and axilla are difficult to bandage without causing other difficulties)
Elizabethan collar (Figure 13.33)	All sites except neck, distal limb and tail
Devices to prevent body flexion (stiff collars, body brace) (Figure 13.34)	Wounds of trunk and proximal limbs
Tranquillizers	Used with caution and often ineffective alone. Long-term use of questionable justification
Topical bitter substances	Sites prone to chewing rather than rubbing or scratching (e.g. not head or perineum)

13.32 Methods of preventing a patient from interfering with a wound.

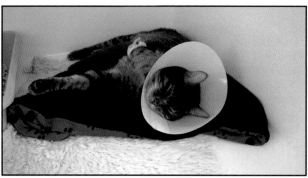

13.33 Elizabethan collar applied to prevent a patient from interfering with a wound.

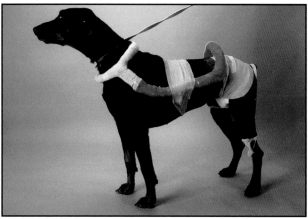

13.34 Body brace applied to prevent a patient interfering with a bandage over the pelvic area.

Routine postoperative checks

The earliest time that veterinary patients can be discharged is when they are able to stand unaided and walk. In addition, before discharge, postoperative pain must be controlled (if necessary, a course of oral analgesia will be prescribed by the veterinary surgeon) and there must be no expectation of immediate postoperative complications. Most patients are discharged on the same day if elective surgery takes place in the morning.

At the time of discharge, the nurse must ensure that the client has received instructions on postoperative care, as decided by the surgeon, and has collected postoperative medication or prescriptions and any special food. It is often better to meet the client and talk about postoperative care before the animal is returned to them.

The client will also be informed of what postoperative checks are required. The timing and number of these depend on practice policy and the procedure performed, but may include:

- Telephone consultation on the day after discharge – to check the general wellbeing of the patient and to ensure that the owner understands the postoperative care instructions
- Early postoperative check at 3–5 days after surgery – to ensure that the patient is making expected postoperative progress (e.g. return to normal appetite, use of the operated limb)
  - Typically, any dressing covering the surgical wound will be removed at this time and the wound inspected
  - There should be minimal swelling, an absence of discharge and little or no local inflammation
  - Limb bandages may be replaced
  - This check is often carried out by the nurse, who should consult the veterinary surgeon if there are any concerns
- Standard postoperative check/skin suture removal – 10 days after routine surgery
  - The patient is re-examined and skin sutures are removed
  - At this time, the wound edges should be firmly adherent to each other, with no wound discharge and minimal local inflammation
  - This check is also often carried out by a veterinary nurse.

Further information on discharging patients is given in Chapter 2.

Skin suture removal

Skin sutures are removed once the strength of the incision is sufficient to prevent it reopening in normal activity.

- Typically the sutures are removed after 10 days if healing has progressed normally, but they may be removed earlier (7 days).
- Delayed wound healing requires sutures to be left in place longer, but rarely beyond 14 days.
- Sutures left in place too long tend to produce more scarring and irritation to the patient.

Sutures are usually removed from the conscious animal, but sedation or anaesthesia is used in some cases, such as: very nervous or aggressive animals; perineal surgery (especially urethrostomy, when it is important that all sutures are removed); ear surgery (because the area is very sensitive); eye surgery.

Technique

■ Sutures are removed with suture scissors or with a stitch-cutting blade. In both cases, one end is held up so that the blade can be passed under the knot and one piece of the suture cut so that as little material as possible is pulled through the skin as it is removed.
■ Ensure that all sutures are removed. This may necessitate bathing off any scabs or exudate that may be present and may obscure the sutures.
■ Skin staples are removed with staple removers supplied with the stapler. In other ways, the same considerations as those for skin sutures apply.
■ Incisions closed with surgical adhesive do not require suture removal. The glue is sloughed once healing is complete.
■ Incisions closed with a subcuticular (buried) suture pattern do not usually require suture removal since an absorbable suture material is used.

Even when techniques are used that do not require suture removal, the animal is inspected at around 10 days to ensure that healing is progressing normally.

Other postoperative checks

These are not required after routine elective surgery but may be scheduled in other cases. For example, follow-up radiography is usually carried out 4–6 weeks after fracture repair. Other checks may be required to monitor the disease process (e.g. neoplasia) or to adjust postoperative medication.

Surgical diseases and their nursing care

This section includes a general discussion of disease processes of surgical importance and subsections dealing with common surgical conditions and specific organ systems.

Orthopaedic injuries
Fractures

Definition

■ *Fracture* is disruption in the continuity of a bone.

Most fractures occur following trauma, such as falls or road traffic accidents. Occasionally bones may fracture following trivial injuries, or even spontaneously. In the latter cases, this is usually because the bone strength is altered by an existing disease, such as a tumour. These are known as pathological fractures.

Fractures are classified in a number of ways (Figure 13.35) and can be treated in several ways, depending on the bone affected, the severity of the disruption, the age of the animal and its size (Figures 13.36 to 13.38). Details of cast application and care are in Chapter 14. Details of complex fracture repair will be found in the *BSAVA Manual of Advanced Veterinary Nursing*.

Classification	Description and comments
Closed	Overlying skin is intact. During first aid and initial management, care should be taken to prevent the fracture fragments pushing through the skin surface, resulting in an open fracture
Open (previously known as *compound*)	Associated with a break in the nearby skin surface. Infection of fracture site more likely and early treatment is important to successful outcome
Simple	Containing a single fracture line and therefore only two fragments. Simple fractures of long bone may be *transverse* (break is across the shaft), *spiral* (break tends to run along the shaft) or *oblique* (break is between these positions)
Incomplete (also known as *greenstick*)	Does not completely disrupt the continuity of a long bone, i.e. one cortex is intact. Usually seen in young animals
Comminuted	Containing more than one fracture line and several fragments
Avulsion	Resulting in the separation of the point of attachment of a muscle or tendon to a bone from the main part of the bone. The pull of the muscle tends to displace fragment from its original site
Condylar	Involving the condyles of a long bone (such as the distal femur or humerus). Needs accurate reduction and internal fixation to prevent interference with joint function

13.35 Classification of fractures.

Factor	Effect on bone healing	Suitable methods
Age of animal	Delayed in older animals	Internal fixation preferred in older animals. External coaptation may be suitable in young animals with greenstick or simple closed fractures
Body size	Greater body weight destabilizes fracture sites	Internal fixation preferred in large dogs
Athleticism	Active animals place greater demands on bones during healing. Working dogs require both early return to full function and optimal long-term results	Internal fixation preferred in active animals. Internal fixation offers early return to function and best outcome in working dogs
Bone affected	Distal limb fractures can be stabilized by external coaptation	Internal fixation preferred for proximal fractures
Severity of disruption	Presence of multiple fragments reduces stability and delays healing. Presence of multiple fragments complicates placement of internal fixation	External fixator may reduce need for complete reconstruction
Stability of reconstructed fragments	Instability of fragments reduces stability, delays healing and can result in deformity	Unstable fractures require internal fixation or external fixator

13.36   Factors in selection of method of fracture treatment.

Method	Application
First aid methods (see also Chapters 7 and 14)	
Cage confinement	Restricting voluntary movement is effective in many cases and is recommended for fractures of spine and of limbs when leg is fractured above stifle or elbow
Dressings	Apply sterile or clean dressing to cover open wounds
Pressure dressing	Haemorrhage controlled by applying firm dressing over the area (tourniquets *not* recommended)
Splint	Fractures of limbs below stifle or elbow can be immobilized by application of commercial or homemade splint
Robert Jones bandage	Fractures of limbs below stifle or elbow can be immobilized by Robert Jones bandage (see Figure 14.22)
Definitive methods	
External coaptation	Splints, extension splints and casts: Suitable for fractures of limbs below elbow or stifle. *Advantages*: cheap to apply; technically simple. *Disadvantages*: limited application; poor healing of unstable fractures (comminuted, spiral); may result in pressure sores; immobilization of limb can cause fracture disease (joint stiffness, muscle wasting)
Internal fixation (IF)	Placement of metal implants to hold fragments rigidly in apposition during healing. *Advantages*: applicable to a wide variety of fractures; potentially allows rapid return to function; avoids fracture disease. *Disadvantages*: relatively expensive in terms of materials and instrumentation; can be time consuming; requires greater technical skill
	Intramedullary pin (Steinman pin) (Figure 13.38a): Long straight pin placed within medullary cavity across fracture line to fix fragments in alignment. Placed at surgery (open pinning) or percutaneously (closed pinning) using Jacob's chuck. Widely used for long bone fractures in cats and smaller dogs. *Advantages*: little specialist equipment required; implant relatively inexpensive. *Disadvantages*: not suitable for fractures prone to collapse in length or rotation; less suitable for big dogs than other internal fixations
	Rush pins: Less commonly used method of IF. Used in pairs to stabilize supracondylar fractures
	Kirschner and arthrodesis wires (Figure 13.38b): Similar to Steinman pins and may be used in a similar way in small bones. Used with other techniques to fix small bone fragments
	Cerclage wires (Figure 13.38c): Flexible surgical steel wire used to supplement other forms of IF. Supplied in reels and cut to length as required. Typically used to repair avulsion fractures, osteotomies and long bones
	Bone plates and screws (Figure 13.38d,e): Plates attached to bones across fracture sites and held in place with screws. Traditional types of plate (Venables, Sherman) attached with self-tapping screws (i.e. screws cut threads within bone as they are placed). Compression plates (e.g. ASIF DCP) can allow greater stability and faster healing; attached with screws placed into holes in which threads have already been cut (tapped). Plates are a relatively expensive and technically demanding method of fracture repair
External fixation	**Kirschner–Ehmer apparatus or Ilazirov fixator:** Pins placed through skin into fracture fragments; pins are linked together externally by frame or bolts and rods (Figure 13.38f,g). Increasing use for complicated fractures and for repair of limb deformities. Placed open or closed (i.e. with or without a surgical approach to fracture site)

13.37   Methods of fracture treatment.

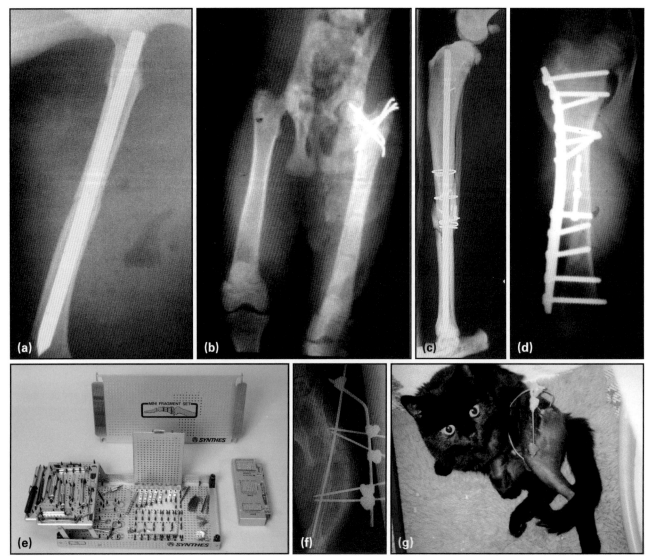

13.38 Equipment for fracture treatment. **(a)** Radiograph of intramedullary pin positioned to repair a long bone fracture (lateral view of femur). **(b)** Radiograph of Kirschner wires used to reconstruct multiple small bone fragments (fracture of femoral neck and trochanteric osteotomy). **(c)** Radiograph of cerclage wires combined with intramedullary pin to repair comminuted fracture of long bone (feline tibia). **(d)** Radiograph of bone plate and screws used to repair long bone fracture (comminuted canine femoral fracture). **(e)** Bone plate kit, consisting of plates, screws and the specialist equipment used to place them. This is the Mini Fragment set of the AO/ASIF system of internal fixation. **(f)** Radiograph of external fixator used to repair severely comminuted feline femoral fracture. **(g)** Same cat as in (f) with external fixator in place. This will be removed 6–8 weeks after surgery, once the fracture has healed. (All except (e) courtesy of Dr Martin Owen, University of Bristol)

Nursing considerations for fracture repair

Preoperative care

Fractures often occur as a result of major trauma. As a result, the animal is often also in shock and may have concurrent thoracic or abdominal injuries. The nurse must take account of these in establishing a treatment plan that will help to stabilize the patient's condition before treatment of the fracture is carried out. Typically, these injuries are a greater threat to life than the orthopaedic condition. Further information on the assessment and initial treatment of trauma patients and their wounds is found in Chapters 7 and 14.

Fractures and other orthopaedic injuries are painful. The nurse should work with the veterinary surgeon to plan and deliver an analgesic regime (see Chapter 12), which will include both drug therapy and physical means of pain control, e.g. fracture stabilization. It is bad practice and unethical to withhold analgesia in a misguided attempt to encourage the patient not to move.

In order to prevent further tissue damage, movement of the affected body part should be restricted. For compliant patients with distal limb injury, this can be achieved by applying an appropriate support bandage (e.g. modified Robert Jones). In other cases, simply confining the patient to a small cage may be preferred. Struggling with an injured patient is likely to worsen the situation, as may applying a dressing that does not provide useful immobilization but increases the weight of the limb (fractures above the midshaft of the tibia or radius, for example). Restricting movement will also reduce the patient's discomfort.

Skin preparation

Once the patient is anaesthetized, the hair on the affected limb should be clipped extensively to allow the surgeon excellent access and to manipulate the limb whilst maintaining asepsis. The clipped area should be circumferential and typically includes the thoracic wall for fractures of the forelimb above the carpus and the hemipelvis for hindlimb fractures above the tarsus. The surgeon may also ask for separate areas of clipping for bone graft harvesting (over the point of the shoulder or wing of the ilium) and epidural anaesthesia. For hindlimb surgery, a purse-string suture may be placed around the anus and a urethral catheter may be helpful. If the foot is not to be included in the surgical field, it can be covered in a bandage, glove or bag before skin preparation is undertaken. Routine skin scrubbing is carried out before the patient is moved to theatre.

The surgeon should be consulted on how the patient is positioned in theatre. Often a 'hanging limb' preparation is used: the limb is suspended from the toes in moderate tension so that the entire surface can be prepared (see Figure 13.42). This can be done with a bandage around the foot or a towel clip on one toe. This position may also help the surgeon to realign the fracture fragments.

A final skin scrub is carried out after positioning. Infection after orthopaedic surgery is a particular problem and special care is indicated during the final preparation: for example, the use of sterile gloves and sterile scrub solutions, even if this is not the usual procedure in the clinic. The surgeon may also carry out a final skin preparation with alcoholic skin disinfectant and sponge-holding forceps.

In addition to conventional field drapes, linen 'footbags', sterile cohesive bandages or stockinette may be useful for limbs, particularly to cover the toes. When the surgeon is ready to drape the patient, the limb can be lowered on to the drapes or the surgeon may keep the limb in suspension during surgery. To reduce tissue contamination further, the surgeon may also apply adhesive 'incise' drapes over the skin exposed in the surgical field.

Perioperative care

If surgical repair (internal fixation) of a fracture is undertaken, this should follow patient stabilization. Often initial radiographs will have been taken under sedation, but typically the surgeon will require further films to be taken under anaesthesia before surgery, with at least two views of the affected area and of the unaffected limb for comparison. Radiographs of the thorax and abdomen are recommended after significant trauma, to assess for other injuries.

Anaesthesia will lead to loss of muscular support of injured limbs and the nurse should take care to avoid excessive movement of the limb that will worsen tissue damage. Patients with open fractures also require wound care and steps should be taken to avoid further contamination of the tissues during manipulation of the limb.

Postoperative care

At the end of the procedure and before the end of anaesthesia, it is common practice to take further radiographs to confirm that the procedure has been successful and as a 'baseline' for later follow-up examinations. After radiography, the surgeon will often require the limb to be placed in a cast, splint or support bandage; the nurse should prepare the materials for this during the surgery to avoid delay.

Similar principles of nursing care can be applied to other orthopaedic surgery. Frequently, a prolonged anaesthetic is required and the nursing team should be prepared for this, by taking steps to avoid patient hypothermia, for example.

At the time of discharge from the clinic, the nurse should ensure that the client understands the aftercare required, such as the care of the dressing or cast, as well as the exercise regime directed by the surgeon and the necessity for re-examination. Many clinics use written discharge instructions to ensure that the necessary information is available to the client. In addition to the usual suture-removal visit, there are likely to be requirements for bandage changes and follow-up radiographs (e.g. at 4-weekly intervals after surgery).

Luxations

> ### Definitions
>
> - *Luxation* is displacement of joint surfaces from their normal articulation (synonym: *dislocation*).
> - *Subluxation* is incomplete luxation (i.e. some of the articular surface remains in contact).

Some luxations arise from congenital malformations of the joint structures. For example, small breeds of dog often have poorly developed articulations of the femur and patella resulting in patellar luxation. *Congenital luxations* are treated by surgical procedures that aim to reproduce the joint architecture of the normal animal.

Other luxations arise as a result of trauma, causing separation of the joint surfaces, often with damage to the supporting structures of the joint (joint capsule and ligaments) and even fractures of the bones forming the joints. *Traumatic luxations* are treated by reduction of the joint surfaces (restoring to a normal position) and repair of the supporting structures if necessary. Often the joint is supported in a normal alignment after reduction by placement of a splint, bandage or casts.

Common luxations and their treatment are summarized in Figure 13.39.

Surgical nursing for joint surgery

Surgery of the shoulder, hip, elbow and stifle is relatively common in small animal practice. The diseases encountered are summarized in Figure 13.40 and the common surgical procedures in Figure 13.41.

Luxation	Cause	Treatment
Hip (coxofemoral joint)	External trauma (e.g. road traffic accident). Also occurs with minimal trauma in animals with pre-existing hip dysplasia	Recent injuries without bone damage and with normal anatomy can be managed by open or closed reduction. A supporting bandage (Ehmer sling, see Chapter 14) and exercise restriction may be used postoperatively. Recurrent cases may need surgical stabilization (placement of surgical implants to support joint), with additional external support. In animals with hip dysplasia or fractures, reduction alone is unlikely to be successful. These are often managed by excision arthroplasty (femoral head and neck excision), which removes the joint surfaces and allows a false joint to form
Patella	Congenital dysplasia of the joint	Mild cases in small breeds: conservative treatment. More severe cases: surgical reconstruction required (sulcoplasty, tibial crest transposition, femoral osteotomy)
Temporomandibular joint	External trauma to head (e.g. road traffic accident)	In absence of local fractures, managed by closed reduction. Postoperative support (e.g. tape muzzle) may be required
Hock (tarsus) and carpus	External trauma (e.g. long falls or severe athletic injuries) or degenerative changes to joint and supporting ligaments	Rarely amenable to reduction and conservative treatment. Require internal fixation and often arthrodesis (permanent surgical fixation of joint)
Digits ('knocked-up toe')	External trauma, usually during exercise	Pet dogs: digital amputation often most practical. Working dogs: internal fixation or arthrodesis are preferred

13.39 Common luxations and their treatment.

Joint	Disease	Cause and features	Treatment
Hip	Hip dysplasia	Congenital with a genetic component. Presents early in life with gait abnormalities and pain or late in life with arthritis. Common in dogs, rare in cats. Radiographic screening scheme in place for breeding dogs	In young dogs: exercise restriction In the absence of secondary arthritis, joint reconstruction may be considered (e.g. triple pelvic osteotomy). In older dogs with arthritis, managed medically (e.g. with NSAIDs) or occasionally by excision arthroplasty or joint replacement
	Luxation	See Figure 13.39	See Figure 13.39
	Fracture of acetabulum or femoral neck and head	External trauma	Internal fixation if practical. Excision arthroplasty if not possible to reconstruct
	Legg–Calvé–Perthes disease (synonyms: Perthes, avascular necrosis of femoral head)	Often genetic (e.g. in West Highland White Terrier). Rare in cats. Causes lameness in young dogs	Excision arthroplasty
Elbow	Elbow dysplasia (osteochondrosis, elbow incongruity, fractured coronoid process, coronoid disease)	Congenital with a genetic component. Radiographic screening scheme in place for breeding dogs	In young dogs: exercise restriction. In absence of secondary arthritis: arthroscopic treatment or joint realignment (e.g. ulnar osteotomy) may be considered. In older dogs with arthritis: managed medically (e.g. with NSAIDs)
	Fractures of humeral condyles	Traumatic. Particularly common in spaniels, which may have genetic predisposition to poor bone strength at this site. Severity varies: may be one condyle only (usually medial), or both condyles and distal shaft (T or Y fracture)	Internal fixation required for acceptable outcome. Technically challenging for Y fractures in particular
Stifle	Cruciate ligament injury	Occasionally traumatic but most cases in dogs reflect a degeneration of the ligaments. Most common, is cranial cruciate ligament (CCL or ACL) rupture Occasionally, traumatic injuries cause rupture of the cranial and caudal ligaments and of the collateral ligaments concurrently. Often concurrent meniscal damage. Usually develop arthritis later, regardless of treatment	Conservative management may be used in small breeds. In most dogs, surgical exploration of the stifle with stabilization of the joint is appropriate. Various surgeries described: over-the-top technique (OTT), lateral femeropatellar suture, tibial plateau levelling osteotomy (TPLO). For severe disruptions, external fixation is required

13.40 Diseases of the major joints. (continues) ▶

Joint	Disease	Cause and features	Treatment
Stifle *continued*	Patellar luxation	See Figure 13.39	See Figure 13.39
	Fractures of femoral condyles	Traumatic	Internal fixation required for acceptable outcome
	Fracture of tibial crest	Traumatic. Affects skeletally immature dogs	Internal fixation required for acceptable outcome
	Osteochondrosis (synonyms: osteochondritis dissecans, OCD)	Congenital with a genetic component	In young dogs: exercise restriction. In absence of secondary arthritis: arthroscopic treatment or arthrotomy may be considered. In older dogs with arthritis: managed medically (e.g. with NSAIDs)
Shoulder	Osteochondrosis (synonyms: osteochondritis dissecans, OCD)	Congenital with a genetic component	In young dogs: exercise restriction. In absence of secondary arthritis: arthroscopic treatment or arthrotomy may be considered. In older dogs with arthritis: managed medically (e.g. with NSAIDs)

13.40 (continued) Diseases of the major joints.

Procedure	Description	Common application
Arthrotomy	Surgical exploration of a joint	Cranial cruciate ligament rupture
Arthroscopy	Endoscopic exploration of a joint	Elbow osteochondrosis
Arthrodesis	Surgical fusion of a joint	Tarsal luxation
Arthroplasty	Surgical procedure to change the shape of a joint	Tibial plateau levelling osteotomy
Excision arthroplasty	Excision of a joint to leave a soft tissue 'false joint'	Fractures of the femoral head or neck (excision of femoral head and neck)
Joint replacement	Excision of a joint and replacement with an artificial joint (prosthesis)	Total hip replacement

13.41 Summary of surgical procedures of the major joints.

Preoperative care

Unless the disease is traumatic in origin, many of these patients are young healthy dogs and no special care is required.

Skin preparation

Similar comments apply as for fracture repair (above), notably the importance of wide clipping to allow limb manipulation and the particular importance of aseptic technique. For hip surgery and shoulder surgery, the trunk and limb to at least the stifle or shoulder should be prepared circumferentially. For stifle or elbow surgery, the limb should be prepared circumferentially from the hip or shoulder to the foot. In all cases, a 'hanging limb' preparation is ideal (Figure 13.42). Water-resistant disposable drapes are used during arthroscopy because of the requirement for joint lavage.

Perioperative care

Radiographs are often taken during surgical anaesthesia, if not already done. For many joint surgeries, particular instruments (e.g. Gelpi retractors, joint distractor, graft passers) are required and the surgeon must be consulted in good time to ensure that these are available.

If arthroscopy is to be used, the equipment (scope and tower) must be prepared and placed in theatre.

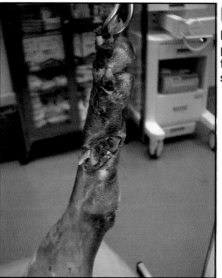

13.42 Hanging limb preparation for limb surgery.

Postoperative care

The requirements vary and the surgeon must be consulted. Often, a support dressing or modified Robert-Jones bandage is placed for a few days postoperatively and the materials for this should be prepared (see Chapter 14). Exercise requirements and physiotherapy regime should be discussed with the veterinary surgeon and owner.

Soft tissue injuries
Hernias and ruptures

> ### Definitions
>
> Hernias and ruptures are defects in the body wall through which organs can protrude (prolapse).
>
> - *Hernias* are enlargements of existing anatomical holes.
> - *Ruptures* are tears that appear where there were previously sheets of tissue.
> - *Reducible hernias* are those where the protruding tissues can be returned to a normal position by pressure, without enlarging the hole.
> - *Irreducible hernias* are those where they cannot.
> - *Incarceration* is the reduction of blood supply to the contents of irreducible hernias so that the tissue is at risk of necrosis.
> - *Hernia ring* is the border of the tissue in which a hernia is present.

Common sites of hernias in cats and dogs are:

- *Umbilical* – abdominal fat or organs protrude through the umbilical canal of the ventral abdominal wall
- *Hiatal* – abdominal organs (usually the stomach) protrude through the oesophageal hiatus of the diaphragm
- *Inguinal* – abdominal organs (such as the bladder) protrude through the inguinal canal of the groin.

Common types of rupture are:

- *Diaphragm* – a tear in the diaphragm, usually as the result of trauma, allows abdominal organs (such as the liver) to enter the thorax
- *Perineum* – degeneration of the muscles of the pelvic floor allows pelvic structures (such as the rectum) to enter a subcutaneous position next to the anus
- *Incisional* – breakdown of a surgical repair of the abdominal wall allowing abdominal tissues to protrude into a subcutaneous position.

Ruptures and hernias are treated to prevent organ prolapse and incarceration. Surgical treatment consists of:

- Reduction of the herniated tissues (replacement into their normal position)
- Closure of the hernia ring (the ring can usually be closed by placing sutures across the hernia ring)
- Occasionally, patching the hole with an implant of synthetic material such as plastic or steel mesh.

Nursing care of patients with hernias and ruptures

This is a wide variety of conditions and no general advice can be given. The care required depends on the site of the rupture and any complications associated with it (see later for nursing care based on different organ systems).

Abscesses

> ### Definition
>
> - An *abscess* is a discrete collection of purulent material (pus). It is often surrounded by a wall of inflamed and fibrous tissue, sometimes known as a *pyogenic membrane*.

Superficial abscesses usually develop after introduction of bacteria into tissue by sharp trauma, such as animal bites or infected surgical procedures. Clinical signs of an abscess include:

- Local swelling (due to the presence of a pocket of pus and local oedema)
- Local pain
- Warmth and erythema of the overlying skin
- Systemic signs of toxaemia (e.g. pyrexia, depression, anorexia, tachycardia)
- Discharge of purulent fluid from the area if the overlying skin bursts (described as 'pointing').

Nursing care of patients with abscesses
Preoperative care

The degree of preoperative care depends on the degree to which the abscess is affecting the patient systemically. Anorectic patients and those with pyrexia may require preoperative stabilization with fluid therapy, analgesia and antibiotics, for example. For uncomplicated cat-bite abscesses, minimal preoperative care is required.

Perioperative care

Superficial abscesses (e.g. subcutaneous cat-bite abscesses) can be lanced by a stab incision in the overlying skin, made with a scalpel blade. Depending on the position of the abscess and the temperament of the patient, this may require local anaesthesia, sedation, general anaesthesia or none of these. The cavity is then flushed (lavaged) with a solution such as sterile saline to dilute and remove infected material or with an antiseptic solution. Many antiseptics irritate tissue and must be used cautiously.

Preparation for lancing a cat-bite abscess

1. Check with the veterinary surgeon on how the patient is to be restrained (manually, sedation, anaesthesia).
2. Prepare:
   - Simple surgical kit (scalpel handle and blade, scissors, haemostats, rat-tooth forceps, needle holders) in case suturing is required
   - Warm bag of sterile saline, sterile bowl and syringes
   - Appropriate dilution of disinfectant, if wished.
3. Clip and scrub an area centred on the point of the abscess, with margins of 5 cm or more, both to maintain asepsis and to prevent contamination of the coat.

4. The abscess is lanced with a stab incision.
5. The cavity is expressed and then flushed copiously.
6. Clean and dry the surrounding skin and hair.
7. Apply a dressing or drain, if required.
8. Check what postoperative care, medication and follow-up are required.

Postoperative care

Although abscesses, such as those arising from cat bites, usually carry a good prognosis and can be managed in a straightforward fashion, in other cases they can be an indication of significant concurrent diseases. Deeper abscesses (e.g. within the prostate gland) may be opened and flushed at surgery, and a soft latex Penrose drain then placed within them to exit through the nearby skin and allow continued drainage of infection. The underlying disease should also be addressed. Abscesses around the face, especially in rabbits, are often an indication of dental disease and local treatment alone is not helpful. Dental surgery is often required and the prognosis can be poor.

Ulcers

Definitions

- An *ulcer* is a full-thickness loss of epithelium at a tissue surface (skin or mucous membranes of other organs).
- *Decubitus ulcers* occur over bony prominences as a result of skin trauma, reduced local circulation, local infection and poor tissue healing. They readily develop in animals that are recumbent and systemically ill.

Loss of epithelium can result from a number of processes, including:

- Trauma
- Local infection
- Neoplasia
- Drug therapy (notably the NSAID class of analgesics, which can cause ulceration of the gastrointestinal tract)
- Foreign bodies (e.g. corneal ulceration as a result of ocular foreign bodies).

Once ulceration has developed, further damage to underlying tissues is possible; for example, perforation of the stomach and local infection is common.
Ulcers are treated by:

- Removing the underlying cause
- Local therapy to improve tissue healing (including wound dressing, see Chapter 14)
- Surgical excision and closure of adjacent normal tissue if necessary.

Nursing care of patients with ulcers

This is a wide variety of conditions and no general advice can be given. The care required depends on the site of the ulcer and any complications associated with it (see later for nursing care based on different organ systems). For patients with skin ulcers, particular consideration should be given to why the ulcer has arisen and to treating the underlying cause (see Chapter 14 for details of wound care).

Fistulas and discharging sinuses

Definitions

- A *fistula* is a connection between two surfaces lined with mucous membrane.
- A *discharging sinus* is an opening in the skin lined by granulation tissue.

Fistulas commonly develop after trauma to tissues and, once established, require surgical repair. One example is the oronasal fistula (see below). Occasionally congenital fistulas are encountered: for example, a connection between the vagina and rectum in bitches (rectovaginal fistula). Congenital clefts of the palate may be considered as oronasal fistulas.

A discharging sinus commonly arises as a result of chronic infection of deeper tissues, often due to the presence of a foreign body. The commonest example is anal furunculosis (see later).

Nursing care

The nursing care depends on the site of the disease process (see later for nursing care based on different organ systems). Many discharging sinuses are the result of chronic infections, often with an underlying foreign body, and are managed with a combination of antibiotic therapy and surgical exploration to identify an underlying cause. Tissue samples may be taken for pathological and bacteriological examination.

Neoplasia and tumours

Definitions

- *Tumour* is a non-specific term usually referring to uncontrolled growth of cells without physiological cause.
- This usually results in swellings which are more correctly termed *neoplasms*.

Neoplasms can affect any tissue of the body and can be benign or malignant ('cancerous').

- *Benign* neoplasms:
  - Tend not to invade surrounding tissues
  - Are often slow growing
  - May be cured by surgical excision.
- *Malignant* neoplasms:
  - Invade surrounding tissues and/or spread (metastasize) via the lymphatics or blood to other tissues
  - Often enlarge in size more rapidly than benign tumours
  - Are more difficult to cure surgically or by other methods.

Tumours are named according to the tissue of origin and their tendency to malignancy:

- *-oma* refers to a benign tumour
- *-carcinoma* refers to a malignant tumour arising from epithelial tissue
- *-sarcoma* refers to a malignant tumour arising from solid tissue.

Specific tumours will be mentioned in the sections on different organ systems below.

Signs of neoplasia may be local or systemic.

- *Local*:
  - Signs caused by the presence of the tumour mass (such as obstruction of viscera, ulceration, impediment of movement).
- *Systemic* (paraneoplastic syndrome):
  - Release of hormonally active substances, such as pseudoparathyroid hormone – this results in hypercalcaemia, a frequent finding in dogs with lymphoma
  - Cachexia – muscle wasting due to increased catabolism and often accompanied by anorexia
  - Histamine release – a feature of canine mast cell tumours (mastocytoma), resulting in anaphylaxis and gastric ulceration.

Determining the prognosis for tumours

The prognosis for a disease is a statement of the way in which it is likely to progress and the way in which it may respond to treatment. The prognosis for tumours of different types varies tremendously and so it is important to determine the tumour type so that the correct treatment can be chosen and the owner can be informed of the likely outcome. Information used in assessing prognosis in neoplasia includes:

- History – some tumours (rarely) affect typical breeds and ages of animal
- Appearance – some tumours (rarely) have a typical appearance
- Presence of attachment to deeper tissues – malignant tumours more frequently adhere to surrounding tissues
- Presence of ulceration – malignant superficial tumours often ulcerate
- Radiography and ultrasonography – to look for evidence of metastasis to other sites (such as the lungs and liver)
- Biopsy – to determine the type of tumour and the prognosis. A piece of tissue is removed from an animal for laboratory examination (Figures 13.43 and 13.44); this is usually the most reliable way in which a prognosis can be made
- Blood samples – to look for evidence of systemic involvement (specific paraneoplastic features, such as hypercalcaemia) or general debility
- Bone marrow biopsy – to assess extent of tumours affecting the haemopoietic system (lymphoma, mast cell tumours).

Treatment of neoplasia

Neoplasia can be managed medically (chemotherapy), with radiation therapy or surgically. Each has a role in cancer therapy in small animals, but in many cases surgery remains the most important approach. The rationale for choice of therapy is outlined in Figure

Application	Advantages and disadvantages
Fine-needle aspirate biopsy (FNAB)	
Any swelling, also bone marrow and solid organs (liver, etc.)	Quick and easy; rarely requires anaesthesia and no special apparatus. Cytological processing also rapid. Limited information on tissue type and prognosis in most cases
Needle core biopsy (Tru-cut, Jamshidi) (Figure 13.44)	
Any swelling or organ that can be reached at surgery or percutaneously	Relatively fast to perform. Often percutaneous samples can be taken without general anaesthesia. Gives more tissue information than above, but still limited by small sample size. Requires specialized needle
Incisional (wedge biopsy)	
Skin masses or organs/masses that can be reached surgically	Usually requires general anaesthesia. No special instruments required. A surgical procedure. Greater tissue mass acquired increases information, particularly on invasiveness
Excisional biopsy	
Any mass that can be excised completely. Reserved for cases when surgical excision requires no special planning or when cure by excision is thought likely	Usually requires general anaesthesia. No special instruments required. A surgical procedure. Greater tissue mass acquired increases information, particularly on invasiveness. Possibly curative

13.43 Types of biopsy.

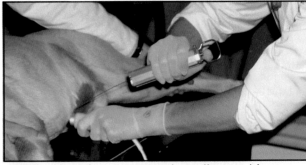

13.44 Use of an automated needle core biopsy device to obtain a sample from the liver of a dog under ultrasound guidance.

13.45. Surgical treatment (excision) is of most value as a sole modality for small to moderately sized discrete tumours with a benign behaviour or where metastasis has not yet occurred.

The size of the surgical procedure is restricted by the surgeon's ability to excise the affected area, including a margin of normal tissue around the neoplasm, and then carry out whatever reconstruction is required to maintain an acceptable postoperative function and therefore quality of life. For skin tumours in areas of low skin tension (e.g. the flank) this means that relatively large procedures can readily be performed. For many invasive tumours this may not be possible, though amputation can be considered for those affecting the limbs.

Type of treatment	Application	Specific examples of use
Surgical excision (extensiveness of surgery should be tailored to tumour type)	Widely available. Commonest form of treatment. Limited use for locally invasive and metastatic tumours	Mammary tumours; solitary lung tumours; isolated skin tumours
Chemotherapy	Less widely used. Commonest use is for tumours of white blood cells. Occasionally used to prolong survival of animals with malignant tumours, particularly after excision (e.g. osteosarcoma of the limbs)	Lymphoma; mast cell tumour
Radiation therapy	Very restricted availability. Sometimes used after excision of tumours without complete removal	Intranasal tumours (as sole treatment); oral tumours (after incomplete excision)

13.45 Treatment of neoplasia.

Nursing care of patients with neoplasia

Preoperative care

The preoperative care required depends largely on the systemic results of the neoplasia, if any. Where possible, this should be assessed and treated before surgery. For example, anaemic patients may require blood transfusion (see Chapter 8) and anorectic patients should have their nutritional status addressed (see Chapter 9). The nurse will also be involved in the assessment of prognosis (above).

In addition, the owners may require particular support before, during and after the treatment of their pet.

Perioperative care

The nurse should be aware of any paraneoplastic effects that may be present so that these can be monitored and treated if they arise (for example, histamine release during manipulation of mast cell tumours). Since many tumours metastasize to the lungs, high quality thoracic radiographs are important before surgery and this will be done under the same anaesthetic as surgical treatment, if they have not already been taken.

Often oncological surgery requires extensive resection of tissues (e.g. skin and subcutaneous tissues). The nurse must liaise with the surgeon as to the extent of surgical skin preparation required, since the development of skin flaps for closure may require larger than usual areas of preparation. This also influences the positioning of the patient.

During resection of a neoplasm, the surgeon, instruments and drapes may become contaminated by the neoplastic cells. To reduce the risk of spread or recurrence of the neoplasm, the instruments used for closure should be from a fresh instrument set. The surgeon may also wish to re-glove and place clean drapes at the surgical site before closure.

Postoperative care

The nursing care depends on the site of the disease process (see below for nursing care based on different organ systems). Although most patients will have surgery as a sole treatment modality, there is a benefit to chemotherapy or radiotherapy after surgery in a number of cases. This may have implications for nursing care and should be considered (see Chapter 9 and the *BSAVA Manual of Advanced Veterinary Nursing*). For example, chemotherapy drugs often have toxic side effects on the patient and represent risks to the safety of nursing staff and owners through excretion in the urine.

At the time of discharge, the client may have questions about the prognosis that should be addressed to the veterinary surgeon. They should also be given information about any follow-up treatment or monitoring that is required.

Common surgical conditions of the organ systems

Upper respiratory tract

The upper respiratory tract comprises the nostrils, nasal chambers, nasal sinuses, pharynx and larynx. Figures 13.46 to 13.49 describe common surgical conditions of these organs.

Group	Condition	Comments
Congenital	Stenotic nares	Commonly seen in brachycephalic dogs – part of the brachycephalic obstructive syndrome (BOS). Suitable for surgical widening (see Figure 13.51) and with a good prognosis
	Cleft lip (harelip)	Less common than clefts of the hard or soft palate, which often occur together with this disease. Obvious at birth and may interfere with nursing. Surgical repair can be undertaken, but is delayed until animal is at least 8 weeks old, when tissues are more mature (may require tube feeding until that time)
Acquired	Neoplasia	Not uncommon, particularly in older cats with non-pigmented tissue. Squamous cell carcinoma (Figure 13.55) is commonest type. These tumours have tendency to recur locally but rarely spread elsewhere. Useful treatments include cryosurgery, radiotherapy and excision of the nasal planum
	Trauma	Can result in obstruction to nostrils. Early wound management necessary to avoid this

13.46 Conditions of the nares.

Condition	Comments
Chronic rhinitis	Relatively common in cats and rabbits, rarer in dogs. In cats, may be associated with chronic viral infections. In rabbits, often associated with chronic upper respiratory tract infection or dental disease. Nasal sinuses also commonly involved. Response to medical treatments can be disappointing, but surgical exploration often not helpful
Foreign bodies (see Figure 13.52)	Important cause of acute sneezing and nasal discharge in dogs. Some dislodge naturally; others require removal by vigorous flushing under anaesthesia, forceps retrieval using endoscopy or, occasionally, open surgery (rhinotomy)
Fungal rhinitis	Uncommon in cats, but important cause of nasal disease in dogs. Usually due to infection with *Aspergillus*, causing sneezing, nasal discharge, nasal pain and nose bleeds (epistaxis). Treatment methods include oral antifungal drugs and topical treatments. Flushing the nose and frontal sinuses with clotrimazole solution, under anaesthesia, is the most common approach
Neoplasia	Important cause of chronic nasal disease (discharge, obstruction and epistaxis) in elderly dogs and cats. Surgery alone not helpful treatment but radiation therapy with surgery in dogs and chemotherapy in cats helpful in reducing signs and prolonging survival

13.47 Conditions of the nasal cavities and sinuses.

Condition	Comments
Congenital	
Cleft palate (see Figure 13.53)	Not uncommon in kittens and puppies. Results in difficulty in feeding and nasal discharge but surgery is delayed until animal is 12 weeks of age, when tissues are more mature. Nursing care and tube feeding are required until then. Many breeders elect to have such animals euthanased if defects are recognized soon after birth
Overlong soft palate	Part of BOS. Causes dyspnoea and stertorous respiration (snoring). Shortening by excision of tip of the palate is effective treatment in many cases, if other components of BOS are not severe
Acquired	
Traumatic cleft palate	Often follows road traffic accidents or falls in cats. Can be repaired by suturing of soft tissues, but many will heal uneventfully. Assessment and treatment of concurrent injuries, which may be severe, is important
Oronasal fistula	Usually follows trauma or tooth removal. Removal of upper canine teeth is common cause, if supporting bone of root socket is fractured. Results in food entering nose and chronic infection. Defect is closed by creation of flap of mucosa from nearby area which is sutured to patch hole

13.48 Conditions of the palate.

Condition	Comments
Laryngeal paralysis	Paralysis of the muscles of the larynx, most importantly those allowing the vocal cords to be opened. Relatively common in dogs, occasionally seen in cats. Elderly, medium–large breed dogs, particularly Labrador and Golden Retrievers, Irish Setter and Afghan Hound. Results in coughing, rasping respiratory noise (stridor), altered bark and most importantly dyspnoea. A result of degeneration of nerves supplying laryngeal muscles. Treated by various surgical procedures that increase size of laryngeal opening, most commonly a 'tie-back' surgery, which is effective even in these elderly patients
Laryngeal collapse	Component of BOS in which structures of larynx become distorted and collapse into airway, causing laryngeal obstruction. These dogs are usually severely dyspnoeic. Treated by excision of obstructing structures from within airway. Guarded prognosis
Neoplasia (Figure 13.50)	Occasionally seen in cats and dogs. In dogs, usually malignant and treatment not successful in cats, most are lymphosarcomas and chemotherapy may produce period of remission
Laryngospasm	Spasm of muscles of larynx produces marked obstruction of airway. Most often seen in cats after endotracheal intubation, particularly if this was difficult to accomplish. Usually resolves after treatment with corticosteroids or local anaesthetics. Avoided by use of topical local anaesthetic and careful technique

13.49 Conditions of the larynx.

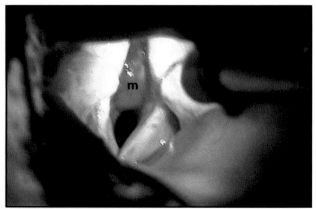

13.50 Laryngeal neoplasia in an elderly dog. Examination with a laryngoscope under anaesthesia reveals a soft tissue mass (m) between the arytenoid cartilages.

Nursing care for upper respiratory tract surgery

Preoperative care

Immature patients with congenital defects require nursing until they are old enough for surgery. The tissues do not heal readily after surgery until the animal is 12 weeks old and so surgery is delayed until that time.

Affected animals have difficulty feeding naturally and require tube feeding by nasogastric or orogastric intubation. Episodes of rhinitis may need antibiotic treatment.

Inpatients with upper airway obstruction (Figure 13.51) must be carefully monitored to ensure that the stress of hospitalization does not lead to a worsening of signs. The environment should be cool and calm. Patients that become agitated should be reassured or sedated and a minimal period of preoperative hospitalization is suggested. Otherwise no special preparation for these surgeries is required.

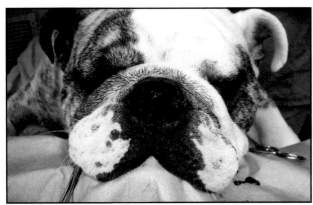

13.51 Stenotic nares in an English bulldog during surgical correction.

Skin preparation

The skin preparation required in these cases varies according to the procedure planned.

■ For surgery of the nasal planum, the local skin is clipped and prepared routinely.
■ For surgery within the oral cavity, often no skin preparation is necessary since the surgeon can place drapes around the lip margins to exclude the skin from the surgical field.
■ The pharynx should be packed around the endotracheal tube to prevent blood, saliva or lavage fluids being aspirated, unless this will interfere where surgical access to the caudal part of the soft palate or to the larynx is required.
■ Prior to oral surgery, it is sometimes recommended that the teeth should be scaled and polished on a previous occasion. This is probably only necessary for animals with marked periodontal disease.

Surgical approaches to the larynx usually do require skin preparation. The commonest of these surgeries is the laryngoplasty ('tie-back') for laryngeal paralysis. For this procedure, a lateral approach to the larynx is usually performed, on the left side. The skin clip is on the left side, from the commissure of the lips to the mid neck and from the ventral midline to the wing of the atlas.

For extensive surgery of the upper respiratory tract, it may also be appropriate to prepare the ventral aspect of the neck in case a tracheotomy is required.

Perioperative care

In general, these surgeries should be scheduled for early in the day, so that the patients can be observed recovering during normal working hours.

Patients undergoing airway surgery (Figures 13.52 and 13.53) require particular care during anaesthesia. The nurse must ensure that spare anaesthetic equipment is to hand, in case of accidental extubation of the patient, for example. Tracheotomy equipment should also be available during and after surgery.

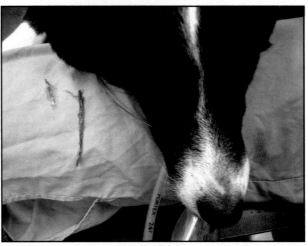

13.52 Foreign body removed from nasal chamber of a dog under endoscopic guidance.

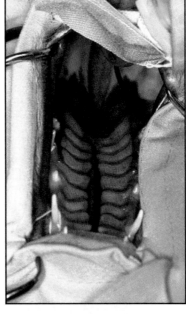

13.53 Cleft of the hard palate in a puppy (under anaesthesia, immediately before surgery).

Postoperative care

Particular concerns in the postoperative period in these cases relate to airway obstruction as a result of surgical swelling or aspiration of oral contents. After surgery of the pharynx, larynx or trachea, postoperative oedema of the surgical site can cause worsening respiratory obstruction. Perioperative corticosteroids are often given to reduce the occurrence of this, but special care is always required in recovery to identify if this develops and to take appropriate action. Brachycephalic dogs in particular should be constantly observed until they are able to stand. During recovery these dogs should be placed in sternal recumbency with the tongue gently extended and the head slightly extended (Figure 13.54).

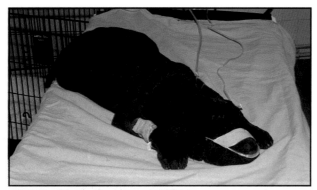

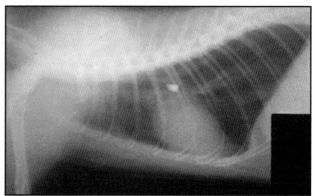

13.54 Sharpei recovering from upper respiratory tract surgery. Note the sternal position the animal is placed in and the use of nasal prongs for supplemental oxygen therapy without causing distress.

Postoperatively the environment should be calm. Patients that become agitated should be reassured or sedated if necessary. Dyspnoea may lead to hyperthermia and the body temperature of patients with upper airway obstruction should be measured regularly. Cooling may be required, for example by using fans or an air-conditioned environment. More extreme measures (e.g. wetting the patient or icepacks) should be used with care because of the possibility of hypothermia.

Feeding may need to be altered during the convalescence period, particularly after procedures that may compromise swallowing or protection of the airway (e.g. pharyngeal or laryngeal surgery). These patients should be offered water only for the first 12 hours and then a soft non-sloppy food for the next 4–6 weeks.

Cats are often anorexic after nasal surgery of any type (Figure 13.55) and need to be tempted to eat, since the sense of smell may be lost and cats tolerate nasal obstruction poorly. Nasogastric feeding is contraindicated after nasal or pharyngeal surgery; alternative routes of assisted feeding (pharyngostomy or gastrostomy tubes) are available, but in practice are usually not necessary since good nursing care (warming the food, cleaning the nostrils and maintaining analgesia) often overcome anorexia.

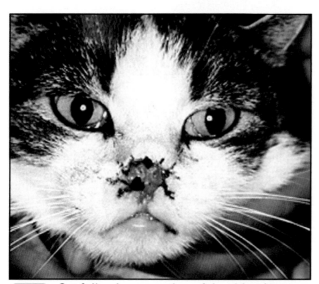

13.55 Cat following resection of the rhinarium for treatment of squamous cell carcinoma (5 days after surgery).

After airway surgery, exercise should be restricted and barking discouraged. After oral surgery, flushing of the mouth with an oral antiseptic solution is sometimes advised, but is often unnecessary.

Lower respiratory tract

The lower respiratory tract comprises the trachea, bronchi, bronchioles and lungs. Figures 13.56 to 13.59 describe and illustrate common surgical conditions of these organs.

Condition	Comments
Tracheal collapse	Yorkshire Terriers commonly affected. Results in characteristic honking cough. Results of surgical correction often poor
Trauma	Following external trauma (RTA, dog fight, stick penetration) or intubation injuries. Mild cases may heal without surgery. Severe injuries require surgical repair
Filaroides infestation	Parasitic worm causing granulomatous masses. Usually treated medically
Foreign bodies (Figure 13.57)	Usually inhaled grass seeds, occasionally pebbles and others. Cause cough and sometimes dyspnoea. Endoscopic retrieval preferred

13.56 Conditions of the trachea.

13.57 Thoracic radiograph of a cat showing a radiodense foreign body in the distal trachea. A pebble was later removed endoscopically.

Condition	Comments
Primary lung tumours (Figure 13.59)	Solitary masses, often occupying an entire lung lobe. Important cause of chronic coughing in elderly dogs. Usually malignant but surgery (pulmonary lobectomy) improves quality of life
Lung abscess	Usually due to chronic inhaled foreign body (see trachea). Lobectomy often required
Metastatic lung tumours	Arise from spread of distant tumours. Surgery rarely indicated

13.58 Conditions of the lungs.

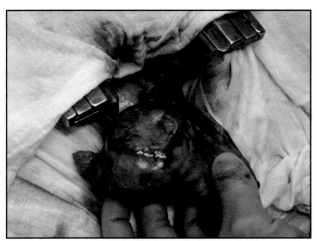

13.59 Primary lung tumour in right middle lobe of a dog, seen during lateral thoracotomy. This was removed by a lobectomy.

Nursing care for lower respiratory tract surgery

Preoperative care

The main consideration is that these patients may be critically unstable. Although they may have adapted to tolerate reduced respiratory function at home, the stress of travel to the clinic, hospitalization and diagnostic procedures may precipitate a dramatic worsening of clinical signs. The animals must therefore be handled carefully and any distress avoided. In particular, nervous animals (cats, rabbits and birds, for example) may benefit from being placed in a quiet dark place to recover from travel before any further handling. The stress of manual restraint for sample collection or radiography can be particularly dangerous and the nurse must consult with the veterinary surgeon so that these procedures are carried out efficiently and without undue distress. It may be better to use sedation or anaesthesia rather than physical restraint.

Skin preparation

Surgery on these cases requires an approach through the sternum (median sternotomy) or the lateral thoracic wall (left or right lateral thoracotomy). Although the exact site of surgery is dictated by the organ and lesion of interest, a large surgical field is always prepared.

- For a lateral approach, the clip and skin preparation extend from the dorsal to the ventral midline and from the point of the shoulder to the mid abdomen.
- For a sternotomy, the area extends from the mid neck to the umbilicus and on each side to include the ventral half of the body wall. It may be necessary to extend this on one or both sides to place chest drains, at the direction of the surgeon.

The final skin preparation is completed in theatre, once the patient has been securely positioned.

- For a ventral sternotomy, the patient is in dorsal recumbency, well supported and restrained to remain immobile during surgery, with the forelimbs gently extended cranially.

- For a lateral approach, the forelimbs are similarly extended cranially, to expose as much of the lateral thoracic wall as possible.

Perioperative care

The key part of intraoperative care in many of these cases relates to anaesthetic management and is covered in Chapter 12. The nurse must ensure that all the equipment that may be required by the surgeon and anaesthetist is to hand so that the anaesthetic period is not unnecessarily prolonged.

In addition, there are often significant postoperative requirements for care of these patients (see below). The nursing staff should ensure that the equipment and other resources required for this have been prepared before the patient leaves theatre.

Postoperative care

Each case must be monitored and have nursing care adapted to suit the individual patient following the particular surgery. The following are general points to take into consideration.

- Consider keeping the endotracheal tube in for as long as possible. It may be useful to remove it with the cuff inflated to avoid debris passing into the trachea. Even after the endotracheal tube has been removed, have a clean appropriate-sized tube and laryngoscope to hand.
- Have oxygen on standby, with a suitable method of administration (facemask or nasal catheter).
- Handle respiratory cases carefully; avoid causing the patient unnecessary distress.
- Regular monitoring is important: constant observation at least until the endotracheal tube is removed and then every 5–15 minutes.
- Watch for any changes in respiratory pattern or colour of mucous membranes.
- Ensure that the volume of air movement is adequate.
- Check the patient's temperature regularly as hyperthermia can develop in animals with respiratory obstruction. Conversely, hypothermia often occurs in patients after open thoracic surgery.
- Have a suitable tracheotomy tube and small surgical kit ready in case of emergencies.
- A patient that has been in lateral recumbency during a lengthy surgical procedure should not be turned on to the other side in recovery. The 'down lung' during surgery will be congested and underventilated and may interfere with respiratory function if it is placed uppermost. As soon as possible the patient should be placed in sternal recumbency.
- Chest bandages can be used post surgery to protect the surgical incision or to hold a chest drain in place. Bandages should be checked regularly to ensure that they are not so tight that they interfere with respiratory function. Two fingers should be held underneath the bandage during inspiration, when the chest is at maximum capacity.

■ Chest drains are usually placed at the time of surgery and a secure system is vital for the safety of the patient. They should be sutured in place and held securely with a body bandage (see Chapter 14); Elizabethan collars may also be used. Any tubing used for chest drainage should be sterile.

■ Patients connected to a drainage system should never be left unattended.

Further details of chest drainage are given in the *BSAVA Manual of Advanced Veterinary Nursing*.

Oral cavity

Figures 13.60 and 13.61 describe and illustrate common surgical oral diseases.

Nursing care for oral cavity surgery

Patient care is similar to that outlined for surgery of the upper respiratory tract.

Dental disease

Figure 13.62 describes common dental diseases.

Condition	Comments
Fractured mandible	Common after RTA, especially in the cat. Often open and comminuted. Also possible complication of dental extraction. Repaired by internal or external fixation or by muzzle support. May require tube feeding during healing
Separated mandibular symphysis	Common after RTA, especially in the cat. Readily repaired by cerclage wiring
Ulceration	Oral ulceration may be caused by ingested irritants, uraemia, liver failure, allergy and viral infections (cats). Biopsy may be necessary to distinguish from ulcerating neoplasm
Epulis	Non-specific term applied to benign masses arising from gums
Neoplasia	Various benign and malignant tumours reported. Prognosis depends on site, size and tissue type. Squamous cell carcinoma most common, particularly in cats. Prognosis poor after traditional surgery but fair after radical surgery (mandibulectomy/maxillectomy, Figure 13.61a,b). Melanoma, fibrosarcoma, osteosarcoma and basal cell carcinoma also occur

13.60   Conditions of the oral cavity (see also upper respiratory tract and dental disease).

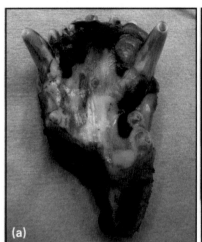

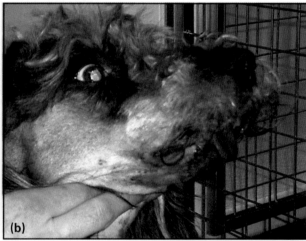

13.61
(a) Excised specimen of a mandibular neoplasm from a dog managed by bilateral rostral mandibulectomy. (b) Postoperative appearance of the dog.

Condition	Comments
Gingivitis	Inflammation of the gums, usually around teeth. Commonest tooth-related disease and usually associated with accumulation of plaque and tartar on teeth and associated infection. Treated by removing accumulated tartar and improving oral hygiene (oral antiseptics, short-term antibiotics, dietary change, tooth brushing). Prevented by attention to dietary hygiene. Also associated with causes of oral ulceration
Periodontitis	Progression of gingivitis resulting in regression of gum-line and pocket formation around teeth. Early cases may be reversed by treatment of gingivitis. Other cases require gum surgery or tooth extraction
Caries	Demineralization and destruction of tooth substance induced by bacteria. Results in defect in enamel and deeper tissue. Rare in animals compared to humans. Treated by extraction or filling
Fractures of crown	Usually traumatic in origin. Canines commonly affected. Often managed conservatively but may be capped or extracted
Feline neck lesions	Also known as subgingival resorptive lesions. Seen exclusively in cats. Cause cavities in tooth substance at gingival margin. Painful. Treated by filling or extraction

13.62   Dental diseases. (continues)   ▶

Condition	Comments
Retained deciduous teeth	Retention of deciduous canines is most significant. Deciduous teeth should be shed by time permanent teeth are beginning to erupt. Retention of teeth after this leads to misplacement of permanent teeth and malocclusion. Retained teeth should be extracted, with care to prevent damage to emerging permanent teeth
Overgrown teeth	Particular problem of rabbits. May affect incisors, which can be managed by burring or occasionally extraction. Less obviously, may also affect cheek teeth, causing damage to soft tissues, facial abscessation, weight loss, nasal or ocular discharge. Cheek teeth can be shortened by burring or may require extraction

13.62 (continued) Dental diseases.

Nursing care for dental surgery

Patient care is similar to that outlined for surgery of the upper respiratory tract. After dental treatment, soft food should be given for 4–5 days before gradually returning to a normal diet. At the time of discharge following dental procedures, owners need to understand the importance of home hygiene care and should have been instructed on how to provide this. More detail on the role of the veterinary nurse in veterinary dentistry will be found in the *BSAVA Manual of Advanced Veterinary Nursing, 2nd edition.*

Oesophagus

Figures 13.63 and 13.64 describe and illustrate common surgical conditions of the oesophagus.

Condition	Comments
Megaoeso-phagus	Loss of muscular tone leading to reduced ability to swallow. Signs include regurgitation, coughing, pneumonia and weight loss. Seen as congenital and acquired disease in both dogs and cats. Well recognized breed predisposition including Siamese cat, Irish Setter and Great Dane. Prognosis variable but can be poor. No effective treatment in most cases. Usually idiopathic condition but underlying cause occasionally identified (e.g. myasthenia gravis)
Oesophagitis	Inflammation following severe vomiting, reflux due to hiatal hernia or under anaesthesia or ingestion of hot/caustic substances
Oesophageal stricture	Stricture (narrowing due to scarring) usually follows episode of oesophagitis. Most commonly develops within few days of general anaesthesia if stomach contents have refluxed into the oesophagus. Animals present with dysphagia and regurgitation. Managed by treatment of oesophagitis and repeated dilation of the stricture (bougienage). Prognosis guarded
Oesophageal foreign body (Figure 13.64)	Various ingested objects may become lodged in oesophagus, most commonly pieces of bone. Terrier dogs predisposed to this problem. Fish-hooks also encountered occasionally. Require removal, by forceps, endoscopy or surgery (oesophagotomy). Complications of oesophageal perforation and aspiration pneumonia may develop
Vascular ring anomaly (persistent right aortic arch)	Congenital malformation resulting in obstruction of oesophagus. Animals present soon after weaning with regurgitation of solid food

13.63 Oesophageal diseases.

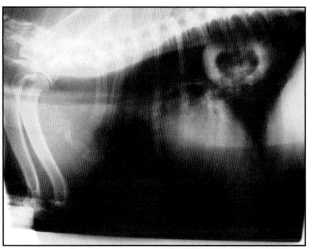

13.64 Lateral thoracic radiograph of a dog with a foreign body (tennis ball) in the caudal thoracic oesophagus.

Nursing care after oesophageal surgery

Oesophageal surgery is covered in the *BSAVA Manual of Advanced Veterinary Nursing.* Following oesophagitis or removal of oesophageal foreign bodies, tube feeding should be considered for 5–10 days to allow the oesophagus to heal. After oesophageal surgery, the animal must be closely monitored for signs of deterioration suggesting oesophageal perforation (increasing pain, shock, dyspnoea, pleural effusion). Oesophageal perforation is a devastating complication of oesophageal surgery.

Gastrointestinal tract

Figures 13.65 to 13.68 describe common surgical conditions of the gastrointestinal tract.

Nursing care for gastrointestinal surgery

Preoperative care

Many of these cases are emergencies and little preoperative care is possible. Nonetheless, the patient should be stabilized as far as possible before anaesthesia and surgery (see Chapters 7, 8 and 12). Before elective surgery of the stomach and small intestine, routine preoperative starvation is usually adequate, but a longer period without food and water may be requested by the surgeon if gastric outflow obstruction is suspected.

In some cases, it can be helpful to ensure that the colon is empty before surgery.

Condition	Comments
Foreign bodies	Indigestible material of various types can lodge in stomach. Signs vary from none to severe vomiting. Diagnosed on radiography or endoscopy. Treated by inducing vomiting (if small and smooth), endoscopic retrieval or surgery (gastrotomy)
Ulceration	Gastric ulceration usually result of systemic disease (liver or kidney failure) or drug therapy (NSAIDs, corticosteroids). Usually managed medically rather than surgically
Neoplasia	Not uncommon in older animals. Signs: vomiting, weight loss, haematemesis. Diagnosed by radiography or endoscopy and biopsy. Most are large and malignant but surgery can be helpful occasionally (partial gastrectomy, Figure 13.66). Poor prognosis
Hairballs	Occasionally affect cats; managed by inducing vomiting or with liquid paraffin administration. Also occur in rabbits; grooming may help prevent formation; administration of papain or fresh pineapple juice can help dissolve
Pylorospasm/pyloric stenosis	Narrowing of outflow of stomach. Causes food retention and vomiting. Diagnosed by radiography. Treated by surgery to widen outflow (pyloroplasty or pyloromyotomy)
Gastric dilatation/volvulus syndrome (GDV, bloat) (see Figure 13.69)	Distension of the stomach with gas and fluid, often with concurrent twisting of the stomach. Typically seen in large and giant dogs with deep chests (e.g. Labrador, Irish Setter, Dobermann, Great Dane). Causes severe shock and can be fatal if not treated rapidly. Diagnosed on clinical examination (gastric distension) and radiography. Requires emergency treatment: aggressive fluid therapy, gastric decompression and surgery to reposition stomach and prevent recurrence of volvulus (gastropexy) (details in text)
Hiatal hernia	Prolapse of part of stomach into thorax through enlarged oesophageal hiatus. Results in oesophageal reflux, dysphasia and regurgitation. Managed medically or occasionally by surgery to prevent herniation

13.65   Diseases of the stomach.

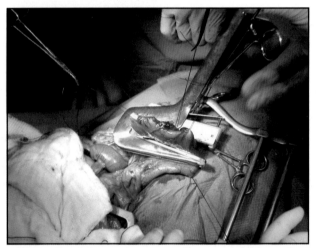

13.66   Partial gastrectomy using a surgical stapler (thoracoabdominal device) to remove a gastric neoplasm.

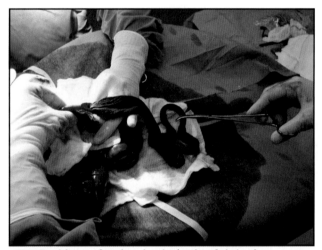

13.68   Linear foreign body (pair of tights) being removed from a dog through an enterotomy.

Condition	Comments
Simple foreign body (FB)	Compact FBs that are ingested can cause varying degrees of intestinal obstruction. Commonest in younger animals and in dogs. Severity of signs greatest when obstruction complete and in proximal intestine. Typical signs include vomiting, shock, abdominal pain but in less severe cases include weight loss and diarrhoea. Diagnosis: abdominal palpation, radiography. Can be managed conservatively if incomplete obstruction and carefully monitored. More commonly surgery required: removal at enterotomy if intestinal wall viable, else resection and anastomosis (enterectomy)
Linear foreign body (Figure 13.68)	Elongated FBs (string, tape, etc.) cause more severe signs. Typically proximal end lodges at pylorus or base of tongue. Intestine becomes plicated along the FB. Causes severe obstruction and often perforation as the FB saws through the intestinal wall. Removed at surgery: often requires several enterotomies and repair of perforations. Prognosis cautious
Neoplasia	Intestinal neoplasia can be focal or diffuse. Focal neoplasms produce obstruction and similar signs to simple FBs (above). Diffuse neoplasms may cause obstruction or malabsorption, weight loss and diarrhoea. Majority are malignant but surgery can be helpful for focal neoplasms

13.67   Diseases of the small and large intestine. (continues)   ▶

Condition	Comments
Strangulation	Intestine can be strangulated/incarcerated by entrapment in a hernia or rupture. Signs of obstruction severe and intestinal compromise also causes pain, toxaemia and shock. Following stabilization, exploratory surgery necessary to relieve strangulation and usually to excise affected area. Surgery to prevent recurrence is also important (e.g. hernia repair). Prognosis is guarded
Intussusception	Condition in which part of intestine invaginates (telescopes) into adjacent part. Present with signs of obstruction (see above, FBs). Often in young animals, after enteritis. Commonest site is ileocolic. Surgery indicated to reduce intussusception if possible or resect it. Recurrence not uncommon and steps to prevent it may be used (enteroplication or antispasmodic drugs)
Megacolon	Loss of tone in colon resulting in constipation. Commonest in cats and may follow pelvic trauma or be idiopathic. Managed conservatively with stool softeners and periodic evacuation or by subtotal colectomy

13.67 (continued) Diseases of the small and large intestine.

- Starvation of patients undergoing large bowel surgery may need to be longer than the normal 8 hours to ensure that the gut is as empty as possible at the time of surgery.
- A low-residue diet fed for 3–5 days before surgery may reduce the volume of large intestinal contents.
- The day before surgery food may be withheld and an enema given.
- On the day of surgery another (non-irritant) enema can be given if necessary.

However, these steps can result in liquid rather than solid colonic contents, which the surgeon may find more difficult to control than normal firm faeces.

Recovery after surgery will be improved if the patient is not lacking in nutritional requirements at the time of surgery and therefore prolonged pre- or postoperative starvation should be avoided as a routine. The technique of giving oral antibiotics before surgery to reduce intestinal bacterial load is no longer considered good practice.

Skin preparation

For all abdominal procedures, the nurse should prepare the patient to allow a full abdominal exploration. A midline approach is routine and the clip and skin preparation should extend from the mid sternum to the perineum so that the incision can be extended from the xiphisternum to the pubic brim if necessary. The lateral limits of the prepared area extend halfway to the dorsal midline. The patient must be securely positioned so that it remains in true dorsal recumbency throughout surgery. In male dogs, it is often helpful to place a urethral catheter connected to a collection bag, and to position the prepuce outside the surgical field (it may be clipped to one side with a towel clip).

Perioperative care

For abdominal surgery of this type, the surgeon may request the provision of additional surgical instrumentation:

- Self-retaining abdominal retractors (e.g. Gosset's or Balfour's)
- Intestinal forceps (Doyen's)
- Atraumatic thumb forceps (DeBakey's).

The nurse should also give consideration to the surgical supplies used. Water-resistant gowns and drapes are of particular value since lavage fluids are commonly used during the surgery. In addition, large surgical swabs (laparotomy swabs) or sterile towels (Huck towels) can be useful to isolate the intestinal tract and reduce abdominal contamination.

Postoperative care for gastric surgery

Patient care following gastric surgery will be adapted according to the reason for surgery and the type of surgery performed. As with the care of any patient that has undergone surgery on the alimentary tract, fluid therapy, electrolyte balance and nutritional support are very important during the return to normal function.

- Offer very small amounts of water on recovery from anaesthesia.
- If water is retained by the patient and no problems are encountered for 12 hours post surgery, small amounts of a bland diet can be offered.
- Give little and often and gradually increase over several days.
- Return to a normal diet over approximately 3–5 days.

Particular concern after surgery is the risk of dehiscence of the gastric or intestinal closure. Indications of this complication include anorexia, abdominal pain, vomiting, pyrexia and abdominal distension.

Postoperative care for intestinal surgery

Following surgery on the intestinal tract consideration should be given to fluid and electrolyte balance, nutritional support and return to normal function of the alimentary tract.

The feeding regime after intestinal surgery can be accelerated compared with gastric surgery, since vomiting is much less likely. Although the traditional approach has been to withhold oral intake for 12 hours or more after surgery, most patients can be offered small amounts of water and bland food once they have recovered from anaesthesia and then returned to normal diet over 2–3 days if there are no complications. Early return to oral intake will reduce the risk of ileus (see below) and improve intestinal healing.

Assisted enteral feeding may be necessary in patients that refuse food and total parenteral nutrition (nutritional support via an intravenous catheter) could be considered in vomiting patients. However, it is expensive and technically difficult to do in a safe and effective manner.

Early signs of ileus (lack of significant peristaltic activity) are difficult for the nurse to observe, but may be signified by abdominal distension due to the retention of gas, abdominal pain, vomiting, anorexia and absence of defecation. When defecation occurs, note the consistency, colour, signs of blood and whether any straining is present.

Gastric dilatation/volvulus syndrome (GDV)

This condition (Figure 13.69) will be covered in more depth since the veterinary nurse may have to assist with emergency treatment.

Treatment of GDV

■ Aggressive intravenous fluid therapy (100 ml/kg/hour initially, to rapidly restore circulating blood volume).
■ Gastric decompression, carried out concurrently with fluid therapy – several methods are in use:
  – Orogastric intubation (stomach tube): possible without sedation in many cases, but may be difficult to enter the stomach if grossly distended or if volvulus is present
  – Trocharization: passage of large-gauge needles through the most distended flank into the stomach; advised in cases where intubation is not possible
  – Flank gastrotomy: when decompression is not possible by other means, a limited surgical approach to the stomach under local anaesthesia may be used, but is rarely required.
■ Gastric lavage: flushing of the stomach with warm saline is often recommended.
■ Treatment of shock: continuation of fluid therapy and correction of acid–base and electrolyte disturbances until patient is stabilized.
■ Treatment of arrhythmias: cardiac arrhythmias are common in affected dogs and should be

monitored by electrocardiography and treated if necessary – lidocaine by intravenous bolus or infusion is the treatment of choice.
■ Additional drug therapy: antibiotics are indicated because of the danger of septicaemia; corticosteroids may be used in the treatment of shock.
■ Radiography – may be used to confirm the diagnosis and assess the position of the stomach.
■ Surgical exploration of the abdomen under anaesthesia – recommended once the patient is stable, to allow repositioning of the stomach and spleen if displaced, inspection of tissue viability and resection if necessary (the spleen and stomach may be partially necrotic) and surgical fixation of the stomach (gastropexy) to prevent future volvulus (twisting).

Advice to owners to reduce recurrence of GDV

Owners of breeds prone to GDV, and in particular owners of dogs previously treated for the condition, should be advised on how to recognize the disease and the steps that they might use to reduce the risk of recurrence. Owners should watch for:

■ Restlessness and discomfort up to 3 hours after eating
■ The animal retching but not able to vomit
■ Abdominal distension
■ Respiration rapid and laboured
■ Pulse rapid and weak.

GDV can occur in any breed, but it is more common in large deep-chested dogs such as the Irish Setter or St Bernard. To reduce the risk of recurrence:

■ Avoid feeding large meals
■ Avoid exercise immediately before or after eating
■ Feed a mixed diet, rather than a complete dry diet fed alone.

Anorectal and perineal surgery

Figures 13.70 and 13.71 describe and illustrate common surgical conditions of the rectum, anus and perineum.

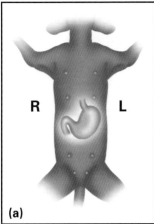 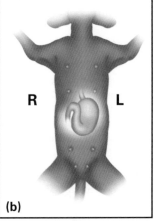 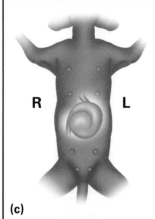 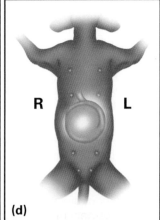

(a) (b) (c) (d)

13.69 Ventral view of 180-degree rotation of stomach. **(a)** Pylorus moves ventrally from right to left. **(b)** Pylorus and body of stomach move clockwise. **(c)** Pylorus lies to left of stomach. **(d)** Pylorus moves more dorsally. (Reproduced from *BSAVA Manual of Canine and Feline Abdominal Surgery*.)

Condition	Comments
Rectal tumours and polyps	Present with dyschezia, urgency, tenesmus and haematochezia. Prognosis varies according to tissue type. Various surgical approaches used: most are accessible by iatrogenic rectal prolapse, which allows conservative surgery
Rectal prolapse	Commonly seen in young animals after diarrhoea. Occasionally also seen after perineal surgery (e.g. perineal rupture repair) and parturition. Prolapsed tissue must be protected from self-inflicted trauma and desiccation. First aid measures are patient restraint and application of lubricant creams. Treated by replacement and purse-string suture if possible. Traumatized tissue requires resection. Recurrent cases treated by colopexy
Anal sac impaction	Common condition of dogs and occasionally cats. Retention of anal sac secretions causes local irritation resulting in licking or chewing at perineum and 'scooting'. Usually managed by expression, occasionally by anal sac removal (sacculectomy)
Anal sac abscessation/ sacculitis	Less common anal sac disease. Bacterial infection causes discomfort, purulent discharge and sometimes systemic signs. Managed by expression, lavage of sacs and antibacterial therapy. Sacculectomy may be used for recurrent cases
Anal furunculosis (Figure 13.71)	Almost only seen in German Shepherd Dogs. Ulceration of perineal skin around anus (less commonly other sites: perivulvar, lip folds, foot pads). Causes local irritation, malodour, dyschezia. Usually managed medically, sometimes by local excision, but guarded prognosis
Perineal tumours	Commonest is benign perianal gland adenoma of elderly entire male dogs, managed by local excision and castration to reduce recurrence. Other tumours of skin, subcutaneous tissue and anal sacs occur less commonly
Perineal rupture (also called perineal hernia) (see Figure 13.72)	Breakdown of muscles lateral to anus resulting in loss of support to rectum, bulging of perineum and dyschezia. Common in middle-aged and older entire male dogs. Managed with stool softeners or by surgical repair. Concurrent castration often recommended

13.70 Diseases of the rectum, anus and perineum.

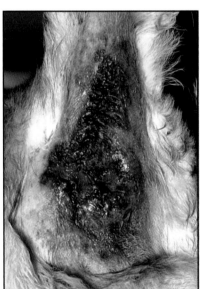

13.71
Extensive anal furunculosis on the perineum of a German Shepherd Dog.

For most of these procedures, the patient is positioned in the perineal position (Figure 13.72): in sternal recumbency at the end of the operating table. The hindlimbs are extended caudally and supported by firm sandbags to tilt the pelvis dorsally. The tail is drawn cranially and maintained in a symmetrical position with ties to either side of the table. It can be helpful to tilt the table by up to 15 degrees in a head-down position to improve surgical access, but a more extreme position will interfere with respiration and should be avoided.

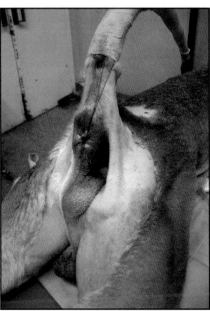

13.72
A dog placed in the perineal position for repair of a right-sided perineal rupture (the rupture has been reduced and appears as a large depression). A purse-string suture has been placed in the anus.

Nursing care for anorectal and perineal surgery

Preoperative care

In general the considerations given for gastrointestinal surgery also apply in these cases. For surgery carried out in the terminal rectum via the anus, the surgeon may wish to pack the descending rectum with swabs or bandage to keep intestinal contents away from the surgical site. During perineal surgery, a purse-string suture is usually placed in the anus for the same purpose. The nurse should establish whether the surgeon requires access to the rectum through the anus; if not, placement of a purse-string suture will reduce the possibility of contamination of the perineal skin during surgery. The nurse must ensure that a purse-string suture, if placed, is removed at the end of surgery.

Skin preparation

The extent of skin clipping required will depend on the extent of the surgical approach.

■ For surgery carried out via the rectum (e.g. excision of rectal polyps), 5–10 cm of skin is prepared around the anus.

■ For procedures requiring a skin incision (e.g. perineal rupture repair, Figure 13.72), a more extensive surgical field is required: the incision for this procedure extends vertically just to one side of the anus, from just dorsal to it to the level of the ischial tuberosity, and the skin clip should therefore extend dorsally to include the base of the tail and ventrally to the caudal scrotum.

It is helpful for all of these types of surgery to place a bandage around the tail to avoid clipping of the tail during skin preparation. Postoperatively, the bandage can be kept in place for 24 hours to reduce soiling of the tail.

In patients undergoing perineal rupture repair and removal of common perineal skin neoplasms, castration may be used to prevent recurrence and the surgeon should be consulted as to whether skin preparation for this procedure should be carried out and whether castration is to be carried out before perineal surgery or following it. Performing castration first reduces the risk of faecal contamination of the castration incision.

For large surgeries in this region, an epidural anaesthetic technique may be used as part of a multi-modal analgesic regime. If this is planned, the nurse must also prepare the skin over the lumbosacral space.

Perioperative care

Depending on the surgical procedure planned, the surgeon may require particular surgical instruments, such as self-retaining retractors to open a perineal skin approach (Gelpi retractors). In other cases, the surgeon may use multiple stay sutures to prolapse the rectum and a scrubbed assistant is often required to manipulate these. Often a probe is useful to identify the anal sac ducts or explore the lesions of anal furunculosis.

Postoperative care

Postoperative analgesia is important particularly to reduce any tendency to tenesmus postoperatively. This is achieved by systemic analgesics (opiates and NSAIDs), epidural anaesthesia and topical local anaesthetics, used in combination depending on the extent of surgery. Continuing topical anaesthesia after recovery from anaesthesia is difficult, but applying topical lidocaine gel to the rectal mucosa at the end of surgery can be helpful.

Discomfort and excessive straining on defecation after surgery is minimized by manipulating faecal consistency to ensure soft but formed faeces. This is achieved by the addition of fibre to the diet for 2–4 weeks after surgery. In dogs, proprietary fibre granules can be added to the food. These are unpalatable to cats but this species will often tolerate lactulose solution for the same purpose. Small amounts of blood may be seen on the faeces for the first 24 hours after surgery but should not continue after that time. The rectal temperature should not be measured in animals after surgery in this region.

Liver and spleen

Figure 13.73 describes common surgical conditions of these organs.

Nursing care for liver and spleen surgery

Preoperative care

Particular concerns are the systemic effects of these diseases. Patients with chronic liver disease may have neurological dysfunction (e.g. hepatic encephalopathy), hypoproteinaemia and reduced blood clotting function. These may all affect the anaesthetic management of the case (see Chapter 12). In particular, plasma protein levels and clotting times must be assessed preoperatively and a blood or plasma transfusion may be required. The patient may also benefit from a period of medical stabilization before surgery to address these issues (e.g. dietary modification, vitamin K administration).

Disease	Description	Treatment
Hepatic tumours	Relatively common in older dogs. Signs usually non-specific (weight loss, anorexia, vomiting)	May be surgically treatable if discrete but usually malignant
Portosystemic shunts	Abnormal blood vessels joining portal vein to systemic circulation. Result in signs of liver failure, particularly neurological signs (hepatic encephalopathy)	Medical management often helpful. Surgical ligation of anomalous vessel possible in some cases (advanced surgical technique)
Trauma to liver or spleen	May result in severe haemorrhage. Falls, crush injuries and car accidents are common causes	Usually haemorrhage will stop if animal supported with fluids/blood transfusion. Surgical treatment rarely required
Splenic tumours	Haemangiosarcoma most frequent. Common in older large-breed dogs. Result in vague signs or collapse due to intra-abdominal haemorrhage	Splenectomy, but poor prognosis since malignant
Splenic haematoma	Similar presentation to splenic tumours. Prognosis better. Histopathology necessary to differentiate the diseases	Splenectomy

13.73 Surgical diseases of the liver and spleen.

Many patients with splenic disease have undergone intra-abdominal haemorrhage or may have another cause of anaemia and require intensive fluid therapy, including blood transfusion (see Chapter 8) before anaesthesia.

Skin preparation

This is the same as that described for gastrointestinal surgery (above), noting that the surgical incision will be immediately caudal to (and occasionally cranial to) the xiphisternum and ensuring that the caudal ventral thorax is clipped to allow this.

Perioperative care

The surgical nurse should prepare particular surgical instrumentation: self-retaining abdominal retractors (Gosset's or Balfour's) are particularly important for exploration of the cranial abdomen. Surgery of the liver or spleen requires control of large blood vessels and the nurse should provide:

- A variety of haemostatic forceps – right-angled forceps (e.g. cholecystectomy forceps) are useful for liver lobectomy, and splenectomy traditionally requires a large number of Spencer-Wells forceps
- Surgical staplers – thoracoabdominal (Figure 13.74) and ligation devices (Figure 13.75), where available, greatly facilitate liver lobectomy and splenectomy
- Electrosurgery (diathermy) – bipolar diathermy is appropriate for sealing smaller vessels (<2 mm in diameter).

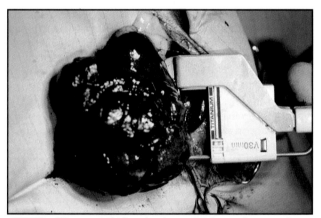

13.74 Thoracoabdominal surgical stapler used to carry out liver lobectomy in a cat.

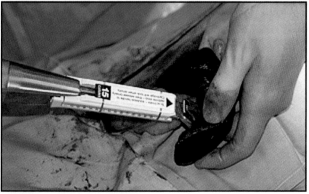

13.75 LDS device (Autosuture) used during splenectomy in a dog.

The surgeon will also require illumination of the cranial abdomen, and sterile operating light handles are useful. Surgical suction and an appropriate tip (e.g. Poole tip) should be provided since there is often peritoneal effusion or haemorrhage present that requires removal during surgery. For the same reason, water-repellent drapes are preferred to linen drapes. Large laparotomy swabs should also be provided.

Postoperative care

The comments made above about care after gastrointestinal surgery also apply in these cases.

Liver biopsy

Biopsy is often required for diagnosis of liver disease. Available methods include:

- Fine-needle aspirate
- Needle core biopsy (e.g. Trucut)
- Surgical biopsy (wedge biopsy)
- Laparoscopic cup biopsy.

A clotting profile should be carried out before liver biopsy since animals with liver disease are at risk of clotting defects. Following biopsy by any technique, there is a risk of severe haemorrhage and the animal must be observed closely for signs of developing shock (e.g. poor recovery from anaesthesia, tachycardia, cool periphery, pale mucous membranes).

Urinary tract

The urinary tract comprises kidneys, ureters, bladder and urethra. Figures 13.76 and 13.77 describe and illustrate common surgical diseases of these organs.

Nursing care for urinary tract surgery

Preoperative care

The most significant patient preparation is required for those animals with renal insufficiency. This can be due to pre-renal failure, such as dehydration, renal failure due to kidney disease and post-renal failure, usually a result of urinary obstruction. Renal disease and pre-renal failure are addressed in Chapter 9.

Management of urinary obstruction

Urinary obstruction is common in dogs, cats and rabbits. It usually occurs in males, because of the relatively long and narrow urethra in this sex. There are various causes, but the most important are feline lower urinary tract disease and urolithiasis (see Chapter 9). Affected animals strain to urinate unsuccessfully and later become systemically affected (shocked, uraemia, vomiting, collapse).

Important steps in management of patients with urinary obstruction before surgery are:

- Fluid therapy – to correct fluid deficits and electrolyte imbalances (typically affected animals are hypovolaemic, acidotic, and hyperkalaemic)
- Emptying of bladder – by cystocentesis or passage of a urethral catheter
- Establishment of diagnosis and specific treatment

Disease	Description	Treatment
Kidney tumours	Uncommon. Signs include haematuria and abdominal mass	Nephrectomy if no gross metastasis
Kidney trauma	Follows blunt abdominal trauma	Kidneys usually recover without surgery. Less commonly surgical repair or nephrectomy required
Ureteral trauma	Occasional consequence of abdominal trauma or surgical misadventure (particularly ovariohysterectomy). Results in accumulation of urine within abdomen or in retroperitoneum, or hydronephrosis	Repair or ureteronephrectomy
Ureteral ectopia	Congenital condition in which ureters insert into urethra or vagina. Causes incontinence	Ureteral repositioning or ureteronephrectomy (Figure 13.77)
Bladder tumours	Cause urinary frequency, urgency and haematuria in older bitches. Usually extensive at time of diagnosis	Rarely amenable to surgical treatment
Urolithiasis (stones)	Most commonly affects bladder but all parts of urinary tract may be affected. In males, usually causes dysuria due to urethral obstruction. In females, usually causes signs of cystitis (urgency, frequency). Several chemical types occur: may be associated with infection	Depends on stone type; includes elimination of infection, surgical removal and dietary manipulation
Feline lower urinary tract disease (FLUTD, FUS)	Syndrome of signs associated with bladder and urethra. May cause frequency, urgency and haematuria in females and males. More common presentation in males is obstruction of urethra by stones or mucus	Dietary and drug treatment often helpful. Males with recurrent obstruction may require urethrostomy to prevent further difficulties
Urinary incontinence	Wide variety of causes	Depends on specific diagnosis. Some cases respond to medical treatment, others benefit from surgical intervention

13.76 Diseases of the kidneys, ureters, urethra and bladder.

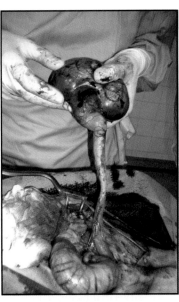

13.77 Ureteronephrectomy to manage a case of ectopic ureter with hydronephrosis.

- Flushing urethral stones back into the bladder and removal by cystotomy
- In recurrent cases, urethrostomy to bypass an area of obstruction or to bypass the penile urethra (narrowest part).

Skin preparation

These surgeries may be carried out through an abdominal approach or an approach to the urethra in the perineum or ventral abdomen. Preparation for an abdominal approach is similar to that required for gastrointestinal surgery, but if the bladder alone is of interest the area prepared need not include the cranial abdomen (prepare only to the umbilicus).

However, for surgeries of the kidneys or ureters, the entire abdomen must be prepared to ensure adequate access for nephrectomy if this becomes required. The nurse should consult the surgeon to establish whether a urethral catheter needs to be placed before surgery and excluded from the surgical field (typically connected to a collection bag), or whether the surgeon will require access to the urethra during the surgery, in which case the catheter will usually be placed following draping. In male dogs, the prepuce is prepared by flushing with surgical antiseptic solution (e.g. povidone–iodine) and not surgical scrub, which contains detergent.

Surgical procedures carried out through the perineum require preparation as described for other perineal procedures (see anorectal surgery, above).

Perioperative care

If abdominal surgery is planned, similar considerations to those for gastrointestinal surgery apply. However, surgery of the ureters or urethra also requires the provision of fine surgical instruments, such as those manufactured for ophthalmic procedures:

- Castroviejo needle holders
- Iris scissors
- Micro-dissection scissors
- Corneal forceps
- Alms retractor.

In addition, the surgeon and assistant may require optical magnification (operating loupes or access to an operating microscope), a fine surgical suction tip (e.g. Frasier tip) and small surgical swabs (e.g. sterile cotton buds).

A selection of urinary catheters should be available in theatre for use in the urethra or ureters. A tube suitable for use as a cystotomy tube (e.g. a DePezzer catheter) may be required.

Postoperative care

After urinary tract surgery the following are important.

- *Maintain fluid and electrolyte balance.* Fluid therapy is covered in detail in Chapter 8, but adequate fluid administration can be maintained by intravenous and/or oral fluid therapy.
  - Initially a high rate of infusion may be used for the administration of intravenous fluids to encourage the production of urine.
  - Oral intake of fluids should be encouraged as soon as possible.
  - Water may also be added to the patient's normal diet to increase water intake.
- *Maintain urine output.* Cystitis is common following surgery of the urinary tract and so the patient should be observed for frequency of urination and the amount passed each time.
  - Observe the patient passing urine for signs of difficulty or discomfort.
  - Check the colour of the urine passed.
  - Watch for the presence of blood.
  - Check the smell of the urine.
  - Note any changes.
- *Maintain indwelling urinary catheters if present.* To reduce bacteria tracking up the catheter, a closed drainage system is preferable. This also enables the nurse to monitor urine production, take samples if necessary and watch for any changes in the type or volume of urine produced. Flushing of the urinary catheter may be required to remove blood clots from the urethra or bladder. If necessary, this should be performed using sterile saline. The patient must be prevented from interfering with indwelling urinary catheters: Elizabethan collars are usually used.
- *Manage the urethrotomy/urethrostomy site.* Prevention of self-mutilation is vital to the success of these cases.
  - Elizabethan collars and possibly sedation in the initial postoperative period may be required.
  - Patients should be given plenty of opportunity to urinate.
  - The area around the wound should be kept clean and petroleum jelly may be applied to surrounding skin to prevent scalding initially.
  - Cats' litter trays should be filled with shredded newspaper or something of a similar consistency for 4–5 days post surgery since particles of conventional litter may irritate the site.

Male reproductive system

Figures 13.78 to 13.80 describe and illustrate common surgical diseases of these organs. Castration is dealt with separately in more depth (below).

Nursing care for male reproductive system surgery

Preoperative care

In most cases, no special care is required, unless urethral obstruction is present (see care of patients with urinary tract disease, above).

Disease	Description	Treatment
Cryptorchidism	Failure of one or both testicles to descend to scrotal position by usual time (typically birth). Usually unilateral. Most are abdominally retained in dog but in cat many are inguinal or subcutaneous. Condition has heritable component	Abnormally located testicles have increased incidence of torsion and of neoplasia, justifying their removal prophylactically. Bilateral castration recommended
Testicular neoplasia	Represent 5% of canine neoplasms. Most are benign, but some are oestrogen secreting and related signs may be seen. Remainder present with testicular enlargement and/or distortion	Castration
Testicular torsion	Uncommon, but occurs principally to retained testicles, especially those having undergone neoplastic transformation. Presenting signs are those of abdominal pain and/or an abdominal mass	Castration
Orchitis	Not uncommon in dog. Acute onset of pain, swelling and local oedema, may be systemic signs (fever, listlessness). Prostatitis may be present concurrently	Castration usually most appropriate treatment. Antibiotics, analgesics and hypothermia may be attempted
Scrotal haematoma (Figure 13.79)	Commonest complication of castration due to patient interference, haemorrhage (from scrotal tissue, septum or testicular vessels) and trauma at surgery or preparation. Particularly a problem in larger mature dogs, for which routine scrotal ablation should be considered at time of castration	Prevention of patient interference and/or scrotal ablation in susceptible animals
Balanitis (infection of penis and prepuce)	Slight purulent preputial discharge is common in normal mature dogs and does not represent disease. Infections of penis and prepuce do occur occasionally, resulting in irritation, copious purulent to serosanguinous discharge and occasionally adhesions	Careful search should be made for underlying diseases (foreign bodies, trauma, neoplasia) before starting treatment with local irrigation and antibiotic therapy. Condition tends to recur

13.78 Diseases of the testes, scrotum and penis.

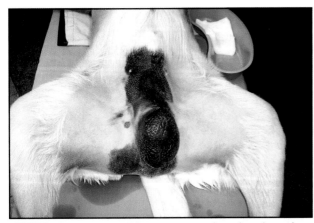

13.79 Large scrotal haematoma that developed during the 24 hours after castration of a dog.

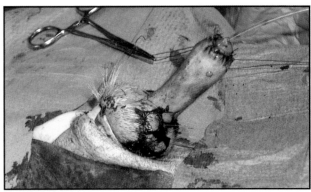

13.81 Intraoperative view of canine penis that has been reconstructed after traumatic partial amputation. The penis has been held out of the prepuce with a Penrose drain tightened around the base and a urethral catheter is in place.

Disease	Description	Treatment
Benign prostatic hyperplasia (BPH)	Common in older entire male dogs. Usually causes dyschezia without systemic signs	Treated hormonally or by castration
Prostatitis	Bacterial infection of parenchyma of gland. Often causes systemic signs of pyrexia, lethargy, etc. Also dyschezia, dysuria, tenesmus and purulent penile discharge	Systemic antibiotics and hormonal therapy or castration
Prostatic abscessation	Often concurrent with prostatitis. Similar signs but mass can also cause pelvic obstruction	Drainage percutaneously or at surgery as well as treatment for prostatitis. Cautious prognosis
Prostatic cysts	Usually accompany BPH	Drainage at surgery or percutaneously as well as treatment for BPH
Prostatic neoplasia	Carcinoma commonest type. Unlike other prostatic diseases, occurs frequently in castrates. Painful enlargement of gland with marked tenesmus and dysuria/dyschezia. Malignant and locally invasive	Not usually attempted. Grave prognosis

13.80 Diseases of the prostate gland.

Skin preparation

This often requires preparation of delicate tissues: the scrotal skin (see castration, below) and preputial mucosa. The nurse should avoid contact of surgical spirit with these areas. The mucosa should be prepared by washing with a sterile solution of povidone–iodine, which does not contain detergent, rather than with surgical skin scrub. If the penis itself is of surgical interest, it may be extruded from the prepuce and exposure maintained by a firm bandage or Penrose drain around the base of the penis (Figure 13.81).

Peri- and postoperative care

In most cases, the care is similar to that described for urinary tract surgery.

Castration

This is the commonest surgical procedure of the male reproductive system and is defined as removal of the testes (orchidectomy, gonadectomy). Chapter 2 gives information on discussing the routine benefits of this procedure with clients.

Indications for castration include:

- Social reasons (undesirable sexual behaviour, dominance, prevention of pregnancy, keeping animals in social groups)
- Scrotal/testicular neoplasia
- Hormonally responsive conditions (perianal adenoma, perineal rupture, benign prostatic disease, stud tail)
- Prophylaxis of the above diseases
- Cryptorchidism – prophylaxis of testicular neoplasia or torsion
- Testicular or scrotal trauma
- Inguinal herniation.

Skin preparation for feline castration

1. Pluck or clip the hair from over the testicles.
2. Give the area a gentle surgical scrub, wiping the fur away from the area of incision.

Skin preparation for canine castration

Care is important as hurried preparation may lead to scrotal dermatitis, which will interfere with postoperative healing.

- Clip under anaesthesia to try to avoid damage to the skin of the scrotum with the clippers.
- Skin that is wet or damp is more difficult to clip and damage to the skin is more likely.
- Povidine–iodine is generally more irritant to the skin, so use chlorhexidine surgical scrub to avoid skin irritation after clipping.

- Some surgeons prefer to minimize preparation of the scrotal skin to avoid dermatitis and instead exclude the scrotum from the surgical field.
- The area clipped will depend on practice policy and surgeon's preference but typically includes the scrotum and extends 5 cm to each side of it.

Castration of other species

The surgical technique for castration in other small mammals is somewhat variable.

- Rabbits and guinea pigs are able to retract the testicles into an abdominal position and can be castrated through a scrotal or abdominal approach. The nurse must liaise with the surgeon as to which is planned and prepare the patient appropriately.
- Preparation of the ferret for castration is similar to that of either the cat or the dog, according to practice policy. Ferrets are also occasionally vasectomized: the nurse admitting and preparing the patient must clarify which procedure the owner has requested.

Postoperative care

Interference with the surgical wound by the patient may cause wound breakdown or worsen scrotal haematoma formation. If some degree of scrotal dermatitis is present after surgery, the patient will be more inclined to lick the area. Elizabethan collars are useful to prevent patient interference. Owners should be advised to look for signs of redness or swelling or bruising at the surgical site, discharge from the wound or discomfort in the patient.

Female reproductive system

Figure 13.82 describes common surgical diseases of the ovaries, uterus and vagina. The commonest surgical procedure of these organs is ovariohysterectomy (OHE) (spay) and this is dealt with separately (below). Caesarean section is also considered separately.

Pre-, peri- and postoperative nursing care

This is similar to that described for the urinary tract and the male reproductive system. Most procedures are carried out through an abdominal approach, though occasionally surgery of the vulva or vagina is carried out from the perineum (see anorectal surgery, above).

OHE in the bitch, queen and doe

It is common practice to remove the ovaries and uterus together, though in many cases ovariectomy alone would produce similar benefits. Routine neutering is additionally discussed in Chapter 2.

Indications for ovariohysterectomy include:

- Prevention/termination of pregnancy
- Social reasons (elimination of oestrus)
- Management of medical disorders (diabetes mellitus, epilepsy)
- Prevention of mammary tumours (see below)
- Ovarian disease (neoplasia, irregular cycles)
- Uterine disease (pyometritis, complications of pregnancy, neoplasia in the rabbit)
- Vaginal disease (hormonally responsive conditions).

Disease	Description	Treatment
Ovarian tumours	Uncommon in bitches (1% of canine neoplasms); rare in cats	Ovariohysterectomy (OHE). Prognosis is limited by potential for metastasis
Pyometra (synonyms: pyometritis, 'pyo')	Disease of mature bitch, most commonly in bitches over 6 years old. Hormonally mediated cystic uterine change accompanied by bacterial infection. Usually in entire females. Occasionally seen in uterine remnants of spayed females ('stump pyometra') under influence of exogenous progestagen treatment or those with ovarian remnants. Disease occurs during metoestrus, typically 5–80 days after oestrus. Association exists between incidence of disease and irregular oestrous patterns and also with use of oestrogens (e.g. for misalliance) and progestagens. Less common in cats and has less distinct relationship with oestrus. Clinical signs of pyometra: depression, lethargy, anorexia; vomiting and diarrhoea; polydipsia and polyuria; purulent vaginal discharge; abdominal distension; pyrexia	OHE is treatment of choice in majority of cases following supportive care
Vaginal neoplasia	Usually present as perineal swelling, in entire bitches of around 10 years, and show oestrus-related growth. Usually benign	Episiotomy and submucosal dissection. OHE is essential to prevent recurrence
Vaginal hypertrophy	Excessive hypertrophy of vaginal mucosa occuring in oestrus. Can cause perineal or vulval swelling, or vaginal prolapse. Most cases occur at first oestrus and regress in dioestrus. Affected breeds include Boxer, Bullmastiff, Bulldog and Sharpei	Tissue should be lubricated and replaced if not devitalized and OHE performed at next oestrus
Vaginal prolapse	Occurs postpartum or associated with vaginal hypertrophy	Submucosal resection indicated if mucosa devitalized. Otherwise reduction and placement of purse-string retaining suture

13.82 Diseases of the ovaries, uterus and vagina.

Timing

- Technically, OHE is feasible from a few weeks old and this is preferred by some rehoming organizations.
- Leaving until after first oestrus in the bitch may reduce the incidence of incontinence, vaginitis, infantile vulva.
- Avoid surgery in oestrus (increased vascularity) and false pregnancy (may be prolonged).
- Ovariectomy early in life reduces the incidence of mammary neoplasia (see below).
- Kittens and rabbits are typically neutered at 4–6 months, bitches during anoestrus after the first season.

Caesarean section

This is the removal of the term fetuses by hysterotomy. Obstetrical intervention in bitches and queens is restricted to drug intervention, limited vaginal manipulation and Caesarean section. Around 60% of canine and feline dystocias are managed by Caesarean section.

Fundamental to successful use of this surgical technique are selection of anaesthetic technique, care of the neonate and careful preparation of the dam.

Preoperative care

- The dam must be handled quietly and as much preparation should be made prior to anaesthetic induction as possible.
- The animal is often exhausted and dehydrated and fluid therapy should be initiated.
- Adequate assistance must be available for preparation, surgery and care of the neonates and additional nurses or helpers should be found before surgery commences.
- The recovery area should also be prepared (see below).

Skin preparation

This can often be started before induction of anaesthesia, to reduce later delay in delivery. The standard approach is a midline laparotomy and the ventral abdomen should be clipped widely, from xiphoid to vulva, to accommodate this. Less commonly, a flank approach is used. Final skin scrubbing is completed after induction and patient positioning.

Perioperative care

The patient is positioned in dorsal recumbency, but lying slightly to the left side to reduce pressure of the uterus on the major abdominal blood vessels. Water-repellent drapes and large laparotomy swabs should be supplied to manage the uterine contents encountered during surgery. Surgical suction and lavage fluids are also helpful to reduce contamination of the abdomen. A surgical assistant is useful to help to exteriorize the uterus and then pass the neonates to unscrubbed assistants for revival.

Postoperative care of the dam

- Gently clean the surgical area before the pups begin to suckle.
- The dam should be put back with her puppies as soon as possible, but should not be left unattended until she has recovered sufficiently from the anaesthesia as she may inadvertently cause damage to the puppies when moving or trying to stand.
- Following surgery, place the dam in a large kennel with clean bedding. Ideally there should a bed or enclosed area where the bitch can lie with her puppies and an area where she can move away to avoid their attentions.
- Environmental conditions are important. The area should be draught-free, the atmosphere should be warm but not so warm that the bitch will become too hot. The bitch should be free to move away to a cooler area if she wishes.

Care of the neonates

- Check the mouth for any debris or mucus that may be blocking the airway.
- If necessary, remove debris from the mouth or nostrils with swabs or gentle suction. Swinging the neonate to remove fluid from the airways is not satisfactory, since it may damage the delicate brain.
- Wrap the puppy in a warm towel and gently rub to dry the puppy and stimulate respiration.
- Have oxygen and a respiratory stimulant to hand in case they are needed.
- Make a quick check for any congenital abnormalities such as cleft palate or imperforate anus.
- Keep the puppy warm until it can be returned to the dam at the earliest opportunity (Figure 13.83).
- Once the puppies have been returned to the dam they should be watched to avoid accidental damage by the dam while she is recovering from anaesthesia.
- Suckling should be encouraged at the earliest opportunity.

Further information on care of neonates is given in Chapter 2.

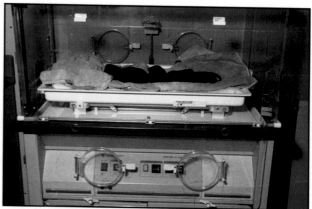

13.83 Puppies recovering in an incubator after Caesarean section whilst surgery is completed.

Mammary glands

Three pathological processes are encountered in the mammary glands:

- *Hypertrophy*, which is a physiological process during late pregnancy but pathological during false pregnancy or following exogenous progesterone treatment
- *Inflammation* (mastitis), which is usually associated with bacterial infection around the time of parturition
- *Neoplasia*, which is the most important surgical disease of this organ.

Mammary tumours represent around a quarter of canine neoplasia and around half of all neoplasms occurring in the bitch. There is an obvious age distribution, with a peak incidence at 10 years, and mammary neoplasia is rare below 5 years of age. Ovariectomy significantly reduces the incidence of mammary tumours if it is performed early in the bitch's life. However, after 2–3 years ovariohysterectomy has no effect on the incidence of later mammary neoplasia, and there is no evidence at present that ovariohysterectomy at the time of mastectomy improves the survival times.

A variety of histopathological types occur:

- Benign (represent 52% of the total)
- Carcinoma (40% of the total)
- Sarcoma (4% of the total)
- Malignant mixed tumours (4% of the total).

The prognosis depends heavily on the histopathological type and thus histopathology should be carried out on the excised tissue so that the owners can be offered an accurate prognosis. The prognosis is excellent for simple and benign mixed tumours or malignant tumours where the tumour is small (less than 5 cm diameter) and local invasion or distant metastasis has not occurred. As with all neoplasia, clinical appearance and examination are not a reliable guide to prognosis.

Mammary neoplasia is also a very common disease in female rats. Many similar considerations to those in the bitch apply, though rats often present with advanced tumours and the prognosis is usually poor, due to extensive or recurrent disease.

Surgical treatment

Surgical excision remains the primary treatment of mammary neoplasia in the bitch. Non-surgical management with chemotherapy and radiotherapy is occasionally of value but is principally indicated for palliation if local recurrent disease occurs.

Surgical techniques include:

- Local excision (lumpectomy)
- Simple mastectomy, i.e. removal of tumour and associated glands
- Partial radical mastectomy, i.e. removal of the tumour complete with the glands associated with it by lymphatic drainage with or without the nodes
- Removal of the tumour with all the glands of that side, with or without the nodes (radical mastectomy, mammary strip)
- Bilateral radical mastectomy, i.e. the removal of all mammary tissue.

The value of each of these techniques remains equivocal and most surgeons would opt for simple excision with small nodules but a more radical procedure for larger nodules, particularly if there was any clinical evidence of malignancy. Overall it is wiser to perform a radical excision at the outset to prevent local recurrence and the need for repeated surgeries.

Preoperative nursing care

These patients are generally well, unless disease is very extensive, and they require little special care before surgery. Preoperative thoracic radiographs are recommended since metastasis to the lungs is relatively common.

Skin preparation

The extent of preparation required depends on the procedure planned, but in any case sufficient skin should be clipped and scrubbed to ensure that no unprepared skin will enter the surgical field during reconstruction of the defect. Radical mastectomy requires extensive skin preparation of the ventrum, from the cranial thorax to the perineum. Closure of this skin defect can be challenging, because of skin tension, and the nurse can help with this by ensuring that all mobile skin is moved from under the patient during positioning.

Perioperative care

No particular issues are usually apparent in these surgeries, though extensive mastectomies may be closed over a wound drain (see above).

Postoperative care

Extensive skin reconstruction can be uncomfortable for the patient and the nurse should ensure that adequate analgesia is provided. Restriction of exercise after surgery is appropriate until the skin has stretched to accommodate the tension (7–10 days). If a drain has been placed, this should be managed appropriately (see above).

Mammary tumours in the cat

The relative and absolute incidence of mammary tumours in the cat is lower than in the bitch, but they do represent the second most common solid neoplasm of this species after skin neoplasia. The prognosis in the cat is poorer than in the dog since 85–90% of tumours are malignant (commonly adenocarcinoma). Intact females are at greater risk than spayed females and Siamese cats may be over-represented.

Eye

This includes the globe, conjunctiva and eyelids. Figure 13.84 describes common surgical diseases of these.

Disease	Description	Treatment
Perforation	Caused by trauma or uncontrolled infection	Enucleation when a non-functional eye is painful or shrunken
Prolapse of the eyeball	Follows head trauma, particularly in brachycephalic dogs with protruding globes. Priority is to prevent further trauma to eye and prevent desiccation	Moisten and lubricate eye with saline and aqueous gel. Replacement is urgent: usually requires general anaesthetic. Restrain animal to prevent self-inflicted trauma
Cataracts	Opacification of lens resulting in loss of vision when severe. May be inherited in some breeds, idiopathic or associated with diabetes mellitus	Intraocular surgery to remove lens is indicated if retina is believed to be functional
Corneal ulceration	Many causes, including: trauma, foreign bodies, infection (especially feline upper respiratory tract viruses), keratoconjunctivitis sicca (dry eye). Risk of perforation of globe if severe	Treat underlying cause if possible. Surgery to promote healing and protect globe may be indicated (third eyelid flap or conjunctival flap)
Eyelid tumours	Relatively common. Particular tumour types are adenoma (benign, usually wart-like in appearance) and squamous cell carcinoma (SCC, locally malignant). SCC most common in unpigmented skin	Adenomas respond well to local excision. SCC require more radical surgery or radiation treatment
Distichiasis	Aberrant lashes growing at margin of eyelids	Often insignificant. If symptomatic, treated by plucking, diathermy or excision of follicles
Entropion/ ectropion	Rolling in or out of eyelid margin. Causes irritation to cornea or conjunctiva. Often associated with conformation of certain breeds (Sharpei in particular, but also others with droopy faces)	Variety of plastic surgical techniques to improve architecture of lids is available
Conjunctival foreign bodies	A cause of severe or chronic conjunctivitis. Grass seeds a common type. Careful ocular examination under local or general anaesthesia important to eliminate in such cases	Removal

13.84 Diseases of the globe, eyelids and conjunctiva.

Nursing care for ophthalmic surgery

Preoperative care

Generally these patients are well, without systemic disease, and little special preoperative nursing is required. An exception is animals with diabetes-associated cataracts, who should be stabilized before surgery (see Chapter 9) and require special anaesthetic management (see Chapter 12).

Skin preparation

The hair around the eye should be clipped carefully following application of an ocular lubricant. Use of small rechargeable clippers with small, fine blades is recommended, to reduce the risk of damage to the eye. The skin must be cleaned carefully with minimal amounts of skin scrub solution, ensuring that none enters the eye. The conjunctival sac is lavaged with a sterile povidone–iodine solution (diluted according to the manufacturer's instructions) which does not contain detergent. Spirit is not used.

Perioperative nursing care

For some procedures (intraocular surgery in particular), muscle relaxants are used as part of the anaesthetic regime and provision for ventilation must be made (see Chapter 12).

Ophthalmic surgery is particularly delicate. The patient must be positioned with the eye uppermost and the head secured firmly. A combination of a conforming sandbag and adhesive tape is useful to achieve this. A fenestrated adhesive disposable drape designed for ophthalmic surgery is ideal. If this is not available, soft drape material that conforms to the head is used. If secured with towel clips, these must be placed with care to avoid damage to the globe (this is true of all surgery around the head).

The surgeon will require excellent illumination and usually optical magnification (operating loupes or an operating microscope). If magnification is used, a scrubbed nurse to pass instruments is extremely useful, to avoid the surgeon having to look away from the surgical field. This surgery is usually carried out with the surgeon sitting on a stool (rather than standing) and provision should be made for the elbows to be supported during surgery.

For intraocular procedures, highly specialized surgical instrumentation is required. For extra-ocular surgery, a fine set of dedicated ophthalmic instruments should be provided, including:

- Eyelid speculum
- Castreviejo needleholders
- Iris scissors
- Corneal forceps
- Micro-dissection scissors
- Mini mosquito forceps.

The surgeon will also require fine swabs (sterile cotton buds or proprietary ophthalmic swabs) and specialized suture material (e.g. 0.5 metric polyglactin).

Postoperative care

The delicate nature of these surgeries and the sensitive tissues of the eye require particular nursing care after surgery.

- Where possible, house patients that have undergone ocular surgery in cages without bars, as the patient may cause damage to the eye by putting its nose through the bars.
- Manual restraint of patients following intraocular surgery should be gentle so as not to cause an increase in intraocular pressure.
- Analgesia for patients following ocular surgery is important as pain or discomfort may cause the animal to rub at the surgical site.
- Foot bandages can be used to prevent damage to the surgical site with the front feet.
- Elizabethan collars can be used to prevent self-mutilation. Some patients may cause more damage by wearing or trying to remove the collar, so careful patient selection is required.
- Monitor the patient carefully for increasing discomfort or change in appearance of the eye and liaise closely with the surgeon to report progress.
- Ensure that the nursing staff and owner understand the postoperative medication requirements and how to apply topical medication effectively without trauma.

Ear

This includes the pinna, ear canal and middle ear. Figure 13.85 describes common surgical diseases of the ear.

Nursing care for ear surgery

The two commonest types of surgical procedure are treatment of aural haematoma and ear canal surgery for otitis externa. Aural haematoma is considered separately and most of this section therefore concerns surgery of the ear canal.

Preoperative care

Particular issues are the pain associated with ear disease and the disorientation of the patient due to loss of hearing or balance disturbances. The animal must be handled with regard to each of these, taking care to avoid pressure around the ears during restraint and reassuring the distressed patient. Provision of adequate premedication with both sedative and analgesic agents will help a great deal during preparation for anaesthesia and surgery.

Skin preparation

Most of these procedures involve the pinna and/or external ear canal. The hair should be clipped from both sides of the pinna and the clipped area should include the entire side of the face, from the dorsal midline to the angle of the mandible. The ear canal may be plugged with cotton wool during clipping to keep the clipped hair out.

The ear canal is often heavily soiled with discharge and can be difficult to clean thoroughly. Repeated gentle scrubbing to avoid skin irritation is required

Disease	Description	Treatment
Squamous cell carcinoma (SCC) of the pinna	Commonly affects tips of ears of white cats (or those with white ears). Pre-cancerous change of actinic keratosis found prior to SCC. Presents as alopecia and crusting of ear tip progressing to ulceration and distortion. Often bilateral	Early cases may respond to reducing exposure to sunlight (confinement and sun block). SCC requires surgical amputation of pinna
Trauma to pinna	Can result in marked haemorrhage	Usually heals well following wound management and bandaging. First aid includes head bandage to control haemorrhage and reduce effects of head shaking
Aural haematoma	Haematoma formation between skin and cartilage of pinna. Usually a canine disease. May indicate ear canal disease (check for this)	Managed by drainage and various surgical procedures. May respond to drainage and corticosteroid administration. Left untreated, distortion of pinna will result
Foreign body within ear canal	Typically grass seeds in summer (usually dogs). Hair accumulations can also cause irritation. Results in head shaking and discomfort	Remove with forceps under sedation/general anaesthetic
Acute otitis externa (OE)	Various causes (yeast infection, bacteria, foreign bodies, ear mites) and underlying conditions (atopy, conformation, hypothyroidism, etc.)	Usually responds well to medical treatment. Further investigation and surgery may be indicated for resistant or recurrent cases
Chronic otitis externa	Usually result of unresolved acute OE. Ear canal tumours, middle ear infection and anatomical abnormalities are also causes	May respond to intensive medical treatment, including ear flushing. Surgery indicated in resistant cases
Middle ear infection	In dogs: usually follows otitis externa and managed concurrently. In cats: seen as primary disease in young cats	May respond to medical management or require drainage at surgery (ventral bulla osteotomy)
Middle ear polyps (nasopharyngeal polyps)	Almost exclusively cats, usually young. Cause signs of middle ear diseases (head tilt, Horner's syndrome, loss of balance), otitis externa (if extending into ear canal) or pharyngeal obstruction (if extending through Eustachian tube into nasopharynx)	Traction and/or middle ear exploration (ventral bulla osteotomy)

13.85 Diseases of the pinna, ear canal and middle ear.

and cotton buds can be useful to wipe around the skin folds. Once scrubbing is completed, any fluid must be removed from the ear canal by suction so that it does not enter the sterile field during surgery.

Perioperative care

The patient's head must be positioned in lateral recumbency with the ear uppermost. The comments made relating to ophthalmic surgery (above) apply: the head must be secure and towel clips applied with care. In most cases, the pinna will be included in the surgical field (Figure 13.86).

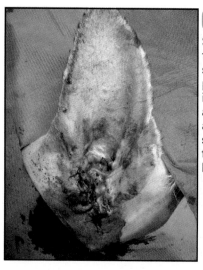

13.86 Surgical field for ear canal surgery. The pinna is included in the draped area (photo taken at completion of surgery and the towel clips have been removed).

Surgical procedures of the ear canal do not generally require specialized equipment, except for sharp Mayo scissors for cartilage resection. However, surgery of the middle ear (e.g. total ear canal ablation with lateral bulla osteotomy, TECA-LBO), requires excellent illumination (operating lights or head lamp), surgical suction and instruments to expose, open and debride the middle ear:

- Frazier suction tip
- Spreull needle
- Osteotome and orthopaedic mallet
- Rongeurs
- Volkman spoon
- Gelpi retractors
- Langenback retractors.

Postoperative care

In the care of patients following ear canal surgery it is important to prevent self-trauma by the patient as this will lead to breakdown of the surgical site. The way in which each case is treated may vary according to the response of the patient following surgical intervention.

Methods of preventing self trauma include the following.

- Elizabethan collars – used to prevent damage to the surgical site by scratching or rubbing. As the collar is close to the area of surgery it must be kept clean. Care should be taken when placing Elizabethan collars on patients following ear canal surgery so that no damage is caused as the collar is passed over the surgical site.

- Bandages – can be applied to cover the surgical wound and protect the ear (see Figure 14.19). However, head bandages can increase patient irritation and should be used with care. Hindfoot bandages can also be useful in the prevention of self-mutilation by the patient.
- Sedation – although less commonly used, sedation of the patient in the initial postoperative period can be used to prevent self-mutilation. This would only be considered in the more extreme cases.
- Analgesia – as with all surgery the patient should be watched for signs of pain or discomfort. As ear canal surgery is potentially very painful, a patient may cause damage to the surgical site by rubbing or head shaking due to pain.

Treatment of aural haematoma

Most cases of aural haematoma are treated by surgical drainage. Several techniques are described. In all cases an incision is made through the skin on the hairless (concave) surface of the pinna to evacuate the haematoma. Continued postoperative drainage is achieved by placing a drain (Penrose or teat cannula) into the cavity or by excising an ellipse of skin. A series of large mattress sutures may be placed through the pinna to eliminate the dead space. The ear is usually bandaged postoperatively to prevent patient interference, protect the drain or wound, reduce dead space and prevent the adverse effects of head shaking.

Some cases of aural haematoma are treated by surgical drainage with subsequent infusion of corticosteroid suspension. Commonly, a bandage is applied after such treatment.

Further reading

Anderson D and Smith J (2007) Surgical nursing. In: *BSAVA Textbook of Veterinary Nursing, 4th edn*, ed. DR Lane *et al.*, pp. 590–639. BSAVA Publications, Gloucester

Brockman D and Holt D (2005) *BSAVA Manual of Canine and Feline Head, Neck and Thoracic Surgery*. BSAVA Publications, Gloucester

Coughlan A and Miller A (eds) (2006) *BSAVA Manual of Small Animal Fracture Repair and Management* (revised reprint). BSAVA Publications, Gloucester

Fossum TW (2007) *Small Animal Surgery, 3rd edn*. Mosby, St Louis

McHugh D (2007) Theatre practice. In: *BSAVA Textbook of Veterinary Nursing, 4th edn*, ed. DR Lane *et al.*, pp. 561–589. BSAVA Publications, Gloucester

Slatter D (2003) *Textbook of Small Animal Surgery, 3rd edn*. Saunders, Philadelphia

Tracy DL (1994) *Small Animal Surgical Nursing, 3rd edn*. Mosby, St Louis

Williams J and Niles J (2005) *BSAVA Manual of Canine and Feline Abdominal Surgery*. BSAVA Publications, Gloucester

Acknowledgement

The authors and editors would like to acknowledge the contribution of Cathy Garden to the *BSAVA Manual of Veterinary Nursing*.

14

Wound management, dressings and bandages

Clare Bryant and Dominic Phillips

> *This chapter is designed to give information on:*
>
> - The normal wound healing process
> - Assessment of the wound patient and wounds
> - Types of wound and wound features; wound classification
> - Types and methods of wound closure; open wound management
> - Types and management of wound drains
> - Complications of wound healing
> - Functions and types of wound dressings, bandages, casts and splints
> - Management of dressings, bandages and casts, and care of the patient

Introduction

A wound is an injury that disrupts the normal continuity and integrity of the external surface of the body or an organ; the term usually refers to injuries to the skin and underlying tissues.

Wounds are a common clinical presentation and often constitute a significant clinical and nursing challenge. Appropriate wound management is critical for effective, timely wound healing and resolution. Wound management is a dynamic process based on the initial assessment of the wound, with subsequent support and facilitation of wound healing processes using a variety of wound treatment, dressing and bandaging techniques, with appropriate responses to developing complications.

The wound patient

When a wounded patient is presented, it is important to make a full examination and assessment of the patient and not to focus inappropriately on obvious but possibly non-critical wounds. Life-threatening wounds must be treated appropriately; however, many

scenarios in which patients sustain wounds have the potential to cause other life-threatening injuries that need to be identified and treated before less critical wounds are attended to. Road traffic accidents, falling, crushing and penetrating accidents can all cause life-threatening injuries to critical body systems such as the head, spine, thoracic organs and abdominal organs. Emergency assessment and treatment of an injured patient may require appropriate analgesia, sedation or anaesthesia if pain and distress make the animal unmanageable (see Chapter 7).

Action priorities are based on assessment of the patient:

1. Identify and treat life-threatening conditions such as cardiorespiratory arrest, haemorrhage, internal injuries (e.g. pneumothorax, splenic rupture) (see Chapter 7).
2. Implement supportive treatment for shock, such as fluid therapy (see Chapter 8), thermal therapy.
3. Implement pain management (see Chapter 12).
4. Start appropriate antibiosis.

Once a patient is assessed as fit and stable, the process of wound management can be started.

Wound management

The objective of wound management is to facilitate the optimal healing of wounds according to the following criteria:

- Patient comfort: to minimize pain and maximize comfort during the wound healing period
- Functionality: to maximize the functionality of the healed tissues
- Time: to minimize the duration of the wound healing period
- Cost: to manage the healing process within any determined financial limits.

Any factor that influences the dynamics of the normal wound healing process (Figure 14.1) and the development of healthy granulation tissue (see Figure 14.8b) will not only affect the speed of wound healing but can influence the functionality of the resulting healed tissues. These factors can work at the patient and systemic level or locally at the wound level. Careful patient and wound level assessment is required to ensure optimal wound management.

Patient assessment

At the patient or systemic level, promotion of wound healing is based on managing influences that have a negative effect on the normal wound healing process, such as immunosuppressant factors or those that compromise the metabolic processes involved in healing. The objective of patient-level assessment is to identify the factors that represent a risk to the wound healing process and thereby manage them as part of the wound management approach (Figure 14.2).

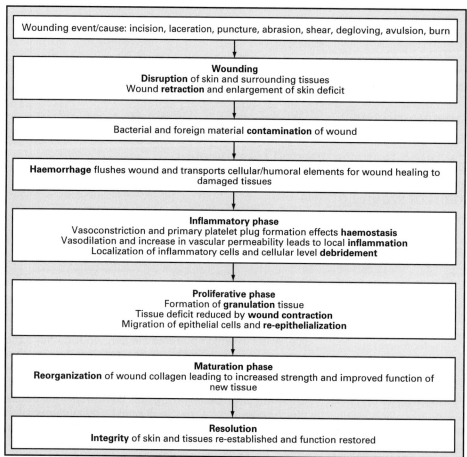

14.1 The normal wound healing process. From wounding to wound resolution, healing follows a series of characteristic phases, each playing a role in the repair and reconstruction of damaged tissues.

Factor	Risk	Risk reduction
Age	Both the biosynthetic capacity and the immune systems of very young and old patients are less effective due to not being fully developed or being compromised by age-related changes	The risks of slow healing and susceptibility to infection in the very young or old patient can be reduced through measures such as more frequent wound dressing changes, and appropriate local and systemic antimicrobial techniques
Nutrition	Patients with malnutrition or with specific nutritional deficiencies (such as protein, minerals, vitamins) are at risk of immunosuppression and impaired biosynthetic capacity	Correction of nutritional deficiencies and maintenance of optimal nutrition are essential throughout wound healing. In some debilitated patients or those unable to eat (e.g. with facial or oral injuries) nutritional support through tube feeding or parenteral nutrition is required. Special critical care diets have been developed specifically for these purposes

14.2 Patient and systemic level factors influencing wound healing. A range of factors represent potential risks to the normal wound healing process; measures must be taken to prevent or reduce these factors having a negative influence on wound healing. (continues) ▶

Factor	Risk	Risk reduction
Hydration	Systemic dehydration will adversely affect the local wound environment and the patient's biosynthetic processes	Correction of fluid deficits and electrolyte imbalances and subsequent maintenance of hydration through appropriate fluid therapy are essential for optimal wound healing. Fluid therapy is particularly important in the debilitated patient unable to meet its own maintenance fluid requirements
Concurrent disease	Concurrent systemic or chronic disease adversely affects the wound healing process through suppressing the immune system, compromising the body's metabolism, competing for limited resources or requiring treatments that deleteriously affect wound healing. These diseases include neoplastic disease, renal disease, hepatic disease, endocrinopathies (such as hyperadrenocorticism, hypothyroidism and diabetes mellitus) and conditions causing cachexia.	Management of pre-existing and concurrent diseases should be reviewed to identify any deleterious effects they may have on wound healing. If required and if possible the management of a condition may be adjusted to ameliorate its negative effect on wound healing. In addition measures are taken to counter any unavoidable negative effects, for example related to immunosuppression or slow wound healing
Drugs and therapy	Any drug or treatment that suppresses the immune system or is damaging to dividing cells will adversely affect the wound healing process; these include corticosteroids, cytotoxic drugs, chemotherapy and radiation therapy	Medication and therapy regimes of patients should be reviewed to identify risks to wound healing and to either adjust regimes or develop measures to counter any deleterious effects they may have. For example, the use of corticosteroids during wound healing may be suspended due to their immunosuppressive effect
Stress	Mental stress (such as that resulting from prolonged hospitalization or pain) or physiological stress (such as hypothermia and chronic pain) have an immunosuppressive effect and adversely affect wound healing processes	Environmental, physiological and mental stressors are identified and specific measures are developed to eliminate or reduce their effect on the patient. Careful control of the patient's environmental conditions is maintained to minimize stress. This is particularly important in patients requiring long-term hospitalization and in easily stressed exotic species

14.2 (continued) Patient and systemic level factors influencing wound healing. A range of factors represent potential risks to the normal wound healing process; measures must be taken to prevent or reduce these factors having a negative influence on wound healing.

In addition to the factors above, other patient-specific factors that should be considered include the following examples.

- Young or exuberant patients may cause subsequent injury to a wound through over-activity and may require the imposition of restraint measures such as cage rest.
- Aggressive patients may require sedation for wound treatment and dressing changes, which may alter the frequency of planned treatments.
- Old or heavy dogs may be more prone to pressure ulcers and require specific bedding and turning during the wound treatment process.

A patient-level review is conducted at each re-presentation of the patient for treatment or a dressing change, with the wound management approach being adjusted accordingly.

Wound assessment

Once the patient-level assessment has been conducted, the wound is assessed. Many patients presenting with wound injuries will have multiple wounds and an assessment must be made of each wound. The purpose of wound assessment is to develop a treatment approach appropriate for the wound. Wound assessment involves the identification of wound characteristics and features that determine how the clinician will manage the wound through the wound healing process (see Figure 14.4). At the local level, promotion of wound healing is based on preventing further tissue damage, establishing a clean and uninfected wound, resolving inflammation and maintaining a healthy wound healing environment. Part of this process is identification and assessment of the local wound factors listed in Figure 14.3 that influence wound healing.

Wound assessment is conducted with the patient appropriately restrained, sedated or anaesthetized (see Chapters 5 and 12). The patient must be handled gently, with care taken not to aggravate existing injuries and wounds. The clinician must maintain aseptic conditions, using sterile gloves, instruments and materials to examine and explore the wound to make a full assessment of its nature and extent. Care must be used when exploring a wound and wound tissues must be handled gently at all times to avoid further injury and tissue damage or inflammation.

Wound assessment should consider:

- Site of wound
- Type of wound
- Infection
- Contamination
- Inflammation
- Tissue viability
- Fluid balance
- Oxygenation
- Tissue movement.

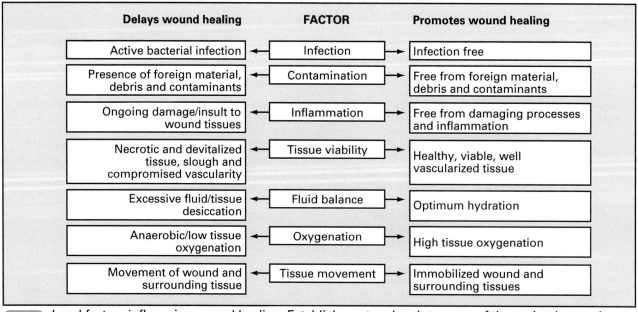

Delays wound healing	FACTOR	Promotes wound healing
Active bacterial infection	Infection	Infection free
Presence of foreign material, debris and contaminants	Contamination	Free from foreign material, debris and contaminants
Ongoing damage/insult to wound tissues	Inflammation	Free from damaging processes and inflammation
Necrotic and devitalized tissue, slough and compromised vascularity	Tissue viability	Healthy, viable, well vascularized tissue
Excessive fluid/tissue desiccation	Fluid balance	Optimum hydration
Anaerobic/low tissue oxygenation	Oxygenation	High tissue oxygenation
Movement of wound and surrounding tissue	Tissue movement	Immobilized wound and surrounding tissues

14.3 Local factors influencing wound healing. Establishment and maintenance of the optimal wound microenvironment is critical to promote normal wound healing.

Site of wound

The site of a wound on the patient's body will influence many aspects of wound management. For example:

- A wound close to a structure such as a body orifice, the eyelids or ears needs to be managed to minimize inappropriate wound contracture, in order to prevent distortion of the structure
- A wound close to the anus, prepuce or vulva will have specific dressing and bandaging requirements so as not to interfere with the function of the structure or become contaminated with faeces or urine
- A wound on a limb or other highly mobile area of the body will require measures such as splinting and bandaging to minimize wound movement in order to prevent disruption of wound healing
- A wound in a dependent site, in an area of loose skin with potential **dead space** (abnormal space within wound tissues containing fluid or gas) or on an extremity will be vulnerable to the build-up of fluid and will require fluid management techniques such as pressure bandaging or drains

- A wound that is easily licked or scratched will require measures to prevent patient interference, such as the use of Elizabethan collars.

Type of wound

There are numerous and diverse causes of wounds; different inciting causes create different wound types. As shown in Figure 14.4, by identifying the wound type it is possible to anticipate characteristic features that are relevant to wound management such as the potential for haemorrhage, the risks of contamination, the extent of tissue damage and the risks of damage to deep structures and surrounding tissues. Assessment of wound type should include identification of tissues and structures either damaged by the injury or at risk:

- Skin involvement (partial or full skin thickness)
- Muscle involvement
- Nerves and major blood vessels
- Tendons and tendon sheaths
- Bones and joints
- Organs.

Wound type	Common causes	Characteristic features
Incisional	Surgical incisions, knife wounds, glass or sharp metal injuries	Clean regular linear wound edges of variable length caused by a sharp object. Variable depth, with possible involvement of deep muscle, tendon and nerve tissue. Significant haemorrhage possible. Minimal trauma to surrounding tissues. Minimal wound contamination
Laceration	Wire injuries, fight injuries	Irregular tearing of epidermis and dermis. Variable depth, with possible involvement of deep muscle, tendon and nerve tissue. Significant haemorrhage possible. Moderate trauma to surrounding tissues. High risk of bacterial and foreign material contamination
Puncture	Bite injuries, gunshots, spike or stick injuries, stab injuries	Perforating (entry and exit wounds) or penetrating (entry wound only) wounds with small skin deficits caused by pointed objects. Variable depth. Low level of haemorrhage. Significant trauma to surrounding and deep tissues possible. High risk of bacterial and foreign body contamination

14.4 Common wound types and characteristics. Different causes of wounding tend to create wounds with characteristic features. These determine the approach to wound management and the potential complications. (continues) ▶

Wound type	Common causes	Characteristic features
Abrasion	Road traffic injuries, cast and bandage wounds	Frictional damage usually to the epidermis and superficial dermis, with high risk of significant skin deficits. Low to moderate haemorrhage. Significant local tissue trauma and tissue loss. High risk of bacterial and foreign body contamination from the abrading surface
Shear	Road traffic injuries	Severe frictional damage, usually to the limbs, involving deep tissues including muscles, ligaments, bones and joints. Features similar to abrasions
Degloving	Road traffic injuries, bandage wounds	Tearing or loss of skin from a limb, through mechanical or physiological processes, often resulting in significant skin deficits. Significant tissue trauma and tissue loss. Initially can be contamination free but risk of secondary contamination associated with infection and devitalized tissue
Avulsion	Road traffic injuries, dog fight injuries	Separation of skin from underlying tissues through traumatic loss of attachments. Significant skin loss possible. Significant local tissue damage with high risk of remaining tissue being compromised. Initially can be contamination free but risk of secondary contamination associated with infection and devitalized tissue
Burn	Thermal, electrical, chemical, radiation burns	Variable damage involving the epidermis, dermis and underlying tissue, leading to potentially significant skin deficits. No haemorrhage. Damage restricted to tissues exposed to the burning agent. Initially contamination limited to persisting chemical agents but risk of secondary contamination associated with infection and devitalized tissue

14.4 (continued) Common wound types and characteristics. Different causes of wounding tend to create wounds with characteristic features. These determine the approach to wound management and the potential complications.

Special measures can be taken to treat damaged structures such as joints or to protect structures at risk of damage or involvement, for example from infection. By defining the wound type the high-level approach to the treatment of the wound will be indicated, such as primary closure or open wound management.

Infection

Increased exudates, wound surface biofilm, discoloration and malodour are signs of bacterial infection (Figure 14.5). If these are present, action must be planned to remove or reduce the bacterial load through lavage, debridement and use of local and systemic antimicrobial treatments.

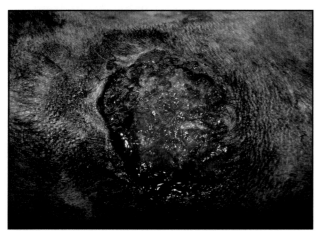

14.5 An infected and contaminated wound. Necrotic wound edges, an irregular wound bed and a surface biofilm are significant.

Contamination

The presence of foreign material (e.g. hair, soil, grit and wood) in a wound acts as a reservoir of infection and a focus for ongoing inflammation. If present, action must be planned to remove all foreign material and contaminants through wound exploration and searching, lavage, debridement and dressing techniques. Assessment of the level of contamination of a wound is an important criterion in the process of deciding when to close a wound. It is critical for wounds to be free from contamination, or to have a level of contamination that is clinically insignificant, before they are closed.

Classification of wound contamination

Clean wounds: wounds with no contamination, created under sterile conditions. Limited to surgical procedures not involving entry into the respiratory, gastrointestinal or urogenital tracts.

Clean–contaminated wounds: wounds with minimal contamination that is readily removed or reduced to a clinically insignificant level. Includes surgical wounds of the respiratory, gastrointestinal or urogenital tracts.

Contaminated wounds: wounds with heavy contamination, usually associated with the presence of foreign material in the wound but not infection. Surgical procedures suffering major breaks in aseptic technique (e.g. spillage of gastrointestinal contents) are classified as contaminated. Acutely presented (within 6 hours) traumatic wounds are considered contaminated on presentation but can be converted to a clean–contaminated state through prompt lavage and debridement.

Dirty wounds: wounds with active infection present, e.g. old traumatic wounds. The presence of purulent and necrotic material is a characteristic of a dirty wound.

Inflammation

The initial trauma of the injury, the presence of infection, contamination and necrotic material all cause local inflammation; action must be planned and taken to eliminate these sources of ongoing inflammation. Measures must be taken to manage the local effects of inflammation, such as drains to remove excess fluid and analgesics to manage associated pain.

Sign	Cause
Redness	Vasodilation
Swelling	Increased vascular permeability, fluid exudation, obstruction of local lymphatic channels
Heat	Vasodilation
Pain	Release of inflammatory mediators, local pressure and tissue stretching
Loss of function	Combined effects of the above changes

Tissue viability

Necrotic and non-viable damaged tissue is non-functional, promotes infection and inflammation and must be removed to allow normal wound healing. Tissue can become non-viable through physical trauma such as crushing, through infection or through blood supply compromise leading to tissue death. It must be remembered that it may not be possible to identify all non-viable tissue for a significant period after injury; tissue death through disruption of blood supply can take several days to be grossly identifiable through examination. Further tissue death will be an ongoing process until infection and inflammation are controlled. Surgical and dressing debriding techniques are used to remove non-viable tissue and necrotic material, leaving healthy and well vascularized wound tissue capable of healing.

Fluid balance

Excessive moisture within wound tissues indicates ongoing inflammation and possible presence of infection; it causes swelling, pain, and tissue maceration and promotes infection. Passive and active draining techniques can be used to manage the risks of excessive fluid, as can absorbent dressings. Dehydration and desiccation of the wound is equally damaging, delaying healing and promoting infection. Optimal wound hydration can be achieved through appropriate wound dressing techniques (see later).

Oxygenation

Wound healing and epithelialization are promoted by high tissue oxygen tensions. The removal of necrotic tissue and debris transforms the wound from an anaerobic (low oxygen) environment, at risk of colonization by anaerobe bacteria, to an environment with high levels of oxygenation that promotes healing. Wound debridement and the use of oxygen-permeable membrane dressings help to maintain appropriate wound oxygenation (see later).

Tissue movement

Wounds to parts of the body subject to movement or wounds of a type where the wound edges are subject to local tension and distractive forces require stabilization and immobilization to enable healing and repair. Closure of wounds using sutures or staples achieves stable apposition of wound edges. Bandaging and splinting techniques are used to provide immobilization (see later).

Wound treatment plans

Based on the assessment of the wound, a treatment plan can be developed for the wound that details actions for each wound factor needing to be managed. Appropriate wound management techniques such as lavage, debridement and drainage can be prescribed to achieve specific wound management goals. These goals can be recorded in the wound management documentation along with the techniques to be employed to achieve them.

Wound assessment needs to be made for each wound on a patient and needs to be conducted each time the patient is re-presented for treatment or dressing changes. This process allows ongoing review of healing progress and allows the clinician to respond to changing wound factors through modification of the treatment plan.

Wound management documentation

Using supporting documentation can aid the process of managing a wound from first presentation to full resolution (Figure 14.6). Documentation captures the mental process that clinicians go through during the management of a wound. Appropriate documentation allows key information and decision-making rationale to be recorded in an easily accessible and objective format, allowing continuity of case management when different clinicians are involved in a case over time. Any documentation used for wound management must be simple, flexible enough to track wound care over multiple re-examinations and easily accessible.

Wound mapping

The main features of the wound assessment can be recorded on a wound map as part of a wound management document. Wound mapping is a useful tool that facilitates the tracking of the wound healing process (Figure 14.6). This reference documentation can be particularly important with slow-healing wounds: over the time period that a serious wound takes to heal, different clinical staff will be involved in its treatment at different times and assessment of progress can be difficult. Wound mapping allows an objective assessment and recording of a wound by one clinician to be compared with that of another.

Features of the wound that can be recorded include:

- Dimensions/measurements
- Wound shape/outline
- Areas of inflammation, infection, necrosis, swelling
- Areas of granulation tissue
- Areas of epithelialization.

WOUND MANAGEMENT PART 1
PATIENT ASSESSMENT

OWNER:	PATIENT:	REF NO:
ADDRESS:	SPECIES:	BREED:
	SEX:	AGE:

TEL:

MEDICAL HISTORY

Current medical conditions:

Current medication/therapy:

WOUND HISTORY   Date of injury:
Cause of injury:

WOUNDS LOG

○   Puncture

| Incision

⟨   Laceration

⫽   Abrasion

▮   Degloving

Right   Left   Right

Wound reference	Site	Type

TREATMENT LOG

Date	Clinician	Next treatment

14.6 Sample wound management document. The wound management process can be documented to allow the accurate and systematic tracking of wound healing, facilitating effective wound treatment from wounding to wound resolution. (continues) ▶

WOUND MANAGEMENT PART 2
WOUND ASSESSMENT

OWNER:	PATIENT:	REF NO:
	SPECIES:	BREED:
ADDRESS:	SEX:	AGE:

TEL:

WOUND REF: DATE OF ASSESSMENT:
SITE: CLINICIAN:
TYPE:

WOUND APPEARANCE/DESCRIPTION:

Infection
Inflammation
Contamination
Necrosis
Fluid/moisture
Granulation
Epithelialization

WOUND MAP/PHOTO

WOUND TREATMENT

Lavage/debridement:

Topical dressings:

Antimicrobials:

DRESSING/BANDAGING

Primary (contact):

Secondary:

Tertiary

NEXT TREATMENT:

14.6 (continued) Sample wound management document. The wound management process can be documented to allow the accurate and systematic tracking of wound healing, facilitating effective wound treatment from wounding to wound resolution.

Digital photography of wounds is a useful development of the wound mapping principle, allowing more accurate recording and evaluation of wound healing progress.

Wound closure

Wound closure is the elimination of the skin deficit and re-establishment of the continuity of the skin. The clinician's decision as to when and how to achieve wound closure is based on the wound assessment process. Two main wound factors will determine when a wound is suitable for closure:

- The level of wound contamination
- The viability of wound tissues.

When a wound is contamination free and the wound tissues are healthy and viable, wound closure can be made. It must be remembered that non-viable tissue can take several days to declare itself and several phases of debridement may be required before only healthy viable tissue is left. It is better to extend a period of open wound management rather than attempt to close a wound before it is free from contamination and non-viable tissue; the presence of either will lead to wound complications and potential breakdown.

Based on the findings of the wound assessment process there are four options a clinician can choose to achieve wound closure (Figure 14.7).

- **Primary closure**: immediate closure of skin edges when no skin tension is present. This is suitable for clean wounds (surgical incisions) or clean–contaminated wounds following immediate presentation, lavage and debridement.
- **Delayed primary closure**: closure of skin edges performed 2–5 days after wounding. This is suitable for clean–contaminated or contaminated wounds with uncertain tissue viability and skin tension. Closure occurs after a period of open wound management based on lavage, debridement and dressing.
- **Secondary closure**: closure of skin edges performed after 5 days or more of open wound management. This is suitable for management of contaminated or dirty wounds that require open wound management to eliminate contamination, necrotic tissue and infection and is based on the presence of healthy granulation tissue.
- **Second intention healing**: healing of a wound through granulation, contraction and epithelialization where surgical closure is not possible or required (Figure 14.8). This is suitable for very small wounds, wounds on extremities or large wounds where there is abundant surrounding skin. This approach requires the application of open wound management techniques until re-epithelialization is complete.

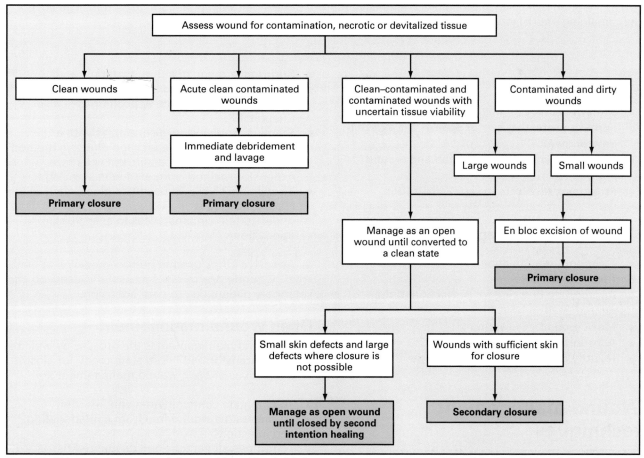

14.7 Wound closure decision making. The initial assessment of a wound is critical in determining the strategy for wound closure. The decision-making process is aimed at ensuring that the wound is free from contamination and that wound tissues are viable before wound closure is attempted.

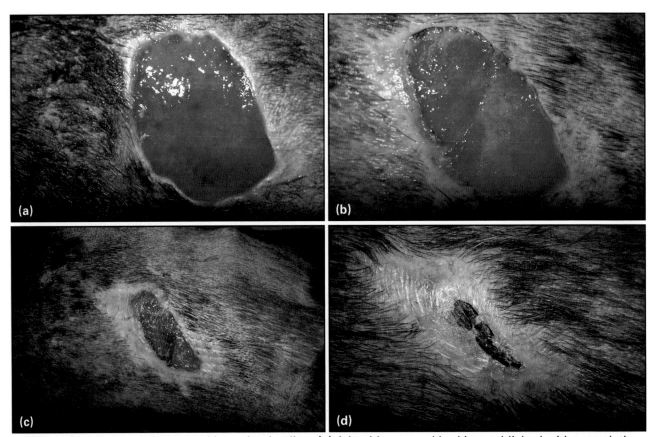

14.8 Wound closure by second intention healing. **(a)** A healthy wound bed is established with granulation tissue. Early re-epithelialization is evident around the wound margins. **(b)** The wound bed of granulation tissue is reduced in size as new epithelium advances from the wound margins. **(c)** A small residual wound bed is surrounded by an extensive margin of new delicate epithelium. **(d)** A thin scab covers the remaining area of wound yet to be covered by new epithelium.

Functions of granulation tissue

- Highly resistant to infection
- Forms a protective barrier against the external environment
- Involved in collagen production and wound contraction
- Provides a substrate for epithelialization

Factors promoting rapid epithelialization

- Freedom from infection
- Absence of a scab
- Appropriate dressing for protection of the wound environment
- Moist wound environment
- Appropriate tissue oxygenation
- Healthy granulation tissue substrate

Wound management techniques

Wound closure techniques

The skin edges of a wound can be brought into stable apposition through three main techniques.

- **Suturing**: a range of suture materials and suture patterns is used in this common and effective method of skin apposition (see also Chapter 13).
- **Stapling**: applying surgical staples with a surgical staple gun is a fast and effective method of achieving skin apposition, but is a more expensive method compared with suturing.
- **Tissue adhesive**: cyanoacrylate glues, such as Nexabond Liquid and Vetbond (3M), can be used under certain circumstances to achieve skin apposition.

Adhesive strips used in human medicine to close small wounds are rarely successfully used on the veterinary patient due to poor adhesion.

Open wound management

Open wound management is the process by which a wound is transformed into a state ready for closure. The objectives of open wound management are:

- To eliminate contamination and infection
- To maintain a wound free from contamination and infection
- To remove all necrotic and devitalized tissue
- To establish and maintain a healthy wound healing environment in terms of factors such as wound hydration and oxygenation.

Wound lavage

The purpose of wound lavage is to reduce the bacterial load of a wound and to remove free foreign material. The effectiveness of wound lavage has been shown to be directly proportional to the volume of fluid used, indicating that physical removal and dilution of contaminants (rather than bactericidal activity) is the key factor in effective wound lavage.

Wound lavage is achieved by flushing a wound with an appropriate fluid.

- Hartmann's and lactated Ringer's solutions are the ideal flushing agents as they are sterile, isotonic, buffered and non-cytotoxic.
- Both normal saline (0.9% NaCl solution) and tap water have mild cytotoxic effects and are therefore not the fluids of choice for wound lavage.

In the presence of severe wound infection an antiseptic agent can be added to the flushing solution: chlorhexidine diluted to a concentration of 0.05% (a 1-in-40 dilution) is the most effect agent for this purpose. Povidone–iodine is considered less effective than chlorhexidine due to its limited residual antimicrobial activity and rapid inactivation by debris, pus and blood. Hypochlorite (Dakin's solution), hydrogen peroxide and cetrimide/chlorhexidine are all irritant and highly toxic to the host cells and are contraindicated for wound lavage.

Initial wound flushing can be achieved by directing a flow of solution from an opened fluid bag over the wound. More active lavage can then be achieved using a 20 ml or 30 ml syringe with an 18 gauge needle, connected to a fluid bag by a three-way tap and giving set (Figure 14.9), to flush the wound with sufficient pressure to dislodge debris. Wound lavage should be performed as a sterile procedure, with appropriate measures taken to minimize the wetting of the patient.

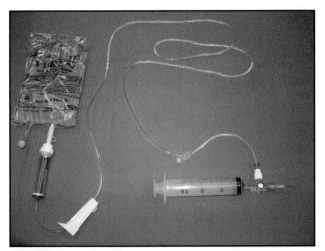

14.9 A wound lavage system.

Wound debridement

Debridement is the removal of foreign material, debris and non-viable tissue from a wound. It is achieved through two processes: surgical debridement and dressing debridement.

Surgical debridement

This involves the sharp excision of gross necrotic and non-viable tissue. It is a surgical procedure requiring aseptic technique and anaesthesia.

To prepare the wound and surrounding area for surgical debridement:

1. Pack the wound with sterile water-soluble gel (IntraSite) or saline-soaked swabs to prevent clipped hair from contaminating the wound.
2. Clip a wide area around the wound. Remove the clipped hair with a vacuum cleaner to minimize contamination risks.
3. Rinse out or remove the wound packing.
4. Surgically prepare the clipped area with surgical antiseptic solution.

Surgical debridement is usually achieved through **layered debridement**, where necrotic and non-viable tissue is removed from successive layers of tissue working from the surface to deeper tissues. **En bloc debridement** is less commonly used and involves the complete wide-margin excision of a contaminated wound, allowing immediate primary closure of the new clean wound created.

Dressing debridement

Once gross debris and necrotic tissue have been removed through surgical debridement, the contact layer of wound dressing can be used for further debridement. Adherent dressings are used for this purpose in the early stages of wound healing when managing contamination, infection and necrosis. Dry-to-dry and wet-to-wet dressing products are designed for this role (see Figure 14.15).

Aids to debridement

Enzymatic debriding agents, cleaning solutions, hydrogels/hydroactive dressings or larval therapy (maggots) can be used as adjuncts to the debriding process (see Figure 14.15).

Prevention and treatment of infection

Systemic antibiotics

These are indicated in the treatment of infected wounds. Ideally their use should be based on wound swab culture and sensitivity results. When not available, antibiotic choice should be based on likely wound contaminants such as *Staphylococcus* spp., *Escherichia coli* and *Pasteurella* spp. The prophylactic use of antibiotics in wound management is controversial; effective lavage and debridement can make their use unnecessary.

Topical antibiotics

These are generally considered to be ineffective and unnecessary when systemic antibiotic treatment achieves rapid and high tissue concentrations.

Topical antiseptics

These are generally considered toxic to fibroblasts and epithelial cells, thereby slowing wound healing more than countering wound infection.

Barrier dressings

Dressings and bandaging provide an essential barrier between the wound and the external environment, thereby preventing contamination and infection of the healing wound. Some contact (primary) layer dressings, such as silver-impregnated dressings, are designed to have antibacterial properties (see Figure 14.15).

Wound dressing

This critical technique in open wound management is described later in this chapter in the section on dressings.

Wound fluid management

The accumulation of blood, serum and exudates is a common feature of the healing wound. These fluids slow wound healing, cause tissue maceration, promote bacterial infection and cause pain through pressure and distension of tissues. Superficial wounds produce and exude fluid on the wound surface; deeper wounds accumulate fluid within dead space. Wound fluid is managed through:

- *Minimizing the production of fluid* through good wound management. Eliminating or controlling haemorrhage, inflammation, contamination and infection removes the underlying causes of fluid production
- *Preventing fluid accumulation* by the elimination or reduction of dead space. This is achieved through surgical techniques, negative pressure generated by active drain systems or by pressure bandaging techniques (Figure 14.10). Until dead space is eliminated, accumulating wound fluid needs to be managed through drainage
- *Absorbing produced fluid* through the appropriate selection of absorbent contact (primary) layers of the wound dressing (see Figure 14.17).

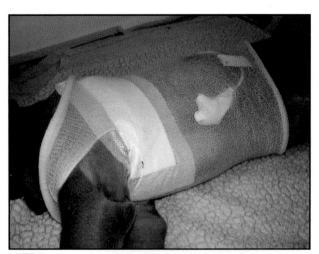

14.10 Pressure dressing applied over a thoracotomy wound. A light pressure dressing consisting of a Primapore dressing covered by an elasticated Tubegauz vest covers a thoracotomy site and chest drain; this protects the surgical site and chest drain and prevents the formation of dead space under the loose skin of the thorax.

Surgical wound drains

Surgical drains (Figure 14.11) are temporary implanted devices that provide a mechanism for the removal of fluids from a wound. Their purpose is to prevent the accumulation of fluid within the wound. The use of a drain is indicated in any wound where there will be the unavoidable accumulation of fluid, the presence of which would have a deleterious effect on normal wound healing. Details on types of drain and their advantages and disadvantages can be found in Chapter 13.

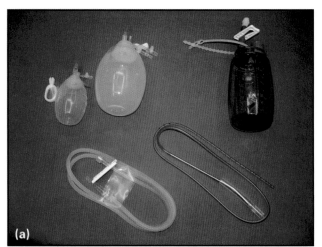
(a)

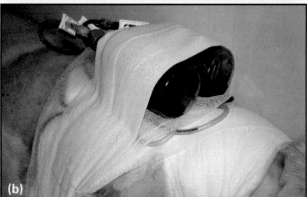
(b)

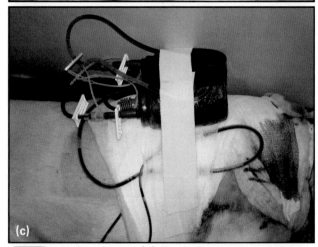
(c)

14.11 Active drains. **(a)** Grenade active suction units (left) and bottle active suction units (right) use negative pressure to drain fluid from a wound. **(b)** Two bottle active suction units in place draining fluid from the surgical site of a large mass resection from the dorsum of a dog. **(c)** Wound fluid striking through a dressing.

Management of drains

- Use aseptic techniques for all postoperative drain care.
- Clip a large area of hair around the wound, especially the area dependent to the wound.
- Use petroleum jelly to protect the skin dependent to the drain exit hole from maceration.
- Clean the exposed drain and skin exit holes twice daily with an antiseptic solution, such as povidone–iodine.
- Empty and change active suction devices as often as required to maintain function.
- Cover with a sterile dressing and light bandage. Change as often as necessary to prevent wound fluid penetrating to the outer dressing layer (strikethrough) (see Figure 14.11c) and to maintain asepsis.
- Prevent patient interference with the drain.
- Drains are kept in place no longer than

necessary, typically 2–5 days, until drainage has almost ceased. Some fluid will always be produced by a wound with a drain due to tissue reaction to the drain itself. The risks of complications increase with the time for which the drain is in place.

Complications of using drains include:

- Wound infection
- Wound dehiscence
- Early loss or removal from wound
- Failure of drainage
- Irritation and pain
- Drain tract cellulitis.

Management of different types of wound

Figure 14.12 outlines management considerations for three different types of wound.

Wound	Wound factors	Examples of wound management
A clean, closed surgical **incision** site	Free from infection and contamination; healthy skin edges closely apposed; mild inflammation; small amount of fluid production possible	To provide short-term protection of incision site and sutures, to pad the surgical site and absorb any fluid produced: apply Primapore or Melolin dressing for 6–12 hours. (Melolin is non-adhesive and requires a secondary layer)
A deep **puncture** wound from a bite	Underlying muscle tissue damaged; significant dead space created; high risk of bacterial contamination; significant wound fluid production likely	To support initial phase of open wound management before secondary surgical closure once wound is infection and contamination free. Careful exploration and assessment of wound, especially deeper tissue: 1. Thorough lavage of wound. 2. Pack cavity with IntraSite gel to aid debridement and exudate absorption. 3. Dress wound with Allevyn to absorb exudates. 4. Cotton wool or Soffban secondary layer to draw exudate from wound contact dressing layer, held in place by a protective layer of Vetrap.
A **degloving** injury in the process of being managed to a healthy open wound	Significant skin deficit from slough of devitalized skin; a generally healthy wound bed with granulation tissue and traces of necrotic tissue; evidence of re-epithelialization	To support wound healing by secondary intention through open wound management with last stages of dressing debridement: 1. Apply Jelonet to support healing and aid debridement of any remaining necrotic or devitalized tissue. 2. Once 100% healthy wound bed established, dress wound with Opsite Flexigrid to maintain a healthy wound environment to support final stages of healing. 3. Add a light secondary layer of bandaging to protect the contact dressings and wound, held in place by a protective layer of Vetrap.

14.12 Examples of three different types of wound, with likely factors to be managed and suggested management.

Complications of wound healing

The main complications of wound healing are:

- Static or non-healing wound
- Haemorrhage
- Seroma formation
- Infection
- Sinus tract formation
- Herniation
- Wound dehiscence.

All the local, systemic and patient factors that influence wound healing discussed above can lead to wound healing complications and failure. These factors must be assessed and corrected as appropriate if they are implicated in disrupting the normal wound healing process (Figure 14.13).

Causes of delayed wound healing and wound complications include:

- Inadequate management of local wound factors (infection, inflammation, contamination, necrotic tissue, moisture imbalance, tissue movement)
- Poor surgical technique
- Drain complications
- Poor dressing and bandaging technique
- Inadequate management of patient and systemic factors
- Patient interference
- Lack of owner compliance.

Wound dressings

A dressing is a material for covering and protecting a wound, commonly understood to be the layer of the dressing/bandage system in direct contact with a wound, known as the **contact layer** (Figure 14.14). Dressings (Figures 14.15 and 14.16) are a critical tool in the management of all wounds, from surgical incisions to large infected skin wounds, and serve a number of different functions. Wound dressing is a particularly important technique in open wound management.

Cause	Complication	Remedial action
Local wound factors, systemic factors, patient factors	Static non-healing wound	Review and correct local wound factors. Wound swab culture and sensitivity. Biopsy. Review and correct patient and systemic factors
Inadequate haemostasis, movement, patient interference, ongoing trauma	Haemorrhage	First aid haemostasis. Identify and stop source of haemorrhage. Prevent patient interference and ongoing trauma
Contamination and infection, inflammation, dead space, poor drainage and wound tissue movement	Seroma formation	Correct local wound factors. Eliminate dead space. Effective wound drainage
Inadequate lavage and debridement, recontamination of wound, ineffective antimicrobial techniques	Infection	Effective wound debridement. Barrier dressing. Systemic antibiotics based on culture and sensitivity
Infection, foreign material/body, suture material and surgical implants	Sinus tract formation	Eliminate infection. Remove foreign material including sutures and surgical implants
Poor surgical technique, patient overactivity	Herniation	Hernia repair. Patient management
Poor surgical technique, infection/wound factors, patient interference	Wound dehiscence	First aid protection of wound. Surgical repair. Correction of wound factor

14.13 Complications of wound healing and remedial actions. Complications during the wound healing process are common. It is important to identify the underlying cause of the complication and to take appropriate remedial action to allow normal wound healing to resume.

Layer	Objective	Functions	Examples
Contact (primary) layer	To support the process of establishing and maintaining optimum wound healing conditions	Wound debridement and decontamination; antibiosis; moisture regulation; wound tissue oxygenation; pH regulation; maintenance and protection of healthy granulation tissue	See Figure 14.16
Padding (secondary) layer	To provide patient comfort	Absorbs and traps exudative fluids away from the wound; pads and protects injured tissues; supports and immobilizes injured parts of the body	Hospital-quality cotton wool, Soffban (Smith & Nephew), Orthoband (Millpledge), Gamgee (Robinson), nappies

14.14 The dressing/bandaging system. The principles of wound dressing and bandaging are based on a functional layering system. Each layer has specific functions in the management of different clinical wound problems. (continues) ▶

Layer	Objective	Functions	Examples
Conforming (secondary) layer	To provide pressure and support	Compresses and holds padding layer in place; supports and immobilizes injured parts of the body; achieves pressure haemostasis; eliminates potential dead space and fluid build-up; prevents blood pooling and promotes venous return from extremities	Knit-fix (Millpledge), Knit-firm (Millpledge), Easifix (Smith & Nephew), Stockinette
Protective (tertiary) layer	To provide support and protection	Holds primary and secondary layers in place; supports and immobilizes injured parts of the body; allows evaporation of moisture; protects wound, primary and secondary layers from external environment, preventing soiling and wetting; protects wound, primary and secondary layers from patient interference	Vetrap (3M), Co-form (Millpledge), Bandesive (Millpledge), Elastoplast (Smith & Nephew), Treatplast (Animalcare)

14.14 (continued) The dressing/bandaging system. The principles of wound dressing and bandaging are based on a functional layering system. Each layer has specific functions in the management of different clinical wound problems.

Type		Description	Characteristics	Examples	Indications
Dry	Dry to dry	Sterile gauze swab	Dry swabs placed on wound to absorb exudates. Adheres to necrotic tissue		Exuding wounds Necrotic wounds Not recommended on granulating wounds
	Wet to dry	Sterile gauze swab soaked in sterile saline	Dry swabs soaked in sterile saline applied on wound. Adheres to necrotic tissue		
	Non-adherent	Perforated polyester film, absorbent, 80% cotton, 20% viscose pad non-woven backing material	Shiny side down on wound. Does not absorb exudates and can adhere to exuding wounds. Needs secondary dressings	Rondopad (Millpledge) Melolin (Smith & Nephew), Primapore (Smith & Nephew)	Dry wounds Postoperative wounds Sutures
		Bleached cotton/rayon cloth impregnated with white or yellow soft paraffin	Paraffin reduces adherence to wound but can dry out if not changed regularly. Needs secondary dressing	Jelonet (Smith & Nephew), Grassolind (Millpledge)	Clean superficial wounds Abrasions Cuts
Interactive	Hydrogels	2.3% modified sodium carboxymethylcellulose polymer, 77.7% water, 20% propylene glycol, 3.5% starch grafted polymer aqueous base, 20% propylene glycol	Available as flat sheets or gels. Have high water content; can rehydrate wounds and ensure moist wound healing. Cool surface of wound. Too much can cause maceration. Can be mixed with topical medications. Needs secondary dressing	IntraSite (Smith & Nephew), Aquaform	Desloughing Exuding wounds Abscess cavities
	Hydrocolloids	Microgranular suspension of polymers – consists of a waterproof polyurethane foam bonded on a polyurethane film that acts as carrier for hydrocolloid base	Absorbs exudates into foam, leading to change in the dressing. Should be 2 cm or more either side of the wound edges. Does not require a secondary dressing	Granuflex (ConvaTec), Tegasorb (3M)	Light to medium exuding wounds
	Foam	Absorbent polyurethane containing either hydrocellular or hydropolymer foam and some carbon. Comes in a variety of forms	Can absorb 6–10 times own weight in exudates. Conforms to cavity. White surface placed on wound. Exudate does not leak through. Works by capillary action drawing exudates from wound. Needs secondary dressings. Can be left in place up to 7 days	Allevyn (Smith & Nephew), Lyofoam (Acme United)	Suitable for all types of wounds that have light to heavy exudates Deep cavity wounds
	Alginate	Made from a variety of seaweeds, some contain calcium. Mixed into a non-woven dressing	Highly absorbent; dressings turn to gel once mixed with exudates. Some have haemostatic properties. Needs secondary dressings. Can be left in place for up to 7 days	Algisite (Smith & Nephew), Kaltostat (ConvaTec)	Infected wounds Exuding wounds Cavities Haemorrhage
	Collagen	Collagen matrix	Binds blood clotting factors XII and XIII. Causes natural wound cleansing. Attracts granulocytes and fibroblasts to the wound and forms an organized structure for basal cells of epidermis	Vet BioSISt (Arnolds), Emovet (Nelson), Collamend (Genetrix)	Most types of wounds Not recommended for full thickness burns or necrotic wounds

14.15 Wound dressings. A wide variety of dressings is available; each has specific characteristics, allowing it to perform specific functions, thereby determining the indications for its use. (continues) ▶

Type		Description	Characteristics	Examples	Indications
Interactive *continued*	Silver-coated dressings	SILCRYST , Nanocrystals	Silver ions released into wound bed Has anti-inflammatory action and kills bacteria rapidly	Acticoat (Smith & Nephew)	Infected wounds
	Vapour-permeable film	Thin conformable adhesive films	Provides thin vapour-permeable film, allowing vapour exchange and maintenance of moist wound environment	Opsite Flexigrid (Smith & Nephew), Tegaderm (3M)	Uninfected shallow wounds Intact skin at risk of pressure or maceration injury
	Barrier film	Spray or foam containing polymer	Sprayed over wound; dries to leave film of polymer that is permeable to moisture vapour and air. Creates a barrier	Opsite (Smith & Nephew), Cavilon (3M), Film dressing spray (Millpledge)	Minor wounds Abrasions Sutures Wound covering on reptiles
Topical	Antiseptics	Dilute chlorhexidine 0.05%, Dilute povidone–iodine 1%	Used as initial cleansing of wounds. These solutions can be toxic to fibroblasts and should be avoided if possible. Contaminated wounds would be better treated with debridement	Hibitane, Pevidine, antiseptic solution	Contaminated wounds
	Aloe vera	Gel	Promotes wound healing by accelerating formation of granulation tissue. Stabilizes fibroblast growth factors and activates macrophages	Acemannan (Forever Living Products)	All wounds
	Maggots	Larvae 1st stage	Used for debriding wounds. Larvae eat liquid protein and feed on exudates, necrotic or infected tissue. They are left in place for a maximum of 3 days. If left longer, 2nd-stage larvae can damage living tissue	LarvE (Biosurgical Research Unit)	Contaminated, necrotic, infected or exuding wounds
	Hydrophilic cream	Hydrophilic cream containing silver sulphadiazine	Inhibits growth of bacteria and fungi *in vitro*. Studies have been carried out to show antibacterial action against methicillin-resistant *Staphylococcus aureus*, *Pseudomonas* spp. and enterococci. Cream must be placed in wound as it will macerate surrounding skin	Flamazine (Smith & Nephew)	Wounds infected with Gram-negative bacteria
	Sugar paste and honey	Paste. Castor sugar and additive-free icing sugar dissolved in hydrogen peroxide and polyethylene glycol 400 has been developed for clinical use	Has been used in wounds for centuries. Paste has lower pH than wound and helps to debride infected or dirty wounds. Not suitable for granulating wounds. Honey must be sterile; has a high osmotic pressure and helps to draw out exudate		Infected dirty wounds

14.15 (continued) Wound dressings. A wide variety of dressings is available; each has specific characteristics, allowing it to perform specific functions, thereby determining the indications for its use.

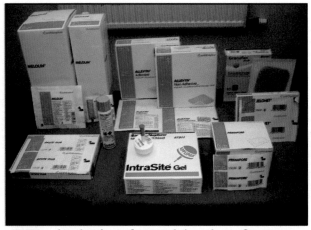

14.16 A selection of wound dressings. Contact layer dressings come in different sizes, suitable for wounds of different sizes and patients of different sizes.

The frequency of changing a dressing will vary through the wound healing process and is determined by:

- The requirement to inspect and treat the wound
- The degree of wound exudate and contamination of the dressing
- The degree of external contamination, soiling and wetting of the bandage
- Dressing or bandage slippage or loss.

Bandaging

A bandage is a strip or roll of material used to wrap or bind part of a patient's body (Figure 14.17). Bandaging forms the outer layers of the dressing/bandage system, known as the **padding**, **conforming** and **protective layers**. Bandaging serves many purposes and is used to achieve a number of different objectives in different clinical contexts (see Figure 14.14).

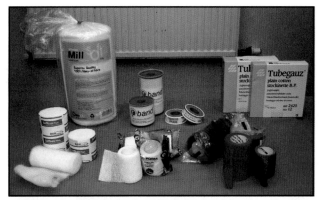

14.17 A selection of materials used for bandaging. Examples of materials for padding, conforming and protective layers.

General bandaging rules

- Always prepare materials and equipment before starting.
- Wash and dry hands.
- Use materials of a suitable size for the patient.
- Carry out procedure in a quiet area away from noise and activity of the veterinary surgery.
- The room chosen must be secure to prevent escape.
- Have the patient restrained suitably by an assistant (Figure 14.18).
- Dress wounds first, using the appropriate dressing.
- Only use a small amount of padding between the toes.
- Apply the bandage in a distal-to-proximal direction so as not to compromise circulation.
- Keep the flat end of the bandage in contact with the patient.

- Check that the bandage is not being (or has not been) applied too tightly by inserting fingers between the patient's skin and the bandage to assess tension.
- Check that the bandage does not interfere with other areas of the patient's body and that hair is not caught up in the layers.

Bandaging techniques

Ear and head bandage

Indications for use:

- First aid treatment for controlling haemorrhage from the pinna
- Postoperative support of the ear following surgery.

Equipment:

- Lister bandage scissors
- Marker pen
- Wound dressing
- Synthetic padding material
- Conforming material
- Protective material.

Technique

This is illustrated in Figure 14.19.

Thoracic bandage

Indications for use:

- First aid treatment for trauma to the thorax
- To hold a chest drain in place
- Postoperative thoracic support.

Restraint method	Bandage type
Lateral recumbency 1. The patient is laid in lateral position (side depends on area to be dressed). 2. The assistant stands with the patient's legs facing away from them. 3. With one hand the assistant holds the foreleg closest to the table and places the arm over the patient's neck to support the head. 4. With the other hand the assistant holds the hindleg closest to the table and places the arm over the hindquarters. This position allows either of the limbs facing upwards to be free to dress	Robert Jones Foot dressing, including casting and splinting Ehmer sling Velpeau sling Thoracic or abdominal dressing for patients that are anaesthetized or sedated
Sitting position The assistant places one hand over the back of the neck and uses the other hand to support the muzzle	Head and ear bandage
Standing position The assistant places an arm under the neck and gently turns the patient's head towards them	Head and ear bandage Thoracic bandage Abdominal bandage Tail bandage
Chemical restraint	Using appropriate anaesthetic agents

14.18 Methods of restraint used for bandaging.

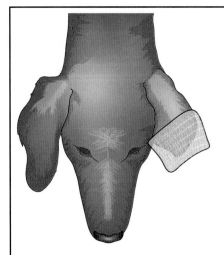

1. Cover any wounds with an appropriate sterile dressing.

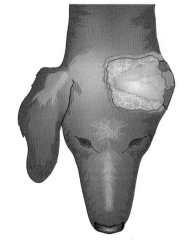

2. Place padding on top of cranium. Pick up ear by tip of pinna and lay flat back on padding; repeat if including both ears. Place padding on top of pinna.

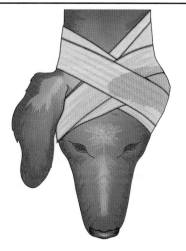

3. Place padding under neck. Wrap conforming layer in a figure-of-eight pattern until the area is covered, using the free ear for additional anchorage.

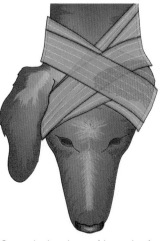

4. Cover the bandage with a cohesive layer following a similar pattern.

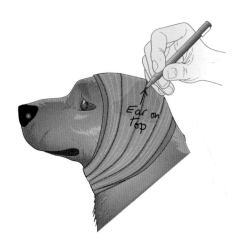

5. Use marker pen to indicate on the outer layer the position of the pinna. Make sure that the bandage does not interfere with swallowing or breathing.

14.19 Applying an ear and head bandage.

Equipment:

- Lister bandage scissors
- Wound dressing
- Padding material
- Conforming material
- Protective material.

Technique
This is illustrated in Figure 14.20.

Abdominal bandage

Indications for use:

- First aid treatment for abdominal wounds
- Postoperative abdominal support for surgical wounds
- Pressure bandage to control intra-abdominal haemorrhage.

Equipment:

- Lister bandage scissors
- Wound dressing
- Padding material
- Conforming material
- Protective material.

Technique
This is illustrated in Figure 14.21.

Robert Jones bandage

Indications for use:

- First aid treatment for immobilizing limb fractures
- To control limb swelling and oedema
- Postoperative limb support.

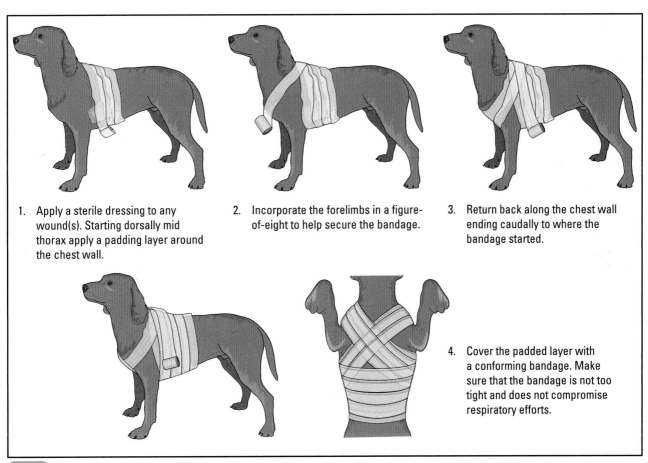

1. Apply a sterile dressing to any wound(s). Starting dorsally mid thorax apply a padding layer around the chest wall.

2. Incorporate the forelimbs in a figure-of-eight to help secure the bandage.

3. Return back along the chest wall ending caudally to where the bandage started.

4. Cover the padded layer with a conforming bandage. Make sure that the bandage is not too tight and does not compromise respiratory efforts.

14.20   Applying a thoracic bandage.

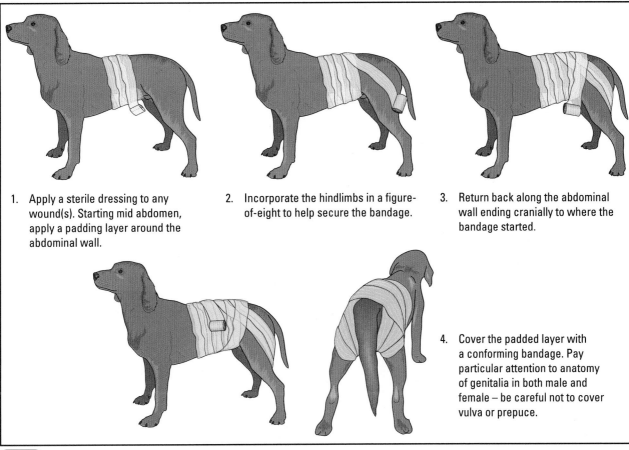

1. Apply a sterile dressing to any wound(s). Starting mid abdomen, apply a padding layer around the abdominal wall.

2. Incorporate the hindlimbs in a figure-of-eight to help secure the bandage.

3. Return back along the abdominal wall ending cranially to where the bandage started.

4. Cover the padded layer with a conforming bandage. Pay particular attention to anatomy of genitalia in both male and female – be careful not to cover vulva or prepuce.

14.21   Applying an abdominal bandage.

Equipment:

- Lister bandage scissors
- Zinc oxide tape
- Padding material
- Conforming material
- Protective material.

Technique

This is illustrated in Figure 14.22.

Foot and lower limb bandage

Indications for use:

- First aid treatment for the control of limb/foot haemorrhage (e.g. cut pad)

- Postoperative limb/foot support following a surgical procedure
- Light dressing for anchoring intravenous fluids
- Protection of a limb/foot wound from patient interference.

Equipment:

- Nail cutters
- Lister bandage scissors
- Padding material
- Conforming material
- Protective material.

Technique

This is illustrated in Figure 14.23.

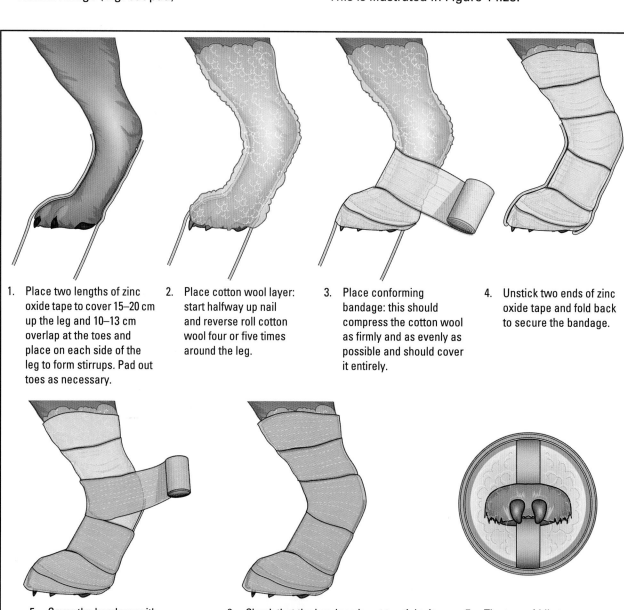

1. Place two lengths of zinc oxide tape to cover 15–20 cm up the leg and 10–13 cm overlap at the toes and place on each side of the leg to form stirrups. Pad out toes as necessary.

2. Place cotton wool layer: start halfway up nail and reverse roll cotton wool four or five times around the leg.

3. Place conforming bandage: this should compress the cotton wool as firmly and as evenly as possible and should cover it entirely.

4. Unstick two ends of zinc oxide tape and fold back to secure the bandage.

5. Cover the bandage with cohesive dressing.

6. Check that the bandage is not too tight: it should be possible to insert two fingers between the bandage and the animal. When flicked, the bandage should sound like a ripe melon.

7. The two middle toes should remain exposed.

14.22   Applying a Robert Jones bandage.

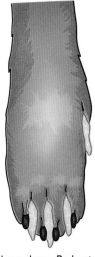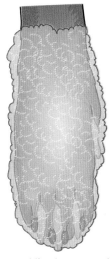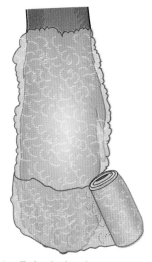

1. Cut long claws. Pad out the toes using a small piece of absorbent dressing.

2. Apply a padding layer over the foot covering the dorsal and palmar/plantar area.

3. Twist the bandage to cover diagonally the medial and lateral aspect of the foot.

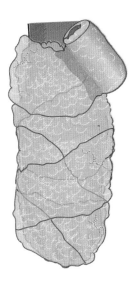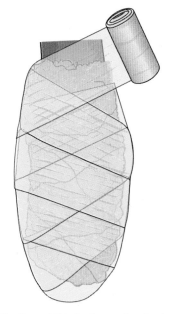

4. Roll the bandage in a proximal direction spiralling up the leg to cover the joint above the area to be bandaged.

5. Repeat this for the conforming layer and the cohesive layer.

14.23   Applying a foot and lower limb bandage.

When applying a pressure bandage on the foot, ensure that:

- Extra padding is applied
- The conforming layer is applied tightly.

To prevent a compromise in circulation, a pressure bandage should not be left on for longer than is necessary.

Velpeau sling

Indications for use:

- To support forelimb following closed reduction of a luxated shoulder joint.

Equipment:

- Lister bandage scissors
- Padding material
- Conforming material
- Protective material.

Technique

This is illustrated in Figure 14.24.

Ehmer sling

Indications for use:

- To support hindlimb following closed reduction of a luxated hip joint.

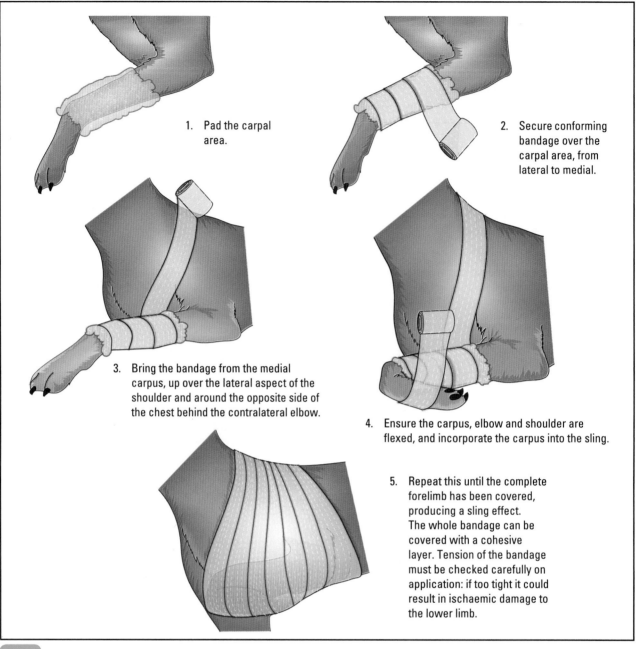

1. Pad the carpal area.

2. Secure conforming bandage over the carpal area, from lateral to medial.

3. Bring the bandage from the medial carpus, up over the lateral aspect of the shoulder and around the opposite side of the chest behind the contralateral elbow.

4. Ensure the carpus, elbow and shoulder are flexed, and incorporate the carpus into the sling.

5. Repeat this until the complete forelimb has been covered, producing a sling effect. The whole bandage can be covered with a cohesive layer. Tension of the bandage must be checked carefully on application: if too tight it could result in ischaemic damage to the lower limb.

14.24   Applying a Velpeau sling.

Equipment:

■ Lister bandage scissors
■ Padding material
■ Conforming material
■ Protective material.

Technique
This is illustrated in Figure 14.25.

Tail bandage

Indications for use:

■ Postoperative protection for a tail tip amputation
■ First aid treatment for tail haemorrhage
■ Protection of tail following anal or perineal surgery.

Equipment:

■ Lister bandage scissors
■ Wound dressing
■ Padding material
■ Conforming material
■ Protective material
■ Syringe case for protection of tail tip.

Technique
This is illustrated in Figure 14.26.

■ A syringe case can be used for protection of the bandage.
■ An adhesive section may be necessary to anchor the bandage in place.
■ Lightweight plastic tail splints are commercially available in three sizes. These can usefully help splint and provide additional support to the tail.

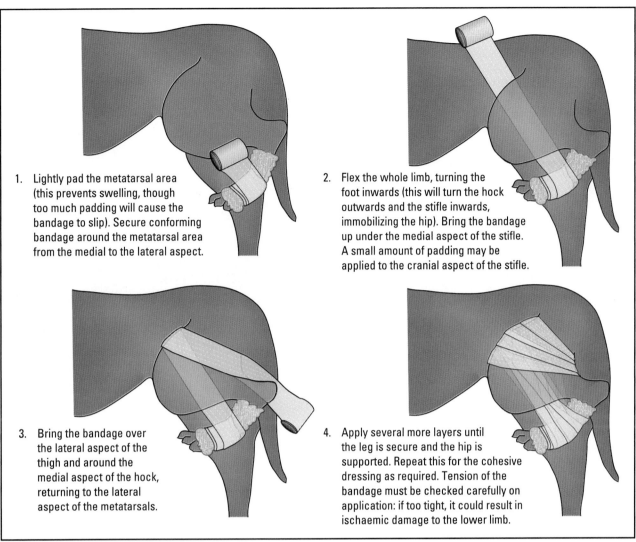

1. Lightly pad the metatarsal area (this prevents swelling, though too much padding will cause the bandage to slip). Secure conforming bandage around the metatarsal area from the medial to the lateral aspect.

2. Flex the whole limb, turning the foot inwards (this will turn the hock outwards and the stifle inwards, immobilizing the hip). Bring the bandage up under the medial aspect of the stifle. A small amount of padding may be applied to the cranial aspect of the stifle.

3. Bring the bandage over the lateral aspect of the thigh and around the medial aspect of the hock, returning to the lateral aspect of the metatarsals.

4. Apply several more layers until the leg is secure and the hip is supported. Repeat this for the cohesive dressing as required. Tension of the bandage must be checked carefully on application: if too tight, it could result in ischaemic damage to the lower limb.

14.25 One method of applying an Ehmer sling.

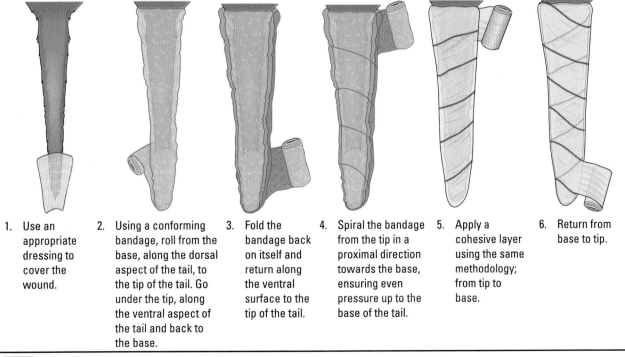

1. Use an appropriate dressing to cover the wound.

2. Using a conforming bandage, roll from the base, along the dorsal aspect of the tail, to the tip of the tail. Go under the tip, along the ventral aspect of the tail and back to the base.

3. Fold the bandage back on itself and return along the ventral surface to the tip of the tail.

4. Spiral the bandage from the tip in a proximal direction towards the base, ensuring even pressure up to the base of the tail.

5. Apply a cohesive layer using the same methodology; from tip to base.

6. Return from base to tip.

14.26 Applying a tail bandage.

Wing bandage for a bird

Indications for use:

- First aid treatment, definitive treatment and postoperative support for a fractured wing.

Equipment:

- Lister bandage scissors
- Zinc oxide tape or masking tape
- Padding material
- Protective material.

Technique

The wing should be positioned in its natural anatomical resting position.

- Fractures of the manus, or of either the radius or ulna alone, need only simple support. This is most easily achieved by taping together the primary feathers of a closed wing. Masking tape or zinc oxide tape is suitable (Figure 14.27a).
- Fractures of the radius and ulna can be supported with a figure-of-eight dressing holding the ulna and radius against the humerus but not including the body (Figure 14.27b). Conforming bandage, such as Vetrap, with the roll cut to a suitable width, is appropriate.
- Fractures of the humerus should be immobilized with a figure-of-eight dressing (Figure 14.27c) but this time including the body (Figure 14.27d), leaving the opposite wing free. When taping the wing to the body, care must be taken that it does not interfere with normal respiratory movement.

Foot bandage on a bird

Indications for use:

- Support for a fracture of digits or lower limb
- Protection for bumblefoot.

Equipment:

- Lister bandage scissors
- Bumblefoot pad, donut ring or other variation (see below)
- Self-adhesive material
- Zinc oxide tape.

Technique

1. Place a donut ring or a foot pad on the foot (Figure 14.28).
2. Do not include leg rings or equipment within the bandage. Rings must be pushed up the leg to prevent damage to the skin under the bandage.
3. Conforming or self-adhesive bandage can then be used to secure the dressing to the foot by wrapping around each digit and the foot.

Variations that can be used if a bumblefoot pad or donut ring is unavailable include:

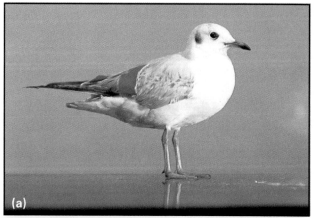

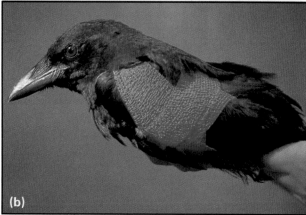

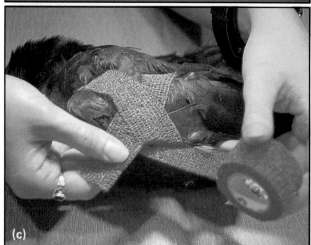

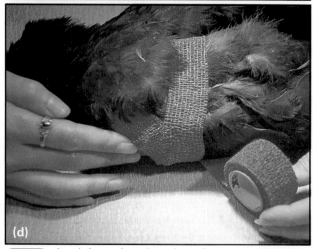

14.27 Applying wing dressings (see main text for details). (Courtesy of R Best; reproduced from *BSAVA Manual of Wildlife Casualties*.)

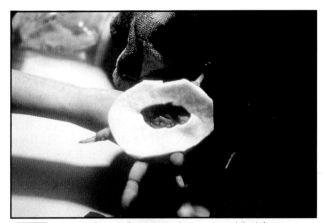

14.28 Applying a foot bandage on a bird (see main text for details). Here, a donut-ring corn dressing is being applied to a lesion on a Himalayan griffon vulture. The dressing is held in place with cohesive bandage wrapped around the foot and between the digits. (Reproduced from *BSAVA Manual of Exotic Pets, 4th edition*)

- Tennis ball cut in half and then taped in place
- Padding material folded to form a protective pad and taped in place
- Allevyn (Smith & Nephew) folded to provide a protective pad and taped in place.

External coaptation – casting and splints

Casting

Casting is a long-established method of repairing fractures. Although its use is now less common in practice as internal fixation has largely superseded it, there is still a place for casting. It can be used on the following types of fracture:

- Easily reducible fractures
- Stable, simple, non-displaced fractures
- Fractures distal to elbow or stifle
- Some tail and neck fractures.

Casting materials

For many years plaster of Paris was the only casting material available for use. Although this is still available, it has many disadvantages and has been replaced by more modern materials (Figures 14.29 and 14.30) and internal fixation. There are new products coming on to the market all the time and it is important to keep up to date with them.

Plaster of Paris

This is traditional and cheap. It consists of a bandage coated with calcium dehydrate (gypsum). The roll of bandage is immersed in lukewarm water for 2–10 seconds to activate the coating. The excess water is squeezed out gently and five or six layers are applied to give enough support. The setting time is 3–5 minutes but the cast will take at least 8 hours to dry completely.

The casts are not waterproof and must be kept dry at all times.

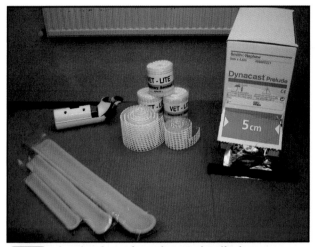

14.29 A selection of casting and splinting materials. Centre back: Hexalite/Vet-lite, a thermoplastic casting material; right: Dynacast, a fibreglass resin-impregnated casting and splinting material. Various pre-made splints are available, such as gutter type (left front) and complete limb splint systems (left back).

Casting material	Advantages	Disadvantages
Plaster of Paris	Cheap, easy to apply, conforms well to leg	Takes several hours to dry, heavy, radiodense, messy
Thermoplastics (e.g. Hexalite/ Vet-lite (Cox))	Light, waterproof, strong, can be reused	Needs high temperature of water to soften, difficult to mould to leg
Resin-impregnated (e.g. Dynacast (Smith & Nephew))	Light, waterproof, conformable, radiolucent	Expensive, requires special equipment to remove

14.30 Advantages and disadvantages of different casting materials. A range of casting materials is available; each case requiring the use of a casting material must be assessed and an appropriate material selected according to the case requirements.

Thermoplastics

These are stronger and lighter than plaster of Paris but require a high initial temperature to mould and do not really mould to the leg very well. Placing the cast material in hot water (70–75°C) for 2–5 minutes softens the plastic. It can then be moulded to shape and will harden as it cools down (hairdryers can be used for this). The setting time is usually between 3 and 5 minutes.

These casts are waterproof. The materials can also be reheated, allowing for removal and reapplication. Hexalite and Vet-lite (Cox) are examples of thermoplastic casting material.

Orthoboard (Millpledge) takes a higher temperature (80–120°C) and also takes longer to reach full strength (15 minutes).

Resin-impregnated materials

These are fibreglass or polypropylene bandages covered with a polyurethane resin. They are activated by warm water (20°C), but will harden in air. Only three or four layers are needed to provide adequate support, so they are lighter. They are also waterproof. Gloves must be worn when applying to prevent resin adhering to the skin.

The properties vary according to type and make of material. The setting time is 3–6 minutes and the material is fully set within 20 minutes. This may vary if the water is warmer.

Once the cast is on it will require sawing to remove it. This can be achieved by an electronic oscillating saw, or by incorporating a gigli saw into the cast when it is applied.

Dynacast (Smith & Nephew) is an example of a fibreglass-based material; it can be used as a cast or as a splint.

Basic principles of casting

- Appropriate anaesthesia should be used when applying a cast to aid with reduction.
- The joint above and below the fracture *must* be immobilized by the cast.
- Cast padding should be snug. Excessive padding results in the cast loosening and rubbing.
- The distal extremity may be exposed or covered, depending on personal preference. If the distal end of the cast is left open, only the middle footpads should be exposed for inspection. If too much of the foot is left exposed, swelling will occur.
- Sometimes a walking bar can be included in the cast to prevent excessive wear on the distal end; this is normally an aluminium bar.
- The cast should be changed within 2 weeks following reduction, as soft tissue swelling will start to decrease. This could cause the cast to start rubbing. Younger animals will need the cast changing sooner as they are growing faster.
- The owner should ensure that the cast is kept dry and should check the cast daily and report any signs of discomfort, smells, rubbing, cast wear, etc.

Technique for applying a cast

- Gather and prepare all equipment.
- Wash and dry hands.
- Ask assistant to restrain the animal in lateral recumbency.
- After reduction of the fracture, the leg is covered with a layer of padding.
- Put on gloves.

1. The cast material is immersed in water for a few seconds until air bubbles cease to rise.
2. The cast material is removed from the water and squeezed gently to remove excess water.
3. The cast is applied from distal to proximal limb.
4. Once the layers of cast are in place it can be smoothed and moulded to shape to fit the limb.
5. Once dry, it can be covered with a cohesive dressing.

Splints

In first aid treatment for fractures, the injury can be immobilized by the use of splints. Splints can also be used following surgery. The different types of splint that can be used include: zimmer splint; gutter splint; Altman splint; cast materials (e.g. Dynacast, Smith & Nephew).

If any of the above splints are unavailable in a first aid situation, temporary splints can be formed from rolled-up newspaper, ice-lolly sticks or even broom handles.

The criteria for a successful splint are that it should be:

- Long enough to immobilize the joints above and below the fractured bone
- Rigid (so that it will not bend and allow movement of the injured limb)
- Smooth (so that there are no parts that can rub or cause further damage to the limb)
- Conforming (so that it holds the injury in position and is comfortable).

Zimmer splint

This is made from malleable aluminium and has a foam backing (which is placed towards the patient). It can be shaped to conform to the limb and can be incorporated into a dressing. It can also be cut to length.

Because of its make-up, the Zimmer splint is really only suitable for small dogs, cats and other small animals; it is not strong enough to provide any support for larger animals.

Gutter splints

These are straight, non-malleable splints of rigid plastic and have foam cushions (see Figure 14.29). They can also be incorporated into a dressing and they provide more support than the Zimmer splint. They are available in different sizes.

Altman splint

This is used for birds as a splint for the tibiotarsus: two pieces of zinc oxide tape are placed on either side of the joint and then stuck together. This will prevent rotation of the joint.

Postoperative care of bandages, casts and splints

When an animal is discharged, its owners should be made aware of potential complications with casts and splints. Written instructions are very helpful and the following points should be covered.

- The bandage, cast or splint should be checked daily for the following signs:
  - Swelling around the cast in either the limb or the toes
  - Signs of rubbing at the ends of the cast
  - Odour
  - Patient interference
  - Movement of the cast from its original position
  - Bending of cast at the joint area.

- A waterproof covering should be used when the animal is taken outside.
- House rest is advisable whilst the bandage is in place, to prevent excessive movement.

The owner should also be given advice on when to return to the surgery for the bandage, cast or splint to be changed.

Complications of casts

- *Pressure sores* (decubitus ulcers) can be caused if the cast does not have enough padding material or is applied loosely.
- *Delayed union, malunion and non-union* can be seen if the fracture is not suitable for casting or if the cast has been applied incorrectly.
- *Swelling of limb* can be caused if the cast has been applied too tightly so that it restricts circulation, resulting in oedema.

Removal of bandage, cast or splint
Bandages

- Bandages should be changed as frequently as required. This can be up to several times a day in intensive wound management cases. Initially a bandage should be changed at the latest within 2 days of application to determine wound healing. After this the time can be variable, depending on type of dressing and wound.
- Bandages should also be removed if there are any of the complications described previously.
- Lister bandage scissors (Figure 14.31) should be used and care taken not to cut skin.
- If soiled, all dressing material should be disposed of in the clinical waste bin.
- When removing bandages, wash hands and wear gloves.

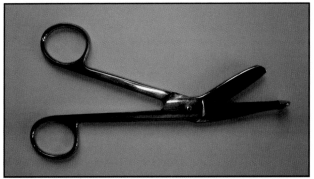

14.31 Lister bandage scissors, designed to cut through bandage layers with the blades kept safely away from the patient's skin.

Casts

- Casts can be left in place for 4–6 weeks.
- A radiograph should be taken periodically to determine callus formation and bone healing.

- The animal should be sedated for cast removal if using a full cast.
- An oscillating saw is used for removal of a full fibreglass splint.
- The cast is cut in two places avoiding bony prominences. The saw should not come in contact with the skin.
- The cast can then be removed and the padding layer removed using bandage scissors.
- Plaster shears can be used: these are inserted at the distal end of the cast and cut in small steps.

Protection of bandages, casts and splints

It is important to protect the bandage from patient interference and from environmental contamination. There are a variety of ways in which this can be achieved, including:

- Elizabethan collar
- Bite-Not collar
- Lotions and sprays (e.g. Bitter Apple spray)
- Bandaging the hindlimbs with a light dressing to prevent the patient from scratching the dressing and to provide protection for the claws
- Protective boot (e.g. Mikki Boot) for when walking outside
- A used fluid bag, attached with a white open-weave bandage, for protection when walking outside (Figure 14.32). Non-breathable coverings should only be used as a short-term measure to protect the bandage.

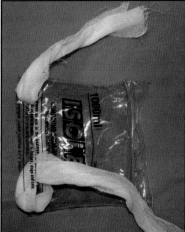

14.32 A fluid bag used to protect a limb/foot dressing. Cutting a section of appropriate length from a fluid bag provides a strong and waterproof 'boot' for a foot dressing. The fluid bag is held in place by a tie made from open-weave bandage material.

Further reading

Anderson D and Smith J (2007) Wounds. In: *BSAVA Textbook of Veterinary Nursing, 4th edn*, ed. DR Lane *et al.*, pp. 595–603. BSAVA Publications, Gloucester

Anderson DM (2003) Wound dressing unraveled. *In Practice* **25**, 70–83

Anderson DM (1996) Wound management in small animal practice. *In Practice* **18**, 115–128

Aspinall V (2003) *Clinical Procedures for Veterinary Nursing.* Butterworth-Heinemann, London

Chandler S (2007) Bandaging and dressings. In: *BSAVA Textbook of Veterinary Nursing, 4th edn*, ed. DR Lane *et al.*, pp. 247–251. BSAVA Publications, Gloucester

Fowler D and Williams JM (1999) *BSAVA Manual of Canine and Feline Wound Management and Reconstruction.* BSAVA Publications, Cheltenham

Morgan DA (2004) *Formulary of Wound Management Products, 9th edn.* Euromed Communications, Surrey

Schultz GS, Brillo DJ, Wozingo DW *et al.* (2004) Wound bed preparation. A brief history of TIME. *International Wound Journal* **1**, 19–32

Swaim SF and Henderson RA (1997) *Small Animal Wound Management, 2nd edn.* Williams and Wilkins, Baltimore

Index

Numbers in *italics* indicate figures; numbers in **bold** indicate boxes.

Index

Index